BEYOND GLUTEN INTOLERANCE

GIS - Gluten Inflammatory Syndrome

BEYOND GLUTEN INTOLERANCE

GIS - Gluten Inflammatory Syndrome

A comprehensive health book that explains how the body works, gives guidelines back to wellness while answering the question of what gluten is and how it affects every person - child and adult.

Karen A. Masterson Koch, Clinical Nutritionist

BookMasters®, Inc
Ashland, Ohio

BookMasters®, Inc

30 Amberwood Parkway,
P.O. Box 388
Ashland, Ohio, 44805

Medical Disclaimer
The information contained in this book is intended to be educational and not rendering professional advice or services to an individual. It is the result of years of research and practice experience by the author and both author and publisher are in no way liable for any misuse of the information. It is not the intent to diagnose, treat or cure any disease or to substitute for seeing your physician for proper evaluation and treatment due to matters of health may require medical supervision.

Mention of specific companies, organizations, or authorities in this book does not imply endorsement by the author or publisher and contrary it does not imply that they endorse the book, author or publisher. Internet addresses and telephone numbers referenced in this book were accurate at the time the book went to press.

Managing editor: Karen Masterson Koch
Copy editor: Lacie Schreiber
Proof reader: Kelly Cappasola
Book design: Mighty Jungle Media

Books may be ordered by writing to Friends Helping Friends, PO Box 710759, Santee, CA, 92072 or by Internet at www.beyondglutenintolerance.com.

Library of Congress Cataloging-in-Publication Data
First Paperback Edition 2012
Masterson Koch, Karen Masterson
Beyond Gluten Intolerance GIS: Gluten Inflammatory Syndrome - health and gluten information plus recipes and supplements / Karen Masterson Koch
Includes research references and index.
2011946078

ISBN-13: 978-0-692-01650-3

Printed in the United States of America

Dedication

Dedication goes to all of the brave souls who have dared to make choices outside of mainstream medicine's definitions of health and disease. While in the process they won their health freedom and in some small way it lessens the pain and regret of those too weak or innocent who have lost their lives not due to the disease but to incompetent care.

Deep felt appreciation goes to all of the patients and clients I have worked with personally and their compliance which reinforces the principals of health that apply to everyone. Also thanks to all of the health professionals that have dared to practice and prescribe the truth that supports the divine design of the body that includes; nutrition, health supplements and a healthier lifestyle.

I thank the Lord of my soul for delaying the writing of this book so I could understand the entire story behind the gluten epidemic. God's wisdom and timing surpasses any technology that a human may ever possess.

Special thanks to my family, friends and staff for their patience, support and co-operation in the evolution of this book over the past 20 years of discovery. Love is ever healing and Beyond Gluten Intolerance!

Contents

- Triggers are Co-Conspirators with Wheat

- Why does Gluten cause health challenges?

- Research Pinpoints Poor Digestion as the Weak Link

- The History of Wheat On Planet Earth

- What is the Goal Concerning Gluten?

- HIGHLIGHT 1: Sprouting & Fermented Foods

- Simplifying Bowel Disease

- History of Bowel Disease

- Research of IBS & IBD - Bowel Health Requirements

- What is the Ultimate Solution for Bowel Disease?

- HIGHLIGHT 2: Probiotics is the First Step To Wellness

- Requirements for Healthy Mental Behavior & Happiness
- GIS III Theory: Inflammation, Mal-Nutrition & Toxicity Share in Disease Development
- Glossary of Conditions
- HIGHLIGHT 5: Essential Fatty Acids for All – Anti-Inflammatory & Structural for Brain and Body Health

- The Body Signals for Help with Fatigue, Mental Distress, Illness & Pain!
- Health Success Takes Learning & Action
- 20 Healthy Focus Factors

- Successful Diet Protocols for GIS and Bowel Disease
- GIS Dietary Guidelines; Zone 1 – Low (Maintenance), Zone 2 - Medium & Zone 3 - High; Low and Gluten Free Suggestions
- Foods & Lifestyle Choices for All Zones
- Menu Suggestions, Shopping Lists for Breakfast, Lunch, Dinner, Desserts and Snacks!
- Healthy TIPS
- Tasty & Delicious Gluten Free and Low Gluten Recipes

- Why is it important to eat well and take vitamins?
- Foundational – Essential Core Nutrients (ECN) That We Die Without!

Acknowledgements

Beyond Gluten Intolerance: GIS – Gluten Inflammatory Syndrome, is not the first book to be written about bowel disease. My goal is to enlighten and connect the pieces of information that are available, include the credible research of others with my own clinical observations while explaining the best options for a solution which I believe resides in health.

My praise extends to all of the organizations around the globe that offer dietary guidelines and support to people suffering with health challenges and bowel disease related to gluten. Hundreds of peer reviewed and repeatable research papers on gluten have been collected by these diligent organizations. Some have come from scientists employed by private agencies and a fairly large amount from foreign government departments of health and agriculture that gives collegial support to this book. Unfortunately even with the impressive research from other governments, the U.S. has remained reluctant to shift from a pharmaceutical focus treatment of bowel disease to a more natural complimentary approach.

Acknowledgment and gratitude must also go to our forefathers for giving their very lives for freedom and the writing and signing of the U.S. Constitution and Bill of Rights. This document gives each U.S. citizen the freedom of press and the freedom of speech to tell the truth that many countries do not enjoy. The Salem Communications Inc. also receives my overwhelming thanks for allowing my voice to join the "Truth Sayers" around the globe equipping individuals and families to discover health for themselves!

Preface

Health is not understood by most individuals. Every person who finds the immense value health plays in ones life has a story of how they arrived at that pinnacle of truth. My health story or awakening took place in 1970 at the young age of 20. The moment, when I first made the big connection to cause and effect of our daily actions - came from a 75 cent pamphlet. It explained that what I ate on a daily basis actually affected the health of my body and how I thought – my mind. It made perfect sense!

I came across this unassuming small pamphlet in a health food store called Jack's and the pamphlet was titled, *Nutrition from A – Z.* As I read about nutrients; vitamins, minerals, essential fatty acids and proteins which the book pointed out came from foods and food supplements, the puzzle pieces began to fall into place. The pamphlet explained how the design of the human body, depends on these nutritional basics to support life itself. To create a healthy body, reduce stress and help a person think more clearly called upon nutrition for the answer. I was amazed and instantly hooked. It was like someone had given me a key to life itself. I quickly began to learn how to stop the roller coaster of emotional ups and downs and was eager to learn more. And I might add this epiphany took place years before I understood my own gluten intolerance.

I grew up like most kids eating for taste and not because food had some special nutrients my body required for health. Oh yes I had heard that carrots were for good eye sight and you needed to drink milk to grow properly for its calcium. And looking back on my young years our family did eat from the four food groups – protein, starch, dairy, a cooked vegetable (canned or frozen, rarely fresh) and it usually included a salad. The salads were marginal and generally consisting of iceberg lettuce with tomatoes with a bottled dressing and sometimes blue cheese sprinkles. We had fruit available yet I ate sugary desserts of cookies, box cereals, ice cream, candy, chips and donuts whenever I had a chance. Sometimes that meant saving up my milk money from school to buy candy and on occasion even stealing money out of my Moms wallet. Yep you guessed it - I was a blooming sugar addict from an early age!

Knowing now as an adult about the pockets of poverty our nation has, I am thankful I had three meals a day growing up and fairly clean water to drink. My heritage was from the south and we traditionally drank iced tea at dinner meals. From my viewpoint today of being a health educator and knowing the need the body has for nutrient dense foods for health - it is truly amazing how my body survived the nutritional abuse it received from my sweet indulgences. As scientists have revealed maybe the black tea I drank gave me the antioxidant protection I needed for survival. Kids of my generation also got a lot of exercise of playing outside whenever we got a chance which undoubtedly kept our bodies leaner and healthier.

My parents did their best in raising me and my three siblings. We were not allowed to have sodas unless it was a special occasion yet Kool-Aid was on tap. The overcooked, fried and processed luncheon meat like baloney were laden with processed fats, sugar and excessive salt tasting yummy yet most likely one of the reasons I didn't feel so good much of my growing years. My older brother was not as fortunate as I to survive unscathed. He developed cancer in his teens. My brother Patrick was unfortunately diagnosed with an aggressive melanoma skin cancer which eventually took his life.

Why I share this tragedy today, as sad as it is for any young person to lose their life prematurely, is to acknowledge that this family loss - became a catalyst for me to look for answers of why people develop Cancer. Patrick, even as a young man of 18, dared to think beyond the mainstream protocol of chemotherapy and radiation for cancer treatment. He experimented with eating healthier and shared with me how research ascertained particular foods to help reverse cancer. *The Grape Cure* was one of the books he read and now many years later in the 21st century, scientists are revealing Resveretrol from red grape skins is helping to reduce disease including cancer in the body and extend life.

On a trip to Mexico Patrick purchased Laetrile, known as B17, extracted from the apricot pit, to spark immune function. Research later confirmed that B17 truly does have good benefits for certain individuals suffering immune deficiency. My brothers pioneering spirit led him to additionally experiment with the mental aspects of Cancer. He attended support groups to reduce unhealthy stress in the body. The facilitators explained how negative stress reduces ones immune system to function. This early theory later developed into the field of Psycho-Neuro-Immunology taught at UCLA Medical University. Its validity has been confirmed in multiple scientific studies. Excessive stress for prolonged periods of time holds disastrous effects on the body's immune system. My brother sparked my curiosity in so many areas of health which led me to purchase foods at the local health food store where I found the pamphlet that lit the fuse of health for me. That was over 30 years ago and I have been connecting the puzzle pieces of health and disease ever since.

I now share with you, after 25 years of intense study and working in medical clinics and private practice, with men, women and children; the health education and guidelines of living a healthy life with Gluten Intolerance. I am not the first to write about this factor that influences health in such a profound way. Yet I do hope you will find this book – ***Beyond Gluten Intolerance: GIS – Gluten Inflammatory Syndrome*** helpful in your life. Your appreciation will best be shown by sharing what you learn with others paving the way for a healthier world.

Introduction

Understanding health takes a good understanding of disease. Disease in the body is when the body is not at ease and is no longer functioning the way it was designed.

Disease can be present at birth due to DNA damage which affects chromosomes and in turn influences how the cells of the body grow and develop from one's heredity. The heredity comes from the biological parents of the child from conception. Scientists have also demonstrated through years of research that nutritional deficiencies can bring about mutation at birth or anytime during ones life [1] [2].

Disease or imbalances of the body's systems and brain function are in direct relationship to all factors in our internal and external environment. They either support or interfere with the brain and nerve transmission, digestive and absorption duties, immune function and tissue renewal of the trillions of cells that make up the body. If the body receives the nutrition it requires and can eliminate waste (both internal and external toxicity) and further protect itself from toxins, pollution and microbial attack through balancing inflammation and detoxification it reduces disease and premature aging.

Health of the stomach and the digestive tract and what we put into the body on a daily basis – affects the health of the entire body including the way we think, look and the illnesses we may develop. To enjoy a life with minimal pain, disease and optimize our longevity and enjoyment we must give the body the health support it demands by its divine design.

I believe in the Maslow's hierarchy of needs for the human body that requires; clean air, water, sunshine, a variety of nutrient dense foods and exercise along with emotional and spiritual nurturing to thrive [3]. As similar as human beings are in our daily requirements for a healthy body - each of us also have some characteristics that are influenced by our genetics and environment.

Factors Influencing Health:

- Environment
- Dietary & Exercise
- Attitude & Mental Wellness
- Obesity & Eating Disorders
- Addictions & Pharmaceutical Drugs
- Genetics

Our genetic code blueprint is made from the template of DNA that we receive from our biological parents. The DNA is responsible for our inheritance that creates genes which give us our strengths, weaknesses and physical characteristics at birth [4]. As you learn about the potential of nutrition and health to improve the profile of the DNA - you will understand the opportunity awaiting you to improve your overall genetic code weakness and deficiencies from your birth parents. Only when you become aware of your genetic flaws as with Gluten Intolerance - can a person strive for a better quality of life. By altering some of the daily eating patterns and making healthier lifestyle choices on purpose you can feel your daily best and protect the important DNA.

Gluten intolerance and to the degree of reaction an individual experiences to gluten are predisposed by both a genetic weakness and the nutritional status of the body at birth. We can be born with a severe sensitivity to the gluten protein and its influence on our health can be much greater than most people have identified [5]. Also, events affecting our health can alter our biology and give way to a heightened sense of gluten reactions. An example of this would be getting hit by the flu. Upon having this illness one takes a series of antibiotics and thereafter begins experiencing more pronounced digestive complaints. Other insults to the body like a car accident or surgery can also be catalysts to gut problems.

Gluten intolerance symptoms can be classified into two major related conditions known as Irritable Bowel Syndrome (IBS) and the advanced state of Crohn's / Celiac known as Inflammatory Bowel Disease (IBD). Both diseases can be recognized by the traditional symptoms to include; digestive complaints of gas, constipation and or diarrhea for a prolonged period of time. The advanced stage of IBD has more intensity and severity of the reactions and may result in intestinal bleeding, scarring of the intestinal tract and set up more mal-absorption than IBS. IBD also requires more intervention at times with pharmaceutical drugs to save lives in advanced cases. In both diseases however the same health regimen is recommended.

In fact some people respond so well to health and the dietary guidelines they follow that even though blood tests result in a positive diagnosis of IBD (advanced) the person only experiences very slight symptoms of bowel distress. The opposite can also be found with an individual having a variety of digestive ailments and the laboratory testing may result in a negative reading. Chapter 4 will explain the unreliability of current testing methods.

Common Symptoms of Gluten Intolerance:
- Gas & Bloating
- Diarrhea & Constipation
- Abdominal Pain & Ulcers
- Nausea & Hemorrhoids
- Allergies & Fatigue

Children can be born with symptoms of IBS and if parents are aware of the warnings signals, they can intervene to avoid years of unnecessary sickness and even stunted growth due to the gluten intolerance. I have found most adults have experienced years and sometimes a lifetime of living with different symptoms of gluten intolerance unaware of the cause. Many people just stop going to doctors with complaints because they offer no solutions to their daily digestive battle.

History of Clinical Observation

Over the past 25 years of counseling thousands of individuals with health conditions from multiple origins the puzzle pieces of how gluten intolerance affects digestion and disease have now come together. When I began back in the early 80's the symptoms of irritable bowel syndrome were thought of as every day food allergies.

During the one on one consultation, I would teach our clinic patients the value of foods and how to incorporate a healthier diet to rebuild their bodies. They would fill out intake questionnaires that gave intimate insight into how their digestive systems worked. Many people fighting cancer or living with other chronic illnesses like diabetes, CVD, allergies and a gamut of other conditions from rare to ordinary - lived with digestive decline not aware that they were dealing with gluten intolerance.

Digestive deficiency was confirmed with testing for levels of proper acidity in the stomach called Hydrochloric Acid (HCL) which is needed for a healthy digestive system. Some patients had no other physical symptoms except a lack of HCL along with their failing health. With other patients I observed symptoms to include; heartburn, diarrhea, constipation, bloating, diverticulitis, ulcers with an occasional combination of all of the above. This clinical on the job observation of health and disease confirmed what I learned in school yet taught me volumes about the association of factors leading up to disease states for children right on through to adults. Without a doubt years of unhealthy bowel habits and a lack of proper digestive ability and nutritional neglect leads people into disease.

I was grateful to learn these important lessons so early in my career. I taught the patients the mechanics of chewing foods well, drinking water between meals, taking digestive supplements to assist the body (as needed) and altered diets to eliminate offending foods.

Dairy and grains were the two food categories often dropped which left the person feeling much better. The grains thought to be most offending at that time were wheat, barley and sometimes corn. As the years passed I added more foods to the offending list that have been included in this book and adopted the phrase gluten intolerance which led to the phrase Irritable Bowel Syndrome or IBS.

I continued to observe the relationship between IBS symptoms and poor digestive health that developed into increased inflammation in the body. What emerged was a pattern of related symptoms setting off a fuse of other inflammatory disease states.

The symptoms of gluten intolerance vary greatly from individual to individual and are compounded with the amount of gluten foods and other offending food products that a person eats. Because of the confusion over what contains gluten or irritants I find people are often eating foods they think are gluten free only to discover from my work that they are ingesting many offending foods products.

Today the good news is IBS patients can now be validated and keep their dignity by not being labeled crazy. I have counseled many patients back in the early 80's and even present day that were given two prescriptions. One prescription to see the staff Nutritionist myself and the other one to see the staff Psych! In 1999 IBS received the diagnosis status of a true disease state that had always been deserved. It is a real bowel disease just less severe than that of Celiac's and Crohn's Disease. This has led the way for better treatment even though diet and the offending foods have still not been fully understood by most professionals and lay people alike.

In the first chapter I explain the history of grains and foods on planet Earth and how the evolution of cultivating grains and the manufacturing of them have precipitated the gluten sensitivity explosion we are now seeing in the 21st century. I also carefully reveal the entire family of gluten based foods (as research has confirmed) called Gliadins and Glutelins along with the rest of the Gluten Triggers that can ignite physical symptoms into advanced symptoms.

The origin of a disease must be identified before an effective protocol can be outlined for maintenance and even reversing the condition. Frequent bathroom visits can be a nuisance living with IBS or wishful daily regularity of the bowels. As the facts are revealed they will show that IBS is responsible for not only unfulfilled lives but also a catalyst for unnecessary suffering even responsible for cutting a life short for both children and adults [6].

What a dangerous catalyst Gluten can be that actually allows other disease states beyond the normal digestive complaints of the bowels to manifest. I call this chain reaction that gluten compounds the Gluten Inflammatory Syndrome (GIS). Chapter 5 will reveal the impact of disease development that is quite devastating in many instances. The relationship Gluten has in exhausting and weakening the body just may explain why many ancient civilizations avoided wheat and ate gluten free grains over the ages as in China where they still primarily eat only white rice [7].

To peak your interest as we begin the gluten story I wish to share with you the pearl of discovery revealed to me during this study. Ready – Set – Go; we are all gluten intolerant! *Gluten Intolerance* is actually a human condition of not being able to properly digest the gluten compounds. The only question that remains for each of us to determine is to what degree is our individual gluten sensitivity? Once I began to follow my own GIS program in its entirety, I have continually felt better than each previous year. I look healthier and younger and my energy is great! Health is truly our greatest wealth especially once we understand the full story - Beyond Gluten Intolerance!

What is Gluten?

"What is wrong with me I kept asking myself? My bowels were never regular during my entire life! I can still remember my parents giving me enemas as a young child. I also battled with my weight right through into my twenties. Weight has always been so much harder for me to shed than other women that I grew up with. Looking back over the years I reflect on what a messed up world I have lived in feeling sick so much of the time and not having a way out! The doctors had no definitive answers and never once did they mention the words gluten intolerant."

— *Kelly, Texas*

Gluten is the most highlighted culprit in the digestive disorder called Irritable Bowel Syndrome (IBS). It causes inflammation which leads to the development of increased bowel distress [1]. Other factors also come to play in IBS and together with the Gluten they ignite the digestive symptoms that include but are not limited to; cramping, gas, bloating, heartburn, diarrhea, constipation and mucus. Mucus in the digestive tract and the stool is very common with IBS besides being very annoying and a symptom not to be overlooked [2].

As you delve deeper into health you will learn how *inflammation* is greatly associated in many other disease states of the body including bowel disease in both children and adults. Known as the "Secret Killer", inflammation is also connected to Heart Disease [3], Cancer, Asthma,

Diabetes, Alzheimer's, Sickle-Cell Anemia, Rheumatoid Arthritis and even neurological diseases like Multiple Sclerosis (MS) and Lou Gehrig's disease (ALS) [4].

Gluten, pronounced glue' tin, describes a *sticky protein compound* having nutritional value, abundant in wheat yet also found in other common cereal *grain-grasses* and food products. A sub-category in the gluten family of grains includes brown rice and oats which have been growing in popularity and promoted in the modern diet. Wheat production has steadily increased over the years due to its nutritional value and in particular its higher percentage of gluten. When yeast is added during the bread making process the gluten from the grain gives the bread the desirable elastic texture and the ability to rise and retain its shape after baking.

The term gluten comes from the Latin word for glue and was first written about in the mid nineteenth century around 1850. The gluten plant protein is not soluble in water and people must extract it through a laborious process of washing the grain with water and solvents to remove the pale yellow-gray substance if they wish to use it as a thickening agent. This method has been used over century's right into present day. Multiple manufacturing applications have been found for gluten as well as fortifying bread and food products. You may be surprised to find out that gluten flour is commonly used today in processed foods.

Gluten was originally identified as the toxic substance abundantly found in wheat, causing symptoms in the advanced bowel condition referred to as Inflammatory Bowel Disease (IBD). IBD was first associated with Celiac Sprue and later Crohn's disease. At last the more common bowel condition, IBS, is also being connected to wheat and gluten intolerance as well. Along with grain intolerance, other dietary sensitivities exist with bowel disease. I refer to these other food catalyst as "Triggers".

Triggers are Co-Conspirators in Gluten Intolerance

One of the better known co-conspirator trigger food groups in bowel disease is dairy products. Cow's milk in particular is directly responsible for the common food allergy called *lactose intolerance*. The reaction to milk and many other milk products cause major digestive symptoms and mild to severe skin rashes. The symptoms can be nausea, vomiting, diarrhea and constipation affecting up to 15% of babies [5]. I find it extremely common and problematic in approximately half of the gluten sensitive individuals I have worked with and to a lesser degree in all adults and children. In fact, milk allergy is the number one allergy among children in the 21st Century [6].

An allergy to milk is defined more precisely as the inability to digest the protein called casein. The other side of the coin is the intolerance to lactose in the milk which is attributed to the lack of the *enzyme lactase*. Lactase is supposed to be secreted in the small intestine and is needed to break down the milk sugar lactose efficiently. So two separate digestive challenges may be taking place simultaneously with an individual having reactions to milk. Both situations call for improved digestive support and to avoid drinking milk.

A better option to drinking straight milk is to use fermented milk products like yogurt, kefir and approved cottage cheese. You can read more on fermented foods at the end of this chapter and also in Chapter 7. As you will discover, the inability to digest cow's milk appears to be ultimately responsible for setting the stage of poor digestion of gluten foods. Two additional partners in crime or triggers that undermine a person's digestion is the abuse of refined sugar [13] and somewhat innocent, a person's genetic weakness [7]. In learning more about gluten we are led to ask the question how does it impact the body so negatively?

How does Gluten Cause health challenges?

The chemistry behind gluten has expanded steadily over the years to help us understand why gluten and associated starch compounds found in wheat, barley, rye, oats, corn and some potatoes cause health challenges for humans. To comprehend why this protein gluten causes such devastating biological reactions and damage to the body we must understand that the body does not digest gluten very efficiently. The gluten molecule which is made up of protein and carbohydrate fractions has an extremely tight molecular bond. This structure has been brought about from years of refining the evolution of the grains genetics through scientific hybrid techniques.

When the body cannot break apart the molecular bond that holds these two food elements together during digestion it remains whole which causes an auto-immune response in the small intestine [25]. This response can be described as a food allergy reaction in the gastrointestinal (GI) tract. The immune system identifies the undigested gluten food particle as a foreign invader and elicits an attack by increasing white blood cells (WBC). The infection fighting WBC's further the response that can be measured in the blood through an increase of serum IgG4 antibodies [1].

This reaction of the immune system towards the gluten molecule results in inflammation of the tissue lining beginning first at the site of poor digestion in the small intestine [8]. As the body becomes more gluten sensitive the reactions can be transferred throughout the entire gastrointestinal tract anywhere from the esophagus to the large intestine even before the gluten or trigger reaches the small intestine.

The site and intensity of inflammation depends on the health of the tissue in each specific area of the GI tract affected. A full gamut of inflammatory responses may occur varying from slight irritation, increased mucus production to an acute response that leads to ulceration of the tissue lining. Ulcerative colitis or irritated pits of ulceration in the intestinal wall found with Crohn's disease demonstrates the acute response [14].

Another key reaction that many researchers are still unaware of is the chain reaction taking place throughout the *Nervous System*. Once the catalyst or trigger enters the body it appears to increase or suspend electrical impulse function upon the inflammatory response. Farfetched some of you may say? It is definitely not hard to comprehend for the person living with Parkinson's who realizes their tremors worsen within minutes upon eating whole grain bread. Once you review the research conducted thus far on bowel disease and learn the neuromuscular reactions that people experience associated with gluten – I think you will broaden your own understanding of just how toxic gluten can truly be [9].

Research Pinpoints to Poor Digestion as the Weak Link

Researchers discovered that the wheat molecule is actually a core of starch wrapped by the gluten protein. Newer techniques in processing grains around 1970 allowed the researchers to extract the gluten protein from the starch element. Their work revealed that the *gluten protein* was made up of smaller fractions primarily called *glutenins* and *gliadins*. The *alpha-gliadin* fraction, even though a smaller percentage in grains was deemed the most toxic to the intestinal cells especially for the sensitive Celiac patient [8].

In 1978 the poor digestive factor, or weak link associated with gluten intolerance, was dramatically proven. The scientists conducted an impressive and conclusive experiment. Researchers chemically separated the gluten molecule from the wheat grain into two separate parts; total carbohydrate and total protein and had the human subjects eat the separated food groups.

The results were unanimous. Upon consuming the separated fractions of the gluten protein not a single subject experienced bowel reactions to either the carbohydrate or the protein eaten apart from one another. Repeating this simple experiment resulted in the same enlightening outcome - no inflammation to the digestive tract was experienced whatsoever! Conversely, when the subjects ate the very same components left tightly bonded in the gluten molecule they developed severe symptoms of gluten intolerance [10]. As you reflect on this very significant finding - let's explore the history of grains more closely and look at the content and percentages of the different gluten containing grains. You will see why some grains can be eaten in moderation and others are best to avoid altogether.

Oats, Corn and Brown Rice Do Not Get a Gluten Free Pass

Historically the wheat grain has been faulted for bowel disease with little attention given to other grains. The reason there has been more referencing and science on the wheat grain is because it contains a higher percentage of gluten irritants than other grains, yet it is not the lone perpetrator.

Disappointing to some of you, oats are very problematic for triggering digestive issues. Researchers believe that this is due to the cross breeding of grains in the fields over many years. This type of natural contamination led to oats becoming more of an irritant in the glutinous category even though oats do not belong to the same family of cereal grasses as wheat, barley and rye [11].

Oats are in a different grain family class called Aveneae yet share several of the subgroup genetic categories with wheat, barley, rye and also corn. Amazingly, oats are still widely eaten by gluten reactive individuals. People need to avoid oats along with the major offending whole grains to stop reactions and regain their health. Corn and even rice, especially brown rice, can also be a challenge for some individuals sensitive in the highest zone of reaction. The bran of the brown rice is where the higher percentage of glutinous protein is found along with other anti-nutrients.

With the grain category being the most widely consumed food group on our planet limiting these food choices can sound threatening and even bordering on ridiculous. The main objective here is to alert people of the entire grain category that brings about varying degrees of inflammation. At this point you may be asking yourself, "What am I going to eat?"

I have gone through the same steps of awareness myself, ranging from shock and denial to gluten sensitivity acceptance. People do not like change yet I encourage each of you to do your best and keep an open mind and a positive attitude. Having already made the switch I testify that truly delicious food awaits you in the low gluten and gluten free world.

The health challenge facing most people of today is that they are flat out eating too much quantity of the offending foods. Gluten and other triggers are abundant in whole grain cereals, bagels, pizza, milk, ice cream and more. Triggers are other food categories that cause similar reactions to grains when eaten that are likened to the gluten molecule in structure. Some triggers that sneak into a person's diet are malt vinegar, hydrolyzed vegetable protein, gluten flour, regular soy sauce, soy products, modified food starch, vegetable gums like carrageenan, milk solids in products and high fructose corn syrup found in sodas and other processed foods. Eating high amounts of fried foods and chips containing a large percentage of Omega-6 Fatty Acids is also considered a trigger because it sets inflammation into motion, bringing on digestive woes due to an imbalance in the Essential Fatty Acids reviewed in Chapter 5.

Large quantities of gluten and triggers cause a greater amount of inflammation and bowel symptoms. A good place to start in a transitional diet is eating less of the offending foods. It does make a difference in lowering inflammation and feeling better. Making other healthy choices in your life outlined in Chapters 6, 7 and 8 along with finding gluten substitutes will bring faster results as well. I must caution you right away though, not to get fooled by over eager marketers that are mislabeling foods - Gluten Free. Chapter 7 will give you lists of low gluten grains and lots of health tips to guide you along the way.

Relax as you continue to learn about grains and I promise there will not be an exam at the end of this chapter. As we continue learning about gluten in the history of grains it can give us a better understanding of how wheat came into its popularity on the planet. Interestingly the largest percentage of the worlds inhabitants thousands of years ago were not eating the wheat grain. Wheat had originally been isolated to the Middle East region and slowly spread throughout the world somewhat recently in history more as an industrial marketing endeavor.

The History of Wheat on Planet Earth

All edible grains of today for human and livestock consumption are classified in the food genetic family called *Gramineae*. There exists thousands of varieties of cereal grains in modern day across the globe, yet the most common cereals you are likely to recognize include; rice, wheat, barley, oats and corn some call maize. Sorghum, millet and quinoa are low gluten grains that have been eaten in many countries for centuries. In the U.S., sorghum has been primarily used in animal feed yet is beginning to develop a following by people. On the other hand millet and quinoa have been incorporated into households for years as gluten alternatives and nutritious choices. White rice plus these three grains are quite tasty and versatile to use in any favorite recipe.

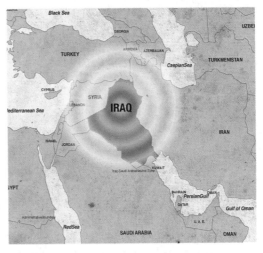

The history of grains goes back to at least 8,000 BC where historians began to record their cultivation [15]. Wheat was traced to first being grown in the Middle East around Iraq and Iran, where it still grows wild today. As researchers followed the cultivation it fanned out to the north and westward regions throughout much of Asia, North Africa and Europe.

From Europe wheat traveled into the southwest of Ireland around 3,000 BC. However the common consumption of wheat did not really emerge until the potato famine in Ireland of 1845 which lasted until 1852. The devastation reduced their population to only 25%. This disaster proved that a variety in food is extremely important to a cultures survival and wheat slowly took over to become a staple in the Irish diet. Ireland is now recording the highest incidence of Crohn's per capita of all the

European countries – coincidence? Its Atlantic neighbor Finland recently reported a doubling of their gluten intolerance in 2000 [12]. The statistics on gluten intolerance are rising all around the globe. History has revealed Celiac Sprue and a bit later Crohn's to be the first diseases directly related to wheat intolerance and you will learn more about the medical history of gluten intolerance reviewing the timeline in Chapter 2 [14].

Following wheat's history revealed that the Egyptians grew the largest amount for exporting. They would ship their finished wheat products from their former capital of Alexandria to many destinations

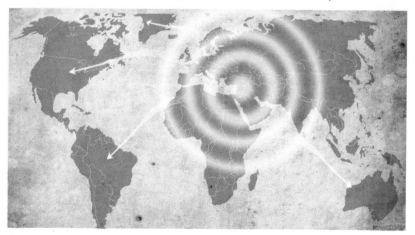

including all the way to Rome. The original idea of making pasta was first believed to have developed in China. The Chinese made noodles from rice developing many varieties and later the idea of pasta trickled down into Italy. The Italian's choice over rice was wheat for their pasta making where it has remained a staple to this very day.

The 7th century Buddhist monks creatively sought out meat-like ingredients for use in their vegetarian diet. They discovered wheat gluten worked most excellently for the imitation meats which they seasoned to taste like chicken, duck, fish, pork and beef. Perhaps this religious practice influenced the 7th Day Adventists religion of today in their use of gluten to make vegetarian mock foods. Historians noted that wheat came to the Americas by way of Christopher Columbus and again by the Pilgrims in 1620. This new grain added variety to the American Indians indigenous food of wild rice, also known as Indian rice and maize. For better or for worse wheat spread throughout the world's population as an expansion to peoples already established diets. Now let's focus on the evolutionary practice of the hybrid techniques of wheat that added to the present day epidemic of gluten intolerance.

Gluten Hybrid Techniques - A Catalyst for Digestive Trouble

Slowly over time the ancient wheat, first named *wild emmers* wheat, began to change. This change occurred through both natural evolution and man's hybrid techniques which changed wheat to closer resemble the modern hard and soft wheat of today.

As difficult as it has been to precisely track the evolving wheat DNA genetics - it is thought that possibly the *emmers wheat* was genetically influenced from the *spelt* variety in Asia before reaching Europe. However some researchers still think the *emmers wheat* came first into Europe and then evolved into the *spelt* variety. Several different varieties of *spelt wheat* have been sprinkled about geographically yet the timeline is not totally clear as to the exact time sequence [15]. The puzzle of how the different grains developed may never be solved yet it does appear that the oldest *spelt wheat* grain seems to be a bit more tolerated by some gluten intolerant people.

A long time ago, approximately 2,500 BC the Egyptians learned how to utilize the gluten of the newer varieties of wheat. They became masters of baking the sturdy leavened wheat breads and that's when exporting took off. Wheat began to be prized as more of a staple than other grains of that era for a couple of important reasons. First, wheat offered much more nutritional value from its higher protein content than other grains. Second and paramount to our discussion is the fact that wheat's are unmatched in their stabilizing characteristic due to the gluten supporting the finished products to hold a firm shape. Oats, millet, rice, rye and barley grains that were originally consumed in Asia and the European cold climates contain some gluten protein yet not in the large quantity that developed in the new wheat varieties.

A modern example of hybridization is the *triticale* grain. A relatively new cereal, food scientists have engineered it by time tested hybrid techniques. They crossed wheat with rye and that doubled the genetic chromosomes and increased the stability of its finished grain products.

Where is gluten located in the grain?

With all the talk of gluten where is it actually located? A single grain of wheat or other grain has the majority of gluten in the outer covering or bran. When milled the outer bran is removed along with the endosperm which contains valuable nutrients including Vitamin E and Vitamin B-Complex. The bran or fiber contains most of the protein, nutritional oils, vitamins, some phyto-nutrients and an array of macro and micro minerals. What is left is primarily a starchy carbohydrate grain with little nutritional value.

Wheat Kernel

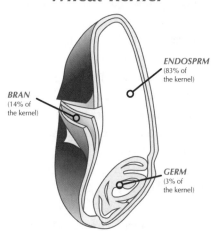

ENDOSPRM
(83% of
the kernel)

BRAN
(14% of
the kernel)

GERM
(3% of
the kernel)

Fortunately, Vitamin E and the B-Complex including minerals can be sourced in significant amounts from; leafy green vegetables, raw nuts and seeds, nutritional yeast and a small amount exist in a variety of other foods reviewed in Chapter 7 and 8 [16].

After milling, only trace amounts of nutritional components are left within the starch carbohydrate, called farina, yet the upside is only a minimal amount of gluten resides as well. 100% white flour is not considered a highly sensitive food for medium to low gluten intolerance. I realize the suggestion to eat refined white flour products is an odd statement with so much emphasis these days on the importance of whole grains. However, white flour and also white rice can add more variety, calories for energy and overall satisfaction to a meal. For most individuals they can enjoy refined wheat and rice without the negative reactions coming from excessive gluten. As a health educator this has become a bit of an oxymoron situation for me to warn people not to eat wholegrain products. I have been well versed on the value of complex carbohydrates, reducing the glycemic spike of blood sugar, as with diabetes and hypoglycemia. Rest assured that the body can control its blood sugar without the addition of whole grains.

Another facet of whole grains you want to make note of is that whole grains contain some other potentially dangerous *anti-nutrients* side by side the gluten. Anti-nutrients interfere with absorption of valuable core nutrients, such as minerals, and are present in other foods besides grains, like soybeans and cooked spinach. The case for eating refined carbohydrates and going back to sprouted and fermented foods is building. The GIS story explains the mystery of why ancient cultures have stayed away from whole grains and included more of the low gluten and refined grain products like white rice [21].

Even though white grain products are somewhat allowable please use caution with persons living with advanced bowel disease. Certain stipulations must be well understood upon eating commercially processed white rice and white wheat products. One important reason to apply caution is the legal mandate of enriching grains of 1900. This federal law which is still in place today requires the practice of *nutritional enrichment* of white grain products in many states of the U.S. The enriching process dictates that manufacturers must add back B Vitamins, Iron and Iodine to refined grains. The problem with this process comes with the fortification of the grain requiring the use of a carrier coating consisting of wheat or corn starch! This may explain why boxed grain products have caused digestive upset for many gluten sensitive individuals. The safer alternative is to purchase organic white grain products from the health food store outlets to reduce the possibility of receiving the enriched grains. Make certain as you do this that you have good nutritional coverage in the diet of the enriched nutrients; B-Complex, Iron and Iodine.

Another shocking situation is the practice of bread manufacturers adding gluten flour into finished products. Manufacturing practices of today are driven by financial gain and the bread companies are sharing in the corporate greed. Wholegrain and white breadstuffs may now contain gluten flour added to help the stability of the finished food. This is happening in regular whole grain breads, sprouted whole grain breads, and even traditional white breads including sourdough bread and white flour and corn tortillas! Some companies claim wheat flour on the ingredients even when the breadstuff is primarily white, as a way to caution the consumer to the addition of the gluten flour.

I am very disappointed to read how many products list gluten flour in the ingredients yet at least they are the honest companies. Other less scrupulous ones are simply adding the gluten flour with no reference on the label at all. Yes you guessed it - there is no way to tell ultimately except by a physical reaction. Also topping it off is the existing federal allowance that approves companies to add trigger thickeners to products like ice cream, catsup, dairy products and more. The government does not require even a notation in the ingredients or anywhere on the label to alert the consumer. It is no wonder that people are having more digestive upset and health challenges than ever before!

Yes - it is very important to become a stealth label reader yet with dishonest companies and loose labeling laws the bottom line is paying attention to the body's symptoms and reactions from eating particular foods. How you react from a certain food will be the best indicator. You also have the option to seek a series of blood tests to measure your inflammation reactions to foods however be warned about blood tests. Some people show a negative result on blood tests to gluten. This is common even though a person can be obviously gluten intolerant. Chapter 4 will review the lab tests available and explain the short comings.

To complete the story of gluten – most people do well eating white rice and white pastry flour products, white tortillas and some corn products in moderation - if no gluten is added. Several alternative grain flours and their products are available and are reviewed in Chapter 7. This will also include the sprouted grain bread products that give a wonderful alternative to cutting out all whole grains in ones diet. I personally love the nutty flavor of whole grains and enjoy incorporating the 100% sprouted variety in moderation and indeed understand the value of their added nutrition when properly processed.

Wheat is not all bad!

Wheat has been called the staff of life because of its excellent nutrition, storability and versatility. Its high nutrition and low cost has gained it a very high status with over 60 countries growing it for their prized crop. Unfortunately and a very important point in our discussion of gluten is the fact that the wheat varieties grown today reflect little resemblance to wheat grown thousands of years ago. It is my belief, due to the ardent work through making the wheat genetically stronger for stability - it is now much harder to digest than ever before!

Another fact to consider is the finished breads made by our ancestors were prepared in a manner that is not practiced by mainstream bread makers of today. Bread flours of yesterday were sprouted and fermented allowing the gluten to change form and lose much of its inflammatory properties. To reap the optimum benefit from all grains as derived with 100% sprouted bread the grain must be sprouted first and then made into flour. The optimal bread recipe needs to allow the kneaded bread to rise for at least 6 - 8 hours. Modern bread makers are baking breads that rise in just 2 hours or less which skips the valuable fermentation process. Sadly the availability of these properly made breads is scarce. Another facet of bread making to keep in mind is that the bran in the breads can be a major source of inflammation in people. Years ago it was a rare situation for breads to ever contain bran [26]!

History has confirmed that the percentage of gluten in the varieties of flours used today has increased. The total gluten content is higher than in the past along with its genetically tighter bound physical property. Of course there is a variance within each type of wheat.

Hard wheat contains the highest gluten content of bread flours with soft wheat approximately 50% less. The cake flour is the lowest in gluten at just 8% average and it makes sense that it is used to produce a light and soft texture in wedding cakes and other confections. Note how high the straight "Gluten Flour" is at 45%. This is the gluten extract being added to many breadstuffs of today. Companies are adding this high gluten flour to increase the durability in white breads, cereals, pizza and manufactured food products. No one eats pizza, right? I am convinced that this fortification with gluten flour is another big factor giving rise to the skyrocketing bowel disease symptoms in kids, adults and even pets of today! As mentioned, some of the manufacturers are not even claiming gluten flour on the ingredients of white bread products. Be aware that also some inflammatory bran is coming from certain seeds along with the grain fibers that are added to foodstuff increasing the total fiber content. These fibers are to be avoided by highly sensitive individuals and that includes what is in the fiber and bran supplements of oat, wheat, psyllium and flax seed fibers.

Percentages of Gluten in Today's Hybrid Wheat:

Gluten Flour	45%
Hard Wheat	13%
All Purpose Flour	10-12%
Soft Wheat Pastry Flour	9-10%
Cake Flour	7-9%

How do people keep their bowels moving and cholesterol in check without the addition of grain fibers?

Since grain fibers are not the best choice due to gluten intolerance the better way to encourage regularity which in itself lowers negative cholesterol is to switch the focus to fruits and vegetables including beans as tolerated. Besides these foods contributing gluten free food fibers they also provide valuable phyto-nutrients for the body to maintain optimum health. By switching you will find the gluten free food fibers will keep the bowels moving better than any grain fiber products without adding to digestive issues!

Breads, bread products and dry snack foods made with alternative low gluten ingredients are popping up in many food store markets and grocery store chains that may possibly work for your level of sensitivity. Review the Healthy TIPS section in Chapter 7 to avoid more confusion. Feeling better and healing the body is all about making the best choices. Some individuals must avoid all grains for a certain period of time to allow the body to heal. Two delicious alternatives to grains that are low inflammatory choices are yams and red potatoes. They are well tolerated by even the most highly sensitive people as discussed in Chapter 7. You are also given complete menu suggestions for any level of gluten intolerance in this chapter along with easy tasty recipes and snack ideas.

Solving the Gluten Puzzle

The first gluten puzzle piece is the realization that "Gluten Intolerance" evolved over the years due to a shift of including more wheat and wheat products in the human diet. Secondly, the hybrid agricultural practices have increased the bond adherence within the gluten molecule and increased the gluten content. The last gluten piece is the onslaught of more and more gluten flour and glutinous triggers being added to processed foods.

Other changes taking place in our civilization has also increased the numbers of people experiencing bowel disturbances. There has been deterioration or in other words a lack of actual digestive ability in people to properly digest food in general. This has come from our fast paced society, food abuse and addictions coupled with an overall neglect of health support for the body.

Taking back responsibility and optimizing the body's health requires improving all digestive capabilities and this is covered in-depth in Chapter 3. Improving ones health of the entire body requires balance and lowering the potential of inflammatory factors from all sources including; diet, stress and lifestyle choices. I believe nature does evolve in a most perfect synergism in our world however the glitches seem to crop up when man changes the natural development of the chemistry of foods or interrupts the chemistry of man with toxins and pollution.

Some individuals suggest that gluten sensitive people can simply take extra digestive enzymes to eliminate their symptoms. I agree that people need to optimize their digestive capabilities. My concern of going for just a "fast fix" is the potential for upsetting the entire digestive tracts chemistry. I have witnessed this outcome in many individuals that by only taking a high potency digestive enzyme resulted in gut aches and long-term digestive challenges not wellness.

A better sequence for individuals is to first take the required Essential Core Nutrients that support all of the systems of the body (see Chapter 8) that supports the digestive metabolism. The second step is to follow the GIS Diet and make improved lifestyle choices that help to rebalance the digestive metabolism and if still needed at that point then experiment with digestive supplements covered in Chapter 8. Digestion is an important part of the gluten puzzle however there are more factors involved in digestion that are equally important to enzymes that demand the health support for the rest of the body's systems. Simply taking a digestive supplement will not provide optimum health.

Delving Deeper Into the Science of Gluten; Triticeae Gluten Grains (TGG)

Learning about the origin and reviewing the scientific data of the family of gluten grains can help you make better dietary choices. Scientists have been busy discovering the biological components from grains that compound bowel distress and other related diseases. A lack of funding unfortunately has limited more specific research into all of the grains [17]. The wheat, rye, barley and oat grains contain the highest amount of protein which is where the gluten compounds are found [18]. Other grains can also be offending foods just to a lesser degree. According to research compiled in the *U.S. Manual of Grasses* by Hitchcock in 1950, the following list can give more perspective. According to Hitchcock the degree of inflammation coming from wheat, rye and barley is the greatest and corn is the least offending grain [22]. Having said this please note that some parents have commented that corn was responsible for the advanced hyperactivity experienced by their children and only through the removal of corn from the diet did their child finally calm down. Review ADD a nd ADHD in Chapter 5 for more details.

Ranking the Inflammation of Grains
1. Wheat, Rye & Barley
2. Oats
3. Brown Rice
4. Wild Rice
5. Millet
6. Sorghum
7. Corn

Family Tree of Sticky Grains Higher in Gluten Gramineae
(Category of all grains)

I. Sticky -Triticeae Glutens Grains (TGG) and [II. Non – Sticky – Triticeae Low Gluten – Not Included]

A. Triticeae Taxa (species) Includes; 1.Triticum aestivum (spring wheat), 2.Triticum monococcum (einkorn wheat), 3.Secale (rye), 4.Triticosecale (wheat, barley, rye), 5.Hordeum (barley), 6.Aegilops speltoides (spelt) and 7.Tauschii strangulatum, 8.Agropyron and 9.Aveneae (oats).

The new terminology used with grains can sound a bit confusing yet give it a read through just for curiosity's sake. There are two protein subsets to focus on; the *Glutelins* and *Gliadins*. It is the *alpha-gliadins* that are the most dreaded inflammatory offenders found in whole grains and wheat contains the highest percentage [19]. For simplicity sake I will continue to refer to the subsets throughout the book as simply GLUTEN.

Delving deeper into the science of gluten the entire large category of grains is called *Gramineae* which includes all of the edible grains. Within this large family are grains with higher seed storage of proteins called *Triticeae Glutens* - also technically called *Triticum aestivum* which bread wheat, durum wheat also known as *semolina wheat* are members. The family tree of grains, focuses on the sticky side of the family and gives a helpful visual which includes all of the sticky species along with the *Triticum aestivum, Triticum monococcum, Secale, Triticosecale, Hordeum, Aegilops speltoides, Tauschii Strangulatum, Agropyron* and *Aveneae*.

Wheat, Rye & Barley

The hybrid techniques used over the years have developed the Triticeae taxa group of grains including the Aestivum varieties which give way to the sticky capacity, from the gluten, allowing the bread to rise and retain its shape during baking. The wheat of today is known as the True Wheat [20]. Wheat as we know it was thought to have developed from three grass species called Aegilops Speltoides to include; Aegilops Tauschii Strangulate and Triticum Monococcum. The True Wheat variety can simply be termed *Triticum*.

The review of sticky gluten containing grains that includes wheat, looks at the high protein of these grains analyzing the content of amino acids (building blocks of protein) that includes; Arginine, Proline, Glutamine and Aspargine. The amino acid Arginine holds another important puzzle piece fueling the inflammatory cycle of GIS. As elaborated in Chapter 6 Healthy Focus Factors Viruses-high Arginine intake stimulates the Herpes Virus which in itself is a secondary trigger evoking bowel disease and other symptoms. Further review of the sticky gluten family includes the species of food barleys *Hordeum* and also food ryes *Secale*. They are lower in gluten than wheat however best to be avoided on a regular basis unless they are sprouted.

Oats

Scientific speculation states that the *Aveneae* known as oats merged into this blood line of grains through cross breeding in the fields therefore it evolved into the family of sticky grains. If you have ever eaten oatmeal you have witnessed this sticky almost slimy characteristic with cooked oats. Some people have speculated that the commercial oat products also may have become contaminated with other gluten flours at the grain mills and for all of the reasons are best left alone unless they are 100% sprouted. Researchers speculate that approximately 8% of gluten sensitive people are extremely reactive to oats even the steel cut. I find the numbers to be much higher. Once you learn to recognize the wide range of gluten symptoms listed in Chapter 2 the chances are you will agree. Why the oat grain has been categorized by many people over the years into the gluten free category is only due to its lower quantity of gluten.

The famous European researcher by the name of Hitchcock found oats to be particularly troublesome in the body. As shown in the ranking list he found wheat, rye and barley in tribe 3, oats in tribe 4, rice in tribe

9 and corn in 14ᵗʰ place or the lowest reaction. I suppose it is because oats have such a sweet desirable flavor that even advanced bowel distressed individuals dread leaving it out of the diet. As tasty as oats are to the palate they can react like a digestive poison to some people. Millet can be a delicious alternative hot cereal with a little added fruit and yogurt, honey and cinnamon - yummy good!

Rice

Rice, especially the brown rice has not been researched to reveal its inflammatory chemistry. I find however that most sensitive people, including myself, feel best eating only white rice perhaps combining it with a little wild rice for added texture and flavor.

The rest of the family of higher gluten grains consists of *Triticosecale, Aegilops* and *Agropyron* which all sound a bit like characters from Greek mythology. As mentioned there is insufficient research on grains including these three therefore they are not included in the chart.

Within the large group of *Triticeae Gluten Grains (TGG)* are four distinguishing *protein groups* that are found in wheat, barley, rye and other grains. The four groups are Albumins, Globulins, Prolamins and Glutelins. It is the Prolamins that contain the **Gliadin** and Glutelins containing **Glutenin** that make up the reactive GLUTEN protein as we know it [23].

The other two protein groups Albumins and Globulins are not directly involved with the gluten response however they do play a role in health. These two groups of proteins found in grains are catalysts for food allergies that can possibly be a secondary reaction for some highly sensitive people. In this discussion gluten is the focused topic yet the GIS diet guidelines and program addresses all allergies from every source.

Four Protein Compounds in TGG Grains:

- **Albumins** - protein isolated from TGG and found in smaller amounts in the first stages of grain development associated with allergies.
- **Globulins** - protein isolated from TGG and found in smaller amounts in the first stages of grain development associated with allergies.
- **Prolamins** - gliadin (smaller units - low molecular weight LMW); Triticum (True Wheat 20% gliadins also containing the *highest quantity of alpha gliadin*), Hordeum (barley), Secale (rye),

Aveneae (oats), Orzenin (rice), Zein (corn). *The gluten protein contains approximately 1/3 of this protein.*

- **Glutelins - glutenin** (larger units - high molecular weight HMW); Triticum (Wheat 35-40% glutenins), Hordeum (Barleys – glutelins; major alpha 3%, minor-beta), Secale (rye glutelin). *The gluten protein contains approximately 2/3 of this protein.*

The *Triticeae Gluten Grains* TGG develops many different protein compounds during a particular growth stage and some are more inflammatory than others depending on their ratio of Gliadin to Glutenin. Significantly 2/3 of the gluten protein compounds are in the form of **Glutelins** containing the **Glutenin.** The smaller percentage of protein compounds fall into the **Prolamins** category of **Gliadins** however this type is much more toxic to the digestive tissue.

Remarkably, scientists have isolated more than 40 different *gliadin protein compounds* that contain slightly different gliadin characteristics which are classed into; alpha (a-), beta (B), gamma (y) and omega (w). Corn and rye both contain more of the y gliadins and according to research other food thickeners contain similar profiles that are used in the food processing industry that will be mentioned later in the trigger category and in Chapter 7.

Scientist Have Isolated 40 Different Gliadin Protein Compounds

- Researchers state that the alpha form of the gliadin protein causes the highest inflammation response compared to the other fractions.
- The alpha form is highest in wheat which is another reason it has been targeted to cause more destructive symptoms in the body besides the highest percentage of total gluten.
- Mammal studies pinpointed the wheat alpha gliadin to be poisonous to young mice [24].
- Secondary in reactions to mammals is the glutenins which are more abundant in grains and foods yet not as lethal to body tissues.

Wheat as listed in the Four Protein Compound TGG list contains the highest percentages in both the gluten Prolamins and also the highest in gluten Glutelins. Because of its higher levels of gluten compounds wheat is best to be avoided in the diet for advanced bowel disease IBD and reduced for IBS along with the rest of the grains if you are to reach optimum health [25]. Sprouting and fermenting grains do offer an alternative to regular flours for all people because as you will read it changes the chemistry of the Gluten molecule.

Sticky Characteristics of Gluten Compounds; Not Good for the Stomach yet are Great in Manufacturing!

Identifying the gluten compounds, regardless of the percentage of glutelins or gliadins can be done in a visual manner along with scientific testing. Most gluten from grains and gluten like triggers display a *sticky gluten physical characteristic*! Regardless of what the source is from plant as with gelatin and grains or animal sources as in the hoofs of mammals, most gluten food products contain a natural occurring "stickiness" characteristic.

The gluten compounds are ultra-radical sticky, so much so that gluten is manufactured for glue. It is used in many industrial applications including; wall paper, fabric adhesives, and fillers for commercial use. It has even been used in making Paper Mache artwork. This sticky characteristic is why cultures over the decades have genetically engineered the varieties of wheat they used in food stuffs for thickening and stability.

Gluten is good on the outside but not on the inside of the body and can be identified quite easily on dirty dishes and cooking utensils. For example it can be spotted in the kitchen by the sticky residue left on a pan from cooking the common Russet potato. A good alternative is the red potato which is significantly less sticky and can be eaten without digestive concern. We have all experienced the cement like coating from oatmeal or spaghetti left in a bowl or hard as nails Parmesan cheese the type that is out of a shaker container. This is due to the manufacturer including extenders in the processed cheese that is laden with milk solids and even wheat protein at times.

Fortunately, most cheeses can be eaten on a gluten free diet. The unprocessed aged Parmesan cheese is great if grated fresh and it tastes better than the box any day! As you become keen at identifying these physical characteristics and adjust your diet accordingly, you will begin to trust your judgment more and more so that eating at home or in a restaurant setting is not a gassy experience. Review the Healthy Tips section in Chapter 7 for eating guidelines. When you experience less of the GIS symptoms - that is an indicator that you are making good choices!

What is the Goal Concerning Gluten?

The goal for people of today is to first identify where the Gluten and GIS triggers are located in one's diet. Our history reveals that the high gluten grains have not always been eaten in the extraordinarily large amounts of today. The modern grains with their hybrid genetics are not the same as the original ancient grains and are prepared quickly, not fermented, and therefore much harder to digest. Experimenting with sprouted and properly fermented grains can allow people to safely add back the nutritious and enjoyable food sources from the grain family.

To take back the responsibility and regain our health we all need to avoid the intake of high gluten, trigger foods and balance inflammatory conditions in the body. Recognizing other inflammatory factors and imbalances in our lives will become clearer as you review the big picture of the Gluten Inflammatory Syndrome (GIS) in the chapters ahead. As you embark on your health path taking steps toward a healthier you by reducing gluten I guarantee that you will begin to feel better than you ever thought possible regardless of your age or state of health!

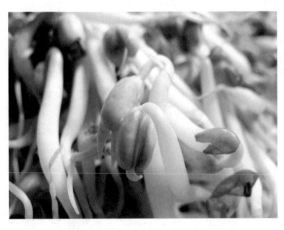

HIGHLIGHT 1:
Sprouted & Fermented Foods

Sprouted and fermented foods are enjoyed today by many people in modern societies yet they were once considered a mainstay by ancient cultures. Evidence suggests fermented foods were eaten as far back as 7,000 years ago in Babylon. Food traditions such as these have prevailed because of providing several significant benefits including health support.

Every culture has adopted some type of sprouting and or fermenting process to make foods more digestible and accessible to the human population. Some grains, dairy products, beans, nuts and seeds and even meats have been processed with these methods. Both practices can enhance a foods nutritional value. The process takes the existing nutrition and develops added health benefits. Fermentation in particular has secured human survival through natural food preservation of otherwise perishable foods. Another enjoyable benefit comes from the addition of the pungent-sour tastes of foods that tantalize the taste buds and compliment other food tastes.

Sprouting & Fermenting Foods Increase;
- *Nutritional Value* – providing more amino acids (protein building blocks), vitamins, minerals and antioxidant constituents.
- *Digestibility* – reduces irritants from sugars (lactose, amylose), starches (amylo-pectins) and gluten compounds changing them to plant proteins – gluten free. Reduction of anti-nutrients in beans and grains that block mineral absorption.
- *Natural Preservation & Health Support* – by creating organic acids (lactic acid bacteria and others) the process reduces the spoilage of foods while increasing health factors that greatly increase immunity in the body.
- *Taste Enjoyment* – adds the pungent- sour taste created by the good bacteria to foods broadening the variety of tastes and flavor.

What is Fermentation?
Fermentation of foods refer to the process of making pickled and cultured vegetables, soured milks, cheeses, yeast breads, bean and meat ferments, fish sauce, alcoholic beverages and even some teas. Coffee and cocoa processes also require fermentation. It actually works by controlling the process of decay using *special bacteria* and *natural enzymes* that create a more stable end product. Some food ferments can even maintain good hygienic standards without refrigeration.

Fermentation can also simplify a food through altering its chemistry. The process lowers the foods pH allowing a type of *pre-digestion* of the sugars and starches found in carbohydrates converting them into simpler forms of alcohols and organic acids that benefit the body as in yogurt. Fermentation also allows for many *anti-nutrients* to be eliminated like natural compounds found in grains and nuts which include; cyanide, phytic acid and oxalic acid. This process can even break apart the gluten molecule. Whole grains are converted to gluten free especially if they are both sprouted and fermented before baking of bread or other cracker like products.

Most fermentation processes require the addition of a *starter culture*. This consists of a special bacteria being added to the food that is to promote the fermentation. You can either purchase this culture or transfer some of the previous batch of fermented food to the new batch. Following the directions or recipe for each type of food ferment is necessary for success. Even though the concept is the same, each particular food or beverage may need to be precooked, sliced in a particular size, soaked for a certain length of time or kept at an exact temperature or other important parameters. If making ferments yourself, take special care to clean all equipment thoroughly, not to contaminate your batches with any bad bacteria that might cause unnecessary spoilage.

What is the Difference of Brine & Vinegar?

A unique type of ferment called *brine solution* is made from salt, water, spices and sometimes sugar. The brine which covers the food allows the naturally occurring anaerobic good bacteria found on the food itself to multiply. The good bacteria, creates acidic acid from the carbohydrate in the food. The acidic acid lowers the foods pH controlling the undesirable aerobic bacteria that would normally spoil a food.

Vinegar is not in itself a ferment catalyst for any foods. Vinegar is made from a fermentation process using apples, grapes or rice. The result is apple cider vinegar, wine or balsamic vinegars and rice vinegar respectively. White vinegar is basically a chemically made product and does not contain any medicinal properties to speak of as does other vinegars.

Natural vinegars add their own flavors to foods and offer some limited health benefits due to their pH and astringent elements. Vinegar can also be used in canning and pickling foods as a natural preservative. If you have fermented or pickled foods open in your refrigerator you can also add extra vinegar to completely cover the contents prolonging the storage by preventing mold growth. Pickled foods do not give the added medicinal value of fermented vegetables that use a brine solution.

Fermentation is the process that allows the growth of colonies of good bacteria. The good bacteria ingested through fermented foods can include hundreds of different species referred to as *Probiotics*. These friendly bacteria live and multiply in the GI tract of a person or mammal if the conditions are just right. Research has confirmed the good bacteria to be advantageous to digestion, fighting infection and helps to heighten one's overall immune system function. Probiotics is reviewed in-depth in the Chapter 2 HIGHLIGHT telling about the important friendly bacteria for reaching optimum health.

Fermented Products Around the Globe

Foods, beverages and seasonings that you can make or purchase that are fermented include; yogurt (goat, cow, other milk), cheese (goat, cow, other) , butter, kefir (cow milk), kumis (horse milk), tempeh (soy-grain burger), buttermilk, prosciutto (ham), salami, pickled herring, fish sauce, miso paste (soy), soy sauce, brined vegetables & relishes, sauerkraut, pickled beets, pickles, vinegar, Kimchi (vegetables), Ogi (millet porridge cereal), Natto (fermented soy cereal), Essene Bread (100% sprouted), Sourdough bread, vanilla extract, hot sauce, olives, coffee, cocoa, black tea, cigars, beer, wine, Sake, whiskey, Kombucha (mushroom family), vodka, mead (honey wine) and varying supplements of Probiotics.

The fermented and sprouted foods have one main common trait. Both types of foods and beverages allow the food to become more easily digested along with developing the stabilizing benefits. Fermented and Sprouted Foods are readily available for purchase in most health food and gourmet food sections of grocery and health food stores. Review Chapter 7 in Tasty & Delicious Recipes for the Homemade Yogurt recipe. It is a fairly easy recipe if your lifestyle lends you a little extra time.

What is Sprouting?

Our ancestors learned how to avoid many of the nutritional pitfalls present in foods to avoid inflammation and the loss of nutrients through several alternatives including *sprouting*. Another way they by-passed the irritants was through the refining of grains. A good example of this is the preference of eating white rice over brown rice. By hulling the brown rice and other grains they avoided the anti-nutrients located in the bran of the grain. Refining the grains solves the challenge of the irritants however it also wastes valuable food nutrients that could be saved through sprouting. Historians have confirmed that early inhabitants of the planet sought out the low-gluten grains, root vegetables when they did not have the fermented or sprouted foods available. Many cultures have continued with the alternative starch choices ultimately because of the health results they receive.

To sprout whenever possible sets in motion a biochemical change of the foods chemistry. The down side of sprouting is the time factor required however similar to fermenting both processes reduce the irritants that come naturally from grain storage foods and provide super nutrition!

Sprouting the grain-seed allows the growth cycle to begin, called *germination*. During the sprouting cycle the molecular structure of the seed changes the original single grain of wheat or other seed into a pre-plant form. The carbohydrate-protein molecule grows into the first stages of the plant. Germination changes the irritating compounds of gluten found in wheat, into green plant compounds which if left to grow develops a blade of grass called wheat grass. Once sprouted and the bran fiber is removed the remaining wheat seed contains zero gluten unable to cause GI distress. The other *anti-nutrient compounds* found in most grain-seed foods are also neutralized by sprouting which allows improved absorption of minerals and proteins. Review Chapter 7 in the Healthy TIPS section under Anti-Nutrients which are Antagonists.

Nutritional Value of Sprouting

All properly sprouted foods can be eaten raw as is the case with most other vegetables. Sprouted beans, seeds and sometimes grains can be purchased in the specialty vegetable section in stores or grown at home. If allowed to fully sprout taking consideration of the size of each bean, they develop into plants no longer require cooking and this is why they can be eaten raw. For some people sprouting is the only way they can eat beans without indigestion. Sprouts also develop extra super nutrition as well, because they manufacture phytonutrients to include Vitamin C while sprouting.

Many people add sprouts to salads, soups, sandwiches, blender drinks and as desired to other favorite recipes. A company by the name of *Kaia Foods*, listed in the Reference section makes sprouts and then dries them for a variety of gluten free snack foods. If inclined to make your own sprouts you can purchase sprouting kits and an instruction booklet. See Reference section for the on-line store called *The Sprout People* to order supplies as desired. Another way to kick up your nutritional status from grains is through a variety of *sprouted grasses* available in manufactured supplement products. These products are known as *Greens*. For example they may include; wheat, barley, oats, kamut and many more ingredients which are 100% Gluten Free. Do not purchase a product in the gelatin capsule form referenced in Chapter 7 Healthy TIPS. Review Chapter 8 as well for more details on *Greens* in the Special Needs Supplements section.

Slow Cooking Your Beans Helps Them Sprout!

To reduce digestive issues from eating beans it is a good idea to first soak them overnight after washing them well and then slow cook the beans to help them sprout. A Crock-Pot or a longer (low heat) cooking method allows sprouting of the smaller beans to take place which reduces bloating and gas. You can even see the small thread like *plant tails* emerge as with lentils, split pea or adzuki beans as they cook. Larger beans may take two full days of pre-soaking with changing the water each day to fresh before this method is successful as with pintos, white or black beans. After sprouting you can cook the beans following your favorite recipe.

Sprouting Grains for Bread Making

If you have already learned to bake bread successfully learning to bake low gluten breads is not an unrealistic learning curve. Time consuming yes, but possible for the patient person. Don't confuse baking with sprouted grains to baking with alternative wheat flours. *Authentic Foods* (see Reference) has a great line of flours in the alternative category. These

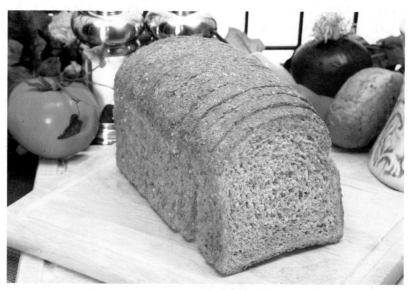

are terrific for people not experiencing advanced symptoms made from rice, sorghum and a variety of grains and foods. Sprouting grains allow the consumption of the offending grains like wheat because it changes the gluten molecule into a pre-plant.

To bake your own sprouted grain bread you first need to decide on the type of grain. Search for organic grains if at all possible to include;

spelt, kamut and or hard wheat varieties. Emmers wheat is a sought after wheat called Farro that contains less gluten content. Most bakers will bake at least three loaves at a time.

Steps for 100% Sprouted Bread

- Requires at least 4 cups of grain. Rinse your grain called berries, and strain through a tiny screen. Large sprouting jars are available that have stainless steel screens for convenience. Two 1/2 gallon jars are needed to soak 2 cups of berries in each to make 3 loaves of bread.
- Soak the berries overnight in clean water. In the morning drain and rinse two more times. After well drained, lay the jars on their sides in an ambient temperature for sprouting and repeat this cycle for two more days. They are done sprouting when a thin tail develops, about 1/8 inch long. The sprouts are then ready for drying.
- Drying is best controlled in a dehydrator set at 95 degrees. Ovens are generally too hot and will over dry the berries. Drying machines have trays covered with a nylon screen that allows the even distribution of the sprouts layering about ¼ inch deep. It takes around 8 hours to dry the sprouts from a moist state to crunchy.
- Once they dry completely you can empty trays to a clean pillow case that you use specifically for bread making or a brand new plastic trash bag. Grind the dried sprouts into a flour consistency ready for making leavened bread after SIFTING thoroughly.
- Follow your favorite bread making recipe allowing the bread to rise over a 6 - 8 hour time period before baking to achieve the best results. *Note:* Each grain choice has a slightly different taste and consistency yet they all taste fabulous. The berries develop a sweeter taste from the sprouting process.

How did the practice of adding high fiber to breads and foods ever get started in the first place?

It's hard to say exactly how the practice began yet a bit shocking to realize that fiber from grains is not our friend. The facts reveal that the outer covering fiber in the bran of grains contains very high levels of gluten! The remedy is to avoid eating sprouted grain breads unless they have been sifted before baking. The addition of bran into recipes for baking breads only evolved over the last century. If you are living with bowel disease stop eating bran in your diet and that includes supplements if you are to have a happier stomach again! Most people (not all) can eat this bread recipe without any GI upset - Enjoy!

CHAPTER 2

Learning about Bowel Disease - IBS, IBD & Celiac

"Thinking back to my childhood I can't remember a time when I didn't have abdominal pains. Allergies were always a problem and my Mom used to take me out on the front porch at night in the cool moist air and give me coffee to calm down my Asthma attacks. The thought never occurred to us that I might be gluten intolerant because my testing came back negative!"
— *Lacie, California*

Bowel disease and digestive disorders like heartburn, ulcers and diarrhea are not new to this world [1]. Writings about health and digestive conditions by the ancients and Greek herbalists, who were the physicians in days of old, go back thousands of years [2]. The records reveal health protocols by the well known Hippocrates who lived around 460 BC [3] Dioscorides [4] and Pliny [5] who came onto the scene around 70 AD. The Greek physician Galen lived from 129-200 AD and also deserves mention. His work carried on the evolution of medicine from these earlier men into the 16th century [6].

These respected men of their day were considered health experts and their work from ancient texts were later translated into English and are now kept in modern museums. They wrote of digestive and constipation complaints along with a myriad of other diseases. The suggestion of

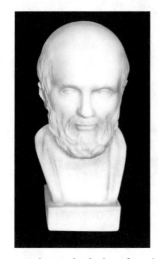

herbs, foods and health practices were included in their patients regimens to reduce symptoms or remedy the ailment altogether. Hippocrates astutely warned physicians to keep wisdom in their medicine, a timeless warning that deserves reflection for all of today's medical professionals.

In the first century A.D., a Greek physician by the name of Aretaeus of Cappadocia reported the first scientific description of bowel disease. He called the condition *koiliakos* after the Greek word for abdomen, *koelia*. This Greek name was later translated into the English word Celiac. Celiac Disease (CD) became synonymous with the intolerance to wheat that is often diagnosed in the first five years of life. Sometimes CD is called Celiac Sprue coming from the Dutch word spruw which is defined as mouth blisters. Three centuries before the definitive connection was made between CD and wheat intolerance another Dutch physician by the name of Vincent Ketelaer in 1669, recognized that mouth blisters were occurring with an elusive digestive disease now known as CD [7].

Simplifying Bowel Disease

There has been far too much confusion surrounding bowel disease in modern times. The perplexed medical community has given way to missed diagnosis, the delay of proper treatment and a multitude of avoidable deaths of both children and adults. For clarity I will review the symptoms and the important factors in the development of bowel disease. Two primary groups of symptoms exist ranging from mild digestive ailments I refer to as Irritable Bowel Syndrome (IBS) and this expands into the more advanced bowel disease group of Inflammatory Bowel Disease (IBD) and Celiac Disease.

The American Medical Association (AMA) clearly states that they do not understand the factors that cause each bowel disease to manifest. The frustration of working and living with bowel disease is only topped off by the AMA's combined enigma of ignorance and stubbornness that prevails even with all of the substantiated research so clearly put before them over the years. Regardless of the copious and significant scientific evidence over the last several hundred years that pinpoint to diet restriction for alleviating much of the suffering, the medical protocols still lack strong dietary restrictions in their treatment recommendations!

History is full of scientists relating bowel disease to the consumption of refined sugar, starch and milk. In fact Dr. Christian Herter a professor at Columbia University and a physician during the early 1900's witnessed firsthand the food to bowel connection. He worked with countless children who had intestinal problems and were experiencing severe diarrhea and underweight. They were able to digest protein foods fairly well yet it was the fats, sugars and starches that were not tolerated by his young patients. He noted that if their conditions reached a stable point and then certain carbohydrates were reintroduced back into the diet the diarrhea returned in full force [36].

Even though this scenario has repeated throughout history over and over again in various cities and countries - dietary restrictions still only receive slight mentions in the medical literature and rarely from the attending physician. Regardless of this great omission there are a handful of doctors across the country beginning to change and to target diet.

One of those doctors advocating diet as a modality with bowel disease is a respected physician who practiced medicine in New York for many years, Ronald Hoffman, M.D. He commented some years ago that even after an article ran in the *Lancet*, a magazine read by physicians, that demonstrated the efficacy of dietary treatment with Crohn's disease, not a single mainstream Gastroenterologist in his area integrated diet with their patients.

The research proved, without a doubt that by removing primarily cereals and dairy products Crohn's patients experienced remission. Dr. Hoffman went on to state that he and some of his nutritionally oriented colleagues put many of their own patients on the Specific Carbohydrate

Diet which is gluten, lactose and refined sugar free to see what results they could observe. They were impressed with the improvements in all symptoms from their patients living with Crohn's, Ulcerative Colitis, Irritable Bowel Syndrome and also Refractory Constipation [8].

Ultimately, our medical professionals need to take a lead in designing appropriate dietary protocols for each group of digestive diseases. Because of this medical boycott that history has confirmed, each individual and family must urgently take action independently of their doctors - to regain their own digestive health while still utilizing any medical support that is beneficial along the way. Diet is the most important focus to begin with yet many other factors influence the ability to optimize bowel health and the health of the body.

As you learn more about the way the body works it will encourage you to choose wholesome foods, reduce gluten, and address any abuse or neglect you may be dealing with. Abuse can come from both addictions and unnecessary pharmaceutical drugs which are undeniably dangerous to ones health.

Potential toxicity to the body not only comes from the food, beverage choices and drugs that are put in the body but also the toxic environment people live in today. There has never been a more critical time in history to understand the impact of how our living environment affects our internal health. We live with massive amounts of toxicity never before experienced by any other civilization.

Even the U.S. Environmental Protection Agency (EPA) is shocked by the unprecedented 88,000 toxic chemicals that invade our water, air and food supply of today. Many people have commented that just by switching to purified water instead of tap or well water their digestive symptoms improved immensely. All of the factors we have just reviewed combined with the assault of our fast pace society allows bowel disease to develop and in turn effect the entire health of the body.

If we are to overcome the sickness associated with bowel disease after learning the factors involved we must also learn the disease profiles of IBS and IBD and their association to other diseases. When you see how much each group has in common then you will also begin to realize just how clear the solution is for all of the conditions.

The RN's Story

A story that shares the gravity of the lack of information in our medical community came from a phone call I received from a registered nurse named Linda. She called my office because she was having digestive issues that included constipation. As I shared the importance of eliminating gluten foods and triggers from her diet to reduce her IBS symptoms I remarked how this same protocol is very effective with IBD. She was shocked to hear my explanation and told me of a patient she had been working with in his home. He was a 12 year old boy with Crohn's. After becoming too sick to go to school the child's parents paid for her to give home care services. I was happy to share with her that I had worked successfully with many people who lived with IBD over the years. The only consideration I remarked is that the recovery tends to take longer for the individual when living in the advanced stages. She was silent on the other end of the phone and I ask if she was still there? Yes she replied and explained that her patient had just died last month of complications and neither she nor the parents were ever made aware of the fact that food restriction was indicated!

IBS & IBD Comparison:

- Symptoms – Same, only different in degrees.
- Cause – Same, other factors complicate symptoms.
- Anatomy Affected – Same, only a few differences.
- Health Program – Same, longer recovery with IBD.

As you read about IBS and IBD pay close attention to the similarities within each group of diseases to include; Gas, Constipation, Diarrhea and Inflammation. The factors affecting both groups have been scientifically proven with peer reviewed research confirming; diet, lifestyle and the environment being faulted. Heredity only raises the frequency of bowel disease a very small percentage approximately 10-15%. Clearly the research has shown that heredity is not a primary cause of bowel disease.

The case I am making is that the primary *symptoms are the same* with a variance to the degree of inflammation that develops. I find the primary *cause is the same* for both groups with a variety of other factors that may complicate or create a particular disease state as with secondary infections. Chapter 4 goes into more detail of each factor that can influence greater inflammation. There are obviously different parts of the anatomy being affected in each disease even though several diseases overlap into the same area of the body. And most importantly for us to embrace is as the symptoms of bowel disease are the same or similar the good news is the *health regimen towards wellness is basically the same* for both categories of bowel disease as well.

Have I oversimplified potentially life threatening diseases too much?

From my viewpoint of working with bowel health I do not think I have oversimplified the review and protocol in any way. I believe it is necessary for the lay person and the professional to take a fresh look at treatment if society is ever going to take hold of the grave situation before us and apply a workable solution. The debauchery of bowel disease has continued and has exploited people for far too long. If we are to stop ruining our civilizations through poor health and leave the confusing framework of present day we must simplify the treatment to heal the masses.

Today we have many of the very same digestive conditions mentioned in the historical writings plus some new unique variations that have developed such as GERD, Gastro-Esophageal-Reflux-Disease. We call this expanding diagnosis Reflux for short and it is further explained in Chapter 5 Glossary of Conditions and Chapter 6. Bowel disease is a growing category of digestive imbalances which affects each person more than most people realize. Before reviewing the medical definitions of the different bowel diseases I offer my suggestion of how to streamline treatment for wellness by condensing many diseases into only two basic treatment groups.

The Definition of IBS-G

For simplicity sake, especially when the conditions are not acute, I am suggesting to group the milder digestive diseases all together. A couple of conditions may share a spot in both groups depending on the severity of a person's disease. The milder group according to severity includes; heartburn, reflux, gastritis, colitis, diverticulitis, stomach ulcers and Irritable Bowel Syndrome (IBS). All of these I refer to as IBS-G. The medical diagnosis criteria, separates each of these diseases into their own class yet because I am revealing their similarity of symptoms, cause and solution, I find it very helpful to umbrella all of these less complicated digestive conditions into one group. I think you guessed that the "G" stands for Gluten.

The traditional IBS is a common condition of the bowel that is primarily described by a variety of milder symptoms including; gas, bloating, nausea, constipation, abdominal pain, diarrhea and hemorrhoids. Many of these symptoms can also be due to a passing cold virus or even food poisoning yet when people experience the symptoms regularly especially daily, you can regard them as the symptoms of IBS, Irritable Bowel Syndrome.

Some people have not yet recognized their own individual symptoms of bowel disease. To explain their digestive issues they refer to themselves as having on-going allergies, perhaps fighting a virus, food poisoning or thinking it is just a lack of proper dietary choices. Of course the latter DIET definitely influences the symptoms one might be experiencing. Fatigue can also accompany bowel disease due to the lack of digestive absorption that develops with IBS-G.

It is important to be preventative even when only mild digestive symptoms are present. If left untreated the mild symptoms of IBS can bring upon failing health. Reality doesn't change just because the connection has not been discovered. IBS may even develop into a more threatening diagnosis of IBD, Inflammatory Bowel Disease or Celiac Disease adding more health concerns even reducing immune function leaving the door wide open to a gamut of other illnesses.

Common Symptoms of IBS (G):

- Gas & Bloating
- Nausea & Constipation
- Mucus & Abdominal Pain
- Diarrhea & Hemorrhoids
- Allergy & Fatigue
- Inflammation

Irritable Bowel Syndrome - IBS

The medical diagnosis of *IBS* according to the AMA criteria includes continuous or recurrent abdominal pain or discomfort for at least 3 months or longer. It also states that at least 25% of the time symptoms are somewhat relieved upon having a bowel movement. The criterion elaborates to include varied bowel habits with loose watery stool which may contain mucus and often paired with hard and incomplete evacuation or bowel movements - we call constipation. Common symptoms of IBS include bloating and abdominal distention. The protocol suggests certain testing recommendations to be carried out according to severity of symptoms and associated clinical features and warns not to over test. The routine testing procedures include; complete blood count, electrolytes (with vomiting or diarrhea), sedimentation rate a urinalysis and stool testing to check for blood. The complete blood count tests are looking for leukocytes called white blood cells (WBC). Also ova and parasites in extended stool cultures may be indicated with diarrhea. Stated in the medical literature are factors that have been found to increase symptoms mentioning both physical and emotional stress, and dietary factors to include dairy, wheat and fried foods [9].

Heartburn is a pressure and or burning feeling in the chest and at times a sour taste in your mouth and is also a symptom for the diagnosis of Reflux. Reflux is the nickname for GERD which is the diagnosis of too much acid. The excess acid makes its way out of the stomach and up into the throat area called the esophagus. The excess acid can actually burn the lining tissue of the throat besides causing inflammation and pain as described in Merck & Co., Inc., 2010.

More naturally oriented health professionals have found Heartburn to not be an "acid-blocking" drug deficiency. Often, Reflux medication does not help the symptoms for the patient and leaves them to struggle to find other answers to their burning. A percentage of patients are helped initially from the burning symptoms however, if a patient continues the medication long-term it has been shown to cause a variety of other side-effects in the body. This is primarily due to decreasing the body's ability to properly absorb core nutrients.

These nutrients may include minerals, some vitamins and proteins that are all required to keep the body healthy. In learning about the digestive system in Chapter 3 you will find that there are two distinct origins that create similar symptoms of heartburn. I find most heartburn is due to not enough proper digestive juices (including acidity) flowing into the stomach. A smaller percentage of heartburn is due to over acidity and the complete answer will be explained in chapter 5 and 6. Heartburn is included in the IBS-G group because many people with IBS also experience heartburn from time to time. People living with heartburn need to follow the GIS guidelines in Chapter 7 to naturally help their intestinal pH rebalance (review in Chapter 6).

Gastro-Esophageal Reflux Disease GERD or Reflux has been sweeping the country with babies, children, teens and adults being given the diagnosis. The medical definition is the muscle sphincter that separates the stomach contents from the throat does not close properly and allows gastric fluids into the esophagus causing burning. Treatment as prescribed includes lifestyle modification with the reduction in coffee, alcohol, fats and smoking. Raising the head of one's bed is helpful and the addition of medication called proton pump inhibitors are given to severely restrict acidity from flowing into the stomach. Read the contraindication sheet in your prescription very carefully. The drug was not designed to take for any lengthy period because of the potential disastrous side effects.

Gastritis is defined as a sudden inflammation of the stomach lining.

Inflammation can be painful and occasionally creates stomach pain which is often traced back to eating irritating foods or drink and or experiencing a stressful situation. I include gastritis as a symptom in IBS because eating gluten or other inflammatory triggers, explained in Chapter 4, can bring on Gastritis. Burping or passing gas can sometimes help the stomach pain to resolve. Acute Gastritis (AG) experienced regularly must be checked out by a licensed physician or health professional. Causes of AG may include; medications from aspirin, Non-Steroidal Anti-Inflammatory Drugs (NSAIDs) like Tylenol, or corticosteroids, alcohol, eating or drinking corrosive substances like soda pop drinks, extreme stress, infections such as the bacteria like Helicobacter Pylori (HP) or other less frequent causes like Cytomegalovirus (CMV) or Herpes Simplex Virus (HSV) -Merck & Co., Inc, 2007.

Colitis is the inflammation of the colon; and there are many types, with a variety of causes. The symptoms are the IBS symptoms. People tend to have occasional bouts of Colitis symptoms that are not taken too seriously which fall more into this IBS group. However, the incidence is rising of Ulcerative Colitis that falls into the IBD category. Sometimes the cause is traced to bacterial or viral infections, drugs such as antibiotics, and radiation from x-rays or other sources. The symptoms may escalate in individuals who develop acute colitis with diarrhea, sometimes bloody diarrhea and cramping alternating with constipation - Merck & Co., Inc. Resource Library 2010.

Diverticular Disease (DD) Many people living with IBS symptoms in their younger years receive the diagnosis of Diverticular Disease *(DD)* or Diverticulitis (active infection) as adults. Statistics show 50% of people that reach the age of 65 years of age have reported some degree of DD, according to the Merck & Co Inc. statistics 2010. The Merck Manual of Geriatrics states that DD has been found with increasing frequency. These sac-like projections develop most commonly in the descending colon and sigmoid colon flexure, the s-shaped turn, directly before the rectum. Infection spikes when trapped stool and liquids cause problems along with the potential of bleeding and rupturing into the abdominal cavity.

Symptoms are similar to IBS states Merck's literature with alternating diarrhea and constipation being relieved after a bowel movement.

Stomach Ulcers develop in a few different areas of the stomach or small intestine. A Peptic Ulcer is erosion of the lining of the stomach but can also be in the first part of the small intestine called the duodenum. If it is located in the stomach it is called a Gastric Ulcer. If the protective lining of the stomach stops working correctly and the integrity of the lining breaks down it results in inflammation and this allows a wound or ulcer to develop. Most commonly the ulcer only occurs in the first layer of the inner lining. If the hole goes all the way through into the stomach or duodenum or into the abdomen it is called a perforation which is a medical emergency. The most common cause of Peptic Ulcers is infection by bacteria such as with Helicobacter Pylori called H. Pylori. However, people can test positive to the H. Pylori and not have an ulcer. Symptoms can be brought on by excessive alcohol, regular use of aspirin and NSAIDS, smoking cigarettes or chewing tobacco, being very ill, radiation treatments and rarely even Pancreatic cancer called Zollinger-Ellison Syndrome. Some people feel daily stress can also bring upon ulcers yet this proposal is not clear to the researchers according to Merck & Co., Inc., Resource Library, 2010.

Inflammatory Bowel Disease - IBD

At the other end of the spectrum is advanced bowel disease referred to as Inflammatory Bowel Disease (IBD) and Celiac Disease (CD). IBD according to the AMA includes primarily Ulcerative Colitis, Ulcerative Proctitis and Crohn's. In general it is a group of diseases that the cause is stated to be unknown. They commonly demand more pharmaceutical drug intervention and hospitalization especially since the importance of diet restriction has not been clearly understood as an important treatment modality.

CD has been kept separate from the IBD category by the AMA because it is considered a treatable disease yet at the same time stated to be incurable. Both CD and the traditional IBD diseases can escalate into advanced

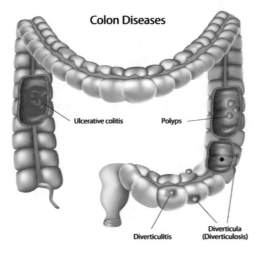

Colon Diseases

Ulcerative colitis   Polyps

Diverticulitis   Diverticula (Diverticulosis)

stages expressing more symptoms to include; infection, inflammation and scarring of the GI tract. Celiac Disease (CD) includes an overactive immune system that may bring about acute intestinal bleeding with advanced malnutrition including anemia and other symptoms.

Crohn's and UC patients may develop deep ulcerations, blood clots, unexplained arthritis, fevers and malaise. There is also a 33% chance of developing the disease called Peri-Anal disease known as Proctitis steaming from UC.

Shared symptoms that may occur with IBD diseases and CD are listed below. You can see how similar the symptoms of pain, gas, diarrhea, constipation and inflammation are and also the similarities to the IBS-G group. This is why I have regrouped the advanced bowel diseases all together with the heading IBD-G designation to include CD. The "G" once again refers to Gluten regarding the fact that all of these advanced bowel diseases do better following the GIS program outlined in Chapter 7.

Symptoms of Advanced IBD-G:
- Acute Indigestion, Diarrhea, Gas & Constipation
- Advanced Inflammation
- Stunted Growth & Weakened Immune System
- Ulcers, Fistulas, Abscesses & Obstructions
- Loss of Villi in Small Intestine Pronounced with Celiac's
- Intestinal Bleeding & Scarring
- Mal-absorption of Nutrients (bloated bellies and flat bottoms)
- Smelly, Hard & Oily Stools

- Potential Hospitalization (blood transfusions) / Elemental Diet (option)

The medical diagnosis of the IBD group includes only a small number of conditions; Ulcerative Colitis, Crohn's Disease and Ulcerative Proctitus (rectum) accompanied by a few subcategories of related conditions [10]. Surprisingly, Celiac Disease (CD) has been kept in a separate class. Once again for simplicity sake I choose to group CD due to its inflammatory symptoms together with the IBD-G group. Each of these diseases exhibit acute inflammation of the bowel with many other shared symptoms. Therefore I believe grouping them together will help both the lay person and the professional alike identify the disease state more frequently and also implement a health protocol to achieve disease resolution.

The medical diagnosis of IBD is a state of chronic inflammation of unknown origin that affects the lining of the colonic wall. *Ulcerative Colitis* can begin in the last segment of the large intestine or the rectum. Recovery is rare according to the medical literature sighting only a 10% of people inflicted go into long-term remission. Another startling statistic of 70% of people diagnosed with UC will have bowel surgery at one time or another. Some people receive multiple surgeries and at times have large portions of the bowel and at times the entire GI tract removed due to the limitation of treatment protocols. Drug therapy offers little to address the cause of the inflammation targeting only the symptoms [11]. Also in this category, *Ulcerative Proctitis (UP)* is the inflammation of the lining of the rectum and it is becoming increasingly more common. UP has several identifiable causes ranging from infection to radiation therapy and actually states that it may be a result from Crohn's or Ulcerative Colitis. Another cause is the result of a sexually transmitted disease including the Herpes Simplex Virus (HSV). Proctitis will generally cause rectal bleeding and mucus to discharge from the rectum [12].

Crohn's Disease shares the IBD diagnosis as well and most commonly is spotted in the distal ileum area which is the last section of the small intestine right before the Appendix and Ileo-Cecal (IC) valve junction.

The IC valve joins the small and large intestine and is supposed to close upon having the contents from the small intestine move into the large intestine. Even though first diagnosed in this area Crohn's can be diagnosed anywhere in the small or large intestine. Crohn's sometimes develops infected sores on the intestinal lining called abscesses. Also occurring may be internal and external fistulas in the colon wall that at times will break becoming a medical emergency. Bowel obstruction may also develop with Crohn's. This type of blockage may arise from years of inflammation and scarring. The general inflammation and abscesses can further develop into small ulcerative pits and develop elongated criss-cross like ulcers that causes swelling in the mucosal lining. Both Ulcerative Colitis and Crohn's share symptoms of pain, tenderness in the abdomen and diarrhea of great magnitude. Dietary restrictions are rarely spoken about and it is more of a question of what mix of pharmaceutical drugs for the doctor to use coupled with the potential of surgery [13].

Celiac Disease (CD) has been kept in its own category of digestive diseases by the AMA. It is directly linked to gluten intolerance from wheat and other offending foods however it too is a disease of advanced mucosal inflammation as is the other IBD diseases we just discussed. The difference with CD is the location. It begins in the small intestine and results in direct mal-absorption of nutrients due to the damaged villi technically called Villas Atrophy. Chapter 4 and 5 will review the Inflammatory-Mal-absorption Cycle. A strict Gluten Free Diet (GFD) is suggested for treatment along with pharmaceutical drugs as needed. If a strict GFD is followed the statistics show lower cancer rates and greater longevity with Celiac's [14]. The weak link coming from Allopathic medicine is the failure to diagnose this disease in early stages and also the vague and weak dietary and health protocol that is given to patients with the milder diagnosis.

According to the Mayo Clinic sometimes people with CD may not show gastrointestinal symptoms at all. Some of the less obvious symptoms include; irritability and nervousness, depression, anemia, bruising, joint pain, stunted growth, muscle cramps, mouth sores, neuropathy, osteoporosis, tooth enamel weakness and a particular type of skin rash called Dermatitis Herpetiformis (DH). The DH rash is easy to miss and shows up in small or large areas of the body usually on the buttocks, back of neck, scalp, elbows, knees or back. The DH rash is characterized by blisters on children or adults which fill with a watery fluid and vary in size from very small up to 1 cm across [18].

The Mayo Clinic goes on to say that other symptoms of Celiac's such as diarrhea, abdominal pain and bloating may mimic those of other conditions such as; Irritable Bowel Syndrome, Gastric Ulcers, parasite infections or even Crohn's. The decrease of absorption of nutrients called mal-absorption that occurs with Celiac Disease can cause vitamin deficiencies that deprive the brain, Peripheral Nervous System, bones, liver and other organs vital nourishment [19]. This can lead to other illnesses and stunted growth in children. This Mayo Clinic reference supports my ground breaking premise of grouping Celiac Disease into the IBD group renaming it "IBD-G".

History of Bowel Disease

In 2010 the United States population was documented by the U.S. Census to be somewhere around 315 million people. This population figure helps us to have a better perspective of just how many Americans are living with a diagnosed digestive condition or bowel disease.

Medical doctors have quantified the reportable numbers of people seeking medical help for Irritable Bowel Syndrome (IBS) to range upwards of 45 million people across the US or approximately 15% of the population. The worldwide figures for IBS have been reported in a similar range between 9 – 23% with respect to each particular country, according to numbers supplied by the World Health Organization [15]. In regards to people being diagnosed with advanced bowel disease the cases have been scantly recorded with approximately one in ten thousand people throughout the U.S. and much greater numbers coming from the European countries.

Past Statistics for IBS & IBD:

- IBS – 15% of the US and 15% Average in the World population diagnosed.
- IBD – 32,000 people in the US diagnosed with even higher percentages from other countries.

These numbers represent a large amount of people who have suffered and have been diagnosed with a specific bowel symptom. However, in my estimation I believe that for every person that goes to the doctor and reports IBS symptoms there is another five sufferers at least that are not being seen by a physician.

Marketers confirm my estimation of the magnitude of people living with bowel issues that are undiagnosed through hard facts [37]. How did I extrapolate this five times multiplier you ask? In my estimation these unrecorded people that are not accounted for through a doctor's visit are simply relying on a variety of over the counter (OTC) products and natural remedies to ease their digestive woes.

Sales numbers of these targeted digestive products that include anti-acids, laxatives and herbals are tracked by the cash register receipts as they are purchased. In just one year the numbers in the U.S. computed a whopping 5 billion dollars of digestive aids alone that people purchased in hopes of effectively treating their endless symptoms [16]. As you can calculate the numbers I used, 5 x 15% (diagnosed IBS) = 75% IBS cases. This brings the incidence of people living with digestive symptoms to include a majority of the population reaching upwards of 75% of people in the U.S. In fact these figures give credence to my clinical research and theory that states all people experience a propensity towards bowel disease. The only question that remains for each of us to contemplate and answer, once we understand the human nature of this phenomena, is to what degree?

Recent Research Supports the Higher Statistics of Bowel Disease

Supporting my findings and theory that all people have some degree of bowel disease which gluten intolerance is a factor, was a study conducted not too long ago in 2003. It was the largest survey completed thus far in North America to establish statistics on advanced bowels disease. The results were a shockingly higher percentage than ever previously estimated. The study was led by Dr. Alessio Fasano, a U.S. researcher and involved more than 13,000 people. For years Celiac Disease (CD) was considered rare outside of Europe with only one person in 10,000 showing the classic symptoms as reviewed. His astounding results in this study found one in every 133 individuals were actually affected with CD. This means that the disease is nearly 100 times more common than previously thought.

Remarkably the team's research also confirmed my theory that considers CD as a potential factor in other auto-immune disorders and disease conditions like Lupus, MS, Arthritis and Asthma. Dr. Fasano's research has estimated upwards of 2 million people in the U.S. are living with CD [17].

IBS and IBD symptoms have clearly been diagnosed in growing numbers of both men and women of all ages and all occupations along with children. IBD has been more commonly diagnosed in white and European descent in the past yet the new research is showing that those statistics may only be due to the diets of other races, not genetics as first thought. Some traditional cultural foods do not contain as many inflammatory GIS agents such as the Asian diet based on white rice.

Present 21st Century Statistics of IBS & IBD:
- IBS – 50 to 75% of the U.S. including diagnosed and undiagnosed population.
- IBD – 60% of the U.S. including both diagnosed and undiagnosed.

With statistics rising across the board we are also seeing more diagnosis among infants experiencing digestive issues. Children are more frequently coming into this world having to fight a digestive battle within the first few months of life. Some symptoms of gas and bloating for infants are normal and as old as Moses with the traditional reference name given of Colic. See Chapter 5 Glossary of Conditions Colic. The infant population is not only having more digestive complications but also experiencing higher premature birth rates opening the door to many more health challenges to include a rise in infant deaths. The need to improve Pre-Natal Nutrition is urgent. This important step for women will reduce all of the health challenges newborns face including digestive ones of gas, bloating, constipation and skin conditions as reviewed in Chapter 9 Healthy Children.

Pediatricians have resorted to prescribing acid blocking medications for infants even before they leave the hospital. This is a drastic measure considering all pharmaceutical drugs come with side effects for the patient and many times leads parents into stronger medication for their newborns. The medications prescribed for infants and young children come with many side effects and may even stunt a child's growth. A natural approach of introducing *herbal bitters* has given newborns relief within minutes and can be reviewed in Chapter 9.

The Modern Allopathic Medicine approach thus far has been to treat the symptoms without finding the cause of bowel disease. This limited mindset has evolved over the centuries and must be reviewed and changed. The "find a bug choose a drug", mentality is based on a crisis management model. If our society is going to reduce medical costs and have healthier children and adults we must all begin to practice more preventative Integrative Medicine. Chapter 7 and 8 outlines the GIS health program that will guide individuals and the whole family on their new health path. The history of bowel research clearly points to the solution people must follow for wellness and it is found in health.

Timeline of Bowel Disease:
- 1500 to 400 BC - Ancient Writings on Digestive Disease – The *Papyrus Ebers* & *The Greek Herbal of Dioscorides*, English translation – 1930-1977.

- 70 AD – Aretaeus of Cappadocia – Greek physician named the first disease of the abdomen *Koiliakos* from the Greek word for abdomen *koelia* associated with eating grains.

- 1887 – Dr. Samuel Gee from England translated Koiliakos to Celiac Disease (CD) associated with wheat intolerance.

- 1904 – Researchers began to focus on Bacteria and Digestive imbalance in CD not only the association of wheat intolerance.

- 1906 – Researchers from 1906 - 1924 isolated certain Bacteria or Bacterial Toxins - that when isolated and then injected back into animals created Ulcerative Colitis. Interestingly it wasn't until 1996 that H. Pylori was proven to create stomach ulcers and was accepted by the medical community as the cause.

- 1920 – Dr. Ilya Metchnikoff proposed Bad Bacteria was producing Toxins, harmful microbes causing Auto-Intoxication. He introduced Fermented Milk similar to Yogurt. His ideas were noted by leading Gastroenterologists and researchers yet not adopted.

- 1932 – Dr. B.B. Crohn introduced the colon disease called Regional Ileitis later named Crohn's Disease. This is most commonly located in the last section of the small intestine, the beginning of the ascending colon and patchy areas in the large intestine before the flexure to the descending colon and sigmoid flexure. Some researchers believed it was due to bacteria and or toxins.

- 1944 – Netherlands doctors noticed a decline in Celiac Disease (CD) after WWII with a food shortage of grains and potatoes. They observed childhood CD dropped from 35% to zero. Once the grains came back into the diet the CD percentage began to soar again.

- 1950 – Dutch researcher, W.K. Dicke, proposed that the protein constituent of wheat, the gluten portion, produced permanent injury to the intestinal cells of people showing symptoms of Celiac Disease. Testing measures were adopted of a series of intestinal biopsy with an instrument to show cellular damage. The cells were viewed before the diet change, after wheat was removed and upon reintroducing wheat back into the diet. Results narrowed the diagnosis of Celiac disease to a small percentage of the larger group of people living with symptoms.

- 1964 – Dr. Donaldson wrote a strong article to the medical community to adopt Dr. Metchnikoff's theory to use yogurt type bacteria calling it the "Beneficial Factor", friendly bacteria, to balance the disease causing bad bacteria types in the gut.

- 1978 – Midwest Celiac Association (MCSA) was formed by Pat Murphy Garst of Des Moines, Iowa. The association wrote the first Gluten-Free cookbook. Later in 1985 the MCSA incorporated into the Celiac Sprue Association / United States of America (CSA / USA). In 2004 they developed a recognition seal trademark for products designating free from Wheat, Barley, Rye and Oats (WBRO).

- 1999 – Irritable Bowel Syndrome (IBS) receives a diagnosis from the AMA to be caused from an "Organic Origin" of unclear factors. This was very important because IBS was at-last not considered originating from a "Psychological Origin".

- 2003 – Dr. Alessio Fasano confirms from his research that (1) in (133) people in North America are now living with Celiac Disease related to the intolerance of wheat. Previously estimated at less than (1) in (10,000) people. The team of researchers stated they felt strongly that gluten intolerance may play a factor in other Auto-Immune Disorders and to Advance Other Illnesses in the body.

- 2009 – *Beyond Gluten Intolerance – GIS Gluten Inflammatory Syndrome* – The puzzle of Gluten intolerance is revealed in this book to show the Gluten Inflammation Syndrome (GIS) connection to health and disease.

Research Highlights of IBS & IBD

Over the last one hundred years researchers have worked diligently to bring light to the cause and the cure for bowel disease. Their discoveries have shown the exact and correct path to follow for decreasing the symptoms of bowel disease and regaining health.

Modern research from around the world abounds with hundreds of confirming papers that support the factors presented from these earlier researchers. The two most important factors that affect bowel health are first the *balance of microbial organisms* in the gut and second, just as important is the *dietary influences*. Once bowel disease begins to advance it is very important to pay attention to the nutritional status of the individual. The diet restrictions must be made to reduce starch, sugar and milk which in turn will *lower inflammation*. Extraordinary efforts must be made to supply proper nourishment through diet and supplementation for the body to reduce the *malnutrition* that may result in children and adults living with bowel disease.

Colon Health Requirements:

- Balance Gut Microbial Organisms
- Dietary Support and Restrictions
- Lower Inflammation
- Reverse Mal-Nutrition

These colon health requirements are effective for prevention and to reverse active bowel disease for both IBS-G and IBD-G. Inflammation leading to mal-nutrition explains the connection of bowel disease to the development of other miscellaneous diseases. The reason this is completely credible is grounded in the fact that the body requires nutrition to build a robust metabolic network. Only when the body receives the essential foundational nutrition can it support the systems to work the way they were designed. When the body does not receive the nutrients outlined in Chapter 7 and 8 it mal-functions or in other words develops a disease. Tufts University in Boston has proven this fact of the direct relationship the body has to nutrition and disease in their ongoing 30 year study on longevity documented in their book called *Biomarkers.*

The Fallacy of the Traditional Bowel Disease Treatment

History has revealed that the traditional treatment of bowel disease has not relied on health of the bowel and nutrition but primarily has focused on pharmaceutical drugs that offer very limited success for remission. Although drug treatments may give temporary relief they come with a long list of damaging side effects. Many times a prescribed medication will cause other issues requiring the attending doctor to add yet another drug which may result in the over-drugging of the body.

Antibiotics in particular have been the go to drug of choice over the years to wipe the colon clean of bad bacteria. Yet in killing off the overgrowth of bad bacteria the good bacteria is destroyed as well. Relying so heavily on this ammunition of treatment has created strains of organisms that become very drug resistant called Super Bugs! These strains of bacteria have mutated and within the over-drugged individual may even threaten their survival.

Trusting only in the limitation of a drug protocol leads the patient into a jungle of medications including; Cortisone, Prednisone, steroid anti-inflammatory drugs, that according to Mayo Clinic may exacerbate; diabetes, heart failure, osteoporosis and hypertension. Also, 70% of Crohn's patients end up with minor to major surgery which sometimes entails the removal of most of the colon! This is an extreme measure that has many stressful side effects impacting ones health and quality of life. I have worked with many individuals who have lost portions of their colon and it borders on cruelty to humans especially when you know as I do that many if not all of these surgeries could have been prevented.

According to the Merck Co. IBD literature a certain percentage of people in every diagnosis also become totally unresponsive to treatment. Physicians are cautioned about serious complications that may develop in treating bowel disease that can lead down the road to the dreaded Toxic Mega Colon which frequently results in death. Choosing to integrate a stronger more assertive health program is the way out of the pharmaceutical jungle. A healthier colon and healthier life awaits you incorporating health. The most important first step to achieve your new healthy goal is to take a quality Probiotics supplement!

Intestinal Balance of Gut Microbial Organisms is the First Step - Think Probiotics!

Taking the important step to permanently regain better health with either IBS-G or IBD-G, demands the use of a good friendly bacteria often called Probiotics. Due to the immense health value Probiotics has shown in the body, it has become one of the most heavily researched health products for bowel health [25, 26].

In 2004 a study confirmed the importance of the friendly bacteria needed in the treatment of bowel disease at the University of North Carolina, Dept. of Medicine - Center for Gastrointestinal Biology and Disease. The study included the normal protocol of antibiotics for the participants to reduce the initial overgrowth of bad bacteria. Most surprisingly to the researchers was that by administering the Probiotics after the drugs the patients did not have the common relapse that was often observed. The researchers clearly stated that the Probiotic agents will likely become an integral component of treating IBD [20, 21, and 22].

Probiotics is the reference name for the valuable good bacteria which naturally keeps the overgrowth of bad bacteria under control in the intestinal tract. There are primarily two groups of the good bacteria that scientists have focused their research attention to and both are categorized as Lactic Acid bacteria. They function by surviving in an acid environment in the bowel and as they multiply the micro-organisms excrete Lactic Acid. This is a natural chemical that further lowers the pH of the bowel (more acidic). Through lowering the pH Lactic Acid naturally causes the gram positive "bad" bacteria to die. It is as simples as that!

One of the friendly Lactic Acid bacteria is called *Lactobacillus* Acidophilus. This one bacteria strain has developed over 100 different species. The other common strain is called *Bifidobacterium* and it also has a large family of species that work very similarly in the bowel. They both guard against infection and sickness that may come from hundreds of potential microbials that include; bacteria, viruses and fungal organisms. New strains of Lactic Acid bacteria have been developed from fermentation of foods including one by Dr. Ohhira from Japan called E. Faecalis -TH10. It is so powerful that it has been found to destroy the virulent staph MRSA, C. difficile, E. coli, H. pylori and other antibiotic resistant strains of bacteria in the gut.

Dr. Ohhira states that there are two main objectives in this growing field of microbiology. First and foremost is the importance to choose a Probiotic that contains a *combination of strains* that are viable and truly work. The next important consideration involves *potency with efficacy.* His work has proven that a product may have billions of colonies yet they must also be able to set up house keeping. Meaning, a Probiotic must be able to implant in the intestinal tract adhering to the lining and grow in the body's environment to get the best results [27]. In this field of Probiotics I have found that the better products on the market get the best results. Also, by incorporating fermented foods in the diet, together with the Probiotics they both create a healthier intestinal environment all around.

Medical History Supports the Importance of Good Bacteria

One of the great pioneers of bowel disease who brought light from the past to modern researchers was Dr. Haas, MD. He discovered that around 1904, researchers in America were busy working with Celiac Sprue in children when they soon began to understand the treacherous role that bad bacteria truly played. These researchers found that the Celiac children had extremely poor digestive ability of both carbohydrates and proteins in their diet. Very interestingly they found that this weak digestive state prompted large numbers of bad bacteria to grow and yeast colonies to also develop. In turn these opportunistic microbials caused fermentation and putrefication of the poorly digested food that was just sitting in the intestines [23].

Dr. S.V. Haas was a pediatrician during the 1920's and as he worked with bowel disease he found that instructing his patients to make dietary changes reduced their symptoms considerably [35]. His protocol included limiting grains and certain starches, lactose and other refined sugars along with advocating the inclusion of ripe bananas and properly fermented yogurt. When you compare the symptoms of chronic constipation and loose stool that existed with his patients at that time to today's patients suffering with bowel disease, the urgency to follow his protocol cannot be ignored if one is to achieve health success.

Regardless of a person's orientation on the physiology of the body the bowels are designed to move daily. If the bowels move less frequently, for example only every few days or less often, this is considered a state of constipation. Just because fewer bowel movements are common in patients - it is irresponsible for a physician to call this normal. The state of constipation is a major health concern and must be addressed. Education and guidance is given for healthy regularity in several chapters because of the critical nature it plays for health of the colon and ultimately health for the entire body.

Another researcher that followed along the same path of bacterial imbalances was Dr. Ilya Metchnikoff who researched health for many years giving speeches to all who would listen. In 1929 he proposed that many of the human illnesses were caused from bad bacteria overgrowth due to their production of harmful *secondary toxins* which bring about a type of auto-intoxication. He introduced *fermented milk* to his followers that resembled the healthy Greek yogurt of today (without fillers). Regardless of the great success that his patients experienced drinking the fermented milk to support bowel health it did not influence the leading Gastroenterologists of his day [24].

To be healthy a healthy colon is paramount. The first priority to achieve this goal is for the *bowels to move regularly* to clear the intestines of stool and microbial debris. Chapter 3 addresses the importance of digestion and regularity and introduces the real culprit that interrupts the normal peristalsis action of the colon. Secondly and paramount for a healthy colon is to regain a state of *Symbiosis* in the colon of good bacteria and the proper food source to insure the colonization of the good bacteria called Prebiotic. Eating a healthier diet of vegetables, fruits, low gluten starches and some dairy products (as tolerated) provides the Prebiotic food. Some of the Probiotic products are astutely formulated to contain this valuable food source Prebiotic such as in the fermented Probiotic by Dr. Ohhira listed in the Reference section.

Paramount to Colon Health:

- *Daily Healthy Regularity* of the bowels is the ultimate goal.
- *Symbiosis Balance* of Probiotics and Prebiotics (food source) for good colonization of friendly bacteria in the colon.
- *Eubiosis* is achieved in the colon by providing a healthy ratio of 85% Good Bacteria to 15% Bad Bacteria.

Thousands of bacterial strains have been cultured in the human body according to the recent work through the U.S. National Institute of Health (NIH). The human intestinal tract in itself contains over 400 different species of bacteria and each of those have hundreds of different stains. If the bad bacterium multiplies into large enough colonies it causes an unhealthy condition called *Dysbiosis* contributing to intestinal illnesses and at times even death. To further broaden the scope of the intestinal environment it can also be the host to multiple viruses and parasites that along with bacteria and yeast may bring about more symptoms including; nausea, bloating, constipation, diarrhea and pain [27].

Modern research has confirmed the great importance of improving the balance of good bacteria colonies in the colon in both IBS and IBD patients that is referred to as *Eubiosis*. Experts agree it is difficult, once a person has experienced many rounds of antibiotics, steroids, birth control pills, eating difficulties and illness to maintain this healthy balance of micro flora without the help of supplementing with a quality Probiotics product daily [25].

The good news is to supplement with Probiotics is easy and safe for infants, children, adults and seniors. The goal for a healthy colon is to achieve 85% Good Bacteria to approximately 15% Bad Bacteria. Once a Probiotic product is started it gets to work quickly eliminating symptoms because it is addressing the cause of bowel distress.

Many strains of good bacteria have been isolated that are beneficial for bowel health including the most well-known group called the Lactic Acid bacteria. Both the traditional Lactobacillus and the Bifidobacterium Lactic Acid species grow easily in milk cultures as found in yogurt and fermented milks like kefir. Some of the modern strains in supplements contain relatively no milk solids in the end product. This is an important consideration for lactose intolerant or milk protein allergic individuals.

There exists a multitude of other important beneficial strains of friendly bacteria. Experts agree that these newer discovered strains are proving to be even more valuable than the L. acidophilus and it is better not to just focus on one strain but incorporate complimentary strains that adhere better to the colon walls. Research has proven them to be extremely valuable for controlling the overgrowth of pathogenic bacterial strains and to help control the overgrowth of yeast in the colon and other health support [28].

It is common to see the overgrowth of the opportunistic yeast in bowel disease. One of the laboratory markers that confirm this situation is the Anti-Saccharomyces Cerevisiae Antibodies often seen in Crohn's [13]. Several different species of yeast can be cultured from the bowel and the body. Yeast has a tendency to greatly impair proper absorption of nutrients in the small intestines along with adding to other health challenges. The overgrowth of yeast can increase inflammation and infection of tissue and add to gaseous symptoms of an individual.

Other undesirable micro-organisms may also thrive in the oxygen starved intestines due to constipation side by side the bad bacteria and yeast. Viruses and parasites are commonly cultured from the intestines and must be addressed for optimum health. To regain health of the colon from all potential microbials it is a matter once again of both regularity of the bowels and *pH balance* to allow micro-organisms to reach the state of

Eubiosis. Attaining Regularity, Symbiosis and Eubiosis will decrease the colonization of all of the opportunistic organisms we have reviewed and often be able to avoid the alternative antibiotics!

Building a healthier *immune system* will also assist in bowel health. Through activating immunity the body's natural fighting forces naturally help to reduce microbials thereby reducing symptoms to occur. Diarrhea can result from multiple origins including viruses, bacteria, parasites and yeast. Clostridium Difficile is one gram positive bacterium that is often responsible for diarrhea and has been greatly reduced with the addition of a quality Probiotics.

Parasites may require some special prescription medications in certain circumstances and often persist for long periods of time before they are completely under control. However, as you learn more about the digestive tract in Chapter 3, 5 and 6 you will begin to understand that health balance in the stomach prevents the reintroduction of parasites and viruses into the gastrointestinal tract all together.

Not only have these live cultures coined Probiotics come to the rescue with reducing yeast and bacterial colonies that cause diarrhea, constipation and gas, research has also shown their effectiveness against the widely seen H. pylori bacteria [29]. This particular strain of bad bacteria that is sweeping the nation has been found to cause stomach ulcers. The significance of research proving a Probiotics to be successful against the H. pylori bacteria is remarkable and the work has been validated in multiple studies [38]. The research gives confirmation to the ability of these natural brigades and credence to my testimony of observing the friendly bacteria resolving the pitted ulcers present in the IBD diseases of Crohn's and Ulcerative Colitis patients who follow the GIS protocol.

A good Probiotics is top on my list to support the body back to colon health and carries with it no side effects except better health. By ingesting a quality multi-strain Probiotics coupled with the GIS Diet people improve regularity and the cleansing of opportunistic debris from the colon allowing healthy detoxification reviewed in the Chapter 2 HIGHLIGHT section.

What is the Ultimate Solution for Bowel Disease?

Lowering Inflammation

More awareness of the inflammatory factor seen with bowel disease surfaced in the US around the 1930's as Dr. Crohn's work with IBD began to go public. This more advanced form of bowel disease could not be missed because it showed more painful symptoms in areas of the large colon than its predecessor Celiac Disease. In 1932 Dr. B. B. Crohn spoke about a new intestinal disorder which he called, Regional Ileitis, later named Crohn's Disease. Crohn's is more isolated in the last section of the small intestine and into the large intestine. It is important to understand that every colon disease from heartburn to Celiac's, including Crohn's and Ulcerative Colitis, all develop a certain level of inflammation of the lining tissue.

By following the GIS health program in Chapter 7 the body's inflammation level begins to gradually lessen and resolve. I have found that the body responds to health 100% of the time as a young seedling thrives when it receives the needed soil nutrients, sunshine and water. Carefully cared for gardens do not develop the same diseases and plight that develop with uncared for plants. Health works for everyone and as you read the testimonials in Chapter 11 your paradigm will shift and you will begin to grasp the importance of health.

Dietary Restrictions of Starches (grains), Lactose (milk) and Sugar (refined sugar)

Celiac Disease was named in 1887 by Dr. Samuel Gee from England. It was declared to be caused by wheat intolerance affecting the entire small intestine. Dr. Gee stated CD disorders cause misery and can take lives at a very young age. Many historical accounts around the world support the fact that gluten intolerance leads to bowel disease in particular CD. One such account came from Holland.

The Dutch citizens had a shortage of grains during WWII (World War) in 1939 and records revealed a drop in bowel disease during this time period. The Dutch pediatrician Willem-Karel Dicke noticed a war related shortage of bread had led to a significant drop in the death rate among children affected by Celiac Disease. The death rate among children with CD dropped from numbers greater than 35% to zero without grains in the diet. After the war when prosperity allowed grains to come back into the diet, the numbers of CD cases rose again. A similar situation also took place in Ireland, during the potato famine of 1845 reviewed in Chapter 1.

The fact cannot be denied that diet plays an enormous role in all bowel disease both IBS-G and IBD-G. The confusion lies in that Allopathic Medicine has limited the diagnosis of CD to inflammation within the small intestine declaring it is due to primarily gluten as the culprit. However, looking at the other IBD diseases and how they can be masquerading as CD must finally be brought to light that they are caused by similar factors. Even the Mayo Clinic has stated that Crohn's, also being an inflammatory disease, may affect the entire GI tract from mouth to anus which would include the small intestine and can be mistaken for CD. It just so happens, that Crohn's disease has been designated to a large percent affecting the very last section of small bowel and into the large colon. By adopting my simple regrouping of diseases as presented can give all people a clearer understanding of treatment.

Multiple worldwide studies on the eating patterns of patients diagnosed with IBD disease have shown that a higher consumption of bread, potatoes, sugar and lactose (found in milk) increase the incidence and severity of bowel diseases [30-34]. It can only be a winning decision to take a 3 month period to follow the GIS program and stop the starches, lactose from milk and refined sugar in the diet no matter what your diagnosis or symptoms may be and evaluate the outcome.

The colon condition of IBS, as shockingly as it may seem now, was first classified as a psychologically based disease right up until 1999. In my work I have realized that stress and mental well-being symptoms are always present with persons living with bowel disease. Chapters 5, explains how inflammation associated with gluten can affect the Neuromuscular System and brain function. This helps to explain why so many people diagnosed with digestive issues also live with psychological disorders. Without exception I have found IBS to be caused from gluten intolerance and other health imbalances.

I celebrated the breakthrough of mainstream medicine to finally give IBS a true physiological diagnosis. However the AMA continues to state IBS is from an unknown origin. IBS can be seen in infants and young children with colic gas, bloating, constipation, diarrhea, skin rashes and even nightmares and bedwetting with toddlers. If dietary changes are not made as children get older you can see these symptoms advancing with more advanced IBD and CD symptoms. These include bruising on the limbs, anemia, stunted growth, acute hyperactivity, scoliosis and more accompanying digestive and skin issues.

Minimize Mal-Nutrition

Being preventative with our health and our families health must be the number one goal in life if we are to avoid pain and suffering of disease now and later in life. There are many reasons why people do not receive the needed nutrition their bodies demand to experience vibrant health. Gluten intolerance is one major factor yet not the only one. The rest of the food factors and challenges will be explained that reduce the ability to absorb the valuable nutrients from our foods. Chapter 3 and Chapter 4 both elaborate factors that may be pertinent in your life that have increased malabsorption. Each area of health must be addressed to optimize overall nutrition for improved mental and physical well-being.

The facts support that inflammation is the primary challenge that causes the development of bowel disease. Inflammation in the body does not always cause pain however it always decreases the body's ability to absorb valuable nutrients from our diets. It might surprise some of you to find out inflammation may be silent.

Inflammation is not all bad. It is actually involved in the natural processes in the body of our immune systems response and healing yet when it comes from chronic irritation in our gut it promotes the disease process to escalate. This inflammation in turn compromises the ability to receive nutrition needed for the support of health in the body. When the body decreases inflammation in the gut it regains health balance to maximize the food, eaten and stops the mal-nutrition cycle.

Getting Out of Denial

Testing for gluten intolerance can be helpful to get out of denial - that is if you are fortunate enough to get a positive on your testing! However as explained in Chapter 4 testing is flawed and false negatives are very common. Most people living with bowel disease never get a diagnosis as you will read in the testimonies in Chapter 11. Chapter 4 will review testing alternatives for bowel disease.

Testing or not testing cannot take away from the fact that people do not like change. I have not been 100% graceful in my own process of getting gluten and inflammatory foods reduced in my life. Fortunately my compliance has been reinforced by continuing to feel better and look better on a daily basis. My increased energy allows me to play with my grandchildren and enjoy other life's pleasures like hobbies and even working in my chosen profession in a more productive way! People comment regularly on how youthful and young I appear even though I am entering my senior years!

Denial runs deep with the topic of gluten intolerance. In fact many of the conversations I have with people concerning gluten go like this: They state that they know someone with gluten intolerance. Yes, is my answer back – I do too! Then I let them know we are all gluten intolerant and a pause of varying lengths follow. Their response is most often - Really? Then I state yes, you and I are both gluten intolerant - it is just a matter of degree. Gluten intolerance is a human condition!

Please review the list of symptoms and conditions that follow to understand just how pervasive gluten sensitivity is in our society. Each of the ailments or symptoms listed, require special foods and or nutrients to help resolve them faster and more completely. Disease in the body is not a drug deficiency but a nutritional one! Disease in the body is closely linked to inflammation. This is a fact and the fact is that both IBS and IBD diseases are both related. Chapter 3 will review digestion and the inflammatory process that leads to symptoms of bowel disease and other illnesses of the body.

Each individual including the entire family and even pets, diagnosed or not, have the opportunity to follow the GIS guidelines in Chapter 7. You will be pleased as you begin to look and feel your very best!

> **Bowel Disease May Manifest in the Following**
>
> Diarrhea • Constipation • Abdominal Pain • Bloating • Irritability & Depression • Inflammation • Auto-Immune Conditions • Anemia • Diverticulitis • Hemorrhoids • Joint Pain • Muscle Cramps • Skin Rash • Mouth Ulcers & Sores • Bone Loss • Neuropathy – Tingling and Pain in Extremities • Impaired Walking • MitroValve Prolapsed • Allergies • Rapid Heart Beat • Heart Attack • Cystic Fibrosis • MS • Accident Prone • Weight Gain or Loss • Fatigue • Foul Smelling, Hard & Oily Stools • Stunted Growth • Neurological Disorders • Failing Immune System • Arthritis • Chronic Illnesses • Diabetes • Scoliosis • Nightmares • Bladder Incontinence • Infertility • Colitis • Ulcers • Thyroid Disorders • Manic Depression • Schizophrenia • Obesity • Cancer • Parkinson's • OCDC • Sneezing • Melancholy • Miscarriage • Menses Pain • Hyperactivity • Skin Conditions • Heart Disease • Seizures • Incontinence • Bed Wetting • Dyslexia

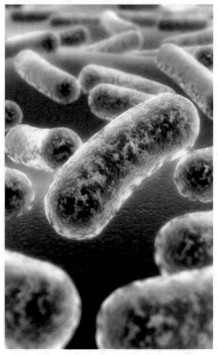

HIGHLIGHT 2: *Probiotics is the First Step to Wellness*

Remarkable in their daily tasks, the micro flora called Probiotics, have become the most important of all food supplements. Probiotics are defined as "Number One - For Life" and develop naturally in fermented foods like yogurt. Friendly bacteria supplements known as Probiotics are paramount for people's bodies to reverse bowel disease and reach optimum health. Once the body receives a quality culture of friendly bacteria it can continue to grow on its own in the gut, through a process called recolonization.

For the good bacteria to thrive the gut demands both viable culture strains and health balance in the body avoiding unnecessary antibiotics and other factors that can destroy them. Antibiotics are defined as "Against Life" and proper discretion must always be used before administering them. Researchers and health professionals alike have found that these tiny protective soldiers Probiotics which are invisible to the naked eye make up a large percentage of a person's immune system. The many different strains together promote the entire body to be healthier for kids and adults.

How do these friendly bacteria work? They reside in the small intestine and throughout the mucus membranes of the body. Each particular species of friendly bacteria carry on specialized protective duties that can in some cases make the difference between life and death. These friendly bacteria are often referred to as Lactic Acid bacteria and work by disarming the bad bacteria that can enter our body through the air we breathe, contaminated foods and water supply as well as secondary toxins made in the body itself. Bad bacteria can cause nausea, gas, tissue damage as with H. Pylori and even create a toxic environment within the colon from pathogenic cells.

The Lactic Acid friendly bacteria naturally excrete a fluid containing an acidic pH. By adjusting the pH in the colon it brings upon death to the bad bacteria. Some other strains of good bacteria contain a different defense mechanism that snuffs out the overgrowth of attackers by engulfing them. The good bacteria can fight against pathogenic cancer causing bacteria, E-coli, antibiotic resistant Staph, H. Pylori and hundreds of other bad bacteria.

The work of the Probiotics extends to even combating the overgrowth of intestinal yeast present in varying degrees in all people especially when a person is diagnosed with a type of Candida. The success and die off of the yeast is a positive step in detoxification yet it can result in temporary intestinal gas and flu like symptoms (see Ch. 6 Detoxification). Considering the immense benefit of the friendly bacteria a little increase of gas is a small price to pay. The detoxifying effect of killing off the yeast can be lengthy for some people yet by following the GIS diet and other supplements (discussed in Ch. 8) you will soon begin to feel the improvement of ones immune system, energy and reduced bowel symptoms!

Who requires Probiotics? Children and adults that have taken antibiotics, birth control pills, abused alcohol, heavy caffeine consumption and over eating of junk foods including sugary treats will all benefit with the daily addition of a quality Probiotics. Both a Probiotic supplement and a variety of fermented foods like Greek style yogurt promote a healthy supply of the friendly bacteria. People who have had surgeries and chronic illnesses that required multiple drugs taken into their system or who take pharmaceutical drugs on a daily basis will significantly benefit with the addition of a good Probiotics and the other core nutrients on the GIS Program. Some of the strains are six times stronger than just relying on yogurt to help the gut. Take a supplemental form daily even when food sources are included in the diet for best health result!

What do they do? The friendly flora bacteria contribute to health in many ways especially with a multi-strain. Their work is confirmed in research to build a stronger immune system, support the metabolic process in the small intestine to make some of the B Vitamins, greatly improve digestion and encourage the detoxification of the body through supporting better regularity of the bowels.

Friendly Bacteria Support

- Stronger Immune System Function
- Manufacturing of B Vitamins
- Greatly Improve Digestion Function
- Encourage Detoxification
- Regularity of the Bowels
- Improved Detoxification

The good bacteria can ease digestive upset, nausea, constipation and diarrhea along with gas in just minutes through their biological defense. The friendly bacteria promote a health balance of good and bad bacteria in the body, a type of homeostasis of the GI tract, called Eubiosis. The common strains reviewed in this chapter are great for the daily digestive challenges and specialty strains are critical to increase the results received from therapeutic products. Some experts state that the good bacteria are responsible for up to 70% of the body's immunity! Hundreds of strains exist throughout the body including a few that are especially indicated for bladder and vaginal conditions. When the body is in health balance the friendly bacteria grows naturally. Valuable food sources of fermented foods are reviewed in Chapter 7 and are encouraged on the GIS program with the regular use of a quality Probiotics supplement for the whole family!

C H A P T E R   3

Understanding the Digestion - Inflammation GIS Connection

"Diarrhea had become such a daily occurrence that I found myself not making plans to leave the house. It began to be more frequent as stress increased in my career and honestly the medications I tried seemed to only make my symptoms worse. I didn't think the GIS diet would work for me because it took months before my bowels began to slow down. Karen you told me it could take a while and it has been almost one year since we first spoke. I was happy to pick the phone up today and make this call. I am truly feeling better than I ever thought possible. Thanks for not giving up on me every time I called for support."
— *Steven, Los Angeles, California*

Many physicians are still in the dark about bowel disease. The general focus of mainstream medicine treatment with (mild) IBS, Irritable Bowel Syndrome has been to increase fiber in the diet and reduce the way a person internalizes stress [1]. Surprisingly, doctors are still writing prescriptions to see a psychologist or psychiatrist for stress induced bowel symptoms without addressing the underlying challenge of the diet [2, 3].

GIS does indeed encompass a brain reaction due to the Central Nervous System being affected by inflammation [4, 5]. However, think about this, if you spent half your life in a bathroom wouldn't you get pretty stressed out yourself? If you are living this scenario presently, do your best to trust in the experience of another - knowing there is a way out of the bathroom!

Depending on the severity of symptoms, most doctors will offer pharmaceutical drug treatment with (advanced) IBD, Inflammatory Bowel Disease and not spend much time on the patient's diet. As mentioned in Chapter 2 bowel surgery is more common than some people may realize with IBD to remove scarred and troubled sections of the bowel when drug therapy is no longer helpful.

The nightmare of colon surgeries also deserves a mention in this chapter. I am talking about the most extreme medical procedure which is the removal of the entire colon! Unfortunately even this radical step does not change the primary cause of bowel disease - Inflammation. The somewhat archaic procedure of partial removal or complete Colectomy is drastic and it greatly alters the quality of ones life. It may be shocking and for some frustrating to learn that most of the surgeries that have been performed could have been avoided all together if only the doctors had understood GIS!

The GIS Program in Action!

One example of how quickly the GIS diet works was a patient who came to see me in the clinic as a pre-op appointment soon to have a resection of the colon. His bowel was markedly restricted at one point to about the size of two pencils in diameter and he was experiencing nausea along with very slow elimination. The surgery would remove the scarred narrowed section. You can imagine his surprise when I presented the GIS program to him and shared that he may be able to delay surgery for a while. It was well worth it to him to experiment with the program for three months because he was living with the Human Immune Deficiency Virus (HIV). Truly he did not want to have surgery at this time if he could avoid it. To his astonishment within days of implementing the GIS Program he started eliminating better and feeling practically normal. At the end of the trial period he felt so good that even the attending physician endorsed his decision to wait.

A Physicians Wait and See Approach Often Offers Limited Success

The medical philosophy has maintained the hope through all of the trial and error with drugs and other procedures that the patient will simply outgrow the disease. Their "Wait and See" approach has offered limited results with select individuals [6]. More often than not the treatments worsen the symptoms and disease in the long run with rebound side effects from the overuse of antibiotics, steroids and prednisone drugs [7]. The repetitive surgeries have also left people with the aftermath of adhesions from scar tissue resulting in slight to major pain. The majority of people living with less pain and fewer symptoms of IBS often out of pure frustration just stop going to a physician altogether and self-medicate.

When health is not a part of a treatment protocol the body is left with an array of negative side effects and unresolved symptoms [8]. Make certain you become informed and read the long term side effects of any drug protocol or procedure you or a family member might be taking or are considering to take. All drugs have detrimental side effects even the OTC's like acetaminophen and anti-acids. The exercise of reviewing any risk of side effects to the benefit one may receive from a drug is known as assessing the "Risk to Benefit Ratio". This can be a great motivating practice encouraging you to choose a more aggressive health path.

Cortisone derivatives for example can help relieve pain temporarily yet if they are used for any length of time may actually cause a depletion of minerals in the body and lead to Osteoporosis. People require minerals in the body as they serve to give structural support for building the skeletal system, teeth, hair and skin. They are also paramount for all metabolic functions of the body including muscle action and healing of cellular tissue. Children may actually experience stunted growth if kept on these prednisone drugs for any length of time [9, 10, and 11].

A variety of nutritional deficiencies, due to prolonged use of pharmaceutical drugs develop that interfere with mineral and nutritional absorption. The wildly used Proton-Pump Inhibitors also deserve major consideration because they delay the uptake of both minerals and protein into the body and are loosely prescribed for the digestive condition called Reflux. Their use may lead to greater symptoms including a reduction in immune function. Let's not forget that these Allopathic protocols are still not addressing the actual cause of bowel disease which has everything to do with poor digestion and inflammation developing into the GIS – Gluten Inflammatory Syndrome.

Digestion - Inflammatory GIS Cycle
- Poor Digestive Ability & Genetics > Reduced Digestion
- Gluten & Triggers > Immune System Activation > Auto-Immune Response
- > Heightened Inflammation > Tissue Damage of Villi > Causes Mal-absorption > Develops Disease > Heightened Auto-Immune Disease Symptoms > Sympathetic & Para Sympathetic Nervous System Irregularities
- Central Nervous System (CNS) Irregularities > Diarrhea > Constipation > Brain Mal-Function > Effects Motor Skills
- Hyperactive CNS > Viral Flare of HSVI & II and other Miscellaneous Viruses > More Inflammation > Lowers Glandular Function > Reduces Immunity > Increases More Disease

Digestion is a Big Deal!
The development of GIS starts with the challenge of poor digestive ability in the body. A good functioning digestive system is a big deal and relies on the total collective of factors working together that includes; diet, metabolism, environmental and genetic strength. The value of optimizing the entire digestive system cannot be over emphasized to decrease bowel disease and optimize health [12].

This chapter explains the digestive process and how the inflammation occurs from eating gluten and the other triggers in particular milk and refined sugar. Once you fully grasp the GIS development you will more clearly understand how improving the efficiency of the digestive process and eliminating the catalysts helps the body heal. This knowledge will also underline the value of adding natural anti-inflammatory herbs and supplements to speed recovery and act preventatively to support health.

We cannot change the fact that people may inherit a weak genetic predisposition to bowel disease. Yet each individual has the ability to reduce ill effects by optimizing all factors in one's environment that effect health including what is chosen to eat and lifestyle choices [13]. Without the understanding of the pinnacle importance that digestion and dietary intervention play in reducing bowel inflammation true recovery remains only a dream.

According to the Webster dictionary the state of inflammation is brought about by injury, infection or irritation and is characterized by redness, pain, heat, swelling and loss of function. In regards to bowel disease - inflammation is brought on by the inability to digest carbohydrates pinpointing milk products, refined sugars, whole grains and miscellaneous other factors that are found in an individual's diet.

Digestive System

Mouth

Liver

Stomach

Small Intestine

Large Intestines

Descending Colon

Normal Digestive Process

Let's review what is needed in a healthy functioning digestive system to better understand what takes place before inflammation strikes with GIS. Knowing the physiology of how the body works will allow us to analyze and take action to revitalize the system for wellness. Every step in the digestive process is important if good health is to be reinstated and endure. An especially important function of the body is its ability to manufacture the required enzymes [14].

Enzymes are specialized compounds that work as catalysts to complete a metabolic reaction in the body. Enzymes along with other digestive juices are needed to achieve success in digestion and they are required at every step of the digestive process. Also, thousands of enzymes play other important roles throughout the rest of the body along with the digestive enzymes to maintain optimum health.

Our focus is on the digestive tract enzymes and digestive juices. Digestion is designed to start in the mouth and move the contents into the stomach and small intestine breaking foods down into their sub-categories. These groups include proteins, carbohydrates, fats and oils along with facilitating vitamins and minerals to be reduced into micro-fractions ready for absorption into the body for wellness.

Mouth

If the body's digestive system is working properly glands in the mouth will secret saliva which contains *alpha-amylase*. Amylase is found in many tissues of the body yet high amounts are needed in the mouth and flowing from the pancreas organ for proper digestion. The alpha-amylase in the mouth is called *ptyalin* and it is crucial to begin the carbohydrate digestion of starch and glycogen which yields glucose, maltose and iso-maltose. Maltose and iso-maltose both disaccharides (double sugars) will require even further digestion as the foodstuff continues through the gastrointestinal tract (GI). Interesting to note that the salivary glands also secrete *lysozyme,* which kills bacteria but it is not classified as a digestive enzyme. It does illustrate however the importance of chewing ones food [15].

Chewing your food is an extremely important digestive step that most people do not spend enough time doing. Children and adults must be taught and reminded to slow down and chew their foods thoroughly which in turn encourages the digestive juices to flow. I often refer to gobbling down food as the Hoover Move (brand of a vacuum cleaner). People actually swallow foods in such large pieces at times they wind up in the emergency room. Besides the threat of dying of affixation due to lack of oxygen when food lodges in the esophagus, by not chewing food properly you skip the first important opportunity to help your body digest your food. Slow down and chew your foods well!

Whatever you do - don't over dilute the contents of foods in the digestive tract by drinking too large a quantity of liquids at mealtimes. Especially iced cold beverages are very detrimental! Ice causes a reduction of enzymatic action. It prevents the enzymes to work as nature intended. A better choice at meals is a small amount of room temperature water or a cup of warm tea or coffee. This first digestive step is very important if you are to experience digestive success at the second step in the Stomach.

Stomach

Pepsin and *hydrochloric acid (HCL)* are both designed to work in the stomach to continue the important job of digesting protein and minerals from food. A small amount of gastric amylase is present in the stomach yet it seems to be of only minor significance for carbohydrate digestion.

Pepsin is the main gastric enzyme in the stomach that is actually made from pepsinogen. *Pepsinogen* is a very large protein compound and consists of 44 amino acids and was designed to flow first into the stomach yet requires two precursors. It needs a specific hormone called *gastrin* and it requires the *vagus nerve* to trigger the release of it as we chew. The gastrin hormone is made in the liver. Chewing also triggers adequate amounts of HCL required for digestive success in the stomach to produce pepsin [16].

This is a great example of the true specificity of the body's digestive process. It takes the chewing action, the liver and the Nervous System all three working properly to support good digestion in the stomach.

PH is Critical for Proper Digestion

The *HCL* must be secreted into the stomach in high enough volume to lower the pH to around 1 -2 which is very acidic. This allows the *pepsin* to activate from the *pepsinogen.* This reaction is a safeguard method which keeps the *pepsin* from digesting the stomach lining since all cells are made of protein. Remarkably, once the needed pH is reached, the pepsin begins its duty to break apart the protein molecular structure from the food that was eaten. This helps free the individual amino acid building blocks to be reused for other compounds in the body later assembled in the liver. Macro and Micro Minerals also rely on the digestive process in the stomach along with protein.

If the pH of the stomach stays at an alkaline pH of 5 or higher and the environment of the stomach is too cold temperature-wise from the result of drinking iced cold beverages, the researchers find that pepsin will not be produced. Other important hindrances to digestion related to low HCL have been researched at Tufts University's nutrition division. In their ongoing 30 year study on longevity they found that a large percentage of adults develop low hydrochloric acid HCL levels as they age. This situation called Hypochlorhydria greatly impairs the digestion of protein and minerals [17].

Their studies related the deficiency of HCL to multiple nutritional deficiencies. Some of the deficiencies were directly related to the consumption of pharmaceutical drugs and others they felt were due to poor nutritional choices or omissions. The numbers of people of all ages who take some form of prescription medicine is rising and I think it is also safe to say that in the greater population both children and adults do not always eat properly adding to the problem of mal-nutrition and inadequate levels of digestive juices. I find the deficiency of HCL in my practice very widespread especially when people are poor eaters or have been experiencing different illnesses requiring excessive drug therapy coupled with their diet limitations.

During the digestive process the food contents may stay in the stomach for up to 45 minutes or longer before the Autonomic Nervous System sends the food on to the small intestine for more digestion. To optimize digestion in the stomach and reduce gas - it is best to allow the meal to "complete its digestive cycle" the best you can which takes approximately 2 – 3 hours before adding more food.

A rule of thumb is that fruits and beverages digest quicker than protein and vegetable meals especially if there is meat. The best waiting period before eating again after fruits would be around one hour or less. Pausing for up to 2 hours is sufficient after eating milk products like cheese, yogurt or nuts and seeds that may have been eaten for a snack or mini-meal.

People who continually eat without allowing the food to digest or overeat at mealtimes put an undo stress on their metabolism and it may lower nutrient absorption. Much more gas and digestive issues are likely to develop including heartburn and headaches by overeating. Experts have estimated that some people greatly reduce absorption from meals due to poor eating habits therefore only receiving a fractional amount of the potential nutrition from the foods sometimes as low as 15% [18]. By simply following the guidelines of proper eating mechanics individuals can significantly reduce digestive woes. Improving your eating habits only requires a little extra time but the return is worth it!

Small Intestine

Digestion in the small intestine has two main objectives. First, it continues the digestive process from the stomach by *adding more enzymes* that come from the pancreas and bile which is stored in the gallbladder plus the enzymes it excretes itself from the villi. The second objective is to *absorb the digested food nutrients into the blood stream*. This takes place through the villi coined the "gatekeepers" that allow the passage on through to the liver.

The eight to nine feet of small intestine is lined with thousands of microscopic size villi called *micro-villi* which have finger like projections. The villi both secrete enzymes and allow the absorption of nutrients into the blood.

At this stage of digestion, if our metabolism has been working efficiently, the food contents will have changed into a liquid called *chime*. This liquid food must be further digested into microscopic size particles ready for absorption. To accomplish this task the chime which is in the duodenum section of the small intestine requires the rest of the digestive juices to be added.

A healthy pancreas is required at this stage in the digestive process. It is designed to secrete digestive juices called *pancreatic enzymes* into the chime which are very specialized. These enzymes are called; *protease, amylase* and *lipase*. They specifically target the digestion of proteins, carbohydrates (starch) and fats respectively reducing them into simple molecular structures.

Bile which is made in the liver and stored in the gallbladder is also needed in the mix. Along with the pancreatic enzymes the bile is delivered through the common bile duct into the chime. The bile further aids in the digestion of fats and oils which we refer to as lipids.

Unbeknownst to many people, bile has a second job once it completes its fat digestive process. It has the important function to adjust the pH in the small intestine to "Alkaline". Proper pH is paramount for the success of each step in the digestive process. Achieving pH balance depends on a person getting the right nutrition into the body.

Four additional enzymes are also required for successful digestion in the small intestine - the first to be highlighted is *lactase*. The ending letters ASE define the enzyme status. Lactase is an enzyme needed to fully digest *lactose sugars* found in milk and milk products. The letters OSE define different sugars.

Intestinal Micro -Villi

Nature designed the villi itself to secrete the *lactase* enzyme along with three other carbohydrate splitting enzymes; *sucrase, maltase* and *iso-maltase*. These latter three are necessary to complete the carbohydrate sugar digestion of refined sugar, potatoes, beans and all grains including corn.

This function of the villi to secrete enzymes is consequential for healthy digestion to continue and unfortunately this appears to be where the body falls short with colon disease. Research has shown that a deficiency of lactase results in poor digestion of the sugar lactose from cow's milk. A lactase deficiency is credited as the initial catalysts of the GIS inflammation. If the villi are found to not make proper amounts of the lactase enzyme you can count that it is also not making enough of the other needed carbohydrate enzymes as well.

Research confirms that the improper digestion of milk, refined sugar and starches which includes the gluten compound all three induce the GIS inflammation. If not halted the inflammation damages the precious villi and prevents them from completing the task of absorbing nutrients from our foods.

The healthier the person, the better their digestive function of the micro-villi works. With a healthy digestive system the villi completes digestion in the small intestine and absorbs the microscopic nutrients into the blood stream. As designed the blood will then deliver the nutrients to the next destination, the liver, where the last step of digestion takes place before going on into the individual cells.

Liver

The Liver has a lot of work to perform before the nutrients extracted from food are ready to be delivered back to the rest of the body. It is an extremely *critical stage of digestion in regards to core foundational nutrients* including; fat soluble vitamins A (beta carotene form), E, D, K and Essential Fatty Acids and the Amino Acids. Amino Acids, which are building blocks of proteins, are processed and synthesized in the liver to *build all the specialized protein compounds* of the body.

The liver is also viewed as a *filter organ* and some speculate it conducts over 4,000 daily duties. *Detoxification and cleansing* of the blood by the liver is so very important to prevent disease. The liver is highly specialized to *make hundreds of antioxidants* such as Super Oxide Dismutase (SOD) that neutralize toxic chemicals. If toxins and free radicals are left unchecked they can lead to damage of the cellular DNA escalating premature aging and may even lead into cancer development.

Another important process conducted by the liver is *cholesterol production* requiring the Omega 3, 6 and 9 lipids. By utilizing cholesterol the liver and other organs of the body can manufacture *hormones* using protein, minerals and other co-factors. Hormones are essential in most of the metabolic processes throughout the entire body required from infancy on through to adults and yes seniors need hormones too!

Also, remember how valuable bile is for fat digestion and preventing over-acidity in the GI tract? The liver is responsible for making bile! Review Chapter 5 and 6 to see the relationship of bile to Reflux.

The liver also handles *storage of nutrients* as with glycogen. Glycogen is used for energy for the vital organs and it works in the *decomposition of red blood cells* and *plasma protein synthesis*. We cannot live without a healthy functioning liver. A sluggish, lazy, fat laden liver greatly hinders all of the systems of the body to work for children and adults. How do we keep the liver working the best we can? The answer is good nutrition and detoxification which demands drinking quality water and exercise. All of these choices are essential to supporting a healthy liver. In turn the liver supports the digestive process, helping people maintain a healthy body weight and reach optimum health.

Large Intestine

The design of the large intestine has two main objectives. The most obvious job is to *eliminate stool* out of the body through the rectum. This natural elimination step is supposed to occur after water and salt is removed automatically from the bulk contents. The daily goal of a healthy body is to have a formed bowel movement not too loose or overly hard once or twice per day.

It is good to become observant of ones stool and be aware of any discharge of mucus, blood or occasionally larger parasites which would call for more medical attention. The stool profile is an important diagnostic tool in health and gives valuable information about the body including the color and texture of the stool. Maintaining a medium brown color with average density, not oily or abnormally smelly are healthy parameters. Alert your health professional with changes in the stool that do not right themselves within a reasonable time table [19]. Also, seeing undigested foods and or supplements coming through the stool is a definite sign that the body is not digesting properly.

The second job of the large intestine is to rid itself of *cellular waste* and impurities that naturally accumulate in the colon tissue. One means of detoxifying its environment begins in the small intestine. The large intestine receives a bacterial mix of both good and bad bacteria from the small intestine accompanying the stool. By encouraging the colonizing of beneficial friendly bacteria called Micro-Flora it helps both parts of the intestinal tract by providing support for detoxification, defense from microbial invaders and help with digestion [20]. Review the HIGHLIGHT 2 Probiotics in Chapter 2 for more information on the role of the Micro-Flora.

The other pathway of safe guarding the large intestines is accomplished through the busy *Lymphatic System*. It is similar to the circulatory system and interlaces with the lymph glands of the tonsils, spleen and liver. Its main objectives are to further the filtration of the blood and also protect the body from microbial attack. White blood cells (WBC) are important infection fighters in the body and are dispersed throughout the Lymphatic System.

The juncture of the Lymphatic System used by the large intestine takes up two-thirds of the rectum. The lymph fluid leaving the colon gets special attention from the largest area of the lymph in the body called the *cisterna chili*. It is located side by side the back bone lumbar section we refer to as the low back [21]. I mention the Lymphatic System at this time because it is an important protector of the body for health that is not often mentioned in the discussion of elimination. Both children and adults require healthy regularity to allow proper lymphatic function in order to feel their very best and stay healthy. Following the GIS Program leads all individuals to experience healthier digestion and elimination which reduces inflammation and disease!

Steps of a Healthy Digestive System:
- *Mouth* - Chew Food Contents > Alpha-Amylase called Ptyalin (begins digestion of carbohydrates)
- *Stomach* - Pepsin/Hydrochloric Acid (begins digestion of protein & minerals)
- *Small Intestine (SI)* - Pancreatic Enzymes > Adding Protease (protein), Amylase (starch) and Lipase (fat) Enzymes > Bile (from the Gallbladder begins fat digestion and adjusts Alkalinity pH) , Micro-Villi > Add Lactase, Sucrase, Maltase and Iso-Maltase, Micro- Flora Bacteria > Lactic Acid and other friendly bacteria (maintains balance in the gut of good and bad bacteria)
- *Micro-Villi (Located in the SI)* – Secretes Enzymes > Absorbs Nutrients into the Blood Stream > Blood Travels into the Liver
- *Liver* - Receives Blood with Nutrients > Last Stage of Digestion > Makes Specialized Compounds & All Nutrients Continue Via the Blood to All Cells of the Body Supplying Nutritional Requirements
- *Large Intestine* - Receives Bulk Waste from SI > Removes Salt & Water > Excretes Waste Into Lymphatic > Good Bacteria (provides balance in the colon of good and bad bacteria) > Eliminates Stool from the Body Through the Rectum Daily

Where is the Epicenter of Inflammation?

Describing a healthy digestive system sounds plausible and normal yet the truth about the average person in today's world is that they do not have this text book digestive system at all. Most digestive systems seldom work smoothly as outlined due to changes in ones emotional temperament, dietary choices, eating mechanics and the physical characteristics of the GI tract as with bowel disease. The body's digestive capacity may be further taxed by a current disease like Diabetes or countless other conditions.

With so many factors to contend with challenges in the digestive process can occur at any step along the way. One factor that each person has more direct control over is their eating habits. Dietary and lifestyle choices both profoundly affect digestion and what we eat and put inside our bodies is influenced by a variety of social pressures that includes "Brainwashing"!

The Brainwashing of a Society

As we strive to live a healthier life, if we are wise we develop goals and attitudes to live by through daily disciplines. Our family, friends and co-workers often influence the choices we make. Another big factor of influence to food and lifestyle choices is not driven by a conscious decision but by subtle and even direct brainwashing. The dictionary defines brainwashing as to indoctrinate so intensely and thoroughly as to effect a radicle transformation of beliefs and mental attitudes.

Brainwashing through the media and certain professional outlets has been a hurdle for all societies. Due to a busy lifestyle or just a lack of interest to study health, the *TV, internet* and even the *back of cereal boxes* are where a large percentage of families receive their greatest nutritional education.

Sounds a little absurd to think the masses have all been brainwashed but who hasn't heard these sound bites, "Every Body Needs Milk?" And then the newer version that followed that was plastered everywhere, "Got Milk?" Advertisers want you to think that drinking milk is necessary and critical to one's survival! How about the Ads that demonstrate that making chocolate chip cookies or giving other sugary treats to your children is the most loving action a mother or father can do? The brainwashing that really irks me most is the continual preaching about the virtues to eat whole grains from cereals to snack bars as often as possible if you are to be healthy. And how about all the commercials for regularity edifying psyllium seed and bran products that many of you know only add to your colon problems! I must admit that until I understood the entire truth behind gluten foods and GIS that I too was one of those preaching the virtues of brown rice, oats and whole grains!

Friends please understand if you haven't come to the realization already - many people including some that have impressive credentials are only partially informed on the real facts concerning food and health. In fact many representatives are very motivated by an ulterior motive agenda fueled by money $$$$ [22]. Unfortunately, when it comes to a product being sold to the millions of consumers across the globe the outcome of a so called "Scientific Study" may be altered to reflect results that are not necessarily in the best interest of people. The facts have revealed that numbers and facts can be selected to reflect an outcome from a study dealing with health or disease to achieve power and or financial gain over others.

Also, lobbyists, who represent the corporate giants of the milk, sugar and the grain industries, have a choke hold on our health and nutrition sectors of the government. They influence the available information coming into people's lives through the media and educational outlets literally fed to them on a daily basis.

Fraudulent advertising has also been coming from the drug industry as they rush through drug approvals with incomplete and or incorrect data to cash in on sales. Lately, every year has fingered more dangerous pharmaceuticals that have been used by unsuspecting citizens who developed dangerous side effects and even untimely death for some. People must not assume that any drug is safe. You need to do your own research to discover if the benefit truly out-weighs the risk. To help give a voice to Americans, consumer groups and responsible health professionals have developed websites that give reports on pharmaceutical drug side effects and other important health information on foods and personal care products that may pose a health problem.

We must also include the pharmaceutical corporations in this brainwashing of society with its unending advertisements and their many parasitic lobbyists [23]. The truth of the matter is that most people are not born with drug deficiencies or require them for survival on a daily basis at all! Yet the brainwashing teaches that if we develop a disease we have a matching drug to alleviate it. The scientific facts prove that humans do not require drugs but nutrients accessed from foods and food supplements to fuel the body and prevent the development of nutritional deficiencies. Further research confirms that nutritional deficiencies if not corrected will then lead to disease development in the body [14]!

Physicians, whom we have placed our trust, thinking they know all there is about staying well, have been some of the least educated when it comes to the health of the human body and how to best care for it [24]! They have perpetuated the brainwashing on many levels thinking perhaps they were doing their job. We need our physicians, however it is time that they join the ranks of integrative health professionals, through educating themselves about nutrition, so they too will encourage responsible pharmaceutical drug use and support optimum health.

The road to understanding GIS has been a humbling experience for me as a health educator yet the truth is so exciting to reveal at last. What I have learned and reinforced in my life is that we must each think for ourselves, learning from one another yes and good dependable science but do not turn over important decision making solely to others. Let the old paradigms fall away and be replaced with the new as we strive for what truly works! Keep in mind above all else that you absolutely do not have to listen to the advertisements - Ha!

What Prevents A Healthy Digestive System?
- Eating Fast & Too Much
- Not Relaxing at Meals
- Emotionally Upset
- Drinking Large Quantities of Liquids at Meals including; Iced Beverages, Sodas, Alcohol & Milk
- Eating High Sugary, Fried & Starchy Meals (whole grains)

- Nutritional Deficiencies & Illness (GIS and other) that Reduces Digestive Juices and Enzyme Production
- Brainwashing that Influences Our Food & Lifestyle Choices

The Food You Eat Today Makes or Breaks Your Digestion Tomorrow

Many individuals who have eaten poorly during the first years of their life and young adulthood without a varied diet but relied on milk as a main-stay, have developed allergies and other illnesses. The common practice of eating sugary carbohydrate starches like box cereals and processed foods also share in speeding the development of digestive issues and failing health to include; constipation, diarrhea, frequent colds and other related illnesses. This scenario can transpire even when people do not inherit strong genetic weakness of Celiac Disease or other advanced bowel diseases.

Dietary abuse or neglect always compromises the body's systems including the digestive system giving way to heartburn, reflux, diverticulitis and other bowel disease. Keep in mind that the weakening of the body and the GIS damage that leads to poor digestion can often be silent. This means that an individual may not experience any particular obvious symptoms of pain yet the body may still be deficient, not receiving the valuable nutrients it needs to build health and maintain the body.

For many people poor digestion only shows up with a diagnosis of a chronic disease like anemia, scoliosis, osteoporosis or even cancer. Review Chapter 5 for conditions related to poor digestion and GIS. Nutrition and digestive stamina is essential to build a healthy body and mind whether you are diagnosed with bowel disease or not!

Having reviewed some of the more obvious factors that lead to digestive challenges, now let's look at the junction that's referred to as the "Epicenter of Inflammation" that allows the opportunity of GIS to develop. Even though several other secondary factors influence the level of inflammation in the body which is outlined in Chapter 4, there exist three primary culprits held responsible at the core of the initial GIS inflammation – Milk, Refined Sugar and Grains (Gluten & Starch).

GIS Inflammation Core Pinwheel

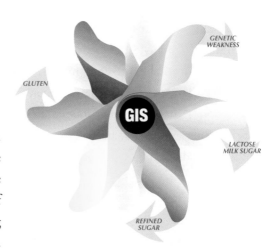

The "Epicenter" of GIS is in the Micro-Villi of the Small Intestine

The Micro-Villi also called the "Gate Keeper Cells" have been the illusive site of inflammation sparking GIS and colon disease. When digestion is incomplete due to all of the factors mentioned the foodstuff is left in larger particles. Upon reaching the small intestine the marginally digested food requires greater digestive capacity coming from the pancreas, liver and the Micro-Villi. Yet often due to the body not working properly the digestive help it needs does not come and inflammation becomes more and more damaging to the tissue at this site [25, 26].

GIS I Theory: Improper Sugar Metabolism Leads to Bowel Disease

GIS inflammation comes from a reaction to eating carbohydrates found in sugars and starchy foods. We know that people living with bowel disease have both a weak digestive system and because of this they experience mal-absorption. The inflammation that occurs with gluten and other triggers develop from the body's inability to digest carbohydrates especially the complex carbohydrate molecules called disaccharides meaning two sugars and the polysaccharides defined as many sugars. Monosaccharide carbohydrates are the easiest to digest being single simple sugars and they do not require any extra digestion from the Micro-Villi [27]. However, each disaccharide and polysaccharide does require the Micro-Villi to secrete; lactase, sucrase, maltase or iso-maltase to complete their digestion. You will see it has less to do with genetics and a lot to do with the unnatural overindulging addictive tendencies of the human being. Understanding this fully means that by honoring the limitations of digestion and improving its function a person can truly lower inflammation and the symptoms of GIS and feel good again.

Carbohydrates; Monosaccharide, Disaccharides & Polysaccharides

To understand GIS the focus is on the digestion of carbohydrates. All sugars and starches are carbohydrates. The sugars are divided into three categories; simple, double and many (poly) also called complex sugars. Foods that contain carbohydrates include; fruits, vegetables, dairy products, potatoes, beans and grains. Some are also found in processed foods in the manufacturing ingredients as in thickeners and extenders.

Monosaccharide

Fruits and honey require very little digestion because they are already largely composed of simple sugars referred to as a *monosaccharide*. These single sugars are primarily fructose and glucose and are easily absorbed illustrating that nature knows best in food selection.

Disaccharide

Enzymes have the important job in the body to reduce the double and complex carbohydrates known as *disaccharides* and *polysaccharides* into the simple sugars of glucose and galactose for absorption. The *disaccharides* (double sugars) found in refined sugar are called *sucrose* and in milk sugar are called *lactose*. The other double sugars are called *maltose* and *iso-maltose*. These last two are the result from polysaccharide starch digestion that takes place in the mouth and from pancreatic enzyme metabolism in the small intestine - that is if digestion is working up to par.

Dairy products especially milk contain the double sugar lactose. When digested properly with enough lactase enzymes, or through the fermentation process or hydrolysis of milk, the result is a simple sugar of glucose and one of galactose ready for easy assimilation into the body. Galactose is a very mild tasting simple sugar only present in animal's milk

Polysaccharide

The most complex carbohydrates are called polysaccharides and must be digested into double sugars first before the body can attempt to reduce them further into two simple sugars for complete digestion. As reviewed in the healthy digestive system section, it requires many different enzymes found in the mouth, a small amount in the stomach, the pancreas and the small intestine to fully digest complex carbohydrates found in grains, beans and potatoes into simple sugars of glucose and fructose.

Understanding Amylose & Amylopectins Starch and Glycogen Poly-saccharides

These larger complex carbohydrates (polysaccharide starch sugars), *amylose* and *amylopectins* are found only in starch foods and glycogen (glucose storage in the body) not in dairy products. All grains, potatoes, beans and other vegetables contain varying percentages of these starches with approximately 25% amylose (starch sugar) and 75% amylopectins (which is a type of fiber).

Glycogen is a polysaccharide carbohydrate of glucose storage in human beings and other animals and contains a large percentage of Amylopectins. It is stored primarily in the liver and muscles and used by the body for quick energy and on demand for brain and cellular metabolism. Researchers have not completed extensive work in the digestive ability of this polysaccharide compound. The investigative work has been more in the manufacturing arena for binding capacity of starches used in prepared foods and in building materials as with gluten that is used in wall paper discussed in Chapter 1.

Glucose   Complex
               carb

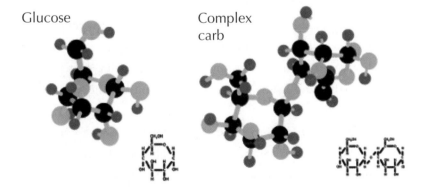

Because the *amylose* starch is in a more linear configuration like a pearl necklace it is easier to break the glucose bonds during digestion than in the amylopectin starch. The *amylopectins* are like a multilayered cabbage leaf design that requires an abundance of enzymes to break the glucose linkages apart for good digestion.

Enzymes that are needed to break these complex starches down are called *maltase* and *iso-maltase* and the process is referred to as "Reducing". Remember that the letters ASE designate an enzyme.

As previously mentioned the enzymes must first reduce the polysaccharides to double sugars and next must further reduce them into small single sugars called *mono-saccharides* of glucose, fructose and or galactose. Only in this single or simple sugar state can they be absorbed through the Micro-Villi into the liver and other cells easily to provide energy.

Types of Carbohydrate Sugars:

- *Monosaccharides* - Simple Single Sugars; Glucose, Fructose, Galactose. Sources; Honey, fruits, vegetables and yogurt are good sources. Easy to digest because it is the end product of digestion of a double and or complex sugar starch compound or found in nature as a single sugar in fruit and honey.

- *Disaccharides* - Double Sugars; (a) Lactose, (b) Sucrose, (c) Maltose and Iso-maltose (from starch digestion). Sources; (a) milk products, Mother's Milk, ice cream, processed cheeses and whey products (requires lactase), (b) refined sugar, processed foods, beverages and desserts (requires sucrase), (c) corn, confections (added maltose sweetened candy) and starches (includes grains, beans and potatoes requiring amylase enzyme in the first step, this complex sugar is difficult to digest and it is the second step in starch digestion.)

- *Polysaccharides* - Compound Sugars (found in starch not Aloe); (a) Amylose 25% (single strands of glucose requiring amylase in first step and maltase in second step), (b) Amylopectin 75%

(complex cabbage like branches of sugars requiring amylase in first step and iso-maltase in second step). Sources; (a) rice, beans, grains and potatoes (b) sweet potatoes, yams, corn, grains, beans and pectin. Both starches require two steps of digestion. Most vegetables including whole grains contain both types of starch in various proportions. Research has been very limited to the exact percentages in grains and other starches. What is known is the Amylose starch is easier to digest. The Amylopectin is more difficult to digest containing a larger matrix of starch protein compound that are in a branch cabbage leaf matrix shape.

The dilemma in health is that the body requires a variety of foods to thrive and feel satisfied within the chosen diet selected from the food groups; proteins, fats and carbohydrates. We do have the alternative choice to sprout and ferment grains for better digestion as explained in Chapter 1.

The question still remains why over the ages did it become so difficult for the body to digest carbohydrates? It appears from reviewing the research with bowel disease, that over the last few hundred years, the inability to properly digest carbohydrates first began from the early introduction of dairy products into the diet. Dairy products meaning more specifically cow's milk seems to have set the stage for GIS development. The challenge is due in part to low production of the enzyme *lactase* specifically required to digest (reduce) the double milk sugar. If the amount of lactase enzyme is flowing properly from the villi then milk digestion appears to work fairly well however there may be some other factors that also affect milk digestion.

Why is milk so difficult to digest?
- Reduced Lactase Enzyme Availability
- Cow's Milk is Not Mother's Milk
- Over consumption of Milk
- Pasteurization and Homogenization of Milk
- Nutritional & B-Complex Deficiency
- Genetics or Cultural Predisposition

ENZYME DEFICIENCY

Exactly why the lactase enzyme deficiency occurs is a bit unclear however several explanations seem to share the blame. In regards to milk it appears that many developed countries including the US have resorted to the over consumption of cow's milk and dairy products in the diet of adults, children and babies.

Statistics show that in 2001 each person drank approximately 23 gallons of milk per year. Even though this figure is down from 1945 of 45 gallons per year the daily consumption of ice cream has consistently increased since 1909 and has maintained a high consumable dairy product since the end of WWII with the average consumption of 23 pounds per person each year. Also, the consumption of cheese has soared to 30 pounds of cheese for each year for every American. With the US in the top three countries producing milk products today it is fair to say from reviewing the statistics that Americans are consuming an exceptionally large amount.

Milk products do contain a fair amount of somewhat absorbable protein yet the calcium it contains is not easily absorbed in fact experts agree that a person can receive much higher quality and quantity of calcium from broccoli or kale greens! Optimum and balanced health is

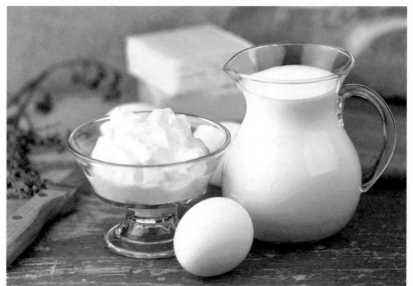

only achieved by eating a variety of different protein and mineral sources and not relying on excessive milk. Cow's milk is limited in nutrition and besides falling short with Calcium it lacks the important mineral Iron! Also, people need to consider the fact that cow's milk was designed for the baby cow [28] and it is not the perfect food for humans especially since most people do not digest it very well.

Humans were meant to begin life drinking their own Mothers milk which is perfectly digested by most babies. During the year 1970 statistics revealed that 75% of infants were bottle fed primarily on cow's milk instead of being breast fed. Review Chapter 9 Raising Healthy Children and the highlights of Breast Feeding.

The addition of cow's milk rose in popularity for babies formula as the practice of nursing infants became unfashionable and time consuming. The most popular baby formula was made with not only cow's milk but also with the addition of refined sugar to provide the needed calories for the growing child. The challenge with this practice is refined sugar is another stimulus in GIS. Supporting this connection to GIS is the fact that babies that are breast fed have a much lower incidence of advanced bowel disease.

Another theory contends that as cow's milk began to be highly *pasteurized*, due to the potential of dangerous pathogens and also *homogenized* to keep the fat from separating, it became increasingly more difficult for humans to digest. Milk is actually a very complex food to metabolize in the first place for any mammal. If including it in the diet as a food source it has been suggested to drink it alone as a separate mini-meal and only drink it in smaller amounts.

Research Reveals B-Complex is Needed to Produce Valuable Enzymes

Scientists recently linked a nutritional deficiency to milk intolerance [29, 30]. This may ultimately explain why children are sometimes born with lactose intolerance. They found a deficiency in B Vitamins prevent the body from producing the required lactase enzymes as well as other digestive juices. In this light it stands to reason that if a mother does not ingest or absorb enough quantity of B-Complex during gestation it would cheat not only herself but the unborn baby.

A deficiency of lactase enzyme may also be the result of a fungal overgrowth in the GI tract known as Candida Albicans. This fungus, one of over 200 species, may decrease absorption of valuable core nutrients to include B-Complex into the body. The overeating of starchy carbohydrates in older children and adults can further deplete the B-Complex stores.

Healthy Villi

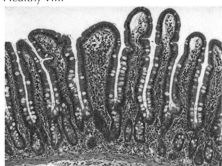

This is one more important reason why junk food and refined carbohydrates, including alcohol is not good for the body.

Lastly, genetics may set up a discrepancy of the lactase enzyme production from the villi. Research has not yet confirmed the fact that lactose intolerance, as commonly seen in African Americans for example, is due to a genetic flaw. It may just be the result of that particular race of people eating more cultural foods that predispose a larger percentage of the people to the lactase enzyme deficiency.

Damaged Villi

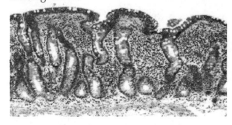

Whatever the exact reason is for milk intolerance the fact remains that many children and adults do not secrete enough quantity of the lactase enzyme to digest the lactose sugar bonds in cow's milk. When the body cannot reduce the double bonded sugars, disaccharides, into the two separate simple sugars of glucose and galactose, the body identifies the sugar molecule as a foreign invader.

At that point the immune system is called upon to attack the double bonded sugar molecule resulting in inflammation. When this reaction occurs over and over again it damages the micro-villi cells leading to varying degrees of mal-absorption in the body.

The damage to the villi can be minor causing mild symptoms or more severe causing a flattening effect of the villi cells compromising absorption. The more damage to the villa the more advanced symptoms of bowel disease that will be experienced. The reaction also affects the Central Nervous System (CNS). If it continues for long periods of time it appears to predispose people to other disease states. With acute inflammation the villi can be destroyed and actually appear to be missing altogether!

Mal-absorption with advanced IBD requires medical intervention along with the GIS program as tolerated. Even with advanced bowel disease, health works. I have worked with some very severely affected individuals who gradually improve. Health always needs to be part of the solution.

Experiment with alternative food choices in recovery that may be easier to digest such as natural fermented milk products like Greek style or homemade yogurt. The fermentation process converts the complex lactose sugars into simple sugars as in aged cheeses which are also easier to digest. Preventatively look for lactose content on all dairy products. People who are aware of their lactose intolerance generally stay away from milk products yet it is important to also understand that eating large amounts of refined sugar can be just as inflammatory and damaging.

Inflammation Compounds from a Deficiency of the Sucrase Enzyme

The second assault to the villi comes from the inability of the Micro-Villi to digest refined sugars like white sugar. Why? Because refined sugar is a double bonded sugar or disaccharide sugar, needing to be reduced through digestion [31].

When the consumption of refined sugar is high in ones diet even for people already avoiding milk the lone perpetrator sugar will cause plenty of inflammation on its own. Proper amounts of the enzyme *sucrase* must be manufactured in the small intestine micro-villi to accomplish the digestive task of complex sugars. The challenge just like lactase is that the enzyme sucrase is often in short supply. When the two part sugar cannot be broken apart to form glucose and fructose the result is increased inflammation at the micro-villi site. I must admit I was shocked to learn that refined sugar was a culprit in bowel disease.

I was aware of how refined sugar caused major B-Complex deficiencies in the body along with unhealthy weight gain, low blood sugar and glycemic reaction with diabetics. As I honed in on bowel disease the research made it vividly clear. Refined sugar was just as damaging as gluten from grains is to the body if not worse because it is so addictive.

Recent research has also connected refined sugar to the dangerous oxidation cycle leading to premature aging of the body called Glycation. The *Longevity Solution: Breaking the Glycation Connection* by Frederic J. Vagnini, M.D. 2010, explains this new health concern of refined sugar in addition to the damage it creates to the villi.

Refined sugar consumption in our populations has increased at a gigantic rate! One hundred years ago refined sugar was found in the diet only in small amounts with an individual consuming about 4 pounds of sugar per year. Today an adult may consume close to 300 pounds per year. Children are receiving an abusive amount at times starting sugar in infancy! Many formulas given to babies over the years and even today contain a significant level of refined sugars and the most widely chosen formula is still from cow's milk so they receive a double punch of disaccharides to attempt to digest! Some parents pervertably pour soda pop right into their baby's bottle! That is such an outrageous act of abuse yet a good example of how our young may become addicted to sugar even before they can walk or talk. Researchers have shown that the increased consumption of sugar by individuals worldwide is proportional to the increase in bowel disease.

Villi in the Small Intestines Supposedly Produce Maltase and Iso-Maltase Enzymes

According to the World Health Organization the WHO developed countries like the US, UK, Canada, Germany and others rely on complex carbohydrate foods for over 50% of their nutritional support. Developing countries are still relying on these valuable food sources for up to 75% or more of their food supply. Because the complex carbohydrates from grains, beans, corn, potatoes and dairy products play such an important role in survival it is important to underline how the digestion of these valuable starch foods can be optimized. The micro-villi must be able to produce adequate levels of not only lactase and sucrase but also the integral maltase and iso-maltase to finish the complex carbohydrate digestion job!

If *amylase* flows properly into the mouth through chewing well and the pancreas assists with digestive help with more amylase flowing into the small intestine then the amount of *maltase* and *iso-maltase* secreted by the *micro-villi* can digest all the starches more appropriately [32]. When digestion is working fairly well the body can digest the complex carbohydrate polysaccharide starch.

The complex carbohydrate polysaccharides as in the gluten containing whole grains called *amylopectins* can still be harder to break down because it takes more protein digestion along with increased starch digestion to reduce the gluten compound molecular structure. It requires more of all digestive enzymes including the HCL flowing well into the stomach even before reaching the small intestine digestive stage. All of the digestive enzymes from the mouth to the intestines are required to optimize digestion of whole grains. Optimizing the digestive process through following the GIS Program makes a big improvement on one's digestion.

Even still for some people that have inherited weaker genetics they must take further steps to avoid or ferment certain foods to feel their best. If individuals continue to eat the gluten containing grains even when their body is not digesting the starch in the small intestine the micro-villi will receive further damage. The damaged villi will escalate the mal-absorption of nutrients and cause bowel fermentation in the intestines of undigested food causing even more advanced symptoms. Research has been very supportive for individuals to take the steps of reducing inflammation in the small intestines which allows them to optimize digestion and regain health again.

Science Supports the GIS I Theory

Several Scandinavian studies written by Dr. O.D. Kowlessar and published in *Acta Pediatrica* Scandinavia in the 1960's and 1970 linked wheat intolerance to poor digestion of milk. Further more, Finnish medical researchers found that problems with gluten in children were connected with assimilating sugar. D.C. Heiner wrote in the *Journal of Pediatrics* during this same time period, problems with wheat, milk and sugar seem to appear fairly often all together. A couple of other interesting studies conducted in Canada and Belgium confirmed that sugar intolerance found with Diabetics was associated with a higher incidence of wheat intolerance.

Dr. Bernard Jensen, PHD, O.D., stated he often saw the association of digestive ailments coming from the over-indulgence of sugar, milk and wheat products working with thousands of patients that came seeking health at his health ranch in California. Dr. Jensen wrote in his book *SURVIVE this day*, "Excessive consumption of processed foods often leads to intolerance of many foods."

Crowning Research Confirms Gluten's Role in Escalating GIS!

As explained in Chapter 1 gluten is a protein-carbohydrate molecule found abundantly in whole grains with wheat containing the highest percentage. Researchers conducted an excellent experiment that revealed the digestive deficiency that takes place with wheat intolerance.

The researchers first confirmed that upon eating wheat the Celiac patients in the study experienced the common reaction including; gas, bloating, diarrhea and or constipation. The second part of the study was remarkable! The researchers separated the gluten molecule into two separate portions; one consisting of protein and the second portion the carbohydrate. The subjects consumed the food at the same time and if you read Chapter 1 you already know what happened? They consumed both portions separated from one another and remarkably by eating the same food yet separated and even at the same time – no significant inflammatory reaction occurred! This obviously confirms that the main problem with wheat is the lack of digestive ability of the body to cleave or reduce, meaning to break apart the protein-carbohydrate molecule during digestion!

Join the Health Resolution: Improve Digestion by Reducing the Catalyst of Inflammation from All Sources

Milk, refined sugar and high gluten complex carbohydrates must be reduced or avoided completely to regain optimum health in the first phase of the GIS Diet. Chapter 4 goes on to review the secondary factors in the larger inflammatory cycle of GIS. Each factor warrants consideration as you rebuild your body back to total health balance.

How to Reduce the Catalyst of Inflammation?

- Stop Drinking Cow's Milk & Replace with Greens, Sesame Butter, Yogurt and other food sources and supplements.
- Stop Refined Sugar & Replace with Honey, Xylitol, Stevia and other simple sugar sources.
- Stop Grains for 6 weeks & Replace with Red Potato, Yams and Low Gluten Grains as tolerated on the GIS Diet reviewed in Chapter 7.

Today I suggest that you stop drinking cow's milk to lower inflammation or at least greatly reduce it. Review Chapter 7 to find suggestions of other healthy alternatives to cow's milk for children and adults. As you go through this process of health transformation remember that the body doesn't care where you get your protein and minerals from but it must have them. Once you supply the nutrients your body requires the cravings for the milk go away. Personally I like the taste of milk yet I rarely have an actual craving for it. Remember milk was designed for babies not adults!

Refined sugar is the next hurdle because this condiment can be considered a keg of dynamite with a slow burning fuse for all people. Entire books have been written on the disastrous effects of refined sugar to ones health. A classic book addressing the sugar addiction is called appropriately, *Sugar Blues*. Another more recent book is even more direct called, *Suicide by Sugar*, written by Nancy Appleton, PhD. Allow your family and yourself to get healthy again by taking the sugar challenge for a 6 week trial and then continue as you see it possible reserving the eating of sugar for only special occasions.

Chapter 7 will give you some healthy alternatives for recipes like using honey or other natural sweeteners. Please understand you can eat a small amount of refined sugar in the future yet most people are very addicted and need to go off of it entirely for a while to break the addiction. Chapter 6 reviews Addictions and gives some very helpful guidelines. It may become possible to indulge in the future for example, if you choose to celebrate a birthday or a special occasion. I find the longer I am off sugar and keep seasonal fruits and alternative healthy desserts around I don't feel deprived. I love the health side effects of staying low on sugar like dropping another pants size and my skin has never looked more youthful!

Suggestions for replacing the gluten grains and starches can also be reviewed in Chapter 7. The more bowel symptoms and illness a person is living with tells you where to begin Diet Zone 1, 2 or 3. All people feel better when they stop the regular whole grains for 6 weeks and stick to the simpler carbohydrates that are listed. After the first 40 days addictions and habits are easier to replace and leave alone. See the Healthy Focus Factors section in Chapter 6 for more great support.

Fast Fixes are Limited for GIS

Some people attempt a Fast Fix of just adding a digestive enzyme during their meals to alleviate inflammation. Getting healthier or being preventative to disease takes more than a bottle of enzymes. Review Chapter 8 GIS Supplements. Other people suggest that you only need to find a replacement for wheat in your diet to alleviate your colon troubles. Wheat is definitely a challenge in GIS however over time and experience has also shown that eliminating wheat will only give partial relief and it is not the hoped for Fast Fix. Reaching optimum health requires the entire

GIS health program including supplements, diet and creating a healthier lifestyle – one day at a time - and people are doing it all over the world.

I suggest that you stop the sources of inflammation first. Adding more nutritious food choices you will begin to balance and rebuild your body. Next add the foundational core nutrients and special needs supplements reviewed at the ends of each chapter (the best you can) which are elaborated in Chapter 8. If you already take supplements simplify your program and make certain you are including the highlighted products. A short cut for supporting health is the addition of foods that contain the Vitamin B-Complex, with an added supplement of B-Complex and B12 that speeds the renewal process in the body. The dictionary definition of vitamin means to support life! It is a substance that the body cannot make and therefore must be supplied either from a food or food supplement. Research abounds with why and how B-Complex works for health!

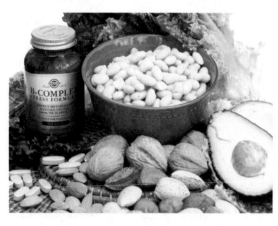

HIGHLIGHT 3: *B-Complex Is Essential for Healthy Digestion & So Much More!*

B-Complex is not only essential to digestion but to life itself for children and adults! Research confirms it to be an integral catalyst to all metabolic processes besides the digestive system, necessary for the repair of tissue and it works behind the scenes to lower all inflammation in the body. Many other nutritional co-factors work together with B-Complex to support the body's health and it just may be one of the core nutrients human beings as a whole wind up most deficient in!

What is the B-Complex? The B-Complex is made up of a family of B vitamins that encompass eight isolated members including; B1 (thiamine), B2 (riboflavin), B3 (niacin), B5 (pantothenic acid), B6 (pyridoxine, phyradoxal, pyridoxamine), B12 (cobalamin), Biotin and Folic Acid (folate, folacin, pteroylglutamic). These nutrients are grouped together and called the B-Complex because of their close relationship and functions in the body.

The other three compounds that are now separated called the non-B vitamins are Choline, Inositol and Lipoic Acid. These nutrients are coenzymes that aid in our metabolism and are found with the B-Complex yet were ruled out not to be essential as with the rest of the B-Complex. The word "Essential" in the discussion of supplements means that a vitamin or nutrient is required by the body because it cannot be manufactured by the body from any other pathway. If the body does not receive the "Essential Nutrients" in large enough quantity a deficiency leading to a disease can manifest and death can follow! Some other co-enzyme nutrients that are not essential have been mistaken to be part of the B-Complex as with Para-Aminobenzoic acid (PABA), Laetrile (B17), Carnitine (BT) and the once called B15 now referred to as Pangamic acid. Bioflavonoids called Vitamin P and Ubiquinone is known as Coenzyme Q10 are two other important co-enzymes that were also thought to be in the B-Complex family at one time or another.

Deficiency of B-Complex

A deficiency of the B-Complex can develop from several factors to include; eating a poor diet as with junk foods, eating a high carbohydrate diet, GIS bowel disease, use of pharmaceutical drugs (including birth control pills and antibiotics), fungal overgrowth (Candida), pesticides (commercially grown foods and household products), high stress and an excessive consumption of alcohol, sodas or caffeine.

The B Vitamins are heat sensitive so cooking and oxidation that occurs during storage of foods will destroy a certain amount of the Vitamin B value. They are also water soluble vitamins and some potency may be lost by drinking an excess of diuretics that include once again alcohol, sodas, caffeine drinks or eating chocolate. A person experiencing lots of perspiration may also wind up dangerously low on the B-Complex as well.

B-Complex Precautionary

Research has found there to be no bad side effects from taking B-Complex. However, there are a few inconveniences you will want to be precautionary. A darker color may be observed of one's urine which is only slightly annoying if it stains clothing. Taking B3 Niacin separately or including a good source of B-Complex with Nutritional Yeast discussed in Chapter 8 or your supplements may bring upon a temporary flushing referred to as the "Niacin Flush". The flushing causes a heat sensation and reddening of the skin due to a healthy increase in circulation. If you are not aware of this vasodilatation effect it may be a little scary. Just drink some water and stay out of the direct sun for a few minutes and any excess flushing of the skin will pass.

Most people who take it in a multiple supplement or even a separate tablet of the B-Complex find it to be very well tolerated. Yet potency of the B-Complex as it is available in 50 – 100 milligrams may be a concern for some people. Occasionally the metabolic pathway for processing the B-Complex is not working properly in the body. In a small percentage of people they experience nausea if taken in larger amounts more than 10 milligrams (mg.) at one time. The nutritional yeast or low potency supplements appear to be very well tolerated by all people.

It is important to understand that each B vitamin performs special unique duties within the body. Research suggests however that it is important to always supplement with the B-Complex altogether better than taking any single B vitamin alone. The exception to this rule is B-12 because it is much more challenging to absorb. Sources of B12 include; animal products of eggs, meat and dairy products. B-12 may also be found in small amounts in fermented soy products like soy sauce and miso paste. Keep in mind that bowel disease increases mal-absorption of many nutrients. B12 has been found to be significantly deficient in most people suffering with IBS and IBD and is elaborated on in Chapter 5.

What does B-Complex do in the body? B-Complex is responsible for all the metabolic systems of the body to achieve both mental and physical health. I call it the "Happy Vitamin" and it is also essential for energy. Energy production takes place in the body only when carbohydrates, proteins and fats are digested, absorbed and metabolized efficiently into each cell. The B-Complex plays an important role in this metabolic process of each food group.

As we discussed previously in this chapter the B-Complex aids in the manufacturing of digestive enzymes and other digestive juices like hydrochloric acid HCL. The B's are also referred to as co-enzymes as they perform the precursor catalyst job for hundreds of enzymes needed throughout the body to carry out thousands of molecular reactions every day.

Heart Disease

Researchers have confirmed the anti-inflammatory support from B-Complex is experienced in the reduction of allergies of all types and they also lower dangerous inflammation in the vascular system called homocysteine. In fact Tuft's University conducted the first pioneering research in 1993, proving the need for B-Complex specifically Folic Acid, Vitamin B6 and B12 to reduce the development of plaque leading to cardiovascular disease (CVD) due to its help to resolve inflammation.

The inflammation that builds in the cardiovascular system due to the B-Complex deficiency can be measured with a C-reactive protein (CRP) blood test relating to high homocysteine levels. Over fifty years of research have confirmed the importance of B-Complex in relationship to heart disease. There is no mistake that a higher plaque build-up within the arteries is observed called arteriolosclerosis when deficiencies of B12, folic acid and B6 exist.

Allergies

With allergies B-Complex calms the inflammatory histamine reactions that can affect the skin and functioning of the nervous system. An allergic response or intolerance in the body brings on a heightened reaction of the immune system that often shows up on the outer skin especially on the face and neck. The internal skin of the body including the lining cells of the digestive tract and glands can all be affected with GIS and allergies both. The histamine reaction results in inflammation causing redness and swelling of the tissue that carries with it the potential for tissue damage.

Observe how many people live with this condition of red skin inflammation noticeable on the face and neck. It worsens by eating excessive carbohydrates as in junk food, gluten, alcohol and even spicy foods. Review Chapter 5 Glossary of Conditions. The red inflammation is the body screaming out for appropriate nutrition and B-Complex to lower and eventually stop the inflammation.

As critical as the B-Complex is to our topic of GIS through supporting digestive function and lowering inflammation it also is an essential support to the entire Central Nervous System. It, along with other co-enzymes, supports the nerves to function properly. I am convinced that GIS has a pivotal relationship with B-Complex and a direct connection to the neuromuscular reactions of the body. When people eat gluten and gluten triggers that require more B-Complex than a person may have in the body stores the result may be constipation, diarrhea or a reduction in motor skills.

Healthy Hormones, Strong Immunity & More

Other important support in the body for the B-Complex that deserves mention is healthy hormones, youthful hair, skin and nails. Having a healthy pregnancy and building a healthy baby, restless leg syndrome and even a strong immune system all require folic acid and the rest of the B-Complex. The B-Complex is so important to prevent disease in the body that *PubMed,* which is respected for posting solid research on health, has printed over 111,000 research papers revealing the integral relationship of B-Complex to mental and physical well-being.

As important as B-Complex is in the body it just may be the widest spread nutritional deficiency in the world today! Pharmaceutical giants would like us to think disease and colon health is all about the body's natural aging process. Why else would they keep encouraging people to seek the use of cholesterol lowering statin drugs for CVD and the hundreds of other medications developed each year, even though many disease symptoms are in fact nutritional deficiencies already proven by scientists?

What are the sources of B-Complex? Green leafy vegetables (raw salads, green juices, green supplements), raw nuts & seeds (fresh), nutritional yeast, B-Complex supplements, beans, grains, dairy products, eggs, meats, vegetables and fruits (bananas). The easiest source to be assured of the absorption of B12 is in a shot form. Liquid or in a tablet absorbed under the tongue would be the next best way to give yourself B12 insurance. Small amounts of the B-Complex are manufactured in the small intestine by the friendly bacteria called Probiotics if it colonizes well as discussed at the end of Chapter 2.

Eating a varied diet with many different foods containing B-Complex and including a B-Complex supplement will guarantee you a healthy supply. You can have a blood test for B12 conducted however this is a very limited test procedure. Often B12 will test sufficient in the normal blood supply and reveal a deficiency in the plasma of the blood. Following the GIS program to reduce all the factors of inflammation in our lives will allow the body to improve B12 and B-Complex absorption into the body. It is best to not waste time if you have experienced any of the symptoms for a lengthy amount of time because permanent nerve damage can occur from B12 deficiency. Aloe Vera is an important partner in supporting the digestive process to improve the deficiency quicker than left on its own power and it will be introduced in Chapter 4. Be happier and healthier with getting the digestive system and all the systems in the body working better with B-Complex and B12 daily!

C H A P T E R   4

The Bigger Picture of GIS

*"No, I never ask my patients about their bowel habits or their
digestive system. Why would I ask them unless I was giving them a
medication that I knew for certain might constipate them?"*

*— GP Medical Doctor
Kaiser Permanente Hospital Group*

The Greek Physician Hippocrates, 430 BC, was a wise man with a talent
for communicating to the people of his day about health and science. By
rejecting superstition in favor of scientific observation, classifying diseases

and by creating a set of moral
and professional standards for
physicians, he earned the famous
title, "Father of Medicine".
Hippocrates is also credited for
giving the world the Hippo cratic
Oath even though he may not
have been the author. Physicians
throughout the ages have taken
this oath upon graduating
medical school before beginning
the practice of medicine yet some

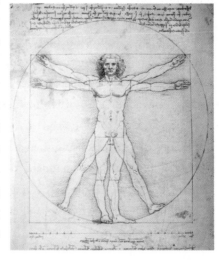

modern schools have dropped this tradition. I think it would be very wise for schools to reinstate the oath because of its important humanitarian doctrine!

Highlights of the Hippocratic Oath, taken from the archives of the National Library of Medicine in Washington, 2002, states [1];

- A physician promises to treat all people equally without corruption or malice.

- Physicians promise to use dietary regimens which will benefit the patient, according to their greatest ability and judgment and do no harm or injustice.

Fortunately for society's best interest the science that drives medicine of today has evolved from ancient times to include a better understanding of the physiology of the human body and the disease process. Bloodletting is a good example of a common medical practice that was performed by doctors from antiquity up until the late 19th century. It was performed on patients with an array of conditions especially for the treatment of hypertension. Even though it sometimes showed a beneficial effect to temporarily lower blood pressure it was at last realized due to the sheer reduction in the volume of blood. In most cases the historical use of bloodletting, practiced for almost 2,000 years, was found to be quite harmful to the patient [2].

The lack of nutritional emphasis in our modern medical system of today originates from both the medical school's limited curriculum and the guidelines communicated to doctors from the American Medical Association (AMA). Although their membership has declined over the years to only about 22% of US physicians and medical students [3] their governing arm is strong. In 1981 they catalyzed the Principles of Medical Ethics directive for practicing medical doctors. It was geared primarily to psychologists updating the standard for behavior in the office setting which was needed. However, the new stringent rules morphed health care into an even more pointed drug focus discouraging doctors from talking about nutrition through panel reviews [4]. Even though there has been some movement into *preventative* and *integrative health care* most professionals are still largely focused on *crisis management of disease* and not relying heavily on *dietary regimens* to prevent illness as in the days of Hippocrates.

The use of pharmaceutical drugs have become like a religion for the modern physician often leaving science and research out of the equation. To even mention to some physicians that the body requires nutrition to reverse disease or toxins like mercury or fluoride might be dangerous and create metabolic irregularity is like blasphemy to many and laughable by others. In my experience of working in medical clinics for almost two decades, a medical doctor rarely talks of dietary regimens, or in other words foods that heal the patient, as mentioned in the Hippocratic Oath. The second insult to the patient is the dietitian who works as an arm of the AMA. They seldom associate the true therapeutic nature of foods and food supplements to the patient for the same restraints experienced by the physicians of today that includes both ignorance and fear.

Modern Medicine has Two Foundational Flaws:

- First, physicians and dietitians of today are very ignorant to certain aspects of health like the body's ability to heal itself. Many doctors flat out don't believe the body can reverse disease. Thousands of scientific studies give credence to this charge that the body can rebuild itself from disease if it is given the nutritional opportunity.

- Secondly, the fear factor is present in the doctor's office. I have come to understand from working with medical doctors and interviewing several of them that they feel intimidated to treat their patients naturally and holistically with food and supplements with the looming risk of a lawsuit or losing their license to practice at all.

The AMA outlines very strict guidelines as to what they will and will not tolerate by the practicing physician or health professional. Health as a modality has all but disappeared from most doctor offices. One might receive a script to talk with a dietitian or take a class on dietary control of their blood sugar yet mainstream health professionals knowledge about the human body is very limited [5]. Further pressures come from the insurance company's acceptance of a doctor's decision for treatment as to what they will reimburse.

A US law that was enacted in 1938 makes any herb or supplement a drug if it is found to reverse a disease state [6]. This ridiculous law prevents most people from endorsing the use of herbs or supplements in a professional setting for fear of litigation. Both the AMA and the US government have together kept the knowledge of foods and supplements from being fully disseminated throughout medical schools and also to the citizens. You ask yourself why would professionals and our government that we are to put our trust in be so deceitful to withhold the truth from us. The answer lies in control of the masses and ultimately in the greed of big business.

Therefore, as you embark on your health journey you must hold fast to the health truth you discover for yourself. As you build a belief in your body's ability to heal you will feel greatly empowered to teach others yet don't hold your breath for your doctors or your senators blessing!

Building a Belief in Your Body's Ability to Heal:

- *Take responsibility for your own health.* Consider your physician's suggestions yet get a second opinion on adding pharmaceutical drug treatment and any surgical procedures or lack of treatment.
- *Stop thinking your medical doctor knows more about health than you do.* Physicians are not taught about therapeutic nutrition in medical school. My suggestion is to work as closely as you wish with the medical community blending what is best for you and your family.
- *Get your yearly checkups as you regain your health.* Our hospitals, doctors and other medical personnel are ultimately paid to work on the patient's behalf yet many have limited knowledge about health and the side effects of pharmaceutical drugs and treatments. One thing you can count on is if you are impatient about the state of your health at any given point most doctors will oblige you with

writing a prescription for a pharmaceutical drug. The average 60 year old takes 6 or more medications!

- *Take action in your own life applying health at least 80% of the time.* You will begin to understand the far reaching capabilities the body has in its design to work by lowering inflammation, increasing circulation and regeneration. This will ultimately translate into less disease of every type.

- *Always research any pharmaceutical drug before taking it.* The goal is to stop any prescription you may be taking that you do not absolutely need after reviewing the pros and cons. This may take place over a few months or even years of research and soliciting a second opinion from another licensed doctor yet take action today!

GIS II Theory: Inflammation Begets Greater Inflammation

All sources of inflammation can ignite one another to create a greater inflammation response experienced throughout the entire body. This is not a far-fetched statement considering researchers have been making a connection for many years of colon Cancer, Alzheimer's disease, Heart Disease and even Polyps growing in the intestines to out-of-control inflammation. Dr. Robert Tepper, president of research and development of a major pharmaceutical company in Cambridge, Mass, stated, "Virtually our entire R & D effort is [now] focused on inflammation and cancer". Cardiologists, Rheumatologists, Oncologists, Allergists and Neurologists are all talking about the inflammation connection to disease in the body. Many factors in our lives can increase the overall inflammation experienced throughout the body including the eating of bread in the intestinal tract [7].

Chapter 3 reviewed the primary core dietary factors that begin the Gluten Inflammatory Syndrome (GIS) inflammation; cow's milk, refined sugar and grains. Chapter 4 further expands the other secondary factors that come to play in heightening the potential pain and tissue damage to one's body from increasing inflammation [8]. The significant contribution of each factor to the GIS cycle in the body is summed up in the second GIS theory that all inflammation effects total inflammation. Chapter 6 in the Healthy Focus Factors section elaborates on each of the secondary inflammatory sources and how to choose alternatives or remedy the situations in your life.

Tina's Story

A good example of the GIS II Theory in action takes place with a woman I worked with for years named Tina. As she strayed from her GIS diet and ate spicy foods, gluten laden pretzels or crackers, processed vegetable dip and indulged in sugary latte coffees containing milk solids her GIS symptoms sky rocketed.

First her bowels would begin to slow up bringing on painful gas alternating with bouts of diarrhea. Heartburn would develop at times along with anxious and hyper behavior giving way to depressive moments edging into panic attacks. After a few days of eating trigger foods bingo a cold sore (Herpes Simplex Virus), showed up on her lip!

I have witnessed this GIS scenario with countless other people besides Tina. Researchers have confirmed this parallel in Celiac Disease patients as well. As they got off gluten they found wonderful relief from Herpes Simplex [9]. Please be warned that if you attempt to caution a person caught in the middle of an inflammation cycle the response you receive can come with mixed emotions. When a neurosis of an individual is triggered in GIS it can be counter productive to talk about the cause during the episode. I have found it is better to wait and discuss options once the health crisis has passed. Chapter 5 elaborates the explanation of the Body-Brain GIS relationship.

An Essential Fatty Acid Imbalance Can Trigger Inflammation

Inflammatory factors affect one's health both mentally and physically. Some of the GIS triggers that bring on reactions to the body are silent such as with the Essential Fatty Acid (EFA) imbalance.

Science has confirmed that the high ratio of the Omega-6 Fatty Acids to the Omega-3's, encourage acute inflammation to develop on varying levels [10]. This is the case in children and adults eating high amounts of vegetable oils abundant in fried and processed foods. Trans-fats also present in processed foods are double damaging because they are often sourced from vegetable oils high in Omega 6's and have also been processed with hydrogen that adds to the difficulty to digest the fats causing even more cellular damage from the free radicals that they create.

In 2009, medical experts together with the Center of Disease Control (CDC) studying the Omega 3 deficiency and Trans-Fat excesses in the American diet felt they were responsible for close to 200,000 yearly deaths! Dr. Hector Lopez, M.D., a specialist in Orthopedic Medicine and Pain Management offices in New Jersey, recently stated he has tested many patients blood work that contained a 17:1 ratio and has even observed higher ratios of Omega 6 to Omega 3's! This illustrates an absolute diet disaster that brings with it more inflammation of the joints, digestion and sets the stage for many diseases.

The solution is to increase foods containing the Omega 3's and add supplements of fish oil and or flax oil to achieve equal or higher levels to the Omega 6's. By experimenting with more Omega 3's you will reap the benefit of lowering inflammation considerably. In over 6,000 research papers the Omega 3 Fatty Acids confirm their value that includes reducing diarrhea frequency and countless other inflammatory conditions as with Asthma, Arthritis, CVD, Depression and unnecessary pain in the body. Many poor health conditions that people experience in life can be attributed to a lack or an imbalance of the Essential Fatty Acids of Omega 3 and 6.

Spicy Foods Increase Inflammation

Keep in mind that as similar as people's bodies are we still have our own individual differences with GIS factors. A good example of this is how food seasonings affect people differently. Hot spices can increase circulation in the body which has healing attributes. Yet for some people living with advanced GIS and perhaps having a congested liver, eating spicy foods can greatly heighten their inflammation response and must be avoided. You can observe this reaction in people living with Rosacea [11]. After eating a meal of spicy and hot foods the face may become very flushed and reddened causing discomfort and even pain to follow. Other triggers include alcohol, sunlight and strenuous activity each increasing the inflammation response on the skin. Review Chapter 5 for Rosacea health guidelines.

All skin conditions respond very favorably to the GIS program. You too may find that it is not always in your best health interest to eat "mucho caliente" hot sauce every night. An easy alternative in a family setting is to reduce the amount of hot spices when preparing a pot of chili or other foods for a group. Each person can then add their own degree of heat and seasoning at the table. I always appreciate this courtesy especially when dining out.

pH a Factor in Inflammation

Tomato and tomato dishes are another common GIS factor that involves pH. Sometimes even eating a small amount of tomato may bring about achy joints and stomach distress. Reducing tomato products also include your favorite hot sauce. Hot sauce is generally made from tomatoes and is an especially important trigger to avoid with the symptoms of Reflux. Review Reflux in Chapter 5. The tomato pH is similar to that of citrus fruits. Each food choice in our diet affects the Acid-Alkaline pH Balance of the body. You can learn more about adjusting pH in the Healthy Focus Factors. Using less of an acidic food or finding an alternative to tomato in your recipes, like using red bell pepper, can significantly reduce inflammation. Red bell peppers can be purchased fresh or bottled, adding red color, taste and are generally better tolerated by most people and add to the alkalinity of the body reducing inflammation.

All Major Secondary Inflammation Factors Increase GIS Symptoms:

- *Alcohol* – Grains (gluten) are used in beer and some liquor production. Alternatives are available in Chapter 7.
- *Capsules and Gelatin Soft Gels* – Made from compounds similar to gluten molecule, very inflammatory and must be avoided.
- *Central Nervous System (CNS)* – An interlaced relationship exists

with nutrition (Omega 6/3 for example), toxins and inflammation response in the body.

- *Colon Health* - Bacterial homeostasis, Candida yeasts, Parasites, Zonulin (protein from wheat) and Leaky Gut (improper absorption of matter into the tissues and blood stream) all may result in a type of infection immune response and more.

- *Dietary Imbalances* - PH acidity, hot spices, tomato products, fats and oils, sugars, molds and chemical sensitivity.

- *Environmental Toxins* – Decrease metabolism efficiency due to multi-factorial issues i.e. mercury which is the second leading nerve cell toxin to the body.

- *Genetic Weakness* – This represents only a 10% influence with environmental factors being a much greater determinate with every type of disease.

- *Mucus Production* – High amounts of mucus in the GI tract is generated from an overactive immune system and cause reduced absorption and increased congestion.

- *Processed Foods* – Manufacturers are bombarding consumers with high gluten flour and gluten triggers in all breadstuffs, soups, dressings, beverages and seasonings.

- *Stress Levels* – Prolonged stress demands high nutritional values such as zinc, B-Complex and Vitamin C plus minerals which if undersupplied increases GIS inflammation.

- *Viral Flare-Ups* – Many viruses exist in our environment and live within our body. Herpes Simplex Virus is common with most adults and many children and is a significant trigger to the GIS.

GIS Daily Goal: Reduce as many Inflammatory Factors as Possible

Food stimulus or triggers that cause symptoms of bowel disease come from many different sources. By simultaneously including more therapeutic nutrition and nutritional supplements, as outlined in Chapters 6 and 7, symptoms will calm down. Once you are aware of the irritants you will want to strive to eat as few triggers in the daily diet as possible to allow the body to heal and feel good.

It may seem like a big understatement when I say it isn't always easy to follow the GIS program. At times you may find yourself hungry and in a situation with few choices to eat. Make the best choice in any given

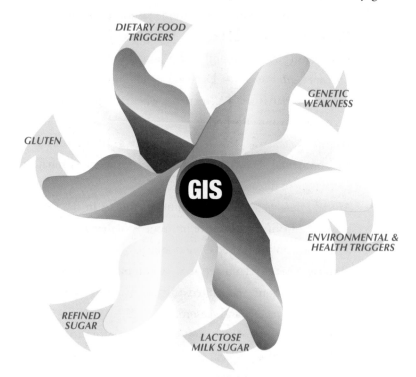

Lactose Sugar Disaccharides
- Milk & milk solids
- Soft cheeses
- Food additives

Refined Sugar Disaccharides
- Cane, beet & malt sugar
- High fructose corn syrup (HFCS)
- Candy, sodas & confections
- Cooking & food additives

Gluten Polysaccharides
- Starch complex – Glutenins & Gliadins
- Whole grains, beverages & food products
- Processed food additives

Dietary Food Triggers
- Gelatin capsules & soft gels
- Hot spices & high arginine foods
- Imbalance of omega 6 & 3 fatty acids
- Molds & other allergies
- Malnutrition

Genetic Weakness
- Human condition (not designed for digesting gluten)
- Poor glandular & digestive health

Environmental & Health Triggers
- Toxic chemicals & pesticides
- High stress levels & pH levels
- Accidents & surgery
- Pharmaceutical drugs
- Viral, bacterial & fungal (yeast) infections
- Colon health status

situation and keep in mind certain supplements will help reduce reactions especially ingesting Aloe Vera with its anti-inflammatory support and help with optimizing digestion. Just knowing you have some natural remedies that can give some forgiveness to your body in a challenging situation may help your mental attitude about getting healthier with gluten intolerance. Let's review some important highlights applying to reactions and symptoms.

GIS Symptom Highlights:

- Symptoms come from an accumulation or quantity of trigger insults which increase inflammation to the intestinal lining and are felt throughout the body.
- Eating less of a trigger is better than eating a large quantity. Become a good label reader to avoid triggers.
- Carry food with you or plan ahead; at work, home and play of non-irritating food choices. Eat foods in their most natural state and avoid irritants found in processed foods.
- Even nutritious foods may be a trigger causing symptoms so customize your GIS program to your own personal needs.
- As the body heals and becomes healthier we experience fewer symptoms with GIS triggers which can allow more flexibility in the diet and lifestyle choices.

Knowing about gluten and GIS triggers is powerful! This knowledge gives you the ability to choose to feel good. The opposite is also true that if you eat the trigger foods you will know why you are not feeling your best. It is all about making the best choices.

Getting into the control seat is exhilarating, a little scary and maddening at times yet freeing. The more advanced your bowel disease is upon starting the GIS program will determine how strict you will want to strive for in the first weeks and months.

With the most sensitive stage of GIS, Zone 3, many people still react to molds on foods along with the gluten and other triggers in the foodstuff. It can literally seem, as if there is nothing you can eat or drink that doesn't cause you GIS symptoms. As you take each day prioritizing your food choices and shopping with a list, you can change for the better. This new healthier life will begin to be easier and easier and you will get the pay off of thinking and feeling better and better. Here are a few of the stumbling blocks that most people face in getting started.

Reduce the Trigger Foods

It is so easy to overeat in trigger foods especially if you are in a party situation or still living with a sugar addiction. If you eat one cookie with regular or whole wheat pastry flour you may not notice any extra stomach bloating or gas. However if you eat 2 or 3 cookies you could be in the bathroom and even need to leave the party and go home because you begin to feel so poorly. Understand that quantity of a trigger food makes a difference and eating foods you thought were good for you can cause a stomachache.

Beware of Natural Molds on Foods

Some healthy food options may still cause painful reactions at times. To be healthy we want to include vegetables in our diets. Vegetables contain lots of good nutritional value however broccoli contains natural molds. If you are very sensitive at first you may experience unwanted symptoms due to molds on cruciferous vegetables and more.

Nutritious Foods Can Be GIS Triggers

Trigger foods that are often included at breakfast include cereals and are promoted as the healthy choice. Raisin bran cereal for instance or the traditional oatmeal both taste yummy yet you will continue having trouble with gas, bloating and more IBS symptoms if you do not choose an alternative GIS choice. A food can be nutritious yet be a horrible trigger food for you.

Find Healthy Replacements for Old Food Rewards

Old food rewards can be transferred to foods that will not cause pain and damage to the body. An example of this would be switching to red potatoes instead of your standby Russet potato. Fruits in season and aged cheeses are good quick treats for young and old alike or peanut butter and bananas. Some snacks are more challenging to replace yet eating regular meals can keep everyone out of heavy snack cravings!

I suggest that you also come up with some good non-food rewards to help in letting go of favorite snack foods that don't have direct replacements. Experimenting with non-food rewards to take the place of a candy bar, favorite dessert or beverage is important when dealing with addictions. I enjoy time out in nature for a walk or time in the garden. Reading a good book or magazine, enjoying a hobby, calling a friend, shopping, cooking, sailing or even taking a bubble bath just to name a few suggestions you can experiment with. People need hobbies to give life more enjoyment and it can take the focus off of eating for a pastime!

Addictions can cause us to stumble as we begin a healthier life. Because this is a very important topic in getting healthier the subject is further covered in Chapter 6. Food Addictions, take time to tackle successfully and require new disciplines to reprogram the body. Setting new health disciplines take approximately 30-45 days for your first goal. You also have the option of adding a support group, counseling when possible or reading positive books on the subject to bring success.

Steps that truly help during your GIS transition:
1. Eat regular nutritious meals.
2. Keep all inflammation down in the body as outlined in the GIS program.
3. Don't give up along your path!

To begin your GIS Program incorporate the knowledge you learn in Chapter 6 while starting the dietary program in Chapter 7. Keeping a Food Diary for 6 weeks and making notes as to how you feel each day tracking your progress and it will help motivate your efforts. Make a note when you experience fewer GIS symptoms. If any trigger causes reactions write it down and do your best to reduce or avoid them for now. Most if not all health challenges are only temporary and in the future you can experiment reintroducing some of the dropped foods and or condiments once again.

In the first 30 days the body begins new cell regeneration building new lining cells of the intestinal tract as the inflammation simmers down. In 3 months greater regeneration takes place in the organs rebuilding larger sections of cellular tissue. Three years as you stay on the GIS Program it allows the skeletal, ligaments and joints to begin rebuilding themselves. After 7 years some researchers view the body as practically brand new with a person experiencing only normal aging.

Each individual has special circumstances that relate to their own eating experience. I encourage you to be as strict as possible at the beginning so you can speed your recovery. When you need some encouragement just read the testimonies of others who have walked in your footsteps in Chapter 11 and throughout the chapters. Health is truly our greatest wealth. As Norman Cousins stated, "Health isn't everything yet without it we have nothing."

Testing for Gluten Sensitivity Has Limitations

Most of the people I have interviewed over the years with their list of health complaints, including some digestive issues, have tested negative to the blood test for gluten. Keep in mind that most doctors are not testing for gluten intolerance and at least some doctors are thinking along the correct lines. The fortunate clients that dared to apply the GIS program regardless of the blood test results understood within just a couple of weeks that the blood test truly does give false negatives. By applying the GIS program they felt considerably better and better!

Stool, Blood, Urine, Tissue Biopsy and Symptomology Tracking

Most of the following tests for gluten sensitivity come with limitations for the individual being tested. False negatives and false positive results definitely occur [12]. I am certain that for you who have been living with the frustration that surrounds bowel disease hearing this is the last thing you were hoping for. So often when I introduce the GIS program to a person to help them understand their symptoms of bowel distress they immediately think of getting tested to confirm the gluten symptoms. As a clinician I relish patients getting diagnostic testing yet unfortunately in regards to colon health and gluten intolerance the results are often not accurate!

People will seek out a physician to order the testing yet the doctor generally does not review the limitations most likely because they don't understand the facts themselves. Nine out of ten times my client calls me back stating profoundly that they do not have gluten intolerance. Ah-huh! Then I must go through the laborious process of informing them the testing methods are out-dated and often inaccurate. I recently read a testimony from a woman who diagnosed herself in 2009. Her name is Destiny and she reminded me of so many clients I have worked with over the years.

Destiny's Story

Destiny spent the first half of her life in and out of doctor's offices. She elaborated that if the doctors would have had their way with her by now she would have undergone neck surgery, still be using three inhalers for Asthma, be vomiting daily and also having her frequent panic attacks! In only one year of getting off gluten she stated that all of her previous health challenges resolved. Her doctors then suggested to her that she now confirm her past challenge of gluten intolerance with the old fashioned testing through the blood looking for inflammatory markers. She knew from her own study on gluten that by getting off the gluten foods already that the testing would have only revealed marginal inflammation if any.

Why is a blood test for gluten often negative?

The challenge of getting a positive test result for gluten through a blood test is that a person must eat as much gluten food as possible for a length of time, perhaps weeks or even months before having the test performed. Then, if the body is truly not digesting the gluten properly as with gluten intolerance, an inflammatory response may then show up in the blood. I use the word "may" because there are more challenges to the accuracy of the test.

The problem lies in that most people are either not making the blood markers in their body (that the laboratory tests are measuring for) or they are not achieving a high enough inflammatory response to show positive at the time the blood test is drawn. Blood tests certainly do not register accurately to whether a person is sensitive to gluten or not as with IBS [13].

If a person is highly sensitive to gluten a tissue biopsy preformed on the villi might possibly show damage after months and years of eating the gluten trigger foods [14]. Judging from Destiny's experience she did not want to put herself back into a disease state just to receive a positive on a blood test nor has anyone else I have worked with over the years!

Some options for testing give more accurate information than others. It is valuable to understand that many of the blood work tests performed are flawed and have potential inaccuracies. The following list will indicate all of the tests available for testing inflammation and or other markers to confirm allergy and bowel disease.

To date, stool testing appears to be the most accurate method and is gaining in popularity. It shouldn't come as too much of a surprise to learn that the medical community has held onto the outdated blood tests to confirm gluten reactions for now - even with the more reliable stool testing available. Individuals can legally have stool testing performed without a prescription from a physician because it is a non-invasive procedure. All blood work must have a prescription written by a physician or other legal medical practitioner.

The main objective in testing, whether through blood or stool is to test for the intensity of inflammation through "protein markers". If the markers confirm a positive to any of the tests then it shows an absolute reaction(s) to food or food products. Receiving a negative to gluten blood testing seems to be a very common inaccurate result.

What are the Blood Tests Limitations?

- The body does not always make the needed markers that the lab test is looking for in order to measure for the gluten response. Malnutrition and poor functioning glands do not always manufacture the required specialized compound proteins needed to build the immune response markers.

- When a test shows positive for gluten immune response it is considered accurate 99% of the time. However, researchers often find that the blood tests come back with a FALSE negative when in fact a person is actually gluten sensitive due to obvious symptoms of bowel disease.

- Doctors rely on a biopsy to confirm advanced bowel disease looking for possible blunting of the small intestine villi yet this does not rule out a lesser gluten intolerance as experienced with IBS.

Stool Testing May Give the Best Results [14]:

- The stool tests may be the most sensitive therefore more accurate than a blood test. The premise is that the inflammation is coming from the intestinal tract therefore the stool will pick up markers first before they are seen in the blood.

- It is very easy to get a stool sample for testing and an individual does not need to have eaten gluten foods in any quantity for more reliable results.

- A physician prescription is not required for stool testing. The reference section will give you contact information to order your own testing and also review the research summary online.

Tips on Test Methods:

- Symptomology tracking your symptoms and progress is best done through keeping a Symptoms Diary of cause and effects coming from foods, drugs, supplements and other factors. Specimen testing is not always 100% yet symptoms do not lie.

Tracking your own health results will always give you the most effective path to follow as you reduce inflammation damage and become healthier.

• Stool Testing [15] has an excellent success rate and is the easiest to have performed for children and adults. An experienced lab will conduct comprehensive tests to check for many food triggers as desired all at one time that includes; multiple food allergens and gluten which together may all be causing advanced inflammation.

• All five Blood Tests can be conducted at the same laboratory with the same blood draw. This may include the foolproof IgG and Total Serum IgA to measure if the individual makes the needed antibodies for several of the blood tests.

• Malnutrition is so common with bowel disease that to test for Anemia plus a complete SMAC Blood Test is important for children and adults with GIS symptoms. Remember B12 testing is most accurate on plasma testing.

• A Tissue Biopsy is only needed in advanced bowel symptoms. Once you get a positive lab test through stool or blood comprehensive testing, a tissue biopsy can be avoided unless health complications require more confirmation to the exact extent of tissue damage in the villi.

Gluten and Food Sensitivity Testing			
Test	**Sub Category**	**Markers**	**Concern / Priority**
Stool	Gluten	Fecal Antigliadin IgA antibody	Inflammation
Stool	Absorption	Tissue Transglutaminase	Villi Damage
Stool	Cow's Milk / Protein-Casein	Fecal IgA	Inflammation
Stool	Malabsorption	Fat Microscopy	Pancreas Under-functioning
Stool	Acute Colitis	Lactoferrin from Neutrophils	Diarrhea Unknown Origin

Stool	Gluten / Celiac's	Genetic Swab of Mouth HLA-DQ	Genetic Possibilities
Stool	Chicken Egg / Protein-Ovalbumin	Fecal IgA	Inflammation
Stool	Dietary Yeast	Saccharomyces cerevisiae – IgA	Inflammation
Stool	Dietary Soy	Fecal IgA	Inflammation
Urine	Peptide Test	Poorly digested proteins-Celiac's	Malabsorption
Urine	Sed Rate	Evaluate Degeneration	Disease
Blood	RAST-Wheat, etc	Allergen-Specific IgE Antibody	Hives, Dermatitis or Asthma
Blood	Celiac's	tTG Anti-Tissue Transglutaminase-IgA Positive	Confirms Celiac's
Blood	Celiac's	EMA Anti-endomysial Antibodies-IgA	Likelihood of Celiac's
Blood	Gluten	AGA Anti-Gliadin Antibody-IgA	Good for Children's Testing
Blood	Celiac's	AGA Anti-Gliadin Antibody-IgG	Good Gluten Foolproof
Blood	Immune Function	Total Serum IgA	Confirm IgA Manufacturing
Blood	CBC	B12, D, Protein, Folate, etc.	Anemia / Malnutrition
Blood	SMAC-25	Protein, Glucose, Minerals, etc.	Malnutrition
Blood	ESR	Erythrocyte sedimentation rate	Inflammation
Blood	CRP	C-Reactive Protein	Inflammation Anywhere in Body
Biopsy	Tissue Samples	Status of Intestinal Villa	Acute Inflammation Damage
Symptomology	Keep a Diary of Cause and Effects	Date	Action Required

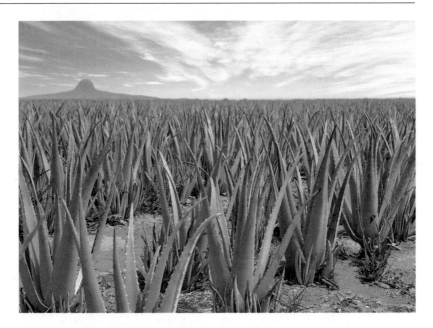

HIGHLIGHT 4: *Aloe Vera to the Rescue; Lowering Inflammation & More!*

The ancient herb Aloe Vera is packed full of powerful active ingredients to support health for people living in the 21st century. Aloe Vera is a succulent in the garlic family and grows all over the world with 300 different species. Aloe is 100% safe to use topically as well as to ingest the juice or powdered products internally as a health drink for children, adults, seniors and pets as well [16]. Research conducted by the US government revealed that among the hundreds of different herbs that people are using medicinally Aloe Vera continues to be the most popular number one choice! To get this type of notoriety the plant must contain some exceptional healing attributes!

Why is Aloe Vera used by so many people around the world? The plant contains over 200 active ingredients researchers divide into 15 compound groups that support the body's healing process from A-Z [17]. Applying Aloe Vera topically to a skinned knee reveals healing resolution in record time. It is no wonder that Diabetics are using it more and more to heal stubborn wounds. Teenagers are finding it to be a best friend for acne and to lessen scarring. Seeing Aloe at work turns you into a real believer. Scientists find Aloe to contain a combination of *five anti-inflammatory agents* coupled with natural *growth factors* and *infection fighters* that stimulate the new skin cells to grow at record speed.

Science Supports Aloe Vera [18]

- Digestion & Regularity
- Bio-Availability of Nutrition; B12, Vitamin C & E
- Anti-Inflammatory Action
- Energy & Relaxation
- Skin Health; Acne, Scarring and Wound Support
- Anti-Microbial; Viral, Bacteria and Yeast
- Immune System; Strengthens and Balances
- Glandular Function; Pancreas, Stomach, Liver and more

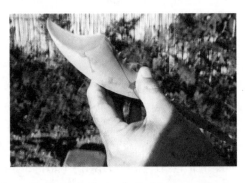

Drinking the juice of the Aloe Vera plant, especially if it still contains the yellow sap, seems to give the digestive system a real advantage. The "Ancients" referred to Aloe as an *herbal bitter*. The bitter yellow sap that is found directly under the outer leaf, called whole leaf, encourages the gastric juices to flow in the GI tract for proper digestion. Within minutes of experiencing heartburn or other discomfort drinking a dose of quality Aloe Vera juice can squelch the pain and even uplift a person to feel much more energetic. The support the juice gives to digestion seems to be the reason behind people experiencing more energy especially if it is taken before meals.

Natural Occurring Anti-Inflammatory Agents Soothe Digestion

Aloe Vera contains *five natural anti-inflammatory agents* that appear to be responsible for another reason so many people drink Aloe Vera for help with all types of bowel concerns. A few of the pain relievers are located in the yellow sap and the rest in the pulp including; *anthraquinones, enzymes, amino acids* and a natural aspirin like compound called *salicylic acid*. Together they work remarkably fast to naturally ease the pain and discomfort inflammation can bring to the body and are important to support the healing process. *Cathartics* are also found along side the anti-inflammatory agents in Aloe that work like prune juice to encourage bowel regularity without dependence, attracting more children and adults as fans.

Immune System Support

Another remarkable area of support from Aloe Vera lies in its ability to *boost immune function* including *fighting off infection*. A natural compound called *Saponins* works as a disinfectant in the bloodstream against impurities in the blood. Ingesting Aloe appears to work through four different pathways to keep immunity strong. One way is through an immune modulation response research shows is dose dependent. This pathway of action calls upon the long chain sugars of 80,000 Dalton size or higher of the *polysaccharides*. These sugars are also referred to as *glyco-mannans* in Aloe that shift the *immune system* into fight mode through macrophage Pac-Man like *phagocytosis*. Research finds Aloe helps to battle against bad bacteria, viruses and yeast microbials alike. Natural *sterols* in Aloe, on the other hand help calm the immune system through balancing lymphocyte T4 to T8 cells as is needed with *auto-immune* support. Taking a maintenance amount is very remarkable coupled with the GIS program. Keep in mind that the quality of the product you choose does make a big difference in the performance.

Quality Aloe Vera makes a BIG difference! Remember when looking for a quality Aloe Vera, there is a big difference in products on the market. I have used the whole leaf and concentrated tablets and juices with great success especially if they contain the ActivAloe logo. Scientists have confirmed that a quality Aloe Vera product assists the body to work the way it was designed with no contraindication when taking it with any medication. Because it works as a mild blood thinner which is beneficial you may wish to stop it ten days prior to any surgical procedures.

A good product will be *cold processed* and not over-heated or fractionated. Excessive heat can denature the valuable active ingredients. Look for a dark yellow color and a rich slightly bitter taste (not too sour) to avoid purchasing an over-filtered or diluted product that will give limited health results. Fractionated means that only part of the Aloe Vera's active ingredients are still present in a finished product. Some products have been so over-processed they taste like water, not an herbal tomato taste, as is found in a quality Whole Leaf Aloe Vera Juice Concentrate. To receive the full benefit from the plant you want products that have the entire spectrum of active ingredients especially the *yellow sap.*

Look for products that state no water or sulfites added and take it before meals for best results. Aloe Vera, along with all the other wonderful applications, is a terrific detoxifier. The sulfur compounds in Aloe are responsible for building exceptional healthy skin, proper insulin and significantly stimulate the liver to make high potency detoxifying antioxidants. These compounds called *Phase II Enzymes*, one being *Super Oxide Dismutase (SOD)* are critical for *reducing inflammation* in the body, *correcting DNA damage* and also supporting *anti-aging effects* we all desire. To avoid diarrhea with detoxification just reduce the daily amount as needed and many find that they can increase the Aloe back to 2 – 4 ounces before long, as desired.

The product I have used for over twenty years can be reviewed at www.aloelife.com. It is concentrated therefore does not demand large quantities of the juice or tablets to be swallowed. It also comes in delicious sugar free flavors for children or for people with sensitive tastes. Once you find a therapeutic Aloe take it regularly to support your digestive stamina and it will give you many added health extras to include; digestion, glandular, energy, skin, anti-fungal, allergy, immune, autoimmune and anti-aging support to the body.

The first person I ever saw the remarkable wonders of Aloe at work with was in a clinic patient's husband who had an under-functioning immune system. In less than two weeks after he began to drink 4 ounces of a therapeutic Aloe Vera juice a tumor the size of a walnut in his lung resolved! This experience opened my eyes to the fact that Aloe was a divinely given plant that had more to offer the human population than I ever imagined [18]. Since that first incidence many other clients have given testimony to Aloe Vera's powerful regenerative support of the human body.

Hundreds of repeatable studies have been conducted around the globe to prove Aloe's therapeutic action on the body including; anti-inflammatory, anti- microbial, Immune System balancing and tissue healing in record time. Recent research showing Aloe's bioavailability factor revealed that humans drinking one ounce of a quality Aloe Vera with meals experienced an increase in bioavailability of core nutrients Vitamin C, E and B12, up to 300% greater. These studies explained why my patients and clients, to the amazement of their attending physicians, have gone into remission with many chronic illnesses so much faster than those not drinking Aloe Vera.

Learning the history of herbs can teach valuable lessons as the "Ancients" were well aware of - especially that health is all about building a strong foundation starting with the support of the digestive system. Aloe Vera assists in optimizing digestion and regeneration of the body and it is 100% safe to take for the whole family!

GIS A Factor in All Disease; Mental & Physical

"Knowing about gluten intolerance has made a big difference in my life especially when it comes to feeling comfortable in my own skin. I took anti-depressant medication after the birth of my last child up until I applied the GIS program. I've been drug free for years now. Even my claustrophobic tendencies and other Obsessive Compulsive Disorders (OCD) have greatly improved. Now both depression and paranoia tendencies are all but gone. Staying on the GIS Diet I don't spend so much time in the bathroom with loose stools, constipation or having digestive upset in general. Also, my son who has a tendency for hyperactivity can stay off medication if I keep the GIS food choices and supplements for the whole family!"

— Theresa, California

Counseling people back to health has confirmed not only the relationship of the Gluten Inflammatory Syndrome (GIS) to physical diseases but also to my understanding of the Brain-Bowel connection. I have witnessed the return of mental well-being, hand in hand with the resolution of bowel symptoms in all of my cases.

For decades researchers and professionals have written about the connection of mental health to the diet of people [1, 2, and 3]. Behavioral challenges in children as seen with hyperactivity have significantly improved with strict dietary guidelines [4]. Daily mental confusion, melancholy, varying degrees of depression, anxiety, grouchiness and even bizarre behaviors have all improved and often resolved completely following the GIS Program. Even the more advanced mental disorders including; Obsessive Compulsive Disorder (OCD), Schizophrenia, Bipolar – Manic/Depressive symptoms have remarkably improved to my astonishment, as with this following true life account.

Bi-Polar – Manic/Depressant

A phone call came into my office one day and as I spoke to the mother of a young woman diagnosed with Bi-Polar disease my interest peaked. She called with a question concerning her daughter's digestion and I suggested that she go on the GIS Diet for a 6 week trial. I told her the diet is a bit like the Atkins program, very low in carbohydrates grains with the focus on lean meats and lots of vegetables. Her response to me was very reaffirming of how well the GIS Diet helps with overall brain function.

She said, "You may be interested to hear that my daughter followed the Atkins diet approximately a year ago and her manic – depressive symptoms cleared up for as long as she stayed on the low carbohydrate regimen". Yes, I replied, that result makes perfect sense to me and thanks for sharing. I believe leaving the grains and high starch carbohydrates (that contain the gluten and complex sugars) alone, allows the inflammation to decrease in the body and the brain and sanity to return. Research on Schizophrenia is also beginning to confirm this Brain-Bowel Connection [5].

GIS Impacts All of the Neurological Systems
- Mental & Brain
- Digestion & Elimination
- Cardiovascular, Circulation & Pulmonary (heart rhythm)
- Muscle & Glandular
- Immune & Auto Immune
- Vocal & Hearing

How does GIS relate to mental illness?

Ultimately the connection of mental illness to the Gluten Inflammatory Syndrome (GIS) lies in the relationship of *inflammation* and *mal-nutrition*. Both factors can greatly influence the Nervous System and its efficiency in the body to balance and build mental wellness [6, 7].

There are two parts of the highly complex Nervous System; the *Central Nervous System* (CNS) which includes the brain and spinal cord and the *Peripheral Nervous System* (PNS) which consists of nerves and neurons that extend throughout the limbs and organs. In the brain alone there are over 10 billion neurons and many times more inter-neural connections that develop the superior intelligence of humans compared to other animal species [8].

The brain sends impulses directing function to the body and in turn receives information back that is transferred by way of *neurotransmitters*. These are made from a group of chemicals and are the smallest of informational molecules that transmit an impulse from one nerve cell to another or a group of neighboring cells. The signals are successful if they jump across a junction called a *synapse*. Neurotransmitters are stored in small sack-like containers called *vesicles* at the ends of neurons. They are responsible for all the information to control each facet of the body to include; heart rate, changes in mood, perception and thoughts. Some neurotransmitters and *neuropeptides* interact with other body organs and have a direct relationship between the Nervous System and the Immune System. More and more researchers are beginning to understand that the Nervous System is involved in Auto-Immune Diseases affecting mental and physical disease states.

One such researcher is Dr. V. K. Singh, Ph.D., a former professor at several universities in the U.S. With over 30 years of experience in neurological disorders he is considered a pioneer in this field of Immune and Auto-Immunity and the relationship to the Nervous System. His work encompasses all Auto-Immune disorders including; Multiple Sclerosis, Autism, Obsessive Compulsive Disorder (OCD), Schizophrenia, Alzheimer's disease and Chronic Depression.

In 1997 he published a review article about his research called, "Immunotherapy for Brain Diseases and Mental Illnesses" [13]. His summary related the diseases to an immune system that goes array and wrote that the mechanism involved is the Nervous System exhibiting "Auto-Immunity!" He has published over 100 scientific publications and given numerous presentations of his work worldwide that illustrates; the Nervous System pathway connects Auto-Immune conditions as described in GIS. He too advocates supporting the body to balance its systems through more natural methods. His unique protocol includes helping the immune system through intravenous immunoglobulin treatments (IVIG) and Secretin Therapy that improves digestion. Like the GIS Program he suggests using "Nutraceutical Therapy". Nutraceuticals as defined by the Merriam-Webster dictionary are foodstuffs of fortified food or dietary supplements that provide health benefits in addition to its basic nutritional value. Allergies are another topic Dr. Singh includes in his writing and states that many of his Autistic patients have gotten off gluten or casein which is found in grains or milk and have experienced good over-all general health improvement.

Nutrition and the Brain

Special nutrition is required in order to build, support and maintain the Nervous System's full capacity. To carry out proper metabolic action and balance of this system an individual must include; Amino Acids (from protein), Vitamin B-Complex, Choline, Inositol, Vitamin C, Essential Fatty Acids (EFA) and a variety of Minerals [9]. Minerals are very under-appreciated for their importance in the body especially Sulfur, Iron, Zinc, Magnesium and the other electrolytes Calcium, Potassium, Sodium Chloride, Phosphate and Bicarbonate. In nature there are also over 200 trace minerals found in foods that scientists continue to reveal their importance for health.

Surprising to some Magnesium plays a very important role in the body and is needed in over 300 metabolic processes. Research is pointing to Magnesium for the success of the neurotransmitters especially in hormone related function, to ease depression and support the overall healthy functioning of the Central Nervous System including the Brain-Bowel Connection [10, 11, and 12].

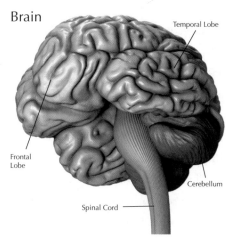

Brain

Temporal Lobe

Frontal Lobe

Cerebellum

Spinal Cord

The Essential Fatty Acid (EFA) research has exploded in the past ten years and you will learn more about its critical role in brain health along with Vitamin B12 found in the B-Complex family and Protein. The National Center for Complementary and Alternative Medicine NCCAM recently published an article in *Brain, Behavior and Immunity*, 2011 that confirmed the Omega-3 Essential Fatty Acids, the types found in fish, lowered anxiety by 20 percent and inflammation by 14 percent in their double-blind human study in only 12 weeks. Another ground breaking study was also just published in the *Journal of Clinical Psychiatry*, 2011 on the coinciding low levels of the Omega-3 Fatty Acids DHA compound in depressed and actual suicide deaths by military personnel. The study was a double blind on 800 random suicides and 800 matched persons of the same age, rank, sex and time period. The conclusion revealed that all of the US military population that took their own life had a very low and narrow range of Omega-3 DHA in their blood compared to the controls. Several observations were discovered during this research that has prompted a review of the role nutrition plays in protecting and supporting the military to include; lowering the stress of combat deployment which manifests in major depression, reducing impulsive violence and lowering the rise in suicides. In fact it was revealed that the number one reason for any medical inpatient utilization of US military (considering all causes) was mental illness; mood disorders, primarily major depression with suicidal risk and adjustment disorders! In light of the enormous challenge facing both the military and also the public sector for mental health research in the *Br Journal of Psychiatry*, 2007 confirmed that when compared to placebo adult subjects taking 2,000 mg of Omega-3 Fatty Acids daily actually reduced their suicidal thinking and depressive symptoms that had been causing them to inflict personal harm.

Inflammation in the Brain

Chronic inflammation appears to disrupt proper circulation in the brain and other organs regardless of the source. Researchers have confirmed that inflammation is present with Schizophrenia even when it is not due to a Folic Acid or B6 deficiency [14] as it does relate in Cardiovascular Disease [15]. Scientists are unclear as to the exact sequence of the reaction yet all of the work confirms a relationship between the Central Nervous System, Auto-Immune and Inflammation as depicted in GIS. It appears to only be a matter of time before the researchers will be able to pinpoint the exact pathway for this relationship.

What has become clear through the research is the existence of a microbial component associated with mental disorders. Some research confirms a bacterial infection and others have shown a viral one that accounts for the escalation of inflammation in the brain [16]. Herpes Simplex I and II has been surfacing as a common virus involved in this cascade of inflammation and is also indicated as one of the secondary GIS triggers [17, 18].

Health Depends on Nutrition

The idea that the body requires specific nutrition to function optimally is scientifically supported yet most professionals and lay people alike still find this fact almost fictional. The analogy of the body compared to a car has often been used because our body is a type of vehicle that we must give to it the designated fuel and make certain that the body can use it to run properly. In the case of the body our fuel is food, which we need regularly if we are to expect the body to perform well. What is also true is the higher quality of nutrients in the food the better the body ultimately works as seen with athletes.

To understand the question of how GIS relates to mental health, it helps to review the factors needed to build a strong functioning mind in the first place. For those of you who view the function of the brain to be more about learned experiences and emotions, coupled with communication skills - it may come as a big surprise that our nutritional stores and physical health play such an integral part in mood and brain function.

It is true that our experiences and communication skills along with spiritual beliefs all color our perception of the world and how we respond to it on a daily basis. However, our moods and the brains ability to function and optimize the IQ have everything to do with nutrition.

To understand the significance of a healthy brain you need only to observe a person who is experiencing Dementia or Alzheimer's disease (AD) which is the advanced state of Dementia. You take a person who has been able to think and carry on a satisfying intelligent conversation and execute daily activities; keeping a happy and optimistic frame of mind, sleeping well at night, able to coordinate daily exercise with stable walking and good talking ability and fast forward them into Dementia.

This same person can become easily depressed with argumentative tendencies. They also cannot keep their focus in a conversation and they forget facts. They may also slowly lose control of their mobility and coordination and even their sleep cycle often becomes very sporadic. Scientists researching the brain damage associated with AD reveal corrosive build-up of plaque in the vascular system that is associated with inflammation and describe it like a neurological jungle of tangles.

Dr. Mark Heyman, MD a Neurologist from Harvard University has directly connected the development of AD to toxicity and dietary factors. The brains health is so important to life itself that Alzheimer's disease (AD) is actually responsible for the 7th leading cause of death in the U.S. With over 6 million people now living with diagnosed AD today Dr. Heyman states that unless people become more preventative through nutrition and health to avoid dementia and AD the numbers will triple in the next few decades!

If you are surprised with these figures - the experts are also reporting that some form of mental illness is now thought to affect one in four people in the U.S. I take it even further to suggest that the incidence is much higher due to all of the self-medication through drugs, food and alcohol that takes place in today's world - just to help one's self feel better!

Mental health as with physical health is achieved only when the body has the proper nutrition yet this simple explanation is much too vague. The full story is that the body must not only receive proper daily nutrition in the correct amounts and variety, it must be able to metabolize the nutrients effectively and each individual cell must be able to absorb these nutrients across the cellular membrane. This is easier said than done especially when you add in the Gluten Inflammatory Syndrome (GIS).

Following the GIS Program will help to optimize your inherited genetic potential - to think, communicate appropriately and use the body and brain to peak performance. Keep in mind what orchestrates the success of the cellular action in the body - beyond the spiritual realm - is the all-important Nervous System along with the health of our DNA!

Other factors definitely come to play in reviewing what truly affects our health status and deserve important consideration in our study. The roadblock list includes each of the factors that influence mental and physical health. You will find many of the topics elaborated upon in Chapter 6 called the Healthy Focus Factors.

Roadblocks to Mental & Physical Health

- The ***Degree of GIS Symptoms*** is determined by the *intensity of inflammation* which decreases the Nervous System, digestion and absorption in the gut leading into *malnutrition and lowering organ* and *glandular function*. The Pancreas gland is a good example of this damaging cycle. As the Pancreas loses its ability to secrete digestive juices and insulin which are responsible for healthy blood sugar metabolism and digestion in turn this *decreases the circulation* even more causing the body to *further malfunctions* (Ch.3).

- *Viral Flare-Ups*, especially Herpes Simplex I & II, increase secondary inflammation as noted in Ch.4 adding to GIS inflammation throughout the body which *exaggerates mental and physical illness symptoms.*

- *Toxins* that are made from *secondary infections* including bacteria, fungus and yeast organisms or *waste residue* as with Lactic Acid within one's own body, can act like poison to the brain cells. *Fungal overgrowth* also blocks absorption of valuable nutrients besides contributing to toxins through die-off residue. Molds can also enter the body and cause infections and toxins. Another category of toxins have emerged called *"Excitotoxins"* found in certain food additives like Monosodium Glutamate (MSG) and artificial sweeteners that researchers have found to be very damaging and even lethal to nerve cells [19]. Chapter 6 reviews the "Excitotoxins".

- Several *Environmental Factors* affect the brain and body's ability to function optimally and are found to cause both birth defects and improper growth and development. Each factor deserves consideration to include; *addictions and voluntary use of drugs and foods, dangerous chemicals* like Mercury, Arsenic and Lead toxicity and even *Electromagnetic Fields (EMF)* have all been associated to increase the disease process including; Diabetes, Low Blood Sugar, Alzheimer's, Arteriolosclerosis, slow learning ability and Mental Illness.

- *DNA Damage* in the body from all factors result in *mutagenic and aging of the genetic code* in every cell of the body thereby impacting newborns and all persons full health potential. Genomic researchers have found the core nutrients (Ch. 8) and antioxidants taken in the appropriate levels can repair DNA damage.

Understanding the Roadblocks

GIS is a big factor in mental and physical illness due to the inflammation it brings to the entire *Nervous System* including the *Central Nervous System* (CNS) directly. Within minutes after eating gluten or GIS triggers a person can experience a reaction in the CNS. Later the GIS will generally affect

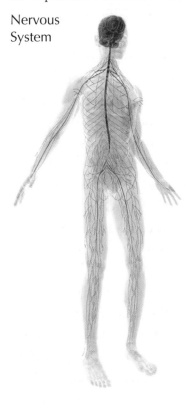

Nervous System

the gut which keeps the heightened auto-immune response active throughout the body. As explained in Chapter 3, Understanding the Digestion Inflammation Connection, the *intensity of inflammation* and the duration of it in the small intestine villi, ultimately leads to *poor absorption* and *malnutrition* of the required Essential Core Nutrients (ECN) including; Vitamins A, C, E, B-Complex, Essential Fatty Acids (EFA's), Proteins and Minerals.

The GIS inflammation causes *varying degrees of malnutrition* in the body depending on each individuals experience from slight to severe. Malnutrition often includes the four brain nutrients directly related to the health of the CNS. A deficiency in these nutrients not only decreases brain function but also affects all the other organs and glandular function of the body. The key nutrients essential for a healthy Nervous System along with the other required ECN and Minerals include; B12, B-Complex, EFA's (Omega 3 & 6 Complex) and Protein which are particularly vulnerable with GIS. Several sections in this chapter explain the value and importance nutrition plays to organ and glandular health which in turn supports metabolic function that ultimately leads to one's full health potential.

GIS reduces the digestive availability of all the healthy fats that encompass the Essential Fatty Acids and fat soluble vitamins even when a person makes the effort to include them in their daily diets. The poor digestive symptoms people may experience when eating healthy fats and supplements include; nausea, burping, heart burn, gassiness and oily stools.

The oil soluble Vitamins A, E, and K depend on good fat digestion and as stated are in jeopardy along with the EFA's with poor digestion due to GIS. An important tip for fat metabolism in general is that all fat digestion requires sufficient fat in the diet in the first place along with proper digestive function to be metabolized efficiently. Many people regard all fats as bad and wind up fat starved! Healthy fats are essential to reach optimum health for babies, children and adults.

A large amount of nutrition is never fully utilized in the body due to poor absorption. Some experts believe that as little as 15% of the possible nutrients from our foods are actually absorbed into the cells of the body. Besides the GIS inflammation in the small intestine reducing absorption, another avenue nutrition is lost is through the stool when diarrhea is present. Especially vulnerable are the water soluble vitamins like Vitamin B and C, along with protein and minerals. Over-consumption in caffeine as with coffee, chocolate, black tea, sodas, energy drinks and alcohol will also deplete the body of these valuable nutrients along with the diarrheic action of the bowel.

Constipation can come from several factors however it is also caused from eating gluten and gluten triggers. Due to the impact on the CNS GIS interferes with the normal peristaltic action of the bowel slowing it down and sometimes brings it to a complete halt. Chronic constipation creates another set of challenges with absorption. An overgrowth of the *opportunistic yeast* condition called *Candida Albicans* arises in the intestinal track with slow elimination. This is a fungal condition as reviewed in Ch. 3, some call "Thrush". Candida literally blocks absorption of nutrients into the intestinal cells like covering a portal with a dense cloth. This fungus along with other yeasts and bacteria also make *internal toxins* during their maturation process. These toxins migrate throughout the blood creating a type of *brain fog* and other potential secondary toxins affecting our brain cells. To combat toxicity from toxins and other *chemical damage* it is important to keep a good supply in the body of Probiotics (discussed in Chapter 2) and a variety of Phyto-nutrients and core supplements having antioxidant capability. Tuft's University recommends a goal of at least 12,000 ORAC (Oxygen Radical Absorbency Capacity) daily for *antioxidant protection*. Research has proven that these natural protectors help to guard against all cellular and *DNA damage* further discussed in Chapter 6.

Researchers have isolated one such toxin damaging the brain cells called *D-Lactic Acid*. Not only have they isolated it as a toxin to the brain scientists have pinpointed D-Lactic Acid to *increase psychiatric disorders*. This toxin which is the same one that is made during exercising the muscles in the body is especially problematic when the liver is congested and cannot properly detoxify the blood. Chapter 6 reviews Detoxification.

Interestingly, larger quantities of the D-Lactic Acid have occurred after surgical procedures of shortening the small intestine and even the removal of the gallbladder and other abdominal surgery. This procedure is called a *"Resection"* and it is a common procedure with advanced bowel disease. *Cholecystectomy* surgery which is the removal of the gallbladder is also becoming very common in the last 30 years, showing how glandular support of the body is undersupplied.

Larger amounts of the D-Lactic Acid have also been observed due to the *over-eating of grains* that are not being thoroughly digested properly. Studies have shown that the effects of the D-Lactic Acid found circulating in the blood *results in more diarrheas*. This in turn triggers a type of brain dysfunction having very similar symptoms to *Schizophrenia or other bizarre behavior.*

Viral Flare-Ups in the body are associated with the ravages of gluten intolerance explained in the GIS II theory introduced in Chapter 4. The GIS II Theory relates that all inflammation affects total inflammatory conditions. With our discussion on both mental and physical disease I find the Herpes Simplex I and II Virus are closely *associated with GIS and*

Mental Illness. Following the guidelines in Chapter 6 in the Virus section especially focusing on Herpes Simplex, will help reduce the symptoms of diarrhea, fatigue, headaches and even mood swings resulting from plummeting blood sugar associated to viral activity. Keep in mind that viruses can be strictly internal and not develop any ulcerous sore or break in the skin yet they may still affect the body's overall health performance.

Organ & Glandular Health especially of the Thyroid, Pancreas, Adrenals and Liver has a big impact on mental health and body wellness. The definition of a gland is a cell, a group of cells or an organ that produces a secretion for use elsewhere in the body. A good example of this is the *Pancreas.* It must manufacture *insulin* to help *maintain proper blood sugar metabolism* besides *secreting pancreatic enzymes* critical to the efficiency of *digestion.* The blood sugar called *glucose* is the *fuel for the brain* and when it drops to a low level without enough insulin for proper use it can cause an emotional roller coaster within minutes. When the blood sugar is unstable it can bring about cross words towards your children, spouse or co-workers. Even greater agitation and confusion may develop and lead into angry behavior and actions. The mineral *Chromium* and the *Vitamin B-Complex* along with *Protein* are all three required for healthy blood sugar metabolism as reviewed in Glossary of Conditions in Chapter 5.

The *Thyroid* and *Para-Thyroid* gland is involved in many metabolic processes including *hormone cycles, mineral absorption,* controlling *energy* expenditure, *weight* and *heat manufacturing* in the body along with *moods* and other body functions. *Iodine* is an essential support mineral required to nourish the Thyroid gland coupled with other Essential Core Nutrients (ECN's).

The *Liver* is an extremely important gland in support of *brain health.* It is responsible for *processing* and *manufacturing of amino acid compounds* and *hormones* specifically involved in regulating mood as with the *hormone Serotonin.* Serotonin is made with sufficient amounts of the amino acid L-Tryptophan ingested into the body. L-Tryptophan is an essential amino acid found in foods like turkey, chicken, bananas and or supplements like 5HTP. Once L-Tryptophan has been processed it is transported to

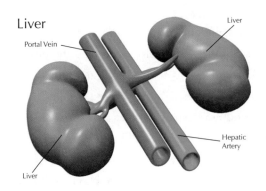

the brain with five other amino acids that can be competitive for uptake. If there is sufficient amount available and the required co-factor nutrients including Vitamin B3 and B6 – the brain will transform L-Tryptophan into Serotonin. A valuable hormone it works as a *natural anti-depressant* supporting the *NS, CNS* and *GI tract metabolism*. It regulates *mood, appetite, sleep* and *muscle contractions*. Even taking a small amount of an L-Tryptophan supplement can support the body's production of natural Serotonin significantly. EFA's are also required to make sufficient hormones including the valuable Serotonin.

Another valuable amino acid is called *L-Glutamine*. It is a precursor to manufacture *GABA* (Gamma-Amino Butyric Acid) in the body that works to *relieve tension* and *anxiety*. At times the brain may experience an abundance of stress, caused by a surplus of *norepinephrine* made in the Adrenal glands or *epinephrine* (another word for adrenaline) also manufactured in the Adrenal glands. To neutralize any extra stress hormones the brain produces neurotransmitters, one being *GABA that helps the nervous system to relax*. Taking a GABA supplement can begin to work within minutes after taking it - giving support for *relaxation* and *calmness*. *Vitamin C* is also a very important essential core nutrient to *reduce unhealthy Adrenaline levels* in the blood due to excessive stress.

Some people have found *immediate stress relief* through addressing another pathway in the body which is through the sense of smell called *Olfactory*. Review the *Bach Remedies* by going to the Reference section for children and adults that includes the *Rescue Remedy* that truly takes the edge off of a challenging emotional situation. Bach Remedies can act like emotional buffers to give temporary or continual comfort likened to smelling a rose or a fresh cut orange!

When the body builds healthy glands they work together as co-regulators to maintain healthy mental attitudes and behaviors even preventing depression. When the Nervous System is not working properly due to GIS it seems to impact all of the organs and glands of the body causing a decrease in the proper hormones and neurotransmitters needed to carry on daily metabolism. This is associated with the lack of brain nutrients as will be discussed. Following the GIS Program and experimenting with supplements allows the regeneration of the body and to reverse mental and physical illness.

Pioneering Psychiatrist Predicts that the Drug Picture will Change in the Future

Case studies from San Francisco psychiatrist, Dr. Michael Lesser, showed that 89 out of 97 patients diagnosed with different types of Psychosis, were found to have abnormally low blood sugar upon testing. Only through stabilizing the patient's blood sugar did his patients once again experience mental stability.

Nutrient therapy has distinct advantages writes Dr. Lesser. He goes on to say, supplements are less expensive than drugs and certainly they are much safer. He states that nutrient therapy is more effective because it is getting at the cause of the problem. With the development of "Orthomolecular Psychiatry" that treats the problem and not just the symptoms, he predicts that the drug picture will change dramatically in the future. For the sake of our future society I certainly hope he is correct!

The importance of eating nutritious nutrient dense foods cannot be overemphasized for the body and the mind. In turn the nutrients from our food support all of the glandular health in the body. Consuming regular meals throughout the day that include quality protein is mandatory to maintain healthy blood sugar balance which is foundational to stabilizing children and adult's moods and behavior.

New research has also shown that *environmental factors* coming from *pollution, toxic chemicals* in our air, food and water supply, *compromise clear thinking* and *physical performance,* of the body for kids and adults. Lead, Arsenic and Mercury are the common *neurotoxins* found in our polluted world of today. Lead is noted as the most lethal neurotoxin often found in people's blood tests, at higher than the EPA allowable levels.

Lead was finally banned in 1996 from the common car fuels with the exception of aircraft, off-road and racing cars, farm equipment and marine engines. Toxic lead content was also banned from modern paints back in 1978 yet extra caution is still needed in our environment. *Lead still exists in large quantities in our soils, older homes, lead pipes, agriculture and public facilities* including some older Day Care and churches lingering from years past. In 2007 the CDC estimated 24 million dwellings still have unsafe levels and 300,000 children may be living with unsafe lead levels in their bodies. Unfortunately, China has also been contributing to more potential lead toxicity through children's toys and or jewelry so buyers please beware. I have often picked up a toy or other item which I do not purchase after noting the country of origin to be China. Lead has also made its way into the food chain and can be found in almost all foods both commercially and organically grown foods.

Arsenic enters our food chain from many sources. It begins as an herbicide to kill weeds around our home, golf courses, and nurseries and is used frequently in commercial agriculture. It is now being found in abundance in common cleaning products, meat, milk and most non-organic foods.

Mercury, the second most deadly neurotoxin next to lead, comes out of the earth naturally in coal. The largest amount of Mercury enters our atmosphere from the *burning of coal* without the proper filtration. Tons of Mercury pollutes our air and food supply every year. Mercury settles in the oceans and streams and that is how our *larger fish like Tuna become more contaminated.* The CDC is well aware of this situation and the rest of the chemical toxicity in the U.S. The clean coal initiative that gets lip service from time to time is extremely past due because of the growing health challenge that mercury toxicity presents to us all. People also receive *Mercury toxicity from tooth fillings.* The alternative *composite materials* can be requested. Ask your dentists for the safer alternatives to the amalgam silver (mercury) fillings. Even though dentists state that young children will not hold still long enough which is needed for the newer fillings to set properly - coming from a safety point of view the Mercury silver fillings need to be discontinued altogether.

Vaccinations are yet another source where people receive *detrimental Mercury*. Slowly the citizen action groups have made inroads through to the government that began new regulation for drug manufactures to offer alternative vaccinations without Mercury. It has been used as a preservative agent in flu vaccines and childhood shots. Regardless as to whether or not Mercury is the sole perpetrator to the higher incidence of Autistic symptoms - it is toxic to the body and must be avoided wherever possible.

Each of these environmental chemicals along with thousands of others is responsible for slower mental and physical development and miscellaneous other metabolic malfunctions in the body. Some experts conclude that higher toxic levels of chemicals are directly responsible for mental psychosis and even violent crimes as seen in criminal behavior. Many of the environmental chemicals are directly linked to the higher incidence of cancer today as well! Detoxification from toxic chemicals is reviewed in Chapter 6.

Another factor that can and does affect overall body wellness is EMF's. *Electromagnetic Fields* (EMF) have been a growing concern on the planet affecting all of our lives. We are living in an unprecedented era known as the "Digital Age" with cell phones, computers and wireless communication. As documented in the book, *Zapped* by Louise Gittleman, 2010, it is an important topic to review within each household and workplace to "Decrease Stray Electromagnetic Fields" that can zap our health. The Central Nervous System and our overall health performance is truly affected by the onslaught of these varied energy fields coming from both plugged in appliances and wireless electronic equipment.

With all of these factors that affect our brain and body wellness the greatest influence on a daily basis is nutrition. As you read about these valuable brain nutrients and deficiency signs I think you will begin to understand why so many people with bowel issues (that cause nutritional deficiencies) also experience a higher diagnosis of depression and other

Psychosis. Hopefully this information answers a lot of the questions surrounding the Brain-Bowel Connection. It can also give light to why in past years and still today doctors write prescriptions to see psychiatrists for many patients suffering with bowel disease thinking it is all in one's head!

Nutrition - Gotta Have It to Remove the Roadblocks!

At every age, starting from conception through senior-hood, nutrition is required and cannot be replaced by any other modality. For brain and body wellness nutrition is paramount, especially the following four that includes; B-Complex, B12, EFA's and Protein.

Over 100,000 Studies Confirm the Importance of B-Complex & B12

The B-Complex is required by the body for life itself. The disease called Beriberi develops from a B-Complex deficiency, in particularly the lack of the B1-Thiamine fraction. The disease has been thoroughly researched since first designated as a deficiency disease in 1901 by a Dutch physician. Beriberi causes fluid retention, nerve damage (associated with mental illness); weakness and pain in the limbs, an irregular heart rate, high Lactic Acid and Pyruvic Acid build up, heart failure and in advanced stages brings about death. Alcoholism, pregnancy, lactation, infections, hypothyroidism, and malnutrition can all bring about the same symptoms as experienced with Beriberi due to the depletion of the B-Complex.

B-Complex which includes B12 is essential to support all of the systems of the body including the Blood Hematological, Gastrointestinal, Psychiatric, Dermatologic (skin) and Cardiovascular Health and is an integral support for the entire Nervous System (NS). In the over 100,000 studies that have been conducted they confirm the importance of the B-Complex underlining the extreme value to the digestive system. For this reason the B's are highlighted at the end of Chapter 3 reviewing digestion. They are required in over 138 important daily functions of the body to include; basic peristaltic action (a bowel movement) of the colon and stimulating all of the required digestive juices and enzymes for healthy digestion.

Falling into the category of "Vitamins", B12 and B-Complex cannot be made in any significant amount in the body therefore it is needed to be supplied on a daily or regular basis through foods and or supplements. A small amount has been thought to be manufactured in the small intestine from a healthy gut however research has not quantified any significant levels.

Anemia, Fatigue, Skin Conditions & GIS

B12 is required for building blood and remember it is a common deficiency with GIS. It works with Protein, Folic Acid and Iron to prevent Anemia. Anemia is the state of low red blood cells and or blood hemoglobin and it brings upon tiredness and sometimes crippling fatigue. Anemia is the most common nutritional deficiency in the world according to both the World Health Organization (WHO) and the Center of Disease Control (CDC) of the U.S. It causes people to feel not only very fatigued but also to have difficulty in thinking and at times causes excruciating headaches. Also, a deficiency of B12 coupled with a Vitamin C deficiency can bring about easy bruising on the skin. Sadly, advanced and prolonged Anemia if not addressed can eventually lead to premature death especially within the senior population!

Pertinent to Anemia is the mineral Iron which is not absorbed very well either in the body due to a lack of B-Complex and other co-factors. What takes place is that a low level of B Vitamins, reduce the production of HCL required in the stomach to break down Iron and other minerals for absorption. Vitamin C, a core nutrient is also a co-enzyme vitamin that is required for proper Iron absorption and it is depleted with diarrhea. Researchers have long recognized that a large percentage of cow milk drinkers in both children and adults develop bowel disease with loose stool symptoms and as a result suffer the deficiency of many nutrients including poor Iron absorption. You can begin to see the relationship with Anemia and GIS and how the cycle of mal-absorption can perpetuate itself.

Pernicious Anemia

Advanced or chronic anemia is called "Pernicious Anemia" which experts relate to a lack of the B12 absorption factor called the "Intrinsic Factor". If this is suspected the suggested protocol is injections of B12 prescribed from a professional to include; 1000 mcg every day for one week, every other day for a second week and then once per month for 3 months and then reduced to every 3 months as a precautionary. Intramuscular injections are best absorbed for an acute deficiency. Many integrative physicians are promoting the methyl-B12 type. The injections by-pass the need for the "Intrinsic Factor" from the stomach which is often insufficient with advanced GIS. B12 deficiency symptoms may mask a second Folic Acid deficiency another one of the B-Complex. For this reason you must make certain that a good supply of Folic Acid is taken regularly and is being absorbed along with a B12 supplement.

Sublingual, under the tongue, B12 supplements are the second best alternative for treatment. Always follow with a strong B-Complex taken regularly by mouth in approximately 50 mg potency as tolerated one to three times per day with meals. If nausea results lower the daily amount and the best alternative to the B-Complex tablet would be Nutritional Yeast powder. Review ECN supplements in Chapter 8 for B-Complex.

B12 is part of the B-Complex and is essential in the metabolism of protein, fats and carbohydrates. The fat soluble vitamins rely on B12 for absorption to carry out hundreds of intertwined activities of the body including maintaining healthy skin and hair. Other vitamins needed for skin health besides the B-Complex include; Vitamins A, E, D, K and the Essential Fatty Acids.

Skin Ailments

Skin conditions are common with GIS. A full range of ailments may be experienced from mouth blisters, rashes, acne, psoriasis and eczema. A cluster of blistery irruptions called Dermatitis Herpetiformis (DH) can be observed anywhere on the torso, back or limbs especially at the joints such as knees and elbows. This flare-up on the skin is caused by an immune response to gluten from the IgA (part of the immune system) attracting WBC (White Blood Cells – infection fighters) which clusters in areas forming the small blisters the size of a pea or larger. At times the DH, also called Celiac Skin is confused for an attack of bug bites. If taking the B-Complex clears the condition you can connect the outbreak directly to GIS. Also, a change in pigment color on the skin with irregular darkening or ulceration in the mouth, patches of dry skin on the elbows and knees all relate to a Vitamin B deficiency.

Research published in 2008 relating B12 and skin conditions showed that even when no Anemia is present a B12 deficiency may still exist. Conducted at the University of Chennai in India researchers revealed that the normal range for B12 was 132 – 875 pmol / L. Even a 19 point reduction allowed skin conditions of hyper-pigmentation of dark skin patches around the toes and fingers to develop. Other skin abnormalities they saw with low B12 levels included Vitiligo (white spots on the skin), angular stomatitis (inflammation of the mucus tissue at the corner of the mouth) and hair changes. They stated that many other skin lesions that would not clear with any other treatment resolved in just weeks of B12 injections of 1,000 mcg.

Both B12 and B-Complex are grossly undersupplied in the U.S. and in other developed countries especially within vegetarian and malnourished populations. Several reasons account for the deficiency including the fact that they are water soluble nutrients that do not store up in the body. They are also heat sensitive and cooking, transportation and storage can destroy much of its nutritional value. Because of these factors and GIS deficiencies replenishing supplies are recommended on a daily basis. Best food sources are eggs, cheese, dairy, meat, liver, fish and nutritional yeast. Leafy greens, Spirulina (algae), sprouts and nuts and seeds are also good sources of the B-Complex but fall short in B12. Miso paste and other fermented soy products contain some B12 yet cannot be relied upon for quality absorbable sources as with animal products. My suggestion is to strive for variety in your diet whenever possible and take B-Complex supplements regardless of your orientation.

Research confirms that when supplementing with B vitamins in order to avoid and reverse deficiencies you must always take a B-Complex as a base - then add the separate individual B vitamin as with Folic Acid or B12 as desired. Testing through the traditional blood test for B12 deficiency will not give reliable levels of B12 in the cells. You may request a more specific test if you are experiencing symptoms as outlined in this chapter. Plasma testing has proven to be more accurate because this test reveals what level of B12 that has actually being absorbed into the cell. You can also safely experiment with B supplements to find what level gives you the best health results because they are water soluble and do not build up in the body as with fat soluble vitamins.

Deficiency of B12 Correlates to the Nervous System Mal-Function & More

The B's are directly related to the health of the *Nervous System*. The Nervous System weaves throughout the entire body and is involved in every function of digestion and elimination, walking and related conditions like Restless Leg Syndrome and very pertinent to mental health as discussed. Overeating in carbohydrates both the bad and good ones including grains use up the body's B Vitamin stores very quickly therefore the body winds up unable to balance and support a healthy Nervous System. This deficiency results in greater inflammation throughout the body and improper functioning of the muscles contributing to severe constipation, diarrhea for some and countless other health challenges that so many people experience with GIS. Review Chapter 6 to learn about Candida Albicans ability to block absorption of B-Complex.

Interestingly a deficiency of *B Vitamins* is primarily why certain people claim to be accident prone and clumsy which is due to the reduction in the Nervous System to function properly. Diminished reflex response, sensory perception, difficulty walking and talking, jerking limbs, memory loss, weakness, fatigue, constipation, insomnia, disorientation, impaired touch or pain perception, neuropathy and burning of the mouth are all due in part to B-Complex and *B12* deficiencies.

A lack of B12 can also manifest in nervousness, neuritis, unpleasant body odor, menstrual disturbances and mental deterioration. Psychosis, depression and dementia are all related to B12 and B-Complex deficiency. The ravages of alcoholism is brought on by many nutritional deficiencies yet the failing mental capacity, fluid build-up and poor walking ability is largely attributed to the lack of B12 and B-Complex. Permanent brain and nerve damage can develop if the deficiencies are not corrected. Research confirms that you cannot regain or retain mental health without a good supply of B12 and B-Complex in the body.

EFA's

Every cell of the body requires the *Essential Fatty Acid* (EFA) Complex which has five fractions yet primarily includes the *Omega-6* and *Omega-3 Fatty Acids*. This core nutrient complex is highlighted in this chapter because of the critical role to the health of the brain and body. Some experts have proposed that 85% of the population is lacking the required amounts of EFA's to thrive and prevent disease.

The EFA's cannot be produced in the body therefore they must also be replenished, as with the other essential core nutrients, on a regular basis through diet or supplementing. They are found in foods both from animal and plant sources however people tend to over consume in the Omega-6 Fatty Acids present in vegetable oils and grains and do not receive enough of the valuable Omega-3's that are required to flourish both mentally and physically !

Excellent dietary choices for the Omega-3's are found in fish, seafood and fish oil products that come with the secondary fractions of EPA and DHA. One must consume very large amounts of vegetable sources of Omega 3's that include flax and walnuts to produce even a fraction of the EPA and DHA received from fatty fish. One of the most important reasons for consuming the Omega-3 Fatty Acids lie in the function of EPA and DHA reviewed in more detail in the HIGHLIGHT section of Chapter 5. Experts suggest individuals to strive for 2,000 mg of EPA and DHA each day with a total of approximately 3,000 – 4,000 of Omega-3's to even out the deficiencies. These fatty acids are key nutrients to healthy nerve transmission and thought processes from the brain throughout the entire Nervous System and back again via the neurotransmitters. To optimize brain function and decrease inflammation, anxiety, depression and other psychosis one must optimize the Omega-3 Fatty Acids, EPA and DHA from all sources. EFA's are also necessary to experience; energy, good memory, healthy heart and cardiovascular health, good circulation, immune strength and balance, reduction in pain, fertility, youthful vibrant skin, longevity, reduction in hyperactivity and even healthy hormones!

Protein

Protein may sound commonly boring yet we fall apart one cell at a time without enough. If the body's metabolism does not have an adequate supply it will slowly come to a painful halt. Next to water, protein is the most plentiful substance in the body. Besides being the main building material it serves as a source for heat and energy.

Humans must have a good supply of the essential building blocks from protein called *amino acids*. There are 8 - 9 essential amino acids isolated from protein foods and food supplements that we require in order to furnish the body with the "Complete Protein" it demands. Only through consuming *complete* and *undenatured* protein, meaning the protein is still viable and intact, can the body make the hundreds of *specialized protein compounds* it needs. Chapter 7 reviews the requirement of a Vegetarian diet to complete the protein and also the value of incorporating a variety of different protein foods for everyone.

A partner in mental health and often undersupplied by children and adults the "PRO" in protein means number one. The name designates the immense importance it plays in building every cell of the 100 trillions of body cells that make up the tissue groups and organs of the body. Besides being responsible for building specialized proteins it makes enzymes, hormones, antibodies and digestive juices that run all the metabolic systems of the body. When the body has enough of its essential amino acid building blocks it will also build sufficient blood cells critical for the transport of oxygen and also build each component of the immune system (with the help from the ECN co-factors).

Besides supplying the body with a variety of protein sources the National Research Council recommends the daily level be .45 grams of protein per pound of body weight. A typical range of protein intake may fall between 30 – 65% of the body weight in grams per day. This equation suggests that the average 150 pound person consume 50 – 75 grams of protein daily. Just take your body weight and divide it in two for the daily protein target for each person. With increased stress and higher daily demands, hard physical labor, athletic performance or post-surgery or illness the body requires extra protein sometimes reaching as much as 100 grams per day. Make certain you are supplying your body and the children under your care with adequate protein every day. A variety of both plant and animal protein is always a good goal. Do your best as well to not overcook your foods which can destroy protein (amino acids) and other valuable nutrients. A food thermometer is very helpful to monitor the cooking time to assure safety with viable protein in each meal.

Researchers have found that essential enzymes and hormones that are manufactured from protein are responsible to carry on thousands of metabolic processes each day. Many of these are often not even being made in the body due to a lack of raw material (protein) and poor metabolism. A good example of the requirement of *protein specialization* is with B12 absorption. The digestive process requires three specialized proteins in its five step process to achieve absorption of B12 into the cells with one of them being the illusive *intrinsic factor*. It is no wonder people are developing massive B12 deficiencies!

A lack of protein can cause symptoms of fatigue, lack of vigor and stamina. Also, mental slowness and depression accompanied with muscle weakness and poor resistance to infection and slow healing can all be due to low protein intake. Stunted growth may go unnoticed in children along with unusually slow development and a loss of hair and pigment color with low intake of protein. Swelling of joints and acute edema (swelling of the abdomen) and a fatty liver may also develop decreasing overall body metabolism even further.

On the other hand excessive protein especially coming from meat in the diet displaces the quantity of valuable nutrient dense foods from vegetables and complex carbohydrates that bring invaluable health support. The high saturated fat in meat can also add to higher LDL cholesterol and excess calories contributing to obesity when overindulging in meat. Excessive meat also increases the body's Vitamin A requirement diminishing eye sight and tips the body's pH into a higher acidity range. See Chapter 6 to review the importance of pH balance in order to avoid Gout, Reflux and Arthritis. Lastly research has found that when people eat high protein it causes a depletion of calcium and other minerals leading to osteoporosis.

Each of these four brain nutrients just reviewed are referred to as *Essential Core Nutrients (ECN)* because we cannot live without them. Learning what happens when a deficiency develops and the myriad of important functions they provide to the brain and body's metabolism is important. Hopefully this knowledge will motivate your actions to follow the GIS Diet eating foods and taking supplements that contain these ECN's as we strive towards optimum health and longevity. Chapter 8 gives more information about the value of the ECN nutrients along with Herbs and Special Needs Supplements (SNS) for wellness.

Richard's Story

This somewhat frantic soul called my office one afternoon with a straight forward question. He had read an article I wrote in a magazine on Aloe Vera helping digestion and wondered how it worked with Reflux which he battled. Richard had a refreshing innocence about him and as he spoke I heard some verbal stammering as if he had Parkinson's disease. He slowly took notes very eager to learn about health stating proudly that he did all of his own food preparation.

As we talked I mentioned that leaving gluten and gluten triggers out of his diet would reduce his Reflux symptoms because it lowered inflammation throughout the entire body including the liver. I told him that it was important to understand that the GIS Diet was going to be the opposite of what he had previously learned about nutrition up until now.

It sounds very kooky, I said, but it is necessary to leave the whole grain cereals and breads alone. I gave him the other common GIS Triggers to avoid which included supplement capsules and soft gels, oatmeal which is a big no-no and shared that even brown rice could be a challenge with his body at this time.

As he relaxed I told him gluten could cause some neurological malfunction as with his shakiness that I detected in his voice. He was surprised to learn this and he said, "No kidding?" "I have been living with a Parkinson's diagnosis for about three years and noticed that after I eat a sandwich made from my favorite whole grain bread my body shakes so badly that I have to stop eating all together and lay down."

I could tell from Richard's acknowledgment in our conversation that he was eager to get started with the GIS Program. Richard was ready to reduce his symptoms from all of his maladies and had not previously made the connection of gluten to Parkinson's. From his excitement I didn't think compliance was going to be an issue for Richard.

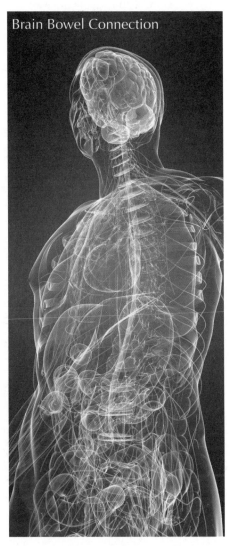
Brain Bowel Connection

The Neuromuscular System includes the Central Nervous System (CNS) and the Peripheral Nervous System (PNS) in the body. Each system is involved and intertwined with mental disorders and physical disease that includes; seizures, epilepsy, tremors, an irregular and racing heartbeat, walking, talking and thinking disorders. Keeping the inflammation down in the body and reinstating health balance through the GIS Program optimizes every function in the body including the Neuromuscular System. I find that even the tendency of a lazy drooping eye responds positively once a person adheres to the GIS guidelines.

The PNS and the CNS is involved in neuromuscular disorders yet also in the reactions of the brain. Scientific research along with clinical observation abounds with confirmation of the Brain-Bowel connection and GIS.

Research Confirms the Brain-Bowel Connection:

- 1966, Dr. F.C. Dohan, Acta Psychiatry Scandinavia; Research points to cereal grains and milk being dietary factors in the intestinal brain connection with mentally disturbed people.
- 1978, Dr. Bruscainos, Italian Neurological Clinic of Naples Reported; Schizophrenics show some form of intestinal disease from psycho toxic factors produced in the intestine.
- 1978, Dr. H. Baruk, French Scientist Summarized 50 yrs of Research in Schizophrenia and Mental Disorders; He stated that one must consider the majority of psychoses or neurosis as reactions to biological factors which are very often digestive in origin.
- 1981, Dr. Dohan, Eastern PA, Psychiatric Institute, USA, Biological Psychiatry: vol.16,no.11; Writes about researcher Cooke who found that a rigorous gluten free diet resulted in the disappearance of Schizophrenia as well as Celiac symptoms in those with both diseases. Dr. Dohan stated he found patients adhering to this diet experienced a 100% faster release from an institution. At three months and also at one year all of the patients

who were followed and complied continued improvements in their overall mental health.

- 1982, Dr. F.C. Dohan, New England Journal of Medicine; Declares his observations of the ill effects of milk on mental health with patients living with Celiac disease.

Compliance is Everything!

I know what some of you may be thinking. How do you get compliance from people with advanced mental disorders? My answer is to make improvements where you can and teach by your own example of following the program. People learn by observing and then experimenting in their own lives. Permanent change occurs slowly with most people. Strive for improvement not perfection!

Remember that with GIS less of a trigger is best. You may wish to review Ch. 4 that gives all of the potential triggers that cause GIS. One of my guidelines is to accentuate the positive with adding the GIS supplements as soon as possible to achieve some quick success. The reality is that the diet may take months and even years to evolve into the 80% or better goal in ones daily regimen.

Mental illness is the most common ailment in the world today yet the least talked about. My hope is that GIS will shed light for mental wellness in the future however we ultimately do not have power over anyone but ourselves especially with certain types of neurosis. This includes our co-workers, relatives and close friends. We can make the best attempt possible to teach the path to physical and mental health freedom while finding as much joy in our relationships regardless of another's compliance. Of course, raising younger children allows parents to incorporate the GIS Program in the easiest of situations. However, change does not come easy for older children, teenagers and adults. Even though many will choose the healthier way and have success, some unfortunate individuals will not survive their own demise.

Once the body slows and even stops the inflammation from GIS and begins to physically feel better, each person has a new challenge and that is to learn better and more effective communication skills that may have been skipped along the way of living with mental illness. A variety of books and programs are available today to teach individuals how to relearn new people skills of talking, listening and responding to others in our lives. One author I find very insightful and helpful to gain mental perspective is Richard Carlson, PhD. He has several books that are enlightening including; *Don't Sweat the Small Stuff and it's all small stuff* and another *You Can Feel Good Again!* I find that just when I think I have learned all I need in communication skills something new crops up that ultimately allows me to learn more about myself and experience more joy and playfulness while living within a family, the workplace and in a community.

Requirements for Healthy Mental Behavior & Happiness:
- *Physical Health Balance;* Nutrition, Glandular & Liver Function, Lowering Toxins & Chemicals, Opportunistic Microbes and more.
- *Environmental Balance*; External Toxins, Pollutants & EMF Fields and more.
- *Reduction in All Inflammation*; GIS, Organic Disease & Pre-Mature Aging.
- *Effective Communication Skills;* Appropriate, Effective, Emotional, Spiritual & Enjoyable (fun), Love

Nutrition cannot be overlooked or down-played as to the importance for supporting mental and physical health in the body. Nutrition is required for both structural health of every cell in the body and to allow the metabolism of our anatomy to work the way it was designed. Thousands of enzymes and catalysts are needed to run the body on a daily basis through approximately 21 essential core nutrients plus an array of minerals to build the cells and tissue systems that allow the transmission of the nerves to signal each body part to work properly called neurotransmission. It is a complex network that is disrupted by poor nutrition, inflammation and environmental factors. Research has confirmed that even our daily thoughts can contribute to how well the body performs its task and heightens overall health. We each have the opportunity to think positively and take health action in our lives regardless of the negative and or lack of support we may receive from our health professionals. You must take an active role in your own health or be willing to live with marginal health potential!

Psyched Out!

Just a few years ago I was flying on a plane and in the seat next to me was a professor of psychiatry from a prominent university in southern California for three whole hours. We got to conversing and I asked her how nutrition was being incorporated into the curriculum? Get ready for a shock! She stated that nutrition was not a subject included in any of the courses! So help me God how can we still be living in the dark ages yet just beginning the 21st century?

Nutrition has been linked to behavior for as long as I can remember. Who doesn't know that when children eat candy they can become hyper and misbehave? Every couple knows to not talk about explosive topics before dinner because both people's blood sugar is at an all time low and emotions can get out of control! Common sense and science must be brought together for our societies greatest good!

Feingold Diet

Researchers have found value in many nutritionally based diets over the years to include the Feingold diet introduced over thirty years ago. This program connects behavior, physical and neurological symptoms to; chemicals of artificial color, flavorings, preservatives, Aspartame (artificial sweetener) and certain salicylates in food products. Moderation of sugar, chocolate and soft drinks are advocated on this program yet not eliminated, although some believers in the program have been surprised at this allowance. The diet accents good wholesome foods omitting certain synthetic chemicals like FD&C and D&C coloring and other additives found in processed foods and the followers rave about the success they have experienced with their children's improved behavior.

Fortunately for Americans, as ridiculous as this may sound, it is not against the law to eat the foods of your choice! You can begin to improve your mental and physical health today from any of the disease conditions you may be living with just by starting to follow the GIS Diet. You have my personal guarantee that following it for 6 weeks to 3 months you will experience better health. The next step on your health path will be to decide with your physician and health professionals how to reduce your pharmaceutical drug intake wherever possible. Don't rush this step yet when the need is no longer required it is good to stop the drugs. Besides reducing toxicity into the body for many people they will save a substantial amount of money from the purchasing of prescription drugs!

The title of this book, **Beyond Gluten Intolerance**, is referencing the inflammation chain of events that develop from gluten and gluten triggers that allow for the opportunity of mental illness and other disorders to develop. In fact, let me be the first to make this bold statement, I truly believe that all disease development in the body including autoimmune conditions relate to the GIS predisposition along with genetic weakness!

Many people are joining this chorus because they have been following the GIS Program and are experiencing disease resolving in their body with each passing day. I am now shouting it, because without a doubt whether improvement is from the more expected bowel disease of IBS and IBD to the more advanced conditions of Rosacea, Eczema and even Diabetes, mental illness and more - people are finding all DIS-EASE conditions are improving with the GIS Health Program.

Listed in the GIS Glossary are small irritating conditions like coughing, bed wetting, nightmares, gas, constipation, acne and depression side by side the more advanced diseases. They include; asthma, osteoporosis, auto-immune, bipolar, schizophrenia and even cancer. All conditions and disease respond excellently following the health program outlined in chapters 6, 7 and 8. Remember to give yourself the time your biochemistry requires to regenerate and regain health. It does not happen overnight yet the process is absolutely certain!

The connection to all disease has become extremely clear in my work with GIS. I hope it is becoming easier for you to understand how the CNS connects to a reduced function of all the glands of the body. Another analogy that may help is looking at the Nervous System likened to an electric cord that plugs in the organs to function! People are only as healthy as their organs and glands and when they under-function due to inflammation and malnutrition all other disease conditions will present more symptoms.

Just reflect upon your own family tree for a moment and the variety of diseases your relatives have experienced. I believe you will begin to see just how penetrating gluten intolerance has affected generation upon generation. Regardless of your age you can experience improved health ahead. The scientific community has confirmed much of the work I have presented here with the Gluten Inflammatory Syndrome (GIS) thus far in both the psychological and the physiology field as it relates to bowel health. Modern research is continuing to discover the catalyst of autoimmune and its relationship to many diseases such as Asthma, Multiple Sclerosis and Rheumatoid Arthritis.

Auto-immune disease arises when the body's immune system becomes overactive (as with GIS) and attacks healthy cells of the body. In other words the body attacks itself including groups of tissues and organs creating more inflammatory diseases. Crohn's, Celiac Disease, Ulcerative Colitis and Pernicious Anemia, pertinent to our discussion in this chapter, are all accepted auto-immune diseases. Shockingly there are also over eighty other diseases that have been confirmed to have strong auto-immune factors to include; Rheumatoid Arthritis, Psoriasis, Schizophrenia, Hashimoto's Thyroiditis, Interstitial Cystitis, Type I Diabetes, Lupus and MS of course. Even Sjogren's that manifest with dry eyes and body fluids and other miscellaneous skin and connective tissue diseases that so many people suffer with needlessly today has an auto-immune stimuli.

GIS III Theory: Inflammation, Malnutrition & Toxicity Share in Disease Development

Genetics has its role in disease development yet keep in mind it is only considered sixth on the list of factors that allow any disease to develop in the body according to good scientific evidence. It is important to understand that the new developing science of "Genomics" have proven that by using nutritional therapy which includes the ECN's of B Vitamins, EFA's, Minerals, Antioxidants and an array of Phyto-nutrients, all working together can repair damaged DNA. By repairing the DNA the researchers have found that the disease process can be reversed! World class scientists have confirmed that DNA damage precedes cancer and other disease conditions of the body without much exception.

Richard's story gave us a glimpse into how GIS plays a factor in causing more symptoms of an existing disease. Thinking a little deeper, who is to say that if Richard had been following the GIS Program preventatively that he just may have been able to avoid Parkinson's disease altogether?

The connection and relationship of auto-immune to GIS has been clear in my work for decades and I am convinced it is not that I am such an exceptional researcher to have discovered the truth. Why then you may ask if this is the truth about health - why has it not been shared with the public? I believe the deception has been disguised in the perpetual lie that begins in the doctor's office. The lie is that aging and disease cannot be slowed down or reversed. This is a complete falsehood and I believe that it has been perpetuated by a cohort from big business, the medical community and some of the governmental agencies at the top.

Raising the Veil of Deception

The denial of therapeutic nutrition by our medical institutions has been pervasive throughout the history of bowel disease, as I have brought light to this fact in the previous chapters. And let's acknowledge all the rest of the deceit that has taken place with every other disease for this discussion! The challenge at hand is that most Allopathic mainstream doctors tend to trivialize or avoid the importance of nutrition and health and its relationship to disease which must stop.

Some physicians are beginning to come clean to the fact that they have not been taught nutrition in medical schools. Because of the thousands upon thousands of peer reviewed research papers now proving the relationship of nutrition and disease resolution medical personnel are practically being forced to accept the role nutrition plays in healthcare. Vitamin D3 is an excellent example of the reluctance of our medical community to drop the pretense and embrace therapeutic nutrition needed by everyone. The research was becoming so redundant over a period of 4 – 5 years confirming the value of increasing D3 by supplementation to the patient that the medical community had to accept it at last!

The abundance of scientific support of dietary nutrients as a factor in auto-immune conditions and other disease like Diabetes, Cancer and Cardiovascular Disease has been strong yet the AMA have kept a death grip on their pharmaceutical drug protocols. After years of feeling perplexed over why nutrition was not getting its due respect I am realizing that the doctors of our world are not stupid people as it has been portrayed. Our professional matrix of health providers on a whole are very astute, capable and intelligent beings. Then if it is not a question of intelligence or knowledge necessarily then what was the reason that good nutritional science has not being incorporated into our medical model? Finally the answer came as to where the challenge lies. Health has been kept in its own separate box because of the tremendous monies tied up in drug treatments and surgical procedures for countless conditions of the body delaying the lifting of the veil of deceit.

What a wrench into the AMA engine nutrition would be if the masses were actually educated to know the truth about food and food supplements and their regenerative powers! When you mix the high emotions of being diagnosed with a disease state - be it Lupus, bowel disease or even Cancer - a roller coaster of confusion and fear can begin the arsenal of pharmaceutical drugs prescribed instead of embracing aggressive therapeutic nutrition.

Absurdly, the chosen treatment for auto-immune disease is toxic drugs that break down a person's immune system so it cannot function.

This treatment helps temporarily however it leaves the individual vulnerable to every other disease that comes along! A look into mental illness brings up the archaic modality now being used again for acute mental psychosis in the 21st century. Some of you may have guessed it – Electric Shock Therapy! It didn't work effectively a hundred years ago and now in such a scientifically drenched society I am more than shocked that intelligent doctors have brought this tortuous treatment back for our loved ones again! Stop the masquerade, I beg you AMA!

On the other hand it would be very irresponsible to not recognize the positive contribution that pharmaceutical drugs bring – of course! Yes, I understand that advanced disease exists and under certain situations of auto-immune, cancer and other disorders it may be prudent, once a person gets in trouble to use pharmaceutical drugs - temporarily. Yet to use them long term or in excessive strength, other than in a life threatening situation of course, can bring damaging side effects with limited value. Each of you must always ask yourself, "What is the benefit to risk ratio of a drug or therapy?"

A small but growing segment of physicians are joining the modern "Integrative Medicine" movement to tell the truth as they learn it. I personally invite all of the medical community to join the health revolution so that each of you can become the healthiest you can be and fight to integrate therapeutic health into your medical practices. You can count on the fact that all roads lead back to health in achieving optimal mental and physical Well - Being!

Common GIS Symptoms and Causes	
Symptoms	**Cause**
Bloating & Gas	Poor Digestion, Constipation, Detoxification
Headache & Flu Symptoms	Lymph Congested, Detoxification, Herpes, Viral
Herpes & Cold Sore Outbreak	High L- Arginine Foods, pH Acidity
Fatigue, Dizziness, Pain in Muscles	Anemia, B12 Deficiency, Herpes, Candida & Blood Loss
Depressed, Anxiety & Anger	Blood Sugar, Viral Infections, GIS
Poor Walking, Speech, Heart Palpitation, Feeling Cold	Poor Circulation, Reduced CNS Function, Mal-Nutrition, Para-Thyroid, GIS
Hair Loss, Fatigue, Depression & Weight Gain or Loss	Low Thyroid, Environmental Toxicity, Blood Sugar Imbalance
Excess Mucus & Coughing	Infection, Bowel Health, CNS-GIS
Slow Healing, Lack of Taste & Smell	Mal-nutrition, Poor Digestion, Candida, Low Immune Function
Sweats Without Fever	Blood Sugar, Secondary Viral Conditions, Thyroid
Failing Health	Low Immune System, Candida, Mal-Nutrition
Not Following GIS Zone Diet 1, 2 or 3	Denial, Lack of Support, Addictions

Glossary of Conditions
Related to GIS - Gluten Inflammatory Syndrome

Accident Prone – People that tend to be accident prone often coin themselves as clumsy. The medical term for this is "Ataxia" meaning bad balance. A large percentage of the lack in muscle control of the body is due to an imbalance of the Nervous System affecting a person's walk, talk and proper body function. Another factor affecting equilibrium can come from a sinus infection or low level congestion of the inner ear. See

Detoxification, Blood Sugar and Candida section in Chapter 6. *Special Needs:* B12, B-Complex, EFA's including Flax & Fish Oil, Minerals - Calcium, Magnesium, Zinc and Daily Greens.

A.D.H.D / A.D.D. – Attention Deficient Hyperactivity Disorder affects many children and even adults. Often the diet will contain a large percentage of wheat, milk, carbohydrates and sugary foods that trigger GIS and hyperactivity. These foods prevent the ability to focus and maintain proper attention and operate on task for work or play. See Ch. 6, Blood Sugar and Addictions. Dyslexia may also be present and is reviewed in this section. Following the Zone 2 & 3 Diet in Chapter 7 and eliminating corn for some people can offer a great head start plus adding the supplements. *Special Needs:* EFA's – Fish Oil (DHA), B-Complex, Aloe Vera, Ginkgo Biloba, 5HTP, Protein, Multiple Vitamin & Mineral (or take separate) and Prevagen (See Ch. 8).

Allergies – The word allergy is often misused to describe symptoms that may be caused from a minor cold or GIS reactions. A true allergy response occurs from certain food proteins to include; eggs, milk, nuts, mold, chocolate and other stimuli in the environment that can be measured in blood tests through an IgA marker or other methods that are even more accurate (See Enterolabs in Reference). Reacting to foods with a heightened immune response even an extreme anaphylactic tissue swelling response can be complicated yet very treatable when applying health. GIS inflammatory reactions may add to protein allergies yet as explained in Ch. 2 they are different and come from the poor digestion of sugars located in the grains, milk and refined sugar. With GIS you may experience a full range of symptoms from fatigue, mental confusion, hives and skin rashes plus digestive disturbances. Whether an allergy or strictly GIS symptoms the protocol is the same. The goal is to proceed in cleansing the body and rebuilding the systems to function without inflammation. Review Detoxification and Candida Albicans in Chapter 6. *Special Needs:* Vitamin C plus Bioflavonoids 500 – 3,000 mg, Aloe Vera, Probiotics, B-Complex, Multiple Vitamin & Mineral, Zinc 50 mg., EFA, Protein, Daily Greens and Liquid Sovereign Silver.

Anemia – Fatigue, headaches, dizziness, chest pains, shortness of breath, tingling along with problems concentrating and constipation can all be associated to anemia. It is generally associated to poor absorption of certain required nutrients that are necessary to carry proper oxygen throughout the body by the blood hemoglobin. B12 metabolism is disrupted with GIS and is an essential vitamin to build blood with sufficient protein, Folic Acid, Iron, Vitamin C and D to avoid anemia. Advanced bowel disease can also cause blood loss resulting in anemia. Eating organic liver is very nourishing to build the blood plus beans, greens, berries, raisins and dates in moderation. *Special Needs:* B-Complex, Methyl B12 (injections or sublingual), Multiple Vitamin & Mineral, Protein, Iron, EFA, Daily Greens and CoQ10 Enzyme.

Asthma – Asthma entails the inflammation of the lungs causing a bronchospasm related to auto immune factors occurring with GIS. Wheezing, coughing, chest tightness and shortness of breath symptoms can be reduced through optimizing digestion and bowel health by making dietary adjustments and minimizing triggers as outlined on the GIS program. One of the important triggers causing inflammation in the body is the imbalance of Essential Fatty Acids (EFA's) having too high of the Omega 6 Fatty Acids and a low level of Omega 3's. Increase the Omega 3's to the same level of Omega 6's ingested daily to lower inflammation. Junk food and fried foods are sources of excessive vegetable Omega 6 Fatty Acids eaten by many people. Other triggers heightening Asthma symptoms can be any of the primary or secondary GIS triggers including; whole grains, gluten flours, cow's milk, refined sugar, fried foods, junk foods, molds, environmental – dust, mites, animal dander, pollen, grasses and other chemicals. Sunshine is an important remedy. Strive to get 30-45 minutes of rays daily or to use a "Full Spectrum Light" to receive both UVA and the important UVB rays needed to make D3 in the skin. Often overlooked is the importance of keeping the bowels regular. Aloe Vera is a special herb for the lungs and regularity of the bowels containing five natural anti-inflammatory agents to ease symptoms. Heating Aloe Vera on a stove and safely breathing the vapors is an herbal remedy to help open up the airways. Drinking a quality Aloe Vera containing the yellow sap has remarkably lowered symptoms. Some individuals even find that drinking coffee is also helpful and tends to relax the constrictions of the lungs as well. Nasal Spray (wash) with Xylitol by Xlear has given relief from Asthma symptoms for adults and children as a preventative exercise. The challenge is that most people are not motivated to act preventatively and use the spray as recommended 2 – 3 times per day unless they have experienced several scary episodes of an Asthma Attack! See Candida and Addictions in Chapter 6 for more preventative steps. Hydrate the body with quality water or herb teas regularly. *Special Needs:* Aloe Vera, EFA's – Fish Oil 3,000 mg including Vitamin A & D, B-Complex, Vitamin C, Bioflavonoids, Vitamin E, Magnesium, Greens, Water, Picnogenol (antioxidant), NAC, Liquid Sovereign Silver, Nasal Spray (Xlear) and Grapefruit Seed Extract. *Note:* Always seek and follow medical advice when breathing is labored.

Athletic Performance – To optimize one's physical abilities of any sport and decrease injury, experiment with the GIS program. It assures better coordination of the muscles and brain performance plus stamina through optimizing cellular nutrition and blood sugar support during recovery. Antioxidants are especially valuable to increase immunity and minimize the cellular tissue damage created through stressing the body from strenuous exercise. *Special Needs:* Protein, Multiple Vitamin & Mineral, Silica, Fish Oils, Vitamin E, Alpha Lipoic Acid, Daily Greens, Minerals (electrolytes), Ginseng and Aloe Vera.

Autism – Special needs children and adults have a history of digestive insufficiency and require exceptional health to compensate, balance and optimize motor skills. Support of detoxification, digestive health and the Central Nervous System are special focus areas. *Special Needs:* EFA's – Flax and Fish Oil, Aloe Vera, Multiple Vitamin & Mineral High Potency, Daily Greens, Protein, Nutritional Yeast, Free-Form Amino Acids, Prevagen and Sunshine.

Auto Immune Conditions – All auto-immune and inflammatory conditions of the body respond well to the GIS program including; skin eruptions and redness, neurological and immune system imbalance. Research shows there are over eighty auto-immune conditions diagnosed including; Lupus, Multiple Sclerosis (MS), Parkinson's, Rheumatoid Arthritis (RA), Asthma, Eczema, Psoriasis, Rosacea, Sjogren's (dryness of body fluids) and more. Detoxification, Candida and pH balancing are all required (Ch. 6). *Special Needs:* Aloe Vera and Pine Bark (both contain Phytosterols), EFA's - Flax and Fish Oils, Barley Greens (Daily Greens), Probiotics, Vitamin E, and Alpha Lipoic Acid.

Arthritis – Arthritis is a family of conditions including; Rheumatoid Arthritis (RA), Osteoarthritis and Osteoporosis. An important fact that is supported by research is that the body has the ability to reverse bone loss without medication. To do so one must lower the percentage of meat consumption and it is critical to stop refined sugar in the diet. Also important is to balance any autoimmune response in the body towards the Thyroid gland (see Chapter 6 Glandular Health). This is helped through following the GIS Program that will reverse malnutrition preventing further bone loss. *Note:* Study the side effects of bone loss medication before deciding on the best route to take. Always make the required dietary improvements regardless of your decisions and incorporate an exercise program that includes weight-bearing resistance training. Minerals play such an important role in avoiding Arthritis symptoms to include the simple addition of taking an alfalfa supplement or formulas containing it (Ch. 8). Some other very interesting research has been conducted in human trials on the Type II Collagen lowering inflammation and joint pain especially through the addition of a liquid product made by the *Bronson Laboratories* by the name of Vital-3. Following the GIS Diet and taking a couple of Special Needs Supplements with the basic supplements will definitely provide big improvements however give it a few months for regeneration. Also review Addictions, Candida and Digestion in Chapter 6. *Special Needs:* Minerals, EFA- Fish Oils including A & D, Vitamin C & Bioflavonoids 1 – 3,000 mg, B-Complex & B12, Aloe Vera, Wobenzymes, Alfalfa and Daily Greens, Type II Cartilage - Vital 3, Chondroitin, Glucosamine, MSM and Hydroxyapatite.

Bed Wetting & Incontinence – Loss of muscle control in children and adults is due to the Nervous System decline and poor absorption of minerals including Calcium and Magnesium. Follow the GIS Diet guidelines in Chapter 7. Hormone replacement may be necessary when the condition is in adults especially natural Estrogen. *Special Needs:* Children's Multiple Vitamin & Mineral (no gelatin), Magnesium, Fish Oils, Aloe Vera, Probiotics, Daily Greens and Bananas.

Bladder & Urinary Infections – It is very important to get off sugar and alcohol and eat "Low Glycemic" foods to reduce Candida fungus often involved in infections of the urethra. Also see I.C. in this section viewed as an auto-immune condition. Review Candida Albicans and pH in Chapter 6. *Special Needs:* Probiotics by *Dr. Ohhira*, FemDolphilus by *Jarrow*, Daily Greens, Fish Oils including Vitamin A & D, Herbs; Uva-Ursi, Chamomile and Aloe Vera.

Boils – Constipation and a poor diet overloads the body's Lymphatic System. GIS adds to this challenge requiring Detoxification of toxins accumulating in the body, coupled with the added nutritional deficiencies. Some waste products attempt to leave the body through pores in the skin causing the boil which is extremely painful until drainage occurs. Hardened waste can also develop attempting to leave the body called a cyst which can linger for long periods of time. A poor functioning Immune System may compound this condition with varying degrees of infection developing in the boils. Hidradenitis Suppurativa (HS) is a type of skin disease developing boils primarily in the groin and underarm areas from small to the size of lemons in some people. All boils including the HS type respond with 100% resolution following the GIS Diet and protocol. See Chapter 6, Detoxification and Addiction. *Special Needs:* Probiotics, Aloe Vera, EFA – Fish Oil and Flax, Multiple Vitamin & Mineral (or taken separately), DetoxPlus Aloe Vera and Daily Greens. Topical application of Skin Gel by *Aloe Life* is supportive.

Bone & Cartilage Loss – GIS can lead to early bone loss and cartilage degeneration. Also common is the "S" curvature of the back bone known as Scoliosis. Reducing sugar is paramount along with proper levels of

Vitamin D3 and Minerals available by following the GIS Diet. Review Thyroid, Auto-Immune and Addiction sections in Chapter 6. Stop eating refined sugar; reduce meat consumption and increase vegetables and fruits by following the GIS Diet. *Special Needs:* Aloe Vera, Alfalfa, Enzymes, EFA's - Cod Liver Oil with A & D (Nordic Naturals), Vitamin C and Bioflavonoids, Vitamin E, B-Complex, Liquid Minerals and or Hydroxyapatite, Type II Cartilage (Vital 3), Calcium, Magnesium, Zinc Citrate and regular Weight-Bearing exercise.

Brain Function – All neurological disorders including healthy thought patterns may be disrupted with GIS advancement (Ch. 5). A condition of slow thinking called "Brain Fog" is a common experience with Candida Albicans overgrowth (See Ch.6). This spacey-ness or brain fog, may accompany a slower overall function or hypo-activity noticeable in Autism and other chronic illnesses. Dementia and Alzheimer's disease will also respond to the suggested protocol. *Special Needs:* Multiple Vitamin & Mineral, Protein & Amino Acids, EFA's - Fish Oil with A & D by *Nordic Naturals*, B-Complex, B12, Ginkgo Biloba, 5HTP, GABA, St. John's Wort by *Herb-Pharm*, Prevagen and Antioxidants.

Bruising of the Skin – Anemia is common with GIS and demands a need for increased nutrition of B12, B-Complex, Vitamin C, Bioflavonoids, Folic Acid, Iron and Protein stores (50 grams or more daily). These nutrients must be supplied through diet and supplementation along with supporting digestion with Aloe Vera. B12 injections may also be needed with acute Anemia deficiency. Testing for other disease conditions may be indicated. *Special Needs:* Vitamin C 500 – 3,000 mg, Bioflavonoids, B-Complex and B12.

Cancer – Cancer is a secondary condition following years of GIS, neglect or contamination of cancer causing agents. Researchers estimate that it takes 10 to 20 years for the body to operate at a reduced function allowing Cancer to develop. Toxic chemical poisoning, radiation, smoking, Obesity and excessive stress in one's life can also increase the incidence of cancer development. Scientists now understand that a healthy immune system has the opportunity to reverse Cancer in the body if it is functioning properly and maintains healthy DNA. Accent is on eating foods, drinking purified water and taking supplements that are high in Antioxidants and high ORAC value plus sufficient protein and core nutrients needed to build immune function. See Detoxification in Chapter 6. Nutrition may be integrated with chemotherapy and or radiation and surgical procedures. Note: Do not take extra Vitamin E with hormone sensitive cancers like breast or prostate types. *Special Needs:* Multiple Vitamin & Mineral high potency (or take each core nutrient separately to avoid high Vitamin E). Also include extra B-Complex 50 mg. 2-3, Vitamin C 3,000 mg. Glutathione or NAC, Aloe Vera by *Aloe Life* (See Highlight Ch. 4), Antioxidants, Selenium Yeast, Liquid Sovereign Silver, Herb - Graviola (leaf & stem), Wobenzymes and Probiotics.

Candida Albicans (CA) – CA is one of several fungal infections that may be present in the body due to constipation and poor nutrition. A coated tongue, vaginal and jock itch, skin conditions, advanced chronic fatigue and other illnesses directly relate to CA. Besides blocking absorption of nutrients like B12 and other valuable life supporting elements, Candida fungus can add to the overall inflammation in the body and is a GIS Secondary Trigger. Detoxification is required to right the challenges caused by constipation that often occurs from GIS. The die-off of the fungus will add temporarily to allergy reactions and GI tract symptoms of gas yet will gradually clear especially once regularity returns even if enemas are required (Review Ch. 12). Also, review Detoxification and Candida section in Ch. 6. *Special Needs:* Probiotics, Aloe Vera, Greens, Essential Fatty Acids (from fish oil is best), Biotin, Liquid Silver - Sovereign Silver, Coconut Oil and Caprylic Acid.

Canker Sores – This type of ulcer is generally due to a viral condition that can be sparked by other inflammation in the gut due to GIS triggers and pH imbalance. Keep citrus, tomato, chocolate and L-Arginine foods low in the diet. See pH balance and Virus section in Chapter 6. *Special Needs:* Probiotics, L-Lysine 500 – 3,000 mg daily, Herbs – Topically Aloe Vera Gel (See Reference *Aloe Life* products.) and Lemon Balm and drink Aloe Vera juice.

Cardiovascular Disease (CVD) – Several factors are responsible for the development of CVD yet the best research points to uncontrolled inflammation and dietary factors that result in plaque build-up called Arteriolosclerosis. Clogged arteries from plaque contribute to the incidence of stroke and heart attacks both. Vitamin C, Antioxidants and B-Complex are critical to avoid certain types of strokes. Review the Dean Ornish, MD Diet and Dr. Sinatra's CVD books. See Detoxification, Liver Health and Addictions in Chapter 6. *Note:* The use of statin drugs disrupts the body from utilizing certain core nutrients and decreases the production of CoQ10 in the Liver that relates to walking and neurological mal-function. *Caution:* If taking blood thinners use caution with the addition of Green Supplements that contain Vitamin K. *Special Needs:* B-Complex 50 – 100 mg daily or Nutritional Yeast, EFA's 3,000 mg daily or more - fish oils are best by *Nordic Naturals*, Vitamin C, CoQ10 Enzyme, Garlic by *Kyolic* 1200 mg, Aloe Vera and Antioxidants.

Celiac Sprue – This is the original bowel disease connected to the reaction of wheat gluten. Celiac is traced back to ancient times and has been found to be very under diagnosed due to archaic testing procedures of today. Review Chapter 2 and Chapter 4 Testing and false negatives. *Special Needs:* Probiotics, Aloe Vera and the entire GIS Program.

Chronic Fatigue Syndrome **(CFS)** – Patients may receive a diagnosis of CFS if they have symptoms of pain for at least 3 months. CFS is caused by mal-absorption from all factors stemming from the Candida Albicans fungus overgrowth in the body and other GIS triggers. Most people living with CFS also have viral flare-ups adding to their fatigue. Get off sugar and follow the GIS Diet. See Chapter 6 Addictions, Detoxification, Candida, Viruses and Immune System. *Special Needs:* B12, B-Complex, Free-Form Amino Acids (protein), Multiple Vitamin & Mineral, NAC, CoQ10, EFA's, Probiotics and Minerals especially Magnesium and Daily Greens.

Crohn's Disease (CD) – First isolated by Dr. Crohn's CD is described in length in Chapter 2 and is found primarily in the ascending colon area attributed to wheat gluten and dairy intolerance. Great success is experienced following the GIS Program. *Special Needs:* Probiotics, Aloe Vera and Fish Oil by *Nordic Naturals.*

Colitis – This condition refers to the spasm of the bowel causing diarrhea or Dumping Syndrome. Colitis can be synonymous with gluten intolerance and the GIS program works brilliantly to reverse it! *Special Needs:* Aloe Vera, Probiotics, B-Complex, EFA's and Daily Greens.

Constipation – Slow elimination and constipation develops from the neurological pathway slowing the peristaltic action of the lining cells in the large intestine due to mal-nutrition and GIS. Slow bowels cause waste products to build up in the body and contribute to the liver congestion referred to as Lazy Liver. A sluggish liver causes more skin conditions of every type on the body including Eczema, Psoriasis and Rosacea and poor hormone production. Detoxification is needed see Chapter 6. See Reference section for "Enema" directions as needed. *Special Needs:* Aloe Vera, B-Complex, Probiotics, Fish Oil, Magnesium Glycinate and a Multiple Vitamin & Mineral as tolerated (Ch. 8).

Cough – Excessive and irritating coughing can be brought about by GIS because it creates an overproduction of mucus in the tissues. This heightened irritation response is commonly experienced in the Esophagus (throat) from GIS. This is due to the auto-immune response to gluten and other secondary GIS triggers. The Central Nervous System may be reacting that links to the condition of Mitral Valve spasms. Normal coughing of the body is good to dislodge waste products being eliminated through the lungs but excessive coughing is directly associated with GIS and or a milk allergy. See Constipation and Detoxification sections. People are designed to eliminate waste through the bowels, skin, kidneys and lungs. Hydrate the body with quality water, herbal teas with honey and drinking Aloe Vera. *Note:* If cough does not resolve in a reasonable time seek medical attention for diagnostic support. *Special Needs:* Aloe Vera, Licorice, Chamomile, Pleurisy Root, Lobelia Tincture by *Herb-Pharm* (use as directed), Eucalyptus Oil, Fish Oils including Vitamin A & D, Multiple Vitamin & Mineral and Daily Greens and Vegetable Juice.

Cramping of the Bowel – Bowel distress with IBS or IBD may include cramping along with other symptoms like diarrhea, constipation or intestinal gas causing the intestinal pain. Minerals like the important electrolytes ease muscle cramping including calcium, magnesium, sulfur, potassium and sodium chloride found in vegetables and fruits. Herbs that can soothe the muscles are aloe, catnip, chamomile, parsley and add some celery and ripe bananas into the diet. A quality Probiotics is extremely important in the daily GIS Program. *Special Needs:* Daily Greens, Alfalfa, Chamomile, Catnip Tea, StomachPlus by *Aloe Life* and Probiotics by *Dr. Ohhira.*

Cystic Fibrosis (CF) of the Pancreas – Documentation is abundant in the relationship to GIS and CF. In 1936 Guido Fanconi, MD, published a paper describing the connection of CF to Celiac disease. Scarring and cyst formation within the Pancreas gland affects the health of the entire body. Difficulty breathing and common lung and sinus infections, poor growth, diarrhea and infertility are common symptoms. The "Sweat Test" and checking for the gene mutation of CFTR gene is recommended. Apply the GIS Program for quality of life. *Special Needs:* EFA's from Flax & Fish oil including A & D, Multiple Vitamin & Mineral, Vitamin E - 1200 IU (micellized or other type), Aloe Vera and a Multiple Enzyme.

Dental Enamel Deficiencies – Nutritional deficiencies from GIS and a poor diet that includes sugary drinks and snacks, promote cavities and poor bone development that leads to more frequent crowding of the teeth. Also required for healthy tooth development are good digestive health (See Chapter 2) and a mineral rich diet of vegetables including dark green and orange selections or vegetable supplements. Adequate protein to build stronger cells is required and fish oil including Vitamin D3 is important for healthy bone development along with daily sunshine as possible. See Addictions and pH in Chapter 5. *Special Needs:* Multiple Vitamin & Mineral, Aloe Vera, EFA's - Fish Oil, Probiotics, Daily Greens, Protein, Calcium, Magnesium and Zinc plus Trace Minerals as age dictates.

Diabetes – Glandular health including the Pancreas is greatly improved by following the GIS Program with proteins, complex carbohydrates from beans and vegetables and low gluten grains omitting the regular whole grains (See Ch. 1 Highlights Sprouting Grains). Following the American Diabetes Association guidelines of incorporating nutritious foods with (3) regular meals and (3) nutritious snacks plus exercise and adequate water intake is almost 100% parallel to the GIS guidelines yet the addition of the supplements are very significant to reach optimum health! Inflammation as in GIS affects proper functioning of the Pancreas relating to both types of Diabetes Type I and II. *Special Needs:* Aloe Vera, Nopal Cactus, Minerals including Chromium and regular Protein.

Digestive Disorders – All digestive conditions respond favorably to the GIS Diet including Reflux, Heartburn, IBS and IBD as reviewed in Chapter 3 Digestion. When the body is given the Essential Core Nutrients and Aloe Vera that encourage the digestive juices to flow properly Dietary Enzymes from a supplement are not always needed on a daily basis if at all. If you choose to ONLY use an Enzyme Complex to help your symptoms people reap limited results - only a portion of their possible health potential! When following the GIS Program it transforms the body on a cellular level and it allows the body to function the way it was divinely designed. *Special Needs:* Aloe Vera, B-Complex, Vitamin E (Entire Complex), Dietary Enzymes (only as needed), Herb Tea – Mint, Catnip and Chamomile and always a quality Probiotics by *Dr. Ohirra's* 12 Strain or another quality product.

Depression & Melancholy – Both of these mental states are common symptoms of GIS and may develop from its nutritional deficiencies, hormone imbalances and or the Central Nervous System inflammatory response. A mood disorder may show symptoms fairly soon after eating gluten or a GIS trigger food and or also with meals having a high Glycemic Index from refined carbohydrates that cause a drop in blood sugar. Review Chapter 6 Blood Sugar. Eat primarily lean meat protein or fish and keep fried foods low in the diet including vegetables with only moderate amounts of carbohydrates as described in the GIS Diet Chapter 7. *Special Needs*: Protein, Multiple Vitamin & Mineral by *Aloe Life*, B-Complex, B12, Mineral - Chromium, 5HTP, GABA, EFA's from

Flax, Borage and Fish Oil, Lavender extracts (Bach Flower - Rescue Remedy) and St. John's Wort (Herb-Pharm Nervous Tonic).

Diarrhea – Chronic diarrhea due to allergy or gluten intolerance including GIS always slows down on the GIS Diet for 90% of people immediately. Most people find diarrhea reduces significantly in just a matter of days and weeks with the addition of the supplements especially Probiotics. For some advanced IBD cases it may take up to one year for total resolution with an occasional bout of loose stool. Other factors like food poisoning from bacteria, viral infection as with a cold or flu, an antibiotic side effect, radiation therapy or taking pharmaceutical drugs can all bring about loose stool. See Chapter 6 Digestion to get the complete list of herbs and foods to include with diarrhea. The BRAT Diet is always a good guideline to follow; Bananas, Rice (white), Apples (cooked) and Tea. *Special Needs:* Electrolytes from Minerals, Liquid or Chewable Vitamin & Mineral, Protein Powder (Hypoallergenic see Ch. 8), Daily Greens (Review in Ch. 7 TIPS & Ch. 8), Herb – Slippery Elm and Probiotics.

Dyslexia – Dyslexia is a condition of reversing letters and words in written matter. Often a child or adult who has been labeled a slow learner in retrospect later discover they were experiencing the brain malfunction Dyslexia. It requires extra nutrition to strengthen the CNS and also to balance the right and left brain pathways of thought. The inflammation igniting from the GIS greatly influences the development of Dyslexia. Following the GIS Program helps to reduce the condition greatly. *Special Needs:* Fish Oils, Aloe Vera, B-Complex, vitamin E Complex 400 – 1200 IU (Ch. 8), Protein, Filtered Water and practice the Special Balancing Exercise called Cross Crawl daily. Review Chapter 12 for Cross-Crawl instruction.

Diverticulitis – Inflamed tissue pockets called pouches form this condition in the large intestine and often they collect body fluids and food debris leading to infection. The pockets are thought to develop from dehydration and with a decreased immune function infection may manifest causing intense pain and or fatigue. To reduce the infection a person must improve their overall health and eating habits. At times a pouch may burrow into the abdomen which is called a "Perforation" demanding immediate medical attention. Occasionally surgery may be required to remove damaged sections of the bowel. Be warned that cancer may develop in the more flattened diverticula cells so preventative steps are strongly recommended. The "Slant Board" exercise reviewed in Chapter 12 is very helpful to drain the pockets. See Chapter 6, Detoxification, Digestion and Candida. *Special Needs:* Probiotics, EFA's including Vitamin A & D, Aloe Vera and to include 6 – 8 glasses of quality purified Water.

   Ear Congestion - Itching and inflammation of the ear canal is generally a sign of allergy and or fungal infection. The Candida Albicans fungal yeast is common in the ear and develops from poor nutrition from eating a high carbohydrate diet and junk foods. Also, the use of antibiotics and poor circulation add to the Candida overgrowth. Due to the yeast mal-nutrition including a lack of B-Complex can contribute to an overproduction of wax in the ear adding to more congestion. Vertigo and dizziness may also develop from inflammation in the ear canal and can increase from either flying or other changes in elevation. Aloe Vera Ear Drops have been very effective for many people to decrease ear conditions. A successful manipulation has also helped from a skilled Chiropractor or Osteopathic doctor when vertigo is present. The adjustment method breaks up tiny mineral crystals that develop in the cranial and ear spaces. See Chapter 6 Immune System, Candida and Addictions. *Note:* Be warned that small children may place objects in their ears or nose and occasionally other organic objects can lodge in the ear canal. *Special Needs:* Probiotics, B-Complex, Aloe Vera Ear Drops and Nasal Spray liquid by *Xlear.*

   Eczema – All skin conditions including Eczema relate to a malfunctioning liver. This is dependable information and the relationship rides in the fact that the liver has the important job of processing the fat soluble nutrients including; Vitamin A & E along with the Essential Fatty Acids. Constipation contributes to a congested liver along with being overweight, eating poorly and sugar or alcohol addiction. The overgrowth of the Candida Albicans in the intestines is another big factor with chronic skin conditions like Eczema. This microscopic fungus grows up the intestinal tract and blocks absorption of the B-Complex vitamins in the small intestine that is also needed for healthy skin. See Chapter 6, Detoxification Addictions and Candida. Besides the requirement of eating healthy foods you must get a minimum of 6 – 8 glasses of water daily and regular exercise to get the liver working well once again. *Special Needs:* EFA's – Fish Oil including Vitamin A & D, Probiotics, Aloe Vera, Milk Thistle, Chlorella, Daily Greens, Niacin 25 - 50 mg and B-Complex 50 mg.

Epileptic Seizures – Neurological disorders require good balanced nutrition with lots of vegetables and fish or EFA's that builds a healthy Central Nervous System. Following the GIS Diet and Program will minimize seizures due to inflammation and malnutrition factors. *Special Needs:* Multiple Vitamin and Mineral by *Aloe Life*, EFA's – Flax & Fish Oil, Minerals especially Magnesium, Aloe Vera, Vitamin E, NAC and Alpha Lipoic Acid needed for chelating toxic metals like mercury out of the body which are associated with seizures.

Fainting Spells – The medical term for fainting is Syncope and is defined as the sudden loss of consciousness generally caused by a lack of oxygen to the brain. Dizziness and fainting is common with advanced GIS especially when the air is stagnant of oxygen below 16%. Many factors contribute to fainting yet the most common includes; lack of blood or oxygen in the blood, Anemia, low blood sugar or pressure, hyperventilation, carbon monoxide poisoning and or poor neurological malfunction. *Special Needs:* Methyl B12 Drops or Injections (prescription required), B-Complex, Protein, Minerals-Iron, Vitamin C & Bioflavonoids and Aloe Vera which supports bone marrow production of Red Blood Cells (RBC's).

Fatigue – General tiredness and weakness can come from malnutrition due to poor absorption of nutrients or a lack of the proper nutrition for the body. This occurs when people are not eating a variety of healthy foods from all categories outlined in Chapter 7. Toxicity can also be a factor coming from a state of constipation or toxins from the environment causing sluggishness and headaches. Low blood sugar can be another common cause of tiredness and emotional ups and downs. Fatigue can also develop from a viral flare-up from Flu, Herpes, Epstein Barr and occasionally Cancer. Don't overlook the obvious that people require approximately 7 - 8 hours of sleep per night to be fully rested. See Chapter 6, Anemia, Blood Sugar, Immune System, Environmental Toxicity and Detoxification. Get a regular physical check up by a health professional   *Special Needs:* Aloe Vera, Multiple Vitamin & Mineral, EFA's, Protein, B-Complex, Probiotics, B12 (sublingual or injectable), Daily Greens, Antioxidants, Melatonin (sleep), 5HTP, Calcium and Magnesium plus Zinc (before bedtime can also be very helpful for sleep) and L-Lysine (viral support – 1 – 3,000 mg).

Fibromyalgia – This diagnosis is linked to muscle pain related to a lack of viable Vitamin B12 in the body. B-Complex and B12 are essential in the body for nerve health and often a deficiency is due to Candida fungal overgrowth blocking absorption of all the B Vitamins. Including green vegetables in the diet is extremely helpful because they contain a high level of Biotin one of the B Vitamins that slows fungal replication. See Chapter 6, Candida, Detoxification and Virus sections. *Special Needs:* Probiotics, Liquid B-Complex, B12 (sublingual or injection), Daily Greens, DetoxPlus or Aloe Gold by *Aloe Life*, Pau de Arco, CoQ10 Enzyme and Magnesium.

Gas – Being gassy is a symptom of not digesting food properly or fermentation of the food contents in the GI tract. Gas is also experienced almost immediately after eating a sugary snack or dessert following a meal. Also, constipation can cause trapped gas which can become very painful. Beginning the GIS Diet can bring on some gas in the first stages of the program as waste begins to be eliminated from the bowel. CVD can mimic digestive stress so follow up with a good check-up to eliminate any possible vascular blockages from heart disease. Chew your foods very well as reviewed in Chapter 3 and include vegetable fibers like celery, carrots and apples to scrub the intestines. Close your Ileocecal Valve located in the GI tract by reviewing Chapter 12. *Special Needs:* Probiotics, Aloe Vera, Papaya Enzymes and Charcoal Tablets (temporarily).

Gastritis – Gastritis is synonymous with GIS and can create over twenty different symptoms to include; stomach upset, nausea, vomiting, pain, belching, bloating, feeling of fullness, burning, blood in the stool, loss of appetite, foul taste in the mouth, bad breath, foul smelly stools, chest pain, gastric erosion, diarrhea and more. Physicians categorize these symptoms under the umbrella diagnosis of Gastritis. See Chapter 3, 6 and 7 for diet guidelines. *Special Needs:* Probiotics, Aloe Vera, Multiple Vitamin & Mineral, Chamomile, Catnip and Mint Tea.

Hair Loss - Poor absorption of nutrients; protein, zinc and B-Complex in particular can lead to hair loss, plus a low functioning Thyroid gland, toxicity, postpartum, hormone imbalance, excessive stress and more. See Chapter 6, Detoxification, Candida and Glandular Function. Apply topical Aloe Vera Skin Gel on scalp and review the herb Saw Palmetto for hormone support. *Special Needs:* Protein, Vitamin E, EFA's, Minerals-Iodine (from sea greens) including Zinc, Aloe Vera and Milk Thistle.

Headaches – Headaches are triggered by many different factors, seven are listed here and they all represent an imbalance in health with the same characteristic – pain. Headache factors include; Anemia, constipation (causing putrefaction in the bowel), viruses, stress (causing muscle tension), high blood pressure, hypoglycemia and dehydration which is common. Drink 6-8 glasses of water daily, right constipation by following a detoxification protocol following the GIS Program. *Special Needs:* L-Lysine, B-Complex or Nutritional Yeast, Aloe Vera, Vitamin C & Bioflavonoids and start the herb Echinacea in a liquid tincture by *Herb-Pharm.*

Heartburn (HB) – HB is very common with IBS and is described as a pressure with a burning sensation in the middle of ones breast bone. Modern diagnosis of HB is Reflux. Doctors are prescribing acid blockers when in fact it is most common to be a state of low acidity that is causing the HB and the body requires higher acidity (proper level) not less. *Special Needs:* Aloe Vera, Probiotics, B-Complex, Digestive Enzyme including HCL (as needed) and Minerals – Calcium and Magnesium taken best at bedtime.

Herpes Simplex **Virus (HSV)** – This viral condition known as HSVI and HSVII can be activated with the inflammation coming from eating too much gluten and gluten triggers. See Chapter 6 Viruses and review Chapter 8 supplements. *Special Needs:* L-Lysine, Monolaurine, Red Marine Algae, Olive Leaf Extract, Aloe Vera, B-Complex, B12 and Liquid Silver – Sovereign Silver.

Irregular Heartbeat – A racing heartbeat has long been connected with an allergy response from foods. Irregular heartbeat also can follow eating Gluten Trigger foods. Reduce stress and caffeine products along with following the GIS Program. *Special Needs:* EFA's – Flax & Fish Oil, B-Complex, CoQ10 Enzyme and Minerals.

Infertility – A high incidence of infertility exists in people with advanced gluten intolerance. Thyroid health is paramount for fertility. Thyroid also controls the body's temperature with the reading of 98.6 degrees as the daily goal. See Chapter 6, Detoxification and Glandular Health and include raw pumpkin seeds, fish roe or caviar, Sardines, Nori seaweed, blanched almonds and wheat germ oil as tolerated to boost glandular health. Review Chapter 9 Healthy Children and fertility is covered in-depth. *Special Needs:* Protein, Minerals - Iodine and Zinc, Multiple Vitamin & Mineral, EFA, Vitamin E 800 IU and Aloe Vera.

Interstitial Cystitis (IC) – Recently IC has been classified as an autoimmune disease which relates to GIS. Women suffer with this self induced condition of indulgence developing inflamed and painful genetalia and urethra tubes. Symptoms include; pain and discomfort with urination, sitting and other daily activities including sexual activity. Some women improve within just a couple of days of starting the supplements and other people require 3-6 months before the pain resolves. The GIS Diet is extremely critical for recovery. See Chapter 6 Addictions and pH balancing. *Special Needs:* Minerals, Probiotics,

Daily Greens, Aloe Vera, Fish Oils including A & D and a Multiple Vitamin & Mineral.

Incontinence – A weak Central Nervous System can lead to under-functioning of the Neuromuscular System reducing the proper muscle action required to retain urine. Incontinence occurs frequently in young overweight women, during pregnancy, seniors and occasionally with small children. Bed wetting with youngsters and accidents during the day generally lessen once an individual follows the GIS program because the diet accents minerals. Muscles rely on sufficient minerals in the body to function properly. Hormones also play a part in incontinence with adults especially valuable is Estrogen. Also, regular strengthening exercises called "Kegels" are responsible for toning the muscle group for urine retention. *Special Needs:* Minerals – Magnesium and Calcium, EFA's – Flax & Fish Oils, Vitamin E Complex, B-Complex, B12 and Aloe Vera.

Kidney Stones **& Infections** – Mal-absorption of minerals is common with GIS and accounts for rogue mineral deposits called "stones" that may form in any organ yet commonly found in the kidneys and gallbladder. Bone spurs on the feet or spine are also due to improper absorption of minerals with GIS. See Detoxification and Digestion in Chapter 3. *Special Needs:* Aloe Vera, B-Complex, Vitamin E, Digestive Enzymes including HCL, Magnesium and Daily Greens.

Lactose Intolerance – A large percentage of people living with bowel disease are also intolerant to dairy products. The symptoms of loose stool, gas and bloating are due to the inability to digest the milk sugar lactose. Special yogurt, cottage cheese and most hard cheeses contain low lactose and are allowable on the GIS Diet see Chapter 7. The research indicates cow's milk to be in the top spot of allergic foods. Wheat gluten is in second place according to the GIS research with peanuts, tree nuts, fish, shellfish and soy following suit. Review Chapter 6 Detoxification. See Chapter 7 for milk alternatives. *Special Needs:* Aloe Vera, Lactase Enzymes, B-Complex, EFA's, Vitamin E Complex, Minerals and Probiotics.

Liver Health – The liver is responsible for thousands of metabolic actions that support the health of the body on a daily basis reviewed in

Chapter 3 Digestion. Eating junk foods, high amounts of carbohydrates including gluten, alcohol, sugar and sodas cause the liver to become fatty and sluggish unable to do its required work. Proper metabolism of Vitamin A, E and EFA's slow down when the liver is congested with fat. The GIS inflammation further reduces the proper function of the CNS required for liver metabolism. When the fat soluble Vitamin E is deficient in the body it retards the capillary strength in the entire body. The capillaries become fragile and break easily resulting in redness on the face, neck and limbs of the body. All skin conditions relate to malnutrition, hormone imbalances and liver disorders. See Chapter 6 Detoxification and Liver health. Eating organic liver is supportive of the liver along with following the GIS Diet. Chapter 12 reviews the Liver & Gallbladder Flush. *Special Needs:* N-Acetyl-Cysteine (NAC), Aloe Vera – DetoxPlus by *Aloe Life*, Milk Thistle, Protein, Minerals, Probiotics by *Dr. Ohhira* and Water.

Loss of Weight – Children can experience underweight tendencies and failure to thrive as infants and toddlers coinciding with GIS symptoms of bloated stomachs and digestive disorders. As described in Chapter 3 the blunting of the villi in the small intestine leads to major mal-absorption that can affect people at any age causing weight loss with young or older children and adults. Any unhealthy weight loss requires medical intervention and dietary recommendations. See Chapter 7 for diet guidelines and eat (6) smaller meals not to overtax the digestion while following the Zone 3 Diet. *Avoid:* sugar, grains including oatmeal, alcohol and cow's milk. *Special Needs:* Chewable or Liquid Vitamin & Mineral, Aloe Vera, Protein Powder (hypoallergenic), Free-Form Amino Acid Complex or Elemental Diet, Probiotics, Micellized Vitamin E, Fish Oil, Daily Greens and Vegetable Juices as tolerated.

Lungs & Labored Breathing – Mucus and congestion may stem from inflammation and neuromuscular dysfunction with GIS. The lung tissue regenerates as do all of the tissues of the body following the GIS program. Asthma, Pulmonary (lung) Disease and other conditions involving the lungs respond to the supplements and diet excellently. See Chapter 6, Detoxification and Addictions. *Special Needs:* NAC, EFA's

- Flax & Fish Oils 1,000 – 3,000 mg or more, DHA & EPA 2,000 mg including Vitamin A & D, Vitamin C & Bioflavonoid, Micellized Vitamin E, Nasal Spray (Xlear), CoQ10 Enzyme, Garlic, Aloe Vera by *Aloe Life*, Liquid Silver – Sovereign Silver and Eucalyptus Oil Tincture (heat and safely breath vapors).

Mal-Absorption – Research confirms that the body develops core nutrient deficiencies with bowel disease. The foundational core nutrients include vitamins, minerals, EFA's and proteins, designed to be absorbed in the stomach, small intestine and liver then pass on through via the blood to the cells. Not eating a varied diet, a poor health status and inflammation in the gut with GIS each reduce the available nutrition for the body. The invaluable nutrients that are eaten are further blocked from absorption by the fungal overgrowth of Candida in the bowel compounding failing health. See Chapter 6 Candida. A higher incidence of cancer and other diseases are attributed to people living with bowel disease especially if action is not taken to improve ones health. *Special Needs:* Aloe Vera, Liquid B-Complex, B12 injections, Digestive Enzyme (full spectrum), Probiotics, Liquid or Chewable Multiple Vitamin & Mineral, Extra Liquid Minerals as needed and Daily Greens in powder form.

Metabolic X Syndrome: Gaining weight around the middle (apple shape), high triglycerides, high blood pressure and sometimes the diagnosis of Diabetes encompass the symptoms of "Metabolic X Syndrome". The condition relates to poor glandular health of the Adrenal Glands in particular. See Chapter 6, Detoxification, Addictions and Glandular Health with the highlight on daily exercise and 6-8 glasses of water. *Special Needs:* Aloe Vera, Nopal Cactus, Aloe Boost by *Aloe Life*, Fish Oils by *Nordic Naturals*, Vitamin E (Entire Complex), 5HTP, Adrenal Concentrate (glandular), Minerals including Zinc 50 mg, Vitamin C and Bioflavonoids 500 – 2,000 mg, Protein and Daily Greens.

Menopause – Hot flashes, depression and other symptoms associated with hormone changes are heightened by the GIS Triggers affecting the glands. The health of the liver and other glands are very important in minimizing Menopause symptoms. Stabilizing blood sugar reduces depression, hot flashes and the other symptoms greatly. Stop eating refined sugar and high glycemic foods. Review Chapter 6 pH Balance, Hormones, Addictions and Blood Sugar. Focus on regular meals with quality protein as described in Chapter 7 including 6 – 8 glasses of water daily and 35 minutes of exercise. Experiment with "Brain Supplements" and Herbs in Chapter 8. *Special Needs:* Multiple Vitamin & Mineral, Vitamin E, Sam E - Antioxidant, FF-Amino Acids, Minerals especially Chromium GTF 200 mcg, EFA's, B-Complex, Herbs – Black Cohosh and Aloe Vera. *Note:* Black Cohosh is effective in relieving symptoms temporarily however monitor liver enzymes every (6) months and stop taking it if they elevate.

Menstrual Cycles – Abnormal and irregular cycles are common with GIS. Healthy glands are needed for hormone health to support the body's biorhythms especially important is keeping the liver functioning well. Some women may experience a thickening of the uterine wall due to liver congestion called Endometriosis. Exercise is critical for balancing out the hormone cycles along with hydrating plus good nutrition. *Special Needs:* B-Complex and B12, Protein, Multiple Vitamin & Mineral, Zinc 30 mg, Vitamin E Complex, EFA's – Evening Primrose Oil & Fish Oil including A & D by *Nordic Naturals* (Omega Woman), Herbs - Red Clover and Aloe Vera.

Mental Illness – All mental illness conditions improve favorably following the GIS Program including; Bi-Polar, Schizophrenic, OCD and more. Review Chapter 5 and 6 Addictions, Candida Albicans and Detoxification. *Special Needs:* Multiple Vitamin & Mineral by *Aloe Life*, B-Complex, B12, EFA's – Flax & Fish Oil, FF-Amino Acids (protein building blocks), 5HTP, GABA, Prevagen and St. John's Wort by *Herb-Pharm.*

Muscle Aches – GIS can increase pain in the body due to inflammation creating a lack of B12 and other nutrients common with gluten intolerance. See Chapter 6 Viral, Candida, Detoxification and Environmental Toxins. The mineral Silica is very important for joint flexibility and also Type II Collagen can be helpful as well. *Special Needs:*

Aloe Vera, EFA's – Flax and Fish oil, Minerals, "EmergenC" - Vitamin & Mineral packs, Wobenzym Enzymes, Alfalfa tablets, FiberMate by *Aloe Life*, Vitamin C, Daily Greens and Sovereign Silver Liquid.

Mitral Valve Prolapse (MVP) – MVP is diagnosed in about 10% of the population. It is associated with autoimmune disorders to include Grave's Disease, an over-active Thyroid, connective tissue disorders and Scoliosis. MVP is when the heart valve does not close properly which may allow blood to flow slightly backwards. Symptoms may be varying degrees of chest pain, difficulty breathing, fatigue, coughing and shortness of breath while lying flat. Healthy neurological function of the body restores improved proper action of all the valves in the body and a regular heartbeat from all challenges. Always seek professional evaluation with symptoms of MVP to rule out any other necessary treatment. MVP events are lessened 99% in most people following the GIS Program! *Special Needs:* EFA's –Flax & Fish Oil liquid, CoQ10 Enzyme, B-Complex, Multiple Vitamin & Mineral (or take each nutrient separate as per Ch. 8).

Multiple Sclerosis (MS) – Symptoms improve significantly on the GIS Diet due to neurological and viral support needed. Research has confirmed a viral factor is present with MS. It is classified as an auto-immune disorder with special circumstances. Methyl B12 injections as tolerated with aggressive natural sterols, fish oils and Integrated Medicine as needed. *Special Needs:* Aloe Vera, B12, micellized Vitamin E, Alpha Lipoic Acid, Pycnogenol-Antioxidant, Barley Greens, Multiple Enzyme, CoQ10 Enzyme, NAC and Liquid Silver – Sovereign Silver.

Mucus – Over-production of mucus in the Esophagus and intestinal tract is both irritating and interferes with the digestive process. The goblet cells are responsible for secreting mucus anywhere in the GI tract and when overactive the mucus not only decreases digestive ability it also interferes with clear speech. Researchers are relating the Central Nervous System slow down to mitral valve malfunction and how that relationship may trigger mucus production in the lungs in particular causing a cough reflex. See Detoxification and Addictions in Ch. 6. The use of Lemon and Lime daily, squeezed into water as an astringent helps to clear the throat. Aloe Vera is also remarkable as an astringent, a disinfectant and it helps to dissipate the mucus while supporting regeneration of the vocal cords and more. *Special Needs:* Lemon & Lime (in water), Aloe Vera, Cranberry Juice Concentrate (no sugar), EFA's – Flax and Fish Oil including Vitamin A & D, Probiotics, Multiple Vitamin & Mineral, B-Complex and CoQ10 Enzyme.

Muscle Cramping – Mal-absorption is responsible for a large percentage of symptoms that relate to poor mineral stores of electrolytes and other minerals including; calcium, magnesium, phosphorus, sodium chloride, zinc, silica and more. Proper glandular support of the Thyroid and Parathyroid gland is also involved in muscle movement which can be reduced by GIS balancing auto-immune. Lastly, the Nervous System must be working properly to allow the contraction and release of the sphincter valves (a muscle group) throughout the digestive tract. Cramping can be alleviated by getting the body back into digestive balance. Review Chapter 3 Digestion and Chapter 7 Diet and Detoxification in Chapter 6. *Special Needs:* Aloe Vera, B-Complex, Minerals-Iodine, Magnesium, Daily Greens, EFA's and a Multiple Vitamin & Mineral.

Neurological Disorders (ND) – GIS decreases the entire Nervous System (NS) function in the body which affects the body both mentally and physically as review in Chapter 5. Research finds that people whose diets are high in polyunsaturated fats (PUFA's), fulfilling the requirements for EFA's and Vitamin E build protection against motor neuron diseases to include Amyotrophic Lateral Sclerosis (ALS), also known as Lou Gehrig's disease. A study noted a 60% lower risk of ALS alone in people with the highest level of PUFA's in their blood also known as EFA's. The GIS protocol reduces symptoms for ALS patients. *Special Needs:* EFA's, Aloe Vera, B-Complex, Lecithin, Methyl B12 injections, Liquid Silver-Hydrosol, NAC and rotate other natural anti-viral supplements as desired.

Neuropathy - The hands and feet are particularly affected by the decrease of circulation due to the CNS and PNS mal-functioning.

Improper sugar metabolism as with Diabetes and Metabolic X Syndrome develop very impaired circulation as does chemotherapy and excess pharmaceutical use. Neuropathy leaves the limbs numb, tingly and painful. This condition is especially difficult for walking. The GIS program helps significantly! Stop all Gluten Triggers for (6) weeks especially NO gelatin capsules or gel caps other than medications. If taking a medication request it in liquid or tablets if possible. *Special Needs:* Methyl B12 injections, B-Complex with Folic Acid 50 mg (1 – 2 times daily) and Vitamin E 400 – 1200 IU, Alpha Lipoic Acid, Chromium GTF, Multiple Vitamin & Mineral, Nopal Cactus and Aloe Vera. Some topical products have been helpful in decreasing pain to include Body Heat by *Aloe Life* see Reference section.

Night Blindness & **Vision** – Most people especially with advanced IBS and IBD lack proper amounts of Zinc in their bodies. Zinc is an important co-factor mineral required for absorption of Vitamin A to build healthy skin, the intestinal tract and ones vision. See Addictions and Decreasing Stress in Chapter 6. Visual purple is also needed and can be acquired by purple foods like blueberries and others. Include as many antioxidant foods in the diet as possible including; Blueberries, Spinach and Greens, Egg Yolk, Carrots and Parsley. *Special Needs:* Multiple Vitamin & Mineral, Vitamin E Complex, Fish Oil -Vitamin A 10,000 IU, Antioxidants – Zeaxanthin, Lutein and Zinc.

Nightmares – The GIS Program has been very helpful in decreasing bad dream states and night terrors that can wake children and adults during the night. Nightmares are common with gluten intolerance and one must stabilize the blood sugar before bed with a healthy snack of protein foods like a good yogurt, a hardboiled egg or a teaspoon of peanut butter as tolerated. It is also important to have adequate minerals to relax the body for restful sleep including; calcium, magnesium and zinc. See Chapter 6, Blood Sugar, Stress, Sleep and Addictions. *Special Needs:* Protein, Minerals, 5HTP, Melatonin, Prevagen (for adults), Bach Flower Essence, Chamomile Tea or Valerian (a strong herb to use as needed).

Nosebleeds – Both nosebleeds and headaches are common with GIS in children and adults. Nosebleeds can be from a deficiency in Vitamin C and bioflavonoids naturally found in fruits and vegetables and other nutrients. Vitamin K is especially important for increasing the clotting factor of the blood and Vitamin E supports better strength of the cell and proliferation. Both are sourced from leafy green vegetables and E can also come from nuts and seeds, beans and grains. Protein along with Vitamin C, Vitamin D and Vitamin E work together building strong Red Blood Cells (RBC) that do not break easily to avoid nosebleeds and reduce Anemia. RBC's are also important to carry oxygen throughout the body. Therefore fatigue and headaches along with fragile RBC's may occur together. Lemons, limes, grapefruits, berries, radishes and bell peppers are all good food sources of Vitamin C and Bioflavonoids. *Special Needs:* Vitamin E, Alpha Lipoic Acid, B-Complex, B12, Protein, Iron, Vitamin C, Bioflavonoids, Daily Greens and Aloe Vera.

Obsessive Compulsive Disorders (OCD) – Nutritional deficiencies can affect the neurological health of the human body as reviewed in Chapter 5. Also, Blood sugar metabolism and a lack of the hormone "Serotonin" has been pointed to as significant factors in OCD often seen in Zone 2 and 3 GIS (Ch. 7). See Chapter 6 for Addictions, Glandular health of Adrenals, Pancreas and the Liver. *Special Needs:* Protein (three meals per day), Minerals including Chromium (GTF type), Vitamin C, B-Complex, 5HTP (increases Serotonin naturally), EFA's – Flax and Fish Oils as tolerated and Aloe Vera.

Obesity – Obesity factors include an "Inflammation Component" adding to the difficulty of controlling one's weight gain. Decreasing inflammation allows the glands to become healthier and in turn work to stabilize the body's weight. See Chapter 6 Digestion, Liver & Glandular Function and Finding Your Healthy Weight. Fish oils surprisingly helps reach a healthy weight through an important biochemistry reaction involving the increase of "Leptin Hormone" activity. At the same time researchers have commented that the fish oil addresses "Obesity Depression" so often a reason for relapse from striving towards a healthier lifestyle. *Special Needs:* Multiple Vitamin & Mineral containing

Chromium GTF by *Aloe Life*, B-Complex, EFA's – Flax by *Flora* and Fish Oil plus A & D by *Nordic Naturals*, 5HTP, L-Carnitine HCL, L-Lysine 1,000 – 3,000 mg, Daily Greens and Aloe Boost Formula by *Aloe Life*.

Parkinson's – Both Parkinson's and Non-Parkinson's neurological conditions respond positively to the GIS Diet and Program. Neurological disorders all benefit by therapeutic nutrition. *Special Needs:* Methyl B12 injections, B-Complex, EFA's – Flax & EFA's Fish Oil, Amino Acids, Aloe Vera and Multiple Vitamin & Mineral.

Polyps in the Colon – Polyps are a bulbous growth in the large intestines remaining either somewhat flat or large and obvious. The flat type is found more often to be cancerous. Often benign the larger polyps may develop into cancer if health steps and or surgery to remove them are not taken. Many people have found Aloe Vera to be effective to stop the body from producing Polyps. Polyps are common with GIS and in people practicing an unhealthy lifestyle including; eating a lot of fatty foods, sugar, smoking and alcohol abuse, not exercising and overweight. Following a healthy diet and drinking 6 – 8 glasses of water daily with an ounce of Aloe Vera added is critical along with the intake of healthy fats, fruits and vegetables. *Special Needs:* Aloe Vera, EFA's – Flax and Fish Oils including vitamin A & D, Daily Greens, Multiple Vitamin & Mineral, Vitamin E and Vitamin C.

Prostate Gland – Experts agree that 50% of men age 60 or above will experience symptoms of an unhealthy Prostate gland referred to as BPH - Benign Prostate Hyperplasia. One in six men will be diagnosed with Prostate Cancer and most of these men have been diagnosed with BPH. Health of the prostate gland will be more preventative to not only Prostate Cancer but all other cancers as well. The GIS program supports all glandular health and immunity. *Special Needs:* Vitamin E, B-Complex, EFA's, Minerals including Zinc, Selenium Yeast and Sterols called beta-Sitosterol from plant sources to include Aloe Vera and Saw Palmetto by *New Vitality* called Ageless Male. *Note:* Research has confirmed that the active ingredient in Ageless Male increases the body's production of natural Testosterone required in many metabolic processes of the body to avoid; hair loss, BPH, loss in libido, a rise in triglycerides, blood pressure and CVD.

Psoriasis – All skin conditions respond positively to the GIS Diet and supplement protocol. Most skin conditions have an autoimmune inflammatory component along with nutritional deficiencies. Review Chapter 6 Addictions, Detoxification and Candida. *Special Needs:* Niacin 50 mg (flushing is normal), B-Complex, Zinc, Magnesium, Calcium, Daily Greens, EFA's – Flax and Fish Oils including Vitamin A & D, Aloe Vera (internally) and Skin Gel Aloe Vera (topically) by *Aloe Life*.

Reflux – GIS interferes with smooth muscle movement in the body required for swallowing and glandular health. Reflux is two-fold including; a lack of bile production in the liver and liver health in general and mal-nutrition that leads to the disease. Many people are misdiagnosed with Reflux to be over-acidic when in fact they are low Hydrochloric Acid requiring higher acidity. True Reflux which is the state of throwing up one's food is only present in a small number of patients. Review Chapter 6 pH, Addiction, Digestion and Detoxification which are all very important factors in the development of Reflux. Focus on eating more vegetables that contain minerals that help buffer and alkalinize the body and stop eating junk foods, caffeine, alcohol, sodas, citrus, tomato and hot and spicy foods until regeneration of the lining tissue takes place. Excess Pharmaceutical Drugs used by adults have been pointed to as a big reason for the rise in Reflux cases. Depending on the individual improvement following the GIS Program requires 30 – 90 days and at times a full year. *Special Needs*: Probiotics, EFA's – Flax and Fish Oils by *Nordic Naturals* containing Vitamin A and D, Stomach Plus by *Aloe Life*, Daily Greens and a Multiple Vitamin & Mineral (or taken separately as outlined in Ch. 8).

Rosacea – A congested and sluggish liver is related to all skin disorders including Rosacea. The constipation that comes with gluten sensitivity in GIS is one cause leading to Rosacea. Reduced circulation and glandular health from malnutrition also slows liver function down. Poor metabolism of Vitamin E in the liver is highlighted as the cause for fragile and broken capillaries that compound the redness on the outer skin of the face and leads to other complications on the skin. Reduce spicy, hot foods and beverages when symptoms are greater. Other triggers to avoid include; alcohol, overeating, gluten, sugar, milk, emotional excess, hormonal imbalance, over exercising, the use of harsh skin cleansers and hot herbs to include; ginger, curry, hot peppers, black pepper and salsa. Review Chapter 6 pH, Detoxification and Liver. *Special Needs:* Aloe Vera, Milk Thistle, Burdock, DetoxPlus by *Aloe Life*, Fish Oil including Vitamin A and D, Vitamin E by *Jarrow*, B-Complex, Probiotics and Daily Greens.

Sinuses – The nostrils which connect to the sinuses have dual purpose in the body. Breathing air into the lungs is an essential function of the nose. Also important is the nose hair located before the sinuses. They act as filters for the breath catching dust particles, pollution and they gently warm the air before it reaches the lungs. Mucus made in the sinuses has infection fighting capacity that can destroy germs. People must keep well hydrated in the body to ensure the nose hairs and sinuses remain moist making certain to not over-dry them by keeping the heater on when not required during the winter months. When the heater is necessary, make certain to refill a bowl of water placed on the kitchen stove that allows moisture to return to the home environment. People often proclaim that their sinuses from allergies are bothering them. Sinuses can become congested and swollen during a cold and allergies can further add to the nasal swelling accompanied by food sensitivities and fungal infections. Drinking good amounts of water daily and avoiding milk, sugar and grains as on the GIS Program will help greatly. Mucus is a response to inflammation therefore GIS is partially responsible and it is also the immune system's natural action too. Acute Sinus infections occur when the swelling reduces circulation to the point that it allows body fungus and bacteria to overgrow as secondary health challenges. Incorporate the Immune System factors and the Anti-Fungal program as outlined in the Candida section found in Chapter 6. Irrigation of the nasal passages with Aloe Vera liquid with added Echinacea and Goldenseal tincture may get relief and speed recovery of the body. A liquid Nasal Spray solution may also help a Sinus condition as well by Xlear. *Special Needs:* Aloe Vera, Golden Seal and Echinacea tincture by *Herb-Pharm* (taken by mouth and put in irrigation with Aloe Vera) and Xlear Nasal Spray 3 times daily, Multiple Vitamin & Mineral, EFA's, Vitamin A 10,000 IU (fish oil), Protein, B-Complex and Vitamin C.

Skin – All rashes and skin conditions respond positively to the GIS Program. From the commonly experienced acne to Hydradenitis Suppuritiva (HS) which is considered an auto-immune disorder follow the GIS Program for a three month trial to allow the regeneration of the skin tissue to take place. Research has documented rashes, along with another form of dermatitis called Dermatitis Herpetiformis (HP), is common with bowel disorders in children and adults and requires the GIS nutritional support. Review Chapter 6, Detoxification, Candida and Addictions. The liver is always congested with skin ailments and in need of cleansing. Stop or reduce smoking, drinking alcohol, eating sugar and junk foods. The supplements can get to work right away while each individual does their best to improve the daily diet. *Special Needs:* EFA's – Flax and Fish Oil 1-3 tsp. daily including Vitamin A & D, Olive Oil, Sesame Oil, Vitamin C & Bioflavonoids 1,000 – 3,000 mg, Minerals - Zinc, Calcium, Magnesium, Vitamin E Complex, B-Complex, Protein, Resveratrol (antioxidant), Daily Greens and Aloe Vera Juice (Aloe Life, Superfruit). *Note:* A Multiple Vitamin & Mineral can help to simplify and consolidate the core nutrients by *Aloe Life* plus extra B-Complex, EFA's, Aloe, Daily Greens and Probiotics.

Sleepy or Lazy Eye – Neurological support from the GIS Program is critical for the body to reduce and at times prevent Lazy Eye. When the condition flares-up it can serve as an excellent reminder that an individual is eating GIS triggers. It results from a slow-down of the Central Nervous System that is required to keep muscle control in the face and body. It is not just a result of the body being tired although you may see more of a droop when fatigued. *Special Needs:* EFA's – Flax and Fish Oil, B-Complex 50 mg (2 – 3 x daily), Niacin (Take separately for 6 weeks, flushing is normal review in Ch. 8.), B12, Minerals - Magnesium, Daily Greens, Multiple Vitamin & Mineral and Aloe Vera taken before meals is best.

Sneezing – The Nervous System is orchestrated by the autonomic nervous system which influences sneezing. The act of sneezing after a meal occurs because it is linked to the bowels and can be a side effect of needing to have a bowel movement or inflammation. Other conditions that relate to this type of Nervous System imbalance are hiccupping, over-sensitive gag reflux and stuttering. Extra supplementing of B-Complex and B12 along with sufficient Magnesium may reduce excessive body reactions. The GIS Program is a type of tune up rebalancing program for all the systems of the body. *Special Needs:* B-Complex, EFA's, Minerals, Daily Greens and a Multiple Vitamin & Mineral.

Sjogren's – An auto-immune disease, Sjogren's is characterized by itchy dryness of the eyes and mouth often resulting in hoarseness, mouth sores and difficulty in swallowing. The body dryness can affect all of the glands in the body resulting in compromised health and annoying vaginal dryness, discoloration of the hands and feet, swollen achy joints and fatigue. People experiencing this must include more quality healthy oils in the diet that facilitate the absorption of all oil based vitamins like the EFA's, Vitamin E and A that are important in building hormones and proper glandular function. B-Complex also supports the metabolism of healthy body lubrication as well. *Note:* If you rely on eye drops you have several nutritional deficiencies. Review the Candida section in Chapter 6 as well. *Special Needs:* EFA's from fish oil 2 – 3 tsp. including Vitamin A & D, Flax, Olive Oil or Sesame Oil 1 – 2 T. daily, Vitamin E 400 IU, Daily Greens, Vitamin A rich foods, B-Complex, Aloe Vera, Zinc 50 mg, Water (6 -8 glasses) and Digestive enzymes that include Lipase.

Swallowing Ability of the Esophagus – Normal neuromuscular action is required to swallow properly and this can be decreased with GIS. Sjogren's may also be present which is common in GIS. Sometimes frightening, difficulty to swallow can occur during any meal which includes Gluten Triggers as with breadstuff. Natural peristalsis action in the throat and intestinal tract all require the Central Nervous System (CNS) to be functioning properly. Avoid medications that slow the CNS and a pharmacist can review your medications if you find it difficult to consult with the prescribing doctor. Review Chapter 6, Detoxification, Digestion, Addictions and Blood Sugar. *Special Needs:* EFA's Fish Oil including Vitamin A & D, B-Complex, Methyl B12 Sublingual or injections, Aloe Vera, Minerals, Daily Greens and Chamomile.

Tinnitus – The name comes from the Latin word meaning to ring. Factors that contribute to the ringing of ears include; earwax, infection, vascular condition (Arterialsclerosis), medication or damage to the ears. If the ear(s) has damage or poor circulation the focus is on managing the condition. The good news is that by experimenting with supplements has shown improvement regardless of the cause. Optimize the body's health by following the GIS Diet guidelines reducing or eliminating junk foods, sugar, alcohol, excessive caffeine and smoking. Drink good amounts of filtered water and exercise. *Special Needs:* B-Complex 25 - 50 mg, Multiple Vitamin & Mineral, EFA's, Ginkgo Biloba, Melatonin, Zinc and Magnesium. *Note:* Ginkgo Biloba can cause headaches so start with just a few drops of a good tincture and increase very gradually to allow the body to adjust.

Thyroid Gland Function - All disorders of the Thyroid and Parathyroid gland, including the autoimmune condition Hashimoto's, is effected by GIS. Symptoms of low or over-active Thyroid include; inability to lose or gain weight, depression, bone loss, infertility, CVD and more. Glandular health in the body slows down with GIS inflammation. When auto-immunity is stimulated the immune system attacks healthy tissue including the Thyroid glands. Anti-Nutrients in the diet can also reduce Thyroid function in particular Soy products. Pollution coming from multiple sources including the rocket fuel Perchlorate and varying sources of radiation reduce Thyroid function in the body as well. Review Chapter 6, Environmental Toxicity and Detoxification. *Note:* Surgery may be required with an overproducing Para-Thyroid gland that causes high Calcium in the blood and urine. This requires a high intake of water and no extra Calcium supplements. *Special Needs:* EFA's - Fish Oil, Aloe Vera, Minerals-Iodine, Thyroid / Parathyroid supplement, Water, Multiple Vitamin & Mineral, Vitamin E, Alpha-Lipoic Acid, NAC, Daily Greens and Seaweeds.

Ulcers – All ulcer conditions relate to an imbalance of pH acidity and alkalinity affecting the health of the gastrointestinal tract lining. The frequency of the bad bacteria known as H. Pylori occurs in the stomach from low Hydrochloric Acid (HCL) levels and poor colonization of good bacteria. Once the environment loses proper acidity the bacteria has the opportunity of attacking healthy tissue which develops into an ulcer. Creating proper acidity in the stomach with rebalancing the HCL levels prevents the overgrowth of bad bacteria and other micro-organisms. Keeping a healthy colony of the good bacteria from Probiotics also regulates any overgrowth of bad bacteria including H. Pylori. Building healthy and strong lining cells in the stomach and GI tract also prevents damage to the lining tissue. *Special Needs:* Aloe Vera, Probiotics, EFA's – Flax and Fish Oils including Vitamin A & D, Multiple Vitamin & Mineral, B-Complex 50 mg. or Nutritional Yeast, Daily Greens, Protein and Deglycyrrhizinated Licorice (DGL) as needed (Ch. 8).

Ulcerative Colitis **(UC)** – UC is a diagnosed condition in bowel disease associated with GIS. It responds most excellently to the GIS Diet and healthy lifestyle choices. Constipation must be addressed and taking the supplements helps speed this condition including the Aloe Vera and Daily Greens. Review Chapter 12 for Enema instructions in the case of Lazy Bowel. *Special Needs:* Aloe Vera, Probiotics, EFA's, Daily Greens, Multiple Vitamin & Mineral, B-Complex 50 mg or Nutritional Yeast and Protein.

Varicose Veins – This condition in the vascular system is directly related to inflammation via the Central Nervous System (CNS) and malnutrition. When the body eats GIS triggers it affects the CNS which in turn causes the tiny flow valves in the vascular system to slow down. This temporary electrical shortage allows the blood to pool back in the veins or arteries causing blood to harden, discolor and bring about pain. A deficiency in structural core nutrients is also responsible for a weak development in the veins causing bulging or premature breaks in the vascular system as well. See Chapter 6 Addictions and Exercise. *Special Needs:* Vitamin E 400 – 1200 IU, Vitamin C & Bioflavonoids 1,000 – 3,000 mg., EFA's Fish Oils & Flax and B-Complex. Topical Leg Gel by *Aloe Life* has been supportive for soothing pain and improving the reduction of spider veins and other vascular irregularities on the face and legs.

Viral Flare-Ups – Herpes is one of many viruses to be found in the body. It is a predominant virus behind many health challenges and is also a secondary trigger in the GIS cycle. Symptoms of viral activity and especially Herpes are headaches around the temples and fatigue. With Herpes the occurrence can come after eating high L-Arginine foods. Fatigue can precede a Herpes ulcer outbreak on the lip, mouth or genitals. Oddly the virus can be active systemically without showing any outward ulcer development whatsoever. Thousands of other viruses are in our environments and can cause miscellaneous health challenges in our body if the immune system weakens. I find it most helpful to stay on a strong core supplement program with added L-Lysine and rotate 1 – 2 special needs anti-viral supplements listed below. You will find what works best to keep viruses in a more dormant state. See Chapter 6 Viruses for more tips and specific dietary guidelines. *Special Needs:* L-Lysine 500 – 3,000 mg, Probiotics, Vitamin C 1 – 2,000 mg., Vitamin E 400 – 1200 IU, Liquid Sovereign Silver, NAC, Monolaurin, Red Marine Algae, Aloe Vera, Olive Leaf, American Ginseng, OTC – Acetaminophen or the prescription drug Acyclovir or others as needed.

Make Today the First Day of a Healthier Rest of Your Life!

Learning what gluten is, the symptoms it creates in the body and the varied connections to other health conditions and diseases allows you to get out of denial and take the next step towards a healthier life. That step is to apply the foundational health principals outlined in the GIS Diet in Chapter 7 in your life and your family's life (the best you can) and reap the health benefits.

Health is a journey and not a destination. Throughout life we have opportunities to improve ourselves and we each learn at different rates and in layers that allow us to adjust our philosophy of life.

Do your best to apply the beginning health steps and create a healthy lifestyle that will carry you through all the chapters of your life feeling well as it unfolds. Health allows us each to Enjoy and Thrive not only Survive!

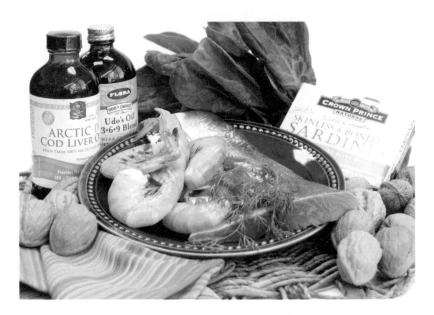

HIGHLIGHT 5: *Essential Fatty Acids (EFA's) for All!*

To attain health and to hold onto it a person must truly understand how the disease process develops in the first place. The body requires all of the Essential Core Nutrients (Review in Chapter 8) including the Essential Fatty Acids (EFA's) highlighted in Chapter 5 to support daily and long term health. The EFA's are critical to every cell of the body supporting its daily biological processes including; cellular membrane function for proper absorption of nutrients, waste removal, detoxification, repair of tissue and proper growth and development. EFA's are also required for cellular energy, reduction in pain, lowering anxiety and depression, brain function and nerve transmission from cell to cell throughout the entire Nervous System of the body. It is what enables people to communicate in a healthy manner and for the body to adequately and optimally function.

The EFA's were originally called Vitamin F when they were first discovered as an essential nutrient class in 1923. In 1930 they were reclassified with the fats rather than with the vitamin category. EFA's are one of the most highly researched classes of nutrients with over 8,000 studies completed and many currently underway. This research-mania is due to their great benefit and significant studies have been conducted around the globe including within the U.S. at respected institutions such as; Harvard University, Georgetown University, Columbia University, the National Institute of Health and many others. All of the research on EFA's has confirmed the diverse health benefits people receive both mentally and physically.

Some of the more pivotal research and applications revealed in the past decade has come from the secondary fractions of EFA's called Eicosapentaenoic Acid (EPA) and Docosahexaenoic Acid (DHA). These two fatty acids have demonstrated support of numerous body functions including blood pressure, blood viscosity, vasoconstriction, immune response and regulating inflammatory function within the body. These pathways have explained and further opened the door for dozens of applications for prevention and maintenance of Heart Disease, Immune and Auto-Immune Support, decreasing Bowel Disease and improving Mental Health.

The term "Essential" infers that the EFA's cannot be constructed in the body from other fatty acids. Their roles are different than fats and oils that provide only fuel for the body. EFA's are required on a regular basis if wellness is to be maintained and because of the EFA's foundational role in one's daily metabolism for maintenance, repair and optimum function they are in the top seven GIS protocol basics.

What is the family of EFA's?

There are many "Conditional EFA's" that the body utilizes for important pathway functions in the body yet scientists agree that there are only two actual EFA's. The Conditional EFA's include; Lauric Acid, Palmitoleic Acid and Gamma-Linolenic Acid (GLA) and each of these hold remarkable credits to their particular fatty acid. GLA for example, has been found to be extremely valuable for healthy skin, hair and hormones. In fact studies have shown that GLA may also be involved in reducing hormone related cancers, promoting balance to the female fertility cycle and calming down an overactive Auto-Immune response. The body can actually manufacture these three fatty acids from EFA's under the right conditions and that is why they are not considered essential in themselves.

The two EFA's of greatest importance that must be supplied regularly to the body is Alpha-Linolenic Acid, Omega-3 and Linoleic Acid referred to as Omega-6. Several other secondary fatty acids are made from the Omega-6's including the Gamma-Linolenic Acid (GLA), the Dihomo-Gamma-Linolenic Acid (DGLA) and Arachidonic Acid (AA). The Omega-3's are required in the synthesis of the other two very important secondary EFA fractions EPA and DHA.

Balanced EFA's are Essential for a Healthy Brain and Body 1:1

- *Omega-3 Fatty Acid* – a - Linolenic acid (ALA) – Fish & sea-foods, flax, raw nuts (walnuts) & seeds, spinach, leafy greens, algae, olive oil (contains some Om-3 yet higher in Om-6) and other sources.
- *Omega-6 Fatty Acid* – Linoleic Acid (LA) – Vegetable oils contain higher Om-6's than Om-3's generally, fried & processed food oils, hydrogenated vegetable oils (also called Trans-fats), beans, grains, nuts & seeds and other sources.

What is the healthiest ratio of Omega 3's to 6's in the body?

The healthier ratio that most experts agree upon is at least a 1:1 ratio of Omega 3's to Omega 6 Fatty Acids. However some people may feel their best to compensate for health challenges at a 2:1 (Omega 3's to 6's) as they strive for optimum health. The facts reveal that most people are receiving excessively high levels of Omega-6 Fatty Acids that contribute to unhealthy inflammation in the body. This plays a big factor in all Auto-

Immune conditions like IBS, IBD, CVD, Asthma, RA, Arthritis and Mental Illness to include Depression, OCD, Bi-Polar, ADD and ADHD. The daily goal of 3,000 mg of Omega-3 Fatty Acids or a greater amount as your health dictates will begin to replenish the body's deficiencies while keeping the intake of Omega's 6 oils appropriately lower in the diet. This is accomplished by reducing the consumption of fried foods, chips, bakery goods, prepared convenience foods and fast foods that will help you meet your goal. Surprisingly even healthy foods may tip the scales towards higher Omega 6's so take note in the review of "Grass Fed" animals. Chicken, turkey, cheeses, milk products, regular beef, eggs, some nuts & seeds, beans and grains generally contain higher Omega 6 Fatty Acids than Omega 3's because the animals are fed grains (higher in Omega-6's) and or the beans for example just naturally contain higher Omega 6's than 3's.

Eating sardines and occasionally other cold water fish are great ways to kick up your Omega-3 intake along with the vegetable sources including leafy greens. Yet to reach the suggested therapeutic levels required with GIS a quality fish oil supplement is encouraged. Flax oil can be used if fish oil cannot be tolerated however make certain you are getting enough quantity for your body's health requirement mixed with other sources. Some experts suggest that the body requires 10x the quantity of vegetable Omega-3's to an animal source of Omega 3's taking at least one tablespoon of flax oil for every fifty pounds of body weight. The conversion of Flax Oil (Omega-3 source) into EPA and DHA fractions is very inefficient in the body and some people may not make any at all due to an unhealthy liver. Detoxification of the liver is important to encourage a more efficient metabolism of vegetable Omega 3's to the conversion of EPA and DHA however fish oil is a great alternative if possible because it comes with EPA and DHA.

The Language of Fats

The category of Polyunsaturated Fatty Acids (PUFA'S) include the EFA's along with other non-essential fatty acids and are sourced primarily from vegetables, nuts and seed oils, fish and sea foods. Vegetable sources of

EFA's contain varying ratios of the Omega 3 and 6's along with some non-essential fatty acids as is the case with olive oil that contains Omega 3's, 6's and 9's. The Omega-9 Fatty Acid is not essential however Oleic Acid an Omega-9 is valuable as found in olives appearing to increase the positive cholesterol High Density Lipids (HDL). Erucic Acid found in Canola Oil is somewhat limited yet is another more well-known food source of Omega-9.

To understand the nomenclature of fats better the Short Chain Polyunsaturated Fatty Acids (SC-PUFA's) are Omega 3 and 6's and they are required for the starting point of creating the Long Chain Polyunsaturated Fatty Acids (LC-PUFA's). They are also called Highly Unsaturated Fatty Acids (HUFA) and include all of the secondary fractions of EPA, DHA, GLA, DGLA and AA. Another class of fats that fatty acids can fall into based on their molecular configuration is partial saturation called Mono-Unsaturated Fatty Acids like butter and some nuts. Animal products contain mostly Saturated Fatty Acids almost exclusively as in eggs, milk, cheeses and meats yet they can contain small amounts of PUFA's as well.

Coconuts are one of the vegetable exceptions with 92% of their fatty acids Saturated, 6% Mono-unsaturated and only 2% Polyunsaturated Fatty Acids. However coconuts are still considered a health food source if not eaten in excess and they contain some very medicinal fats, one called Lauric Acid and another Caprylic Acid that demonstrate both Anti-Viral and Anti-Fungal action in the body. Chapter 8 reviews the health support of using a Caprylic Acid supplement referenced in the GIS Program.

Trans-fats are unnaturally made through the process of taking vegetable polyunsaturated oils and either adding hydrogen as in margarine and some peanut butters or they are created during the deep frying of oils as with French fries. Research has shown Trans-fats along with excessive saturated fats to be extremely destructive in the body increasing the levels of LDL bad cholesterol and lowering the good HDL. Science has made the relationship of a higher intake of the Trans-fats to the higher incidence of Heart Disease. For this reason the FDA has made strong recommendations to keep Trans-fats as low as possible in the diet. The body has tremendous difficulty digesting them and it appears to reduce absorption of the healthy fats from the over-consumption of Trans-fats that also add to unnecessary weight gain, oxidation or premature aging and overall poor health of the body.

What are the food sources of EFA's for both the Omega-3 and Omega-6 Fatty Acids?

Nature has provided both vegetable and animal sources of the valuable EFA's. In vegetables the Omega 3's are found in larger percentages in green leafy vegetables, algae from the sea, nuts especially walnuts and seeds to include; sunflower, sesame, pumpkin and flax. Once again the drawback with the vegetable sources is that they do not contain the important secondary fraction extras of EPA and DHA as found in fish and sea foods. As mentioned they must be manufactured in the body and studies confirm that the amount of EPA and DHA required in the body from vegetable sources is not even feasible because the production can be as low as 2% conversion to EPA and DHA! This is an extremely important fact to consider in optimizing your EPA and DHA level. It is precisely why I encourage the inclusion of fish sources of Omega 3's that help guarantee the body's stores of EPA and DHA for children and adults. Only animal sources of Omega-3 from fish and shellfish contain these secondary fractions without having to rely on the body to work perfectly to synthesize them. Fatty Fish and fish oil products come with varying levels of EPA and DHA. Shrimp is a source however it is lower than the fatty cold water fish that includes; cod, salmon, mackerel, tuna and sardines.

Omega-6 Fatty Acids

Omega 6's is primary found in grains, beans, nuts and seeds and oils. Because animals commonly eat grains in their diets the meat of cows, chickens and turkeys contain the higher Omega-6 Fatty Acids and are relatively void of the Omega 3's. Therefore, eating cheeses made from milk from cows fed grain will also contain the higher levels of Om-6's. The exception would be if animals are "Grass Fed". Grass contains the

Omega 3's so it only follows that the meat of grass eating animals would also contain the Omega-3 Fatty Acids as in "Grass Fed Beef". Avocadoes contain a higher level of Omega 6 to Omega 3's and so do peanuts, Brazil nuts, beans, eggs and turkey! Because the balancing act of EFA's does get a little confusing individuals can order a home test for checking your own level of Omega 3's that is very reliable. The reference section gives you the contact for the reliable testing company and in approximately 30 days after submitting your test you will not have to guess you will know your Omega numbers!

Most people receive an overabundance of Omega-6 Fatty Acids through processed and fast foods that contain high levels of vegetable oil and Trans-fats as well. Some experts have postulated that the intake of Omega 6's may be as high as 16,000 mg. daily due to eating processed and junk foods. New research published in the *American Journal of Nutrition* in 2011 reviewed the eating habits of Americans in the last 100 years and showed a 5% increase in Omega 6's and only a half of percent increase in Omega 3's of the US individual at large. They stated that there has been a 1000 fold increase in soy bean oil consumption and that some people boarder on a 30:1 ratio of Omega 6's to Omega 3's! This excessively high level of Omega 6's have been associated with many disease conditions in the body resulting from the increase of inflammation from the extraordinarily high "6" intake!

Fish Oil Supplements Come with Added Benefits

A bottle of fish oil can make the big difference in giving the body the added extra Omega 3's, EPA and DHA. Some products are also formulated to contain Vitamins A & D which speed-up tissue renewal of the body and other health support. All lining cells of the body both inside and out including the digestive tract, face and skin require generous amounts of Vitamin A along with minerals and protein that together rebuild healthier skin. Review Chapter 8 for more information about Vitamin A & D.

Selecting a quality fish oil product that contains both vitamin A and D is also important because many children and adults do not absorb beta carotene source of Vitamin A from the vegetables they are eating. Beta Carotene requires a healthy liver to efficiently process the Vitamin A as discussed in Chapter 6 in the Healthy Glandular section. Fish oil Vitamin A is absorbed quickly into the blood stream not requiring the liver for digestion as with Beta Carotene. Fish Oil Vitamin D3 - Cholecalciferol is the best source of Vitamin D for absorption as well. Vitamin D reviewed in Chapter 8 GIS Supplements is required for the absorption of minerals like Calcium, Magnesium and Zinc to build healthy tissue, strong bones and avoid Rickets, Osteoporosis, Mental Health, Increase Immunity and other important applications for infants, kids, teens and adults.

What do the EPA and DHA Fractions from EFA's do in the body?

EPA and DHA are linked to a wide range of health benefits revolving around stimulating cell division, cellular function and running the metabolic systems of the body. Ultimately their function relates to health success of the GIS Program and a bonus towards "Healthy Aging".

- *Central Nervous System* – Brain Tissue requires 20% DHA, Glandular Health Improves, Lowers Hyperactivity in Adults & Children, Improves Motor Skills, Reflexes, Athletic Performance and decreases Anxiety, Depression and even Suicidal tendencies.
- *Cellular Communication* – Cellular Function, Reduction in Cellular Oxidation, Weight Loss & Maintenance (Leptin), Tissue Regeneration for Anti-Aging, Total Body Function.
- *Metabolism Support* – Cell Division, Required to Manufacture Hormones (raw material), Fertility, Healthy Fetal & Child Development, Menopause (women) and Andropause (men) and Healthy Aging.
- *Healthy Inflammatory Response* – Colon Health, Reduces Joint Pain, Pain Control, Reduce and Prevent CVD, Asthma, Autism, Skin, Nerve Disorders and Supports Mental Health.
- *Cardio Vascular System (CVS)* – Reduction in Arteriolosclerosis –Plaque & Triglycerides, Reduction of Stroke Factors, Anti-Clotting, Healthy Blood Thinning, Reduced Systolic & Diastolic

Blood Pressure, Lessens Heart Arrhythmias and Increases Survival of Heart Attack Events.

- ***Immunity Balance*** – Regulates the Immune & Auto-Immune System, Reduction in Opportunistic Organisms (fungus including Candida, bacteria, viral), Skin Health and Lowers Allergy Response.

Why choose a Quality Fish Oil product for your GIS "Health" Program?

Researchers estimate that the average American maintains only 24% of the required 50% Omega-3 Fatty Acids needed in their blood for optimal levels. This low Omega 3 numbers coincide with heart disease as the number one cause of mortality in the US. Bill Lands, MD researcher through the National Institute of Health (NIH) as well as his own private research revealed a direct relationship of each country's Omega 3 level in their population to the incidence of Cardiovascular Heart Disease (CHD) mortality. Dr. Land's revealed that the country's population that reached 50% or greater experienced the most drastic reduction in CHD. An impressive high saturation of Omega-3 Highly Unsaturated Fatty Acids was found in the Japanese at 60% who experienced less than a third the mortality from heart disease compared to Americans at 24%. The highest Omega 3 level was in the people of Greenland approaching 70% who cut their CHD mortality even further. He states from his findings that relying on the old fashion blood cholesterol is a poor predictor of CHD worldwide and people need to know their Omega 3 number to remove the guesswork from this equation to reach cardiovascular health. As health educator Stuart Tomc put it, "People need to - Nix the 6 and Eat the 3's – Eat Less [calories] and Exercise More - to prevent mortality due to heart disease!"

It is difficult for most people to reach the suggested level of 50% Omega 3's with diet alone so choosing a fish oil supplement is of critical importance! Fish oil with the added extras of EPA, DHA and Vitamin A & D, balanced with dietary Omega-6 Fatty Acids, supports heart health, colon health and is needed to rebuild and maintain the entire body for optimal health. The EFA's and especially the proper amount of Omega 3's function preventatively to discourage disease development in the entire family at every age and for athletes too!

In choosing a quality fish oil product there is a big difference in EFA's and fish oil products on the market today. With the concern of water pollution in our oceans and also with the GIS challenge of poor fat digestion, the importance of choosing a fish oil product that will satisfy both of these needs leads to the recommendation of the *"Nordic Naturals"* product line - Pure and Great Tasting Omega Oils.

Nordic's passion to exceed the world standard of purity through distillation methods of their fish oils can give all individuals the security of safety to enjoy the health benefits without potential toxicity or carcinogenic chemicals. The Gold Standard processing method by *Nordic Naturals* removes the danger coming from the environment of identifiable plastics of PCB's, Dioxin's and toxic metals including Mercury, Lead and miscellaneous other contaminants. All of Nordic's specialized formulas are made with the same unmatched refining methods for safety and easy digestibility and good taste. Look for published pharmaceutical testing made available by calling the company or visiting their website www. nordicnaturals.com.

The optimum preventative goal for EPA and DHA for adults is 2,000 mg and to reach approximately 3,000 - 4,000 mg total of Omega-3 Fatty Acids to attain excellence. It is not easy to reach the levels through diet alone because living in today's world we are prudently limited on the quantity of fish we can safely eat because of the mercury and PCB pollutants, found in higher amounts in larger fish like salmon and tuna. Smaller fish like sardines and anchovies and others contain less contaminant and may be eaten more frequently even daily. I realize also that many people are not fond of fish. In this case I suggest people consider a quality fish oil supplement because of the unmatched value the body receives compared to the limited vegetable sources – *Nordic Naturals* for All!

Better Digestion of Fish Oil using "rTG" Means Healthier Results!

New research on fish oil absorption has just been completed by the famous pioneer, Jorn Dyerberg. His original work on fish oil and heart disease was published in the *Lancet* and the *American Journal of Clinical Nutrition* in the early 1970's. It revealed that the Eskimo indigenous people of the northern hemisphere who lived on fish and local plant life while eating large quantities of whale blubber fat did not develop heart disease as might be expected. This unique finding led the researchers to discover the unparalleled benefit of eating cold water fish for the prevention of plaque formation. Reducing inflammatory factors from all sources and including fish oil leads people to avoid and reduce Arteriolosclerosis and all other inflammatory related conditions.

Recently Dr. Dyerberg and his Danish co-workers released their finding in September of 2010 that concluded the bioavailability of fish absorption to be 70% greater when the fish oil is processed using "Re-Esterified Triglyceride" over the common processing called "Ethyl Esters Distillation". This new finding was published in the *Journal of Prostaglandins, Leukotrienes and Essential Fatty Acids*. This superior method referred to as "rTG" happens to be the chosen process by the Nordic Naturals company for refining and concentrating their fish oil. The taste is smooth, pleasant (flavored with natural lemon, strawberry, peach and other tastes) and does not repeat as often like so many fish oils do. Children just chew up the little kids gel caps pleasantly and naturally flavored and spit the gelatin out. Don't be surprised when they ask for more!

CHAPTER   6

Healthy Focus Factors

"My life seemed over after losing so many family and friends to accidents and sickness. Drinking the loneliness away stopped working abruptly so I moved to Colorado to start a fresh new life. I checked myself into a 12 step AA program yet my gut was hurting so badly I wasn't sure if I even wanted to live much less stop drinking. After the meeting I went into a health food store and bought Aloe Vera Juice Concentrate by Aloe Life and within minutes of drinking the liquid I felt better. Today with over two years of sobriety I continue to drink my Aloe juice, got on a healthy diet and share with others how much better a person can feel getting healthier!"

— *Charles, Colorado*

Addictions are major stumbling blocks in life! Healthy Focus Factors address "Addictions" first off because all people find themselves with some type of obsession or addiction in life. Some appear to be better than others such as exercise, working, hobbies or shopping vs. eating junk foods, taking drugs or drinking alcohol. However, excesses even with the seemingly healthier obsessions can be taken to extremes and actually destroy families as well as people's health. Balance in life is "Key". Every person needs to strive for balance to achieve not only health and success in life but happiness and fulfillment along the way.

Health is important to build a strong foundation that allows each of us to experience our lives fully. However, health doesn't seem to be on many peoples "to do list" these days until it starts slipping away. Several common tell-tale body signals revealing that your health needs more attention are fatigue, mental anguish, physical illness and pain throughout the body.

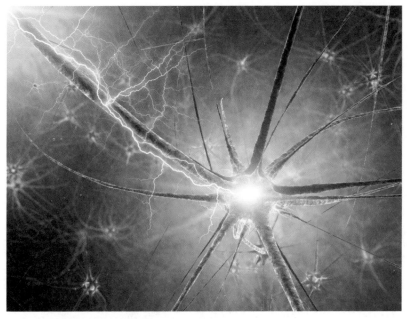

The Body Sends Out Signals for Help!

- Fatigue
- Mental Distress
- Physical Illness
- Pain

Each of these conditions are extremely important to discover the cause in order to minimize suffering in the body but also to ward off pre-mature aging and the potential for an early death – that's all. We talked in length in Chapter 5 about fatigue and mental health and how it often develops from the common conditions of Anemia and Mal-Absorption of nutrients. However, pain in the body is more of a general signal to the brain that can come from a wide variety of causes. We may not always know what is causing the pain yet without a doubt it does signal that something is wrong!

People on the whole try to mask pain instead of finding the cause and alleviate it. Pain and other signals reflect a malfunction or imbalance occurring in the body - similar to a dashboard light on a car panel turning ON. The light is to alert the driver of low oil or other deficiencies in the car needing attention. Pain can develop from physical injury or exertion, infection from viruses, fungus or bacteria or even nutritional deficiencies as in low B12 or protein as discussed in great length in previous chapters.

Daily headaches, stomach pain, pain in the joints or muscles is an alarm telling you that your health needs to be reviewed - covering the basics first; diet, detoxification (especially regularity) or perhaps just a need to drink more water. If the pain is just masked over with an over-the-counter (OTC) medication like Acetaminophen or even a stronger pain medication it may indeed give temporary pain relief yet it does not address the source. The important question to ask yourself is do you know what is causing the pain? If the answer is yes that you do know where your pain is coming from even if it is from an accident, injury or a birth defect a reduction of pain is still possible through lessening overall inflammation in the body. If you don't know where your pain is coming from you need to put on your detective hat and go through a process of elimination.

Pain is not the only signal of a nutritional deficiency in the body. A failing immune system, allergies or even an auto-immune disease or illness each call for action to improve one's health to reduce pain and a poor health status. Being preventative to disease by applying the health principles before a cancer or advanced bowel disease or sickness develops – is the ideal action. Lastly, as much of a warning signal as pain is in the body it is not always present before a devastating disease develops. Many of my patients first awareness of cancer was through an ultrasound test not a pain signal. Sometimes a cancer will create pain yet most often it silently develops from a suppressed immune system. Surprisingly many people also do not experience pain before having a heart attack either! To apply this motto in your life will save you from untold suffering, "An ounce of prevention is worth a pound of cure – Take Action Today to kick up your health another notch!"

Types of Pain in the Body	Common Causes of Pain
Headache	Anemia, High Blood Pressure, Viral, Dehydration.
Muscle, Joints & Nerve	Nutritional Deficiencies; B12, Protein, B-Complex, Minerals, Vitamin C, EFA's, plus Inflammation, Skeletal Misalignment Requiring a Chiropractor or Osteopathic Doctor Manipulation, Stress, Viruses.
Digestive & Gas	Infections, IBS/IBD, Constipation, Detoxification.
Nutritional Deficiencies	GIS (B12 and other), Diet Limitations, Food Abuse.
High Blood Pressure	Mineral Imbalance, Arteriolosclerosis, Stress.
Metabolic Illness	Poor Functioning Immune System, Environmental, Genetics.
Infection - all types	Nutritional Deficiency; Protein, Vitamin A, Probiotics.
Inflammation & Injury	GIS, Accidents, Neglect and Addiction.
Phantom Pain	Nutritional Deficiency; Increase Fish Oils, B-Complex, topical Aloe Skin Gel by *Aloe Life* and drink Aloe juice.

Generally speaking mainstream Allopathic medicine, does not address the cause of the pain or health imbalance, it addresses the symptoms. This is a valuable lesson in "Health 101" so do pay close attention. The cause of your pain or other symptoms of fatigue, mental distress, skin conditions, allergies if not resolved - may develop into a bigger health challenge of disease in the future. You need to be your own health detective and do your best to get the proper diagnoses from an Integrative Health Professional so you can take action to remedy the cause. Some of you know what I am talking about from connecting your own health challenges over the years to nutritional deficiencies and health imbalances. Others of you have sought out professional guidance from trained personnel in complimentary medicine to regain better health. However, too many people have fallen into the trap of adding more and more pharmaceutical drugs in the attempt to gain the allusive gold ring of feeling better instantly! The body does not heal instantly. If you wish to regain permanent resolution of chronic ailments the timeline for the body is days, weeks and even years to rebuild the body's system for permanent health improvement. The following GIS story is an excellent example of the perseverance of a young man looking for the cause of his pain and finding it!

Steve's Unrelenting Pain Led Him to the GIS Program

Answering a phone call in my office one day I met Steve, a young businessman. His call was the first step for his healing process of finding pain resolution. He was living with advanced gluten intolerance symptoms which he was totally unaware of. What comes to mind is the saying, "Necessity is the mother of invention." His GIS condition was escalating with additional side effects coming from his added prescription medication. Each passing day seemed to increase his already excruciating pain in his feet. Steve was becoming desperate to find answers and gave me a call.

Pain in the body has a way of getting a persons attention and if you turn towards health for a solution it will always help. Steve called to find out if drinking Aloe Vera would interfere with his Reflux medication. Apparently he had been on a quest for several years to find the solution to his relentless digestive issues and wound up taking Reflux medication along the way.

His doctor had obliged his cry for help by layering him with several medications to ease his symptoms of heartburn along with high blood pressure, Asthma and his latest challenge burning in the esophagus diagnosed as Reflux. After complying with the prescription medications which didn't seem to help very much he began to develop other symptoms of pain. The newest one that was quickly becoming the worst of all was neuropathy developing in his legs and feet.

Neuropathy develops from the body losing proper circulation to the extremities. This results in a numbness that gradually turns into extreme pain in the feet. As we talked I could hear the fear in his voice as he shared the down turn in his health that was now threatening his very livelihood as a traveling salesman. He announced that he had been turning toward health products and even improved his eating habits yet it all seemed as though it was making him feel worse. I ask him one simple question, "Have you ever consider that you may be gluten intolerant?"

Steve was not happy with my question. His voice was one of frustration to even consider one more diagnosis. For a couple of years now he had been spending hundreds of dollars monthly for supplements and medical costs and the thought of changing anything else in his life seemed unbearable. However, he told me he did feel better when drinking the Aloe Vera StomachPlus juice and wanted to make sure it didn't conflict with his medications. I assured him of the safety and suggested he review my guidelines for a gluten free protocol and follow it for a month. He thanked me and said good bye.

A few weeks later I received another call from Steve. He had stopped eating whole grains and wasn't sure if he was feeling any better from the omission or not. He said it might be helping but he could not say for sure. His neuropathy was still causing major pain yet drinking the Aloe Vera seemed to be helping his digestive burning and improving daily regularity. A further inventory of the supplements Steve was taking was a surprise even for a health veteran as me. Steve was consuming almost 60 supplements every day mostly in the capsule form!

Don't get me wrong, I love food supplements and they can be extremely helpful in rebuilding health. Yet I knew with the shear quantity of gelatin from the capsules he was desperately consuming, that they were compounding Steve's inflammation that linked to his pain. My job now, once I had the whole picture, was to enlighten

Steve. I knew it would be a challenge to make him understand that the supplements he was taking paired with the drugs were actually causing the pain! Steve did not believe me when I told him that he would feel better if he stopped taking the supplements because of the quantity of gelatin he was ingesting.

In fact at that point Steve ended our phone conversation and called the vitamin companies asking them if they contained gluten? It was an understandable question and he called me back to inform me that his cachet of supplements was "Gluten Free". He also added that I should not consider them a health challenge. In turn I shared with him that the company's response was only due to their ignorance and it was not an accurate answer. I also told him that I was absolutely certain he would feel better stopping the gelatin.

Out of Denial at Last

Once again I encouraged Steve to follow the GIS program of diet and supplements which numbered only about six or seven products per day avoiding any gelatin and call me back in a month. A considerable amount of time passed and finally the call came. A tone of kinship and gratefulness flowed from Steve. He told me he had followed my suggestion and after 2 1/2 months the neuropathy was all but gone. He said within days of beginning the GIS guidelines he began to feel better and better. Steve then asked the question about getting off his medication. I told him that was between his doctor and himself. I did offer my opinion that when you don't have the need you don't need the remedy. All medication comes with side effects especially acid blockers if taken for any extended period of time. Just read the medical insert accompanying that medication or any others to confirm the health warnings.

As Steve came to trust my experience and guidance at last - you too can trust the GIS Program. I think you will find the Healthy Focus Factors section crucial to rebuilding body wellness. Learning the foundational truths about the body is very empowering. Applying them is life changing towards a healthier and happier life!

Health Success Involves Learning & Taking Action!

The Healthy Focus Factor topics were chosen because they relate to all people who strive towards optimum health and disease prevention. Pay special attention if you are living with advanced bowel or chronic disease conditions to give you faster health improvements. Searching for the truth about health is a bit like being lost in a jungle with uncertainty as to which way to turn? Once a path of awareness is cut for you in the bush - it will continue to lead you to discovering the "Big Picture" of health – guiding you along for a successful health journey. Gradually you will not feel overwhelmed as you find your way following in the steps of others.

1.) *Education is the First Step to Awareness.* Reading and learning about health challenges that effect all human beings of every age gives you the awareness of what may be preventing you from feeling your very best. As similar as each of us truly are we also have special circumstances, genetics and experiences that demand special nutrients or therapies. You will know what your body requires by reviewing and applying the different sections.

2.) *Applying What You Learn Brings Success.* As an experienced health educator I find the most successful way of improving ones health is to accent the positive health selections in your daily diet first. Choosing to eat the healthy foods in the GIS program in Chapter 7 will give you the best results and help you naturally lose your cravings for junk foods and addictions. Start on the foundational supplements as soon as possible to give you success of improved digestion, more energy in your day and clearer thinking.

Drinking a good amount of water and getting exercise in your day, regularly, will support you to get healthy again and or prevent disease from taking hold in the future. If you do get sick or have a flare-up in your bowel disease in the future you will find that you regain the feel good status much more quickly applying the GIS Program as you become healthier.

3.) *Positive Reinforcement by Keeping a Health Diary/Log.* As you read the Healthy Focus Factors in addition to eating the GIS dietary guidelines in Chapter 7 and starting to experiment with the supplements in Chapter 8 - your health progress will continue in the right direction. By keeping a log or health diary of what you are eating and include in your daily regimen; what you eat, supplements you take or an activity you are incorporating - you become your own health counselor. This exercise of writing it down and how you feel each day will keep you from getting overwhelmed. It also gives great perspective of your weekly and monthly progress.

Review and follow each Healthy Focus Factor for 6 weeks to 3 months as needed to enhance your daily healthier choices of a healthy lifestyle. A diary is also extremely helpful if you choose to work with a health professional which is always an option to pursue yet not absolutely necessary. Most people that I have guided through with a phone call or two have done beautifully being their own life coach. As you learn in turn YOU will become the teacher in sharing GIS with your friends and family as well as any health professional that you might meet. Together we will continue to kick up a Health Revolution that will benefit one and all!

Reaping the Rewards of Health is the result!

As you make the healthier choices outlined in this chapter and Chapter 7 you will reduce all your bowel symptoms and build a healthier more vital immune system. You will not only reduce your bowel symptoms but your body will be able to protect you better against all disease including; Flu & Cold Viruses, Cancer, Cardiovascular Disease along with rebuilding more youthful vibrant skin to avoid pre-mature aging. People respond in different time schedules - so be patient with yourself and others that you may be guiding on their health path. Get moving because exercise is also required to achieve optimum health!

Non-Food Rewards Work!

Rewarding oneself with non-food rewards is a helpful tool as you gain success over addictive habits. Reading positive and uplifting books about health is also a great motivator to keep positive during a more challenging time of improving one's life.

Exercise is an extremely successful tool to utilize during lifestyle transition because it lowers stress, helps the body work better and increases pleasure hormones for the brain! Even doing Cross-Crawl as explained in Chapter 12 Home Health 101 is amazingly helpful to unlock the chains that keep a person from experiencing more health and joy. Giving your own foot massage or trading with a friend, walk in the park or to choose an outing with the family or a friend - anything that does not relate to food or drink can all bring varying degrees of reward and pleasure. Starting a new hobby can also be fun with another person or by oneself and perhaps even taking a class at the local community school or church could be quite entertaining. For you singles I met my husband through taking an adult education class on "Raw Foods Nutrition" many years ago - ha! No matter who you are or what your age – for heaven's sake - allow yourself some FUN whatever may be your choice! When you get your health back the sky is the limit!

20 Healthy Focus Factors
1. Addiction; Sugar, Alcohol, Milk & More

The category of indulgence and addiction is of utmost importance especially the ones linked to sugars. Chapter 3 reveals that sugar is at the crux of inflammation in the body. Alcohol breaks down into sugars and also milk sugar called lactose which is found in cow's milk, adds to the inflammation potential as well. Hopefully you are beginning to see the bigger picture of the importance of addressing addictions to these habits.

Addictions are best described in matter of degrees. Major addictions to pharmaceutical drugs, OTC and Street Drugs and definitely Alcohol can each become much more consuming and dangerous quicker (especially in large quantities) than any minor food addictions. However, drug and alcohol addictions are not the only addictions that pose extreme danger to people. I talk to individuals everyday that are killing themselves with overeating of confections containing white flour, sugar and hydrogenated fats like margarine or other Trans-fats.

Parents mistake the showering of sugary treats on their children for giving them LOVE. Truly loving a family member or nurturing ourselves - whatever the case may be - means offering healthy foods and healthy treats. Love must be tough at times and you are the adult. Keep sugar for an exception – a special treat not the daily or even weekly indulgence if you want to experience optimum mental and physical health.

Children and adults sometimes focus on sugary treats as a type of hobby through baking or being a connoisseur of; candy, bakery goods, ice cream, chocolate, sodas, pies, cookies, junk foods and more. Sugar is a more socially accepted addiction capable of slipping under the radar screen as it creates destruction in the body. Refined sugar sets the stage for inflammatory disease and eaten in excess may bring about digestive illnesses, stunted growth, obesity, bone loss, scoliosis, tooth decay, mental psychosis, weak immune function and premature aging. Not very LOVING is it?

Both categories of addictions to include; drugs, alcohol and the sugars hold potential destruction which I label major and minor. The ultimate damage to one's health depends on the quantity of the substance especially with sugar which is often begun in copious amounts in childhood. Refined carbohydrates in breads and pastries metabolize into sugars adding to the body's nutritional stress and inflammation. Less of a substance is always best yet once an addiction gets a hold of a person whether it is alcohol, drugs, candy or even bread the individual can lose control with any amount and binge. As painful as it may be to hear this word of advice, abstinence is often the only way out of an addiction.

Food & Chemical Addictions

- Major - Pharmaceutical Drugs, OTC, Street Drugs, Alcohol and Smoking.
- Minor (May develop into Major) - Refined Sugar, Dairy Products, Grains – cereals, crackers & bread, Bakery Goods, Ice

Cream, Chocolate, Candy, Sodas, Junk Food, Dessert Coffees, Energy Drinks and Caffeine.

I don't pretend to be an expert in addictive behavior. However, over the years of counseling hundreds of people with health issues, blended with my own addictive tendencies, I have studied and learned volumes on the human addictive experience.

First and foremost we live in an addictive world which condones the addictive lifestyles to a certain extent. You may say to yourself if sugar is so bad for people why do they sell so much of it? Sugar is a mega-industry with lobbyist in Wash., DC just like alcohol. When you study the history of sugar over the ages you truly see that it has been the downfall of many societies because of its disastrous affects on the human body. In the last 100 years the consumption of sugar in the U.S. has gone up from approximately 4 lbs. per year for each person to over 250 lbs. per person yearly. The problem with sugar is people are eating far too much of it because it is so addictive!

Sugar Addiction

The body has a tendency to quickly adapt to the brain stimulation it receives from any stimulant or sedative like sugar and alcohol. It craves for more and more to meet the growing desire in the body. Likened to an emotional Band-Aid – eating sugar can temporarily heighten energy and reduce pain by providing a release of pleasure hormones that are similar to Morphine. They are called Endorphins and the process of eating sugar to increase these hormones becomes very addictive especially when the body is not manufacturing its own healthy hormones. The body can actually make Endorphins naturally when it is in a healthy nutritional balance and getting vigorous exercise. Another way sugars become addictive whether it be from the sugar in candy or the alcohol sugar is its action as a stimulant. The sugars first cause an energy boost and then it causes the body to become depressed as it exhausts its B-Complex supply in the body causing havoc with the blood sugar level. The fact is candy and alcohol are depressants and can really cause a mental downward spiraling affect.

Emotional pain and loneliness are two experiences in life that are not easy to deal with. Humans are wired to be with other humans for companionship, fun and love. When sugar, alcohol and carbohydrate loading fill the emotional and loneliness gap – bingo - an addiction is in the making. Addictions become a best friend! After a while the addiction can become a trap requiring all the support you can conjure up to escape it including; support groups, private counseling, exercise, lots of prayer and above all else a good nutritional program. Many good books are available to help you through sugar and other addictions. Karly Randolph Pitman writes about her binge eating, bulimic and sugar addiction in her series of books. They are entitled, *Overcoming Sugar Addiction, Heal Your Body Image* and *Growing Human (Kind) ness: How to befriend not punish your way to sugar sobriety.* I had the pleasure of interviewing Karly, who was schooled in cognitive psychology and communication and she has developed an educational website. She profoundly states that there is a big difference in people being "Sugar Sensitive" or flat out "Sugar Addicted". The book that first helped her delve into nutrition and break her sugar addiction was called, *Potatoes Not Prozac* by Dr. K. Des Maisons! How's that for a book title giving the content message?

Applying the GIS Program reduces the cravings so the addictions stop ruling your actions allowing you to regain control as the adult takes charge again! It takes approximately 40 days to get a better handle on addictions and to become more comfortable with new healthy habits and a few supplements. In Chapter 7 you will learn about sweet alternatives to refined sugars for desserts that will give the flavor without the "Glycemic (sugar) Rush"!

Breaking the Chains of All Addictions

- Decide to Change! DECIDE – COMMIT – SUCCEED!
- Eat Regular Meals - 3 Times Daily; Protein 20 grams per meal and healthy carbohydrates.

- Take Supplements Stabilizing Blood Sugar (See Blood Sugar section.); Protein Powder, NAC, Aloe Vera and a Multiple Vitamin and Mineral, Chromium GTF and Licorice Tea (as tolerated).
- Exercise Daily; 30 Minutes or more.
- Read POSITIVE & FUN BOOKS, listen to positive or funny TV and other media.
- Seek Emotional Support; 12 Step, Church, Books, Friends, Music, Conviction, Prayer and other support.

Applying health helps greatly along with learning new social communication skills. It is important to learn positive self-talk dialogue with yourself and others that create healthier actions and reactions in your life. Getting enough balance back in your life to break addictions can take several or all of the above suggestions especially adding a good exercise program. Exercising through fast walking, running and other aerobic exercise for at least 35 – 40 minutes gives you the pay off of stimulating more of the pleasure hormones "Endorphins" and helps stabilize blood sugar too! The Cross-Crawl exercise can get a person started or works well for even an experienced athlete. It is basically marching in place to music, the TV, at home, work or outdoors. It encourages deep breathing and as you get warmed up you can begin to lift the knees higher and higher. Start with 7 minutes as tolerated and increase to15 minutes twice per day. You will be surprised with how much better you feel getting more movement in your life. Get busy drinking more water too!

By accenting the positive and maintaining healthy blood sugar - it is easier to reduce addictive cravings. Review the Blood Sugar section. Keep in mind that breaking the chains of addiction involves rebalancing the brain chemistry along with the rest of the body supported through nutrition. *Change Your Brain Change Your Body* written by Daniel G. Amen, M.D., 2010, is a great book that will give you some extra support for your particular needs if you tend to hit a wall. He has worked very successfully I might add, with many NFL football players who became overweight and unhealthy. I know you can experience success just as I have and thousands of others across the globe by forgiving yourself for your short comings and following your health path – One Day at a Time!

Nutrition Highlights: Protein, B-Complex, N-Acetyl-Cysteine (NAC) 1 – 3 times daily, Vitamin C, Alpha Lipoic Acid, Chromium GTF, Multiple Minerals, 5HTP, Herbs; Licorice tea, Chamomile, St. John's Wort, Rescue Remedy and Valerian.

2. Anemia of the Blood

Anemia is becoming extremely common in today's world. As mentioned in Chapter 5 it is the most common nutritional deficiency and effects many children and adults that have poor digestion and gluten intolerance. Once you grasp the fact that all people are living with a certain degree of gluten intolerance within the GIS model you can begin to understand why Anemia affects so many people. Take this opportunity to review your own health status to see if you may be living with Anemia symptoms.

Tufts University completed a study in 2001 that showed when 3,000 men and women were tested the blood results revealed 40% had Anemia with the median age of 60. Anemia was present in the study participants even though they were eating sufficient Protein and Iron from meat in their diets. Anemia is diagnosed when the red blood cells are few in numbers. The missing links leading one into Anemia is the lack of nutritional co-factors largely due to poor digestion and marginal amounts of the necessary Intrinsic Factor required for B12 absorption as reviewed in Chapter 3 Digestion.

Symptoms & Causes of Anemia
- Symptoms; Fatigue, a pale appearance, irregular heart-beat, headaches, breathlessness, hair loss, easy bruising, psychosis, poor motor skills and even dizziness can all be due to Anemia.

- Cause; Injury (blood loss), disease, toxic poisoning (lead), EMF's or unusually heavy menstrual periods for women plus gluten intolerance may all be factors in developing Anemia.

Anemia is influenced by the lack of nutritional co-factors B12, Folic Acid, Vitamin C along with Protein and Iron. When the "Intrinsic Factor" is missing altogether from the stomach, common with gluten intolerance, Pernicious Anemia develops from the failure to absorb B12 (Reviewed in Chapter 5).

Researchers feel that it is the inflammation that develops with gluten intolerance that prevents the Intrinsic Factor from being produced in the required amounts. Plasma testing can diagnose and pinpoint the factor(s) that come to play with this potentially dangerous deficiency. Auto-immune diseases as seen with gluten intolerance and GIS, Thyroid disease and certain types of arthritis are directly linked to the development of Pernicious Anemia. The daily addition of a high dose sublingual (under tongue) Methyl B12, (500 mcg. – 1,000 mcg.), has helped many people rebuild the B12 stores without injections.

B12 injections may however be needed by many people either daily or weekly in advanced cases to reverse the nerve damage and other symptoms that can develop with the deficiency especially present in seniors. Advanced symptoms include; a sensitive and burning tongue, numbness, tingling burning sensations in the limbs, diminished reflexes, fatigue, difficulty walking and talking, stammering, bursitis, muscle and nerve pain, depression and varying psychosis. If the symptoms of B12 deficiency do not improve in a few weeks on the sublingual take steps to start the injections and be diligent.

By following the GIS Program you will begin eating the required food groups and taking the core nutrient supplements that will address nutritional deficiencies like Anemia. Especially important is increasing Vitamin C with Bioflavonoids, B-Complex which includes the Folic Acid, Protein and increase Minerals into the diet including Iron.

The Aloe Vera herb is a very important supplement when dealing with Anemia. It not only contains natural anti-inflammatory properties that support the body to speed healing it also aids in healthy digestion of the blood building nutrients. A fairly recent landmark study reported a significant increase in the bioavailability of core nutrients in humans when an ounce of quality Aloe Vera was included with the meal - in particular Vitamin C, E and B12 were shown to be much better absorbed with the Aloe. Aloe Vera also supports the bone marrow production of red blood cells and lymphocytes for stronger blood and a more robust immune system. Probiotics is another extremely valuable support because it improves the functions of the small intestine. Some experts state that when the small intestines are functioning well the friendly bacteria will actually manufacture a small amount of B12 in the gut!

Nutrition Highlights: Protein, Iron, B-Complex, B12, Vitamin C, Probiotics and Aloe Vera. *Foods:* Beans, Peas, Parsley, Greens, Beets, Kombu Seaweed, Meat, Eggs, Miso Paste, Berries, Raisins, Dates, Raspberry Leaf, Nettle and Greens.

3. Balancing Blood Sugar; Low & High

Blood sugar in the human body is referred to as glucose. Glucose is the main energy source that fuels the cells. Glucose metabolism can become out of balance falling either too low or rising to high levels that negatively affect the body's health and frame of mind.

The goal for a healthy fasting blood glucose level is between 70-80 mg / dL. Another blood test that is quickly becoming the most important laboratory marker for balanced blood sugar is Hemoglobin A1C developed over 40 years ago. This blood test is useful in regulating blood sugar levels for Diabetics and it can also help monitor the aging effect of "Glycation". Glycation can occur from eating too much fruit as well as refined sugar when the body cannot properly metabolize the sugars due to metabolic weakness. Symptoms of low blood sugar are very different from high blood sugar yet they both can effect the body physically and alter a person's mood. Maintaining the glucose level within a healthy range supports the body to feel it's very best and has also been linked in research to living a longer and healthier life into ones 80's, 90's and even 100 years of age.

Low Blood Sugar - Hypoglycemia

Low blood sugar is called "Hypoglycemia" and it is diagnosed when the blood glucose level falls to abnormally low levels. Hunger can be the first sign that blood sugar is dropping and for adults the blood level would generally be classified as low below 55 and children below 60. A drop in blood sugar may leave a person feeling tired, depressed and experiencing mood swings – unless they quickly get some food into their system. If the body is healthy it can even unlock stored glucose from fat raising the sugar level temporarily. Low blood sugar can also bring on headaches, disorientation, weakness of the limbs, sweating and in rare cases a coma and even death. The yawning response is the body's attempt to bring blood sugar into the brain. It is important to eat every 3-4 hours and include a protein source to help balance and stabilize the blood sugar from dropping too soon again.

High Blood Sugar - Diabetes

High blood sugar is the opposite end of the scale and may develop into the Diabetic range of sugar disease. What has occurred over the past 20 years is a gradual rise in the accepted normal range of testing the blood sugar. The high normal is now figured around 120 instead of 80 from just a decade ago. Some labs even push the glucose acceptable limits to even higher at times depending on the lab. The healthy target for glucose is 75-80. When a person's circulating glucose sugar is high it can damage cells and eventually lead to poor circulation in the extremities and cause irreparable tissue and nerve damage.

Symptoms can be unquenchable thirst, fatigue, increased urination, weight loss for some, blurry vision, moodiness, muscle cramps and numbness in the hands and feet. Some people especially with a higher carbohydrate diet will experience more yeast infections with their high blood sugar. Certain individual's including children and adults experience such mild symptoms they are unaware that their body is developing Diabetes. Left without health intervention they can go on to develop advanced symptoms which opens them up to include a higher incidence of CVD, cancer, kidney disease and unfortunately even blindness. Advanced Diabetes can even wind up with amputations of limbs. This can be inevitable due to the development of poor circulation. Be warned that persons living with Diabetes may also experience hypoglycemic symptoms if they are taking too much Diabetic medication. Applying health brings the blood sugar closer into normal and a reduction in one's medication will be required which is a good result. Many people that I have worked with have been overjoyed to let one medication go after another!

Healthy blood sugar is a critical factor in weight maintenance, proper energy in the body, brain health and mental well-being. Healthy longevity is also increased in people who control their blood sugar. The Boston Medical University research team on aging, found insulin levels which regulate sugar to be a significant marker with Centenarians. Centenarians are people who live to be at least 100 years of age and most live to be quite healthy.

Healthy Blood Sugar
- Balancing blood sugar in the body helps energy, brain function, proper mental attitude, neuromuscular function, good behavior, weight maintenance and longevity.
- Body regeneration through the GIS program helps to rebuild the nervous and glandular system including the Pancreas. The Pancreas makes Insulin and Glucagons, needed to regulate the blood sugar.
- Unstable blood sugar is a factor in hyperactivity, weight gain and all psychosis experienced by children and adults.
- Balancing blood sugar prevents degenerative diseases of Diabetes, Blindness, CVD, Arthritis, Kidney Challenges, Cancer, Skin Dermatitis and even Premature Aging.

- Follow the GIS Diet; Reducing refined sugars, lowering bread intake, reducing fried foods and starchy vegetables (too much rice, potatoes, pastas) and increasing lean meats, beans and varieties of vegetables with leafy greens, green beans, turnips, zucchini, broccoli, red potatoes and yams are OK, yellow and green bell peppers, cucumbers and Aloe Vera all support healthy blood sugar.
- Exercise supports glandular health including the Pancreas to make proper Insulin and other hormones needed to regulate blood sugar (30 minutes).
- Drink Filtered Water in between your meals to allow glands to function and to dilute excess sugar in the blood stream.

Low blood sugar may actually first begin with a spike in overall energy from eating sugars, carbohydrates and oils. When the body cannot process the sugar, from poor glandular function and lacking nutritional stores it will then plummet bringing upon Hypoglycemia. A good example of a surge in blood sugar is with a child or adult who eats a piece of cake or even drinks a glass of undiluted fruit juice. The concentration of the sugar can result in animated hyperactivity, perhaps running around, talking back to parents within the first 10 – 15 minutes. As the sugar drops to a low the child can show more defiant behavior with lots of emotions acting totally out of the ordinary. Adults can react in much the same way to include being argumentative, depressed, anxious and even fearful as the sugar level begins to fall. Make certain to dilute fruit juice with water to avoid the natural fruit sugar that plays with the blood sugar just like eating a candy bar. In one 6 ounce glass of orange or apple juice can be the equivalent of fruit sugar from eating 4 whole oranges or apples! Fats and oils in excess can also bring upon similar blood sugar ups and downs. Drinking Coca-Cola and eating potato chips or excessive amounts of caffeine have long been recognized as partners in crime for deviant behavior if the body doesn't have the balance of a nutrient dense protein balanced diet. A bizarre connection some of you may say? Unstable blood sugar can truly bring on radical behavior changes in the body in children and adults.

Poor eating habits and an unhealthy lifestyle lead to exhaustion of the glandular system in the body. This includes the Pancreas and Adrenal Glands that are both involved in balancing the blood sugar levels. Refined sugar found in junk foods, candy and sodas are big offenders because they also bring on more GIS symptoms. All of the sugars from refined sugars and including those from carbohydrate foods located in the starch complex and fruit sugars can be measured for their "Glycemic Index" that effects blood sugar.

Glycemic Index

The rise and fall of blood sugar has been quantified by the Australian born Glycemic Index (GI). A spike in blood sugar coincides with the higher numbers on the Glycemic Index (GI) scale. The carbohydrate foods and additives like refined sugar are numbered from 1 to 100 with the higher numbers representing the highest increase in glucose spike. Refined sugar, white rice, grains, potatoes and sweeter fruits like watermelon are all on the high end of the GI scale at 80 - 100.

People can enjoy the higher glycemic foods in moderation if we focus on a balanced diet as recommended on the GIS Program. Review the Addiction section to reduce the tendency to overeat in the high glycemic sugary foods. Recent studies at Harvard School of Public Health show a direct relationship of the GI to Diabetes and Coronary Heart Disease according to Cardiologist Dr. F. Vagnini, MD. The American Heart Association weighs in on refined sugar and states that to decrease Obesity and CHD men should not consume more than 150 calories (9 tsp.) from refined sugar and woman 100 calories (6 tsp.) per day!

I refer to the easy fluctuation in blood sugar as "Tricky Blood Sugar". It is especially common when a person has abused the body and requires more stabilizing essential core nutrients as outlined in the GIS Program. The bare minimum in supplementing must include quality Proteins, B-Complex and GTF Chromium in higher than RDA levels (Ch. 8).

Vitamin E and drinking Aloe Vera has also helped to stabilize blood sugar long term.

The Pancreas is the most important gland in regulating blood sugar. It is supposed to produce two hormones; Insulin which signals the cells to uptake glucose (circulating in the blood) for energy and second Glucagons. The latter signals the need for glucose to be released from glycogen stored in the liver. This process draws upon a type of glucose reserve. It makes certain that when there is not enough glucose in the blood to fuel the brain and crucial body functions it kicks in and barrows fuel. I think it is a grand design which allows the body to keep functioning even if you miss a lunch break or also in times of famine. The challenge lies in that the body doesn't always work properly or it just may run out of reserves. People must eat preventatively well and exercise to support the Pancreas in order to maintain health.

A Healthy Pancreas Demands a Decrease in Inflammation

The inflammation from the GIS keeps the Pancreas and other organs from functioning properly due to a type of auto-immune reaction involving the Central Nervous System. Because of this relationship it is important to stay on the GIS Diet at least 80% of the time to allow the body to regenerate and balance for glandular health. All the organs involved in proper sugar metabolism benefit including; the Pancreas, Adrenal, Liver and Kidneys.

The exciting fact about low and high blood sugar is that it can be improved and controlled with a healthy diet and lifestyle encouraged by the American Diabetes Association. To support the glands to function properly and be preventative to Diabetes or low blood sugar, Hypoglycemia, eat regular meals that contain nutrient dense foods outlined in the GIS program. Optimum and balanced health is three fold; Body, Mind and Spiritual. The body influences both mental and spiritual health!

Nutrition Highlights: Protein (at each meal & snacks), B-Complex, Chromium GTF 200 mcg 1 – 3 daily, Vanadium, Vitamin E, Aloe

Vera, Nopal Cactus, Antioxidants, Filtered Water, and Exercise. *Foods:* Green Beans, Greens, Low Starch Vegetables, Apples, Berries, Select Raw Nuts & Seeds, Nut Butter, Fresh Vegetable Juices and Green Tea as tolerated. *Reduce:* fried foods, caffeine, sodas, sugar, junk foods and alcohol in the diet.

4. Candida Fungal Overgrowth & Parasites

Intestinal organisms are not the most pleasant topic to discuss however your life hinges on maintaining control over these invaders. It is a fact that a variety of micro organisms can live in the large intestines and throughout the body. They include viruses, bacteria, parasites, fungus and yeast. When the body is working properly with regularity of the bowels, a vibrant digestive system and with proper immunity - these organisms are kept under control. When the bowels slow down and our organs and glands underfunction, as with GIS symptoms, it gives micro organisms the opportunity to overgrow and cause some detrimental effects.

One of the more common micro organisms that can create infections in the body relating to diet and constipation is the fungus called Candida Albicans - a type of yeast. All mammals can develop this opportunistic fungal growth. Humans have greater yeast and fungus infections because of the bombardment and assaults to the immune system with processed and devitalized foods. Also, our Allopathic Medical Model has encouraged the overuse of antibiotics in past years. This abuse has caused stronger drug resistant strains of Candida and other micro-organisms. With some vulnerable people, bacterial strains have become so uncontrollable that even the strongest of antibiotic drugs are not working. This has resulted in a select group of physicians actually turning to natural Probiotics. Yes, you did hear me correctly. Some physicians are resorting to writing prescriptions for the friendly bacteria, needed to boost immunity naturally and restore the gut health called Probiotics. Review Probiotics highlighted in Chapter 2.

Candida a Fungus Among Us

Candida Albicans begins its destruction by overgrowing in the large intestine and travels up the GI tract into the small intestine. Once it infiltrates there it blocks absorption of nutrients from entering the villi causing malabsorption. Depending on how weak the intestinal wall happens to be the Candida yeast, at times, may invade into other parts of the body through the blood stream called "Leaky Gut".

The yeast can travel through the blood and colonize on any of the lining cell tissues when the opportunity allows it to spread especially in areas of low circulation and oxygen deprivation. Common areas include the mouth and esophagus, lungs, genitals, ears, sinuses, feet and fingernail beds. The advanced infection of Candida Albicans and other yeasts that are found throughout the body can be viewed in a specialized blood smear test called "Dark Field Screening". The Candida infection is also common when a person has been eating poorly or living an abusive lifestyle along with individuals that have a weak immune system as with; Cancer, Aids, Diabetes and other Chronic Diseases. The Candida fungus is a common secondary factor in GIS and is responsible for advancing disease or failing health scenarios. This is why whole books have been written about the ravaging effects it can have on the body!

The easiest symptom to recognize with fungal yeast overgrowth is a coated tongue some call Thrush. It can be present in babies, children, adults and even pets. As the Candida matures it can turn to a brownish color showing age of the yeast cells. Brushing the tongue to clean it off is helpful yet only a temporary fix. The goal of a slightly pink tongue in the morning is only achieved as the full program for Anti-Candida is followed very strictly and it takes months and sometimes years to get on top of it. Important to note there are definitely exceptions with people who have extensive yeast in the lower GI tract however they do not develop a coating on the tongue whatsoever.

Other symptoms will include white mucus in the stool, vaginal infections, jock itch, rectal itching and burning, body rashes, acne around the chin area, nail and toe fungus, frequent earaches and more. A test you can do at home is eating fresh garlic and onions. If you develop gas and bloating you have overgrowth of Candida in your gut and need to apply more of the Anti-Candida program. Candida worsens allergies and is a big factor in Chronic Fatigue Syndrome, Fibromyalgia, IBS and Skin Conditions of all types. Also, Cancer and other Chronic Disease conditions appear to all have varying degrees of Candida overgrowth. Even though a few Anti-Fungal pharmaceutical drugs are available if a person is to permanently regain health it is important to apply the Candida protocol and the GIS Program.

What is the Solution? A three-fold Anti-Candida Program within the GIS parameters is required to reduce the yeast back to the large intestine where it belongs to include; Bowel Regularity, the Anti-Fungal Diet and the Supplements. This program will help to *Rebuild a Stronger Immune System* that will better control the yeast along with viruses, bacteria and parasites. It will also begin the process necessary to *Rebalance the Body's pH System*. Review the pH section in Chapter 6. This is valuable because it will explain how the pH balance naturally keeps overgrowth of Candida under control when coupled with the rest of the protocol. Through assisting the body to rebalance the pH in the GI tract the yeast (fungus) goes through a process called "Die-Off" and the individual can experience a type of temporary "Brain Fog" that will come and go as Candida resolves. The result is more intestinal gas at the beginning which shows that the body is working as anticipated. The gas will resolve as you follow the protocol along with clearer thinking once again. It is especially important to make certain the bowels are moving more regularly for proper *Detoxification*. Review Enemas in Chapter 12. Eliminating the waste products created by both normal metabolic function of the body and the detoxification from the immune system and the pH pathway of eliminating the yeast is critical. In fact the most important goal for success of the Anti-Candida program is the regularity of the bowels and the addition of supplements and nutritional foods found on the GIS diet that are essential to rebuilding the gut. By taking health action you will achieve the results of a healthier, stronger and better functioning body for total wellness.

Anti-Candida Program

Bowel Regularity Goal - To reverse the overgrowth requires the bowels to move regularly and that means every day 1 – 2 times. Include; Aloe Vera, Magnesium Glycinate, Enemas, vegetables (bulking foods) and following the GIS Program. If you experience loose stool build up slower with the supplement program.

Anti-Fungal Supplements & Herbs – Probiotics, Multiple Vitamin & Mineral, Daily Greens, Liquid Silver Hydrosol, Glutathione or NAC by *Jarrow*, Garlic, Pau d'Arco, Aloe Vera, Fish Oil plus A & D, Milk Thistle, Caprylic Acid, DetoxPlus by *Aloe Life*.

Anti-Fungal Diet (as tolerated) – Lean Meats & Fish, Vegetables (to include green leafy ones as allowed with blood thinner medications), Cucumber, Radishes (white & red), Lemon, Limes, Coconut oil, Asparagus, Broccoli, Cauliflower, Green Beans, Red Potatoes, Yams, Beans, Zucchini and other squash, Cabbage, Carrots, Avocado, Nuts (as tolerated) and Seeds (better tolerated), low glycemic fruits: Berries, Apples, Banana (as tolerated), Mango & Papaya.

Avoid: Refined sugar, alcohol, grains, rice, yams and red potato (keep low in diet), sodas and junk foods. Keep starchy vegetables and dairy products (eggs as tolerated) lower in the diet.

Parasites - Stomach Acids, Probiotics & Enzymes

Parasites are a much larger organism than fungus with varying sizes. They can infest and colonize in the Gastro Intestinal (GI) tract if a person's stomach acids are low. Stomach acids such as *Pepsin* and the valuable *Hydrochloric Acid (HCL)*, when flowing properly, conduct several very important jobs.

Upon eating foods the stomach juices are designed to flow into the stomach to be able to digest protein and minerals out of the food properly. The second important job of the stomach acids is to kill potential invaders such as parasites and bacteria that can cause food poisoning, H. pylori along with viruses causing colds and flu. See Chapter 3 on Digestion and the importance of friendly bacteria to also help in this regard.

Many children, adults and seniors lack optimum stomach acids and therefore parasites may enter into the bowel from food, water and even the air we breathe. They become a health hazard in some instances and even life threatening at times. Parasites are especially problematic when constipation exists because these organisms are allowed to set up housekeeping living off the waste in the bowel.

The CDC has researched the parasite challenge in the U.S. extensively. The University of Maryland Medical Center states that there are two main types of parasites seen in children and adults called Helminthes and Protozoa's. The first group that is most common in the United States includes; pinworms, roundworms and the larger tape worms. Generally they range in size from (½) inch to 3 inches in length. Tapeworms may be longer yet small sections can break off in the stool so you rarely see one in its full length. Pinworms are also known as thread worms and are smaller in size and white in color.

Adult Helminthes do not multiply as fast as the second type called Protozoa. A more common Protozoan is Giardia, also called the back packers infection. Cryptosporidium is another parasite more commonly diagnosed in individuals with a low functioning immune system. Both types can cause acute diarrhea bringing attention to the condition for treatment. Symptoms include; stomach pain or tenderness, loose stool containing blood or mucus, chronic rectal itching, weight loss and even passing a worm or pod shaped tissue in the stool.

The solution to parasite infection lies in getting the digestive health including pH balance strong in the GI tract to avoid any re-infection of future parasites. Be patient because once applying the Anti-Parasitic program it can take weeks, months and even years to totally rid the colon of infestation. Occasionally medical assistance is needed to stabilize a bowel condition arising from advanced infestation. Chronic diarrhea must be handled seriously by a professional and then the protocol they prescribe may be blending with the GIS Anti-Candida and the Anti-Parasite Program steps to achieve lasting success.

Anti-Parasitic Program - University of Maryland Medical Center

Caution: Work with your health provider to properly diagnose your situation with stool testing. Prescription drugs are given yet natural remedies have found to be important for both types of parasite infections.

- Eat a diet keeping all refined carbohydrates of sugar, breadstuff and excess dairy out of the diet except for honey. (Similar to the GIS Diet)

- Include Anti-Parasitic High Fiber Foods; garlic, (raw) pumpkin seeds, pineapple, Figs, Raw Carrots & Beets, Celery and others to scrub and rid the colon of the parasites as in a daily salad.

- Papaya Seeds & Honey Mixture; One study researchers found this mixture cleared stools of parasites in 23 of the 30 subjects.

- Drink Filtered Water to flush your system.

- Supplements Found Helpful Include; Probiotics, Digestive Enzymes (full spectrum), Vitamin C, B-Complex and Zinc. Herbs; Garlic, Artemesia-Wormwood, Black Walnut, Barberry, Goldenseal, Oregon-Grape and Anise. Aloe Vera on the GIS program is very soothing and works together with the other herbs having Anti-Parasitic properties.

Nutrition Highlights: Cellulase Enzyme (Full Spectrum Enzyme), Aloe Vera, Mugwort, Wormwood - Artemisia (limited time only 6 weeks), Black Walnut, Garlic, Cloves, Betel Nut, Wobenzymes, Enemas, Probiotics and Grapefruit Seed Oil. *Food Fiber:* Raw Carrots, Raw Celery, Raw Pumpkin Seeds, Fresh Pineapple and Figs. FiberMate by *Aloe Life* contains many valuable cleansing and anti-parasitic herbs for prevention and regularity. *Note:* Use pharmaceutical drugs as needed.

5. Circulation, Inflammation & Mucus Formation

Poor circulation is a major health challenge for the body and results from many factors including Diabetes (improper blood sugar metabolism) and has an indirect relationship to mucus formation. Poor circulation impairs proper functioning of the Cardiovascular System (CVS). Review Blood Sugar in Healthy Focus Factors. To have healthy circulation you must support the function of the body's organs especially the Pancreas involved in regulating blood sugar.

Good circulation demands that the entire CVS to function well. This includes the heart and all the blood vessels and arteries that carry the blood throughout the body from the top of the head to all of the organs, fingers and toes. The CVS carries the blood that contains the core nutrients to each cell - required for life itself. Blood also transfers oxygen to the cells and removes the waste including carbon dioxide from them. The blood works together with the Lymph System to discard cellular waste required for healthy cell function and renewal. The blood is also a vehicle to transport critical hormones throughout the body that orchestrate mood and body development.

To understand the total importance of circulation in the body you need to look at all the systems it supports to include; Nervous System (NS), Digestive & Elimination Systems, Lymphatic System, Cardio Pulmonary (lungs) System, Muscular Skeletal System, Immune System and the Organs and Glandular System. Improving the circulation of the CVS not only prevents heart disease but it maintains the health of the entire body!

Varicose Veins & Spider Veins

Beyond poor nutrition and a lack of exercise - what ultimately causes the organs and glands to underfunction, affecting the heart and CVS, is *Inflammation*. As mentioned in other sections GIS creates the inflammation causing the organs and glands to under function. As the glands work slower people develop diseases like Diabetes which further reduces circulation causing more heart disease. Review Chapter 4 which tells more about the relationship of the Nervous System and GIS.

The Nervous System along with core nutrients and minerals are required to regulate all of the valves of the body including the ones in the CVS. We have valves in the heart and veins along with ones in the

GI tract that are required for the digestive process to work smoothly. Proper functioning of the vascular valves support the proper blood flow and prevents the blood from puddling backwards. If the valves are not closing correctly the result is congestion of blood that may darken and become stagnant showing discoloration in the veins. If it puddles long enough it may develop clotting and even cause closures and ulcers in some larger veins and arteries. Besides being painful the veins begin to look a bit unsightly showing dark discoloration on the skin and the potential for a stroke can also become more of a risk. When the CVS works better vascular disease will be reduced. See Chapter 5 relating to CVD and Homocysteine levels.

The exciting news is through following the GIS program you will experience a healthier CVS and a more natural and youthful coloring will return to the skin, legs and face. All vascular challenges improve along with the smaller Spider Veins and it lessens capillary breaks as well. Vitamin E and C both play critical roles in providing greater collagen strength to the entire CVS and they increase the heart to pump more robustly reducing fluid retention around the ankles. Together they also reduce the chances of developing a stroke condition in the body which kills many people every year. Pain and fatigue in the legs may also be greatly reduced as many have experienced.

As time passes following the GIS Program the body goes through more tissue renewal and you will continue to experience reduction of fluid retention in the legs, as well as the ugly Red Spider Veins and the larger Varicose Veins can improve. Especially helpful on the outside is a good topical product that can speed the recovery of the legs and face as I have used called Leg Gel. The spider veins I developed years ago improved over 70%. My legs look better and feel remarkably more youthful!

Nutrition Highlights: Vitamin E Complex including Tocorenols 400 – 1200 mg, Vitamin C & Bioflavonoids 1 – 3,000 mg, B-Complex 50 mg, EFA's, Aloe Vera, Topical Leg Gel by *Aloe Life*, Resveratrol (antioxidant) and Minerals including Silica.

Reducing Mu cus Production

The connection of mucus development to the CVS is surprising. Most people are aware that mucus develops with an infection from a cold virus or a secondary bacterial condition. The way it works with colds is our Goblet cells, which are part of the body's defense mechanism in fighting infection, secrete the mucus to fight the invaders naturally. The darker color of the mucus shows a greater amount of infection was present.

A secondary condition that relates to the CVS causes the mucus to also flow and that is increased inflammation. The interesting fact is that when inflammation does occur in the body as with GIS - it causes an overproduction of mucus in the lining cells of the nose, sinuses, throat, lungs and the intestinal tract. It brings on a type of misfiring if you will when infection is not present!

Experts are now suggesting that this response of over production of mucus is the result of the Nervous System decreasing its electrical charge. Science has not clearly explained why this reaction takes place in all situations however the GIS Triggers are linked to an auto-immune response in the body resulting from inflammation. Stopping the GIS Triggers stops the overproduction of mucus which is a welcome relief for so many.

How to Decrease Excess Mucus in the Body?
- Follow the GIS Diet; Stop Milk, Sugar and Gluten plus GIS Triggers.
- Supplements; EFA's-Fish Oil or Flax, B-Complex, NAC, Aloe Vera, CoQ10 Enzyme and the GIS basics (Ch. 8).
- Immune System Health; Probiotics, Nasal Spray by *Xlear* and Aloe Vera.
- Detoxification; Drink Purified Water, Aloe Vera, Herbal Teas and Enzymes as needed.

MVP, Heart Arrhythmias & Mucus Development in the Lungs

The research has elaborated that the Nervous System is responsible for the Mitral Valve Prolapse (MVP) response of the heart. GIS intensifies the mitral valve reaction and mucus can result from just one of the episodes. Researchers state that this irregular heartbeat, whether it is felt or not, occurs first. Then the body responds with mucus production which causes coughing after the MVP or irregular heart beat event. Some mild to medium MVP events cause understandably anxious feelings due to the obvious rapid or irregular heartbeat. There are various types of MVP conditions known as classic or non-classic. MVP is defined as the thickening of the Mitral Valve Leaflet into the left atrium of the heart and complications may arise if regurgitation occurs, infective endocarditis or congestive heart failure in rare cases that could cause death if severe enough.

Keeping inflammation down in the body is one of the most important goals to promote good circulation and decrease the events and the overproduction of mucus. The GIS program reduces mucus in the lungs, throat, intestines and sinuses regardless of the catalyst; Cystic Fibrosis, Asthma, Allergies or Gluten Triggers.

On a cellular level applying the GIS Program reduces inflammation in the entire body to support health of the CVS and reduces MVP like symptoms. Through applying the GIS Diet and Program cardiac events are greatly lessened in frequency and intensity. Even the temporary irregular Heart Arrhythmias experienced by children and adults can be attributed to GIS. People may be able to avoid the addition of blood thinning medication so widely prescribed in today's world if they can prevent the irregular heartbeat naturally.

Nutrition Highlights: Vitamin E Complex, NAC, Alpha-Lipoic Acid, Vitamin C & Bioflavonoids 1-3 grams, EFA's - Cod Liver Oil, CoQ10 Enzyme, Resveratrol Grape Extract, Curcumin - Turmeric Extract, Multiple Vitamin & Mineral, CoQ10 Enzyme, Garlic, Ginger, Cayenne, Artichoke, Lemon & Lime and Sugar Free Cranberry Juice or Concentrate and Aloe Vera decreases mucus production.

6. Dental Health

Optimum health demands regular care of your teeth and gums. Put dental health on the top of your list if you have NOT been keeping up on your oral hygiene. You can begin today by brushing regularly and flossing after meals. A second generation dentist shared recently that it is helpful to use a small amount of *Hydrogen Peroxide* when brushing to fight potential infection around the teeth. Using a little *Baking Soda* and even *Aloe Vera Gel* has also shown good support to combat bacteria in the mouth and prevent problems from arising. The FDA found clear evidence that toothpastes containing *Triclosan* was able to prevent Gingivitis. The definition of Gingivitis is the inflammation of the gum tissue surrounding the teeth due to improper cleaning. The FDA also confirmed that mouthwash with *Chlorhexidine* or hydrogen peroxide was also effective in fighting bacteria in the mouth. These suggestions will give you some extra natural cleansing support you can incorporate as you catch up with your regular dental cleanings.

Why is it so important to take care of your teeth? If proper care of the teeth is not provided - infection as with Gingivitis can develop in the gums in either the lining or the pockets surrounding the teeth. Most people find that the gums will get worse as the plaque builds up. Dental plague is a sticky colorless film of bacteria and sugars that forms tartar as it hardens on the teeth. If not removed daily it leads to cavities and gum disease. Besides the pain that can develop from the build-up of plague and infection pockets, gum disease may also lead to the development of bone loss in the jaw and the loss of teeth.

The attempt to save your teeth can cost thousands of dollars in deep cleaning procedures. It is possible however to reverse the receding bone with a determined and health minded individual. Cleaning the teeth regularly especially with flossing and the use of a Christmas Tree Brush will greatly help. Also, if possible pick up a Water Pick or other device to optimize the circulation around the teeth. Eating vegetables and other nutrient dense foods is helpful to increase bone density however it is not enough by itself to reverse bone loss. Regular 3 month cleanings from a skilled dental hygienist is required along with your own efforts at home to reverse bone loss. The money it costs for the support equipment and more frequent cleanings will pay you back in savings and ultimately the satisfaction of keeping your own set of choppers!

If you do not heed this warning you may eventually lose your teeth. Just in case you haven't heard, living with false teeth is not an enjoyable experience. Poor fitting especially with weight fluctuations, false teeth come with their own set of pain and discomfort symptoms. I had to learn the hard way about the value of flossing. You won't hear me use this word very often but I was flat out "lazy to floss" and even with my regular brushing it did not keep me from developing gum disease. Yet I fought to reverse the condition by applying the steps in this section and won. I have reversed bone loss to the astonishment of my dentist. My wallet is lighter unfortunately yet I learned my lesson – FLOSS and Take Preventative Action!

The last area of extreme importance linked to dental disease is the connection of the bad bacteria and infection that develops from neglect to other diseases in the body. Researchers have found that the bacteria colonizing in the tooth pockets breed infection associated not only to Cancer but also to CVD, Strokes and even Diabetes. Also, as gum disease lingers and advances it can cause more fatigue and the wearing down of a person's overall health status.

More Inflammation Can Come From Our Teeth?

Researchers have also found diseased gums release a significantly higher level of bacterial pro-inflammatory components, called Endotoxins. They actually travel through the bloodstream causing the liver to make more "C-Reactive-Proteins" – an inflammatory blood marker. This alone may add to an increase risk in Cardiovascular Disease and also compounds the secondary GIS inflammation affecting the entire body's health. The study revealed that people living with gum disease had four times the amount of bad bacteria compared to people with healthy gums and a whopping 30% of adults over 50 live with significant gum disease. It went on to say that people who chew gum cause a release of bacteria four times the normal amount from 6% to 24%. The research team has further linked this bad bacterium to a certain type of deadly heart disease. What else is there left to say but I advise you to take your dental health seriously and do find a dentist in your area to work with you and your family – even if monthly payments are required to set it all in motion!

Save Your Teeth & Your Budget
- Tooth Cleaning ASAP and Regularly.
- Flossing will SAVE YOU BIG MONEY!
- Brush Daily; Mechanical Water Pick or Rotadent are good options.
- Stop Eating Candy, Cookies or Dried Fruit without brushing!
- Eat raw Vegetables and Fruits to rebuild the bone in your jaw.
- Supplement; Calcium, Magnesium, Vitamin D, replacing Xylitol Sugar products for any refined sugar and chew Spry Zylitol Gum by *Xlear**.
- You can reduce and reverse bone loss – I am living proof at 50+ years of age!

Nutrition Highlights: Brushing and Flossing Teeth, Gargle with Aloe Vera, Multiple Vitamin & Mineral, Silica, Calcium, Magnesium & Zinc (for age group), Daily Greens, Vitamin C & Bioflavonoids, Alpha-Lipoic Acid, EFA's – Flax and Fish Oil with Vitamin A & D, Parsley, Raw Vegetables, Cilantro and Alfalfa. * Spry Zylitol Gum by *Xlear* has been supported in research to reduce bad bacteria and cavities significantly if used regularly for prevention. *Caution:* The use of Fluoride in any form may be harmful to your health.

7. Detoxification & Cleansing
Detoxification and cleansing the body is needed on a daily basis to feel good and function properly. It is also essential for the prevention of chronic illnesses and required for the regeneration of health. Consider the process of detoxification in the category of steps to remove the road blocks that prevent the body from healing and maintaining youthful vigor.

Toxins and waste products build up in the body over time. Regardless of whether or not a person is having fast transit diarrhea, constipation or having a regular bowel movement every day toxins still accumulate in the body to varying degrees. The body accumulates waste from many sources.

Sources of Toxins
- Normal cellular metabolism.
- Poor diet and junk foods.
- Improper mineralization and "Glycation".
- Illness and poor sleep.
- Pharmaceutical and street drug abuse.
- Constipation, parasites and fungus.
- Excess mucus from inflammation.
- Environmental toxins like heavy metals, cleaning and personal products.

The body's waste and toxins prevent important metabolic pathways from functioning correctly and increase overall pain in the body including arthritis in the joints and gas build-up in the colon. In regards to pharmaceutical drugs, Harvard Medical University warns that doctors and patients are very ignorant to the serious side effects of taking pharmaceutical drugs. A particular class of drugs function by stopping the Acetyl-Choline pathway known as "Anti-Cholinergic Drugs" that cause a major shut down of the Central Nervous System. They can bring about a slowdown of the entire function of the body adding to more toxic waste. Detoxification is greatly needed for anyone taking pharmaceutical drugs and a reevaluation of use especially (as Harvard researchers suggested) for the following; Paxil, Zantac, Tagamet, Ditropan, Detrol, Elavil, Norpramin, Aventyl and Capoten. Side effects from some drugs are even being associated with fetal birth defects. Seek the guidelines of Dr. Shoshana Bennett, PHD, in her books for pregnancy and anti-depressant medications. Also, review

Chapter 9 Healthy Children for more tips about Detoxification surrounding childbirth.

A newly recognized condition, resulting from sugar abuse, is also emerging which scientists are attributing to body toxicity called "Glycation". Refined sugar is one of the most deadly poisons for the body. Already fingered as one of the major GIS Core Triggers causing inflammation in the intestines, sugar in all of the refined forms including high fructose corn syrup (HFCS), sugar beets and cane sugar are also responsible for adding to the toxic load of the body. Glycation cellular waste is the result of excess refined sugar that actually disrupts the ability of enzymes to bind properly with certain protein compounds. In simple terms refined sugar stops the body from functioning and is directly related to poor circulation, disease development and premature aging.

Symptoms of Toxicity
- Pain in the Joints and Muscles.
- Headaches and Fatigue.
- Bloating, Gas, Constipation and Bad Breath.
- Skin Conditions of All Types.
- Brain Fog, Fuzzy Thinking and Dementia.
- Slow Learning Ability and Bizarre Behavior.
- Lung Congestion and Poor Circulation.
- Weight Gain, Obesity and Weight Loss (due to Mal-Absorption).
- Nervous System Function Decline and the Inability to Conduct Normal Daily Tasks.
- Failing Health and a Shortened Life Span often termed as "Old Age"!

Both the liver and the lymph system are essential in achieving daily detoxification of the body. With advanced toxicity coming from many factors the liver may become overworked from excessive waste and malfunctioning - especially with a history of constipation. See Chapter 3 to learn more about the liver and lymph. The Lymph System found throughout the body processes waste that accumulates - that is if it is functioning properly. It has to work harder when the bulk waste has not been eliminated through the bowel, lungs, kidneys or skin channels of elimination. The other challenge with the Lymph System is when a person is not active or if they are dehydrated the lymph is not very active either. It takes exercise and drinking adequate water to activate the lymph - so make certain to get the body moving and drink half your weight in ounces of water approximately eight 8 ounce glasses per day!

Skin eruptions coming from a congested Lymph System can include Acne flare-ups anywhere from head to toe. Some people not only develop rashes but also boils and infection pockets that will open and drain before and during the detoxification process. Once you start detoxifying and health balance begins to return in the following weeks and months - the skin eruptions, joint pain and headaches lessen and energy and wellness improves greatly.

Detoxification Truths
- The bowels must move daily and have good color and form.
- The cleansing of the liver is paramount to reach optimum health.
- The body detoxifies in layers taking weeks, months and years.
- People cleanse from the inside out and from the present to the past.

The bowels must move on a daily basis for proper cleansing and it is your number one homework assignment. The stool is best when it is medium size (1-1 ½ inches in diameter), medium brown in color and has only a mild odor. Stay away from psyllium and flax meal using only gluten free supplements and food fibers like raw celery, carrot, Daikon and red radish, cilantro, parsley, beets, prunes, raisons and organic apples (peel if necessary).

Reaching your regularity goal may take up to three months or longer. Refer to Chapter 12 for the instructions to do a home Enema or to go to a technician for a "Colonic Irrigation". It will speed the important evacuation process up considerable and even decrease pain in the body. Drinking good water, adding a Probiotic and Aloe Vera juice before each meal, including 2 tablespoons of healthy oils daily and taking the B-Complex as tolerated as you follow the GIS Diet is a must to Detoxify. Add the other Detox supplements when you are ready and as tolerated.

Even with the tendency for diarrhea the need for detoxification is still important. If any of the suggested supplements increase stool frequency - reduce the amount you are taking or stop it altogether temporarily. Stay on a smaller quantity for 10 days if possible to observe if your stool starts to improve. First and foremost is to focus on the diet and second take a good Probiotics. Gradually experiment with the other foundational core supplements mentioned here and in Chapter 8.

The GIS Diet in Chapter 7 actually starts the detoxification process purely by including; water, healthy oils and gluten free food fibers. The Nutrition Highlights in this section suggests some extra Detox herbs and supplements. You will want to include them either individually or in an herbal combination product for 60 - 180 days to help speed up the detoxification process and reach a higher level of health not possible without them.

Daily exercise, stretching and massage are also good tips to eliminate waste from the body as well reviewed in this chapter. Besides loosening tight muscles these activities allow the valuable Lymph System to work more efficiently. Saunas or a warm baths (with added baking soda as directed on the box) or a warm shower allows the pores of the skin to open up and discharge waste. Using a soft skin brush or wash cloth before bathing can both stimulate the Lymphatic System and the body's Immune System function. Brisk towel drying after your bath is also a great way to help the Detox process and it feels rejuvenating!

Herbal Detox Bath Formula: 1 – 2 ounces of Aloe Vera, Sea Salts ½ cups (available at the health food store) and Dried Herbs for the Bath; Red Clover, Peppermint and Yarrow (put in a sachet bag 1 tablespoon of each desired herb). Draw a warm bath and use the ingredients you have for a very soothing treatment which some people remark lowers stress and pain.

Detoxification Steps

- *GI Tract & pH Balancing (see pH section);* Diet, Water, Aloe Vera, Greens & Vegetables, Fruits, FiberMate (psyllium free) and Enemas.
- *Deep Tissue, Liver & Lymph (see Liver Section);* Bentonite Clay, Herbs-Milk Thistle, Dandelion, DetoxPlus (See Ch. 8), Sauna, Hot Baths, Massage, Exercise.
- *Blood Purification & Reducing Opportunistic Micro-Organisms (see Candida);* Probiotics, Coconut Products, Caprylic Acid, Liquid Hydrosol Silver, Enzymes (Ch. 8), Artemisia (herb for 6 weeks), Aloe Vera, Garlic by *Kyolic* and more.

Patience is required with cleansing the colon, body tissues and glands. It is a process that takes months to years as you develop your own individual detoxification lifestyle. Why people stick with it is because it truly works. The body stores waste generally in the fat tissue. As it begins to exit the body you can experience temporary detox reactions that will pass. Cleansing symptoms can feel like a Flu Virus at times to include; fatigue, headaches, muscle aches, skin rashes, boils, scalp dermatitis and increased acne flare-ups before it totally resolves. Don't let the "Flu-Like Symptoms" discourage you! As you achieve better health it will be well worth the "temporary" Detox cleansing symptoms.

Detox Symptoms

- Fatigue
- Headaches
- Muscle Aches
- Cleansing Gas
- Skin Rashes & Boils
- Acne Flare-Ups

How can you tell the difference from Detox Symptoms and Catching a Cold? Just review your actions and if you are eating a good healthy diet and taking your supplements plus living a healthier lifestyle then most likely the symptoms are coming from Detox. The Detox symptoms pass more quickly than colds. They also do not escalate into a greater illness. Once regularity and a healthier stool resumes, all of your efforts toward healing will speed up resulting in looking and feeling better than you ever thought possible!

Let me clear up any misunderstanding about sickness vs. Detoxing. As you get healthier you will still get a Cold or Flu occasionally. When you become healthier and experience a cold however it is different. It is more like the body proving to you that it does have a functioning immune system to fight off invaders by achieving a runny nose, fever or lung congestion. During the non-cold periods you will stop having so many ill health toxicity symptoms as first listed in this topic. Review the Immune System section as well to further understand that some people NEVER GET a COLD yet do wind up getting CANCER. This demonstrates that experiencing a cold shows that you truly do have a functioning Immune System!

Nutrition Highlights: Aloe Vera or DetoxPlus by *Aloe Life*, Daily Greens Supplement, NAC, Probiotics by *Dr. Ohhira*, Liquid Silver -Sovereign Silver, Vitamin C, Bentonite Clay, Artemesia (60 days), Caprylic Acid (Coconut fatty acid), Herbs – Dandelion leaf & root, Milk Thistle by *Herb-Pharm*, Yellow Dock, Oregon-Grape Root (caution with diarrhea), Licorice Tea, Burdock, Turkey Rhubarb, Astragalus, Red Clover Tops, Pau d'Arco, Lemon & Lime, Cranberry Extract, Exercise, Body Saunas, Hot Baths and Massage!

8. Digestion Basics

Children actually come into the world with an under-functioning digestive system to varying degrees. Then during early life other challenges may take place that decrease one's digestive ability even further. Poor eating habits and eating junk foods both deplete the body of core nutrients needed to support the digestive system and can spark the GIS inflammation taking a greater toll on health.

The reasons for the poor digestive downward spiral are many besides one's intentional and unknowing food abuse including; genetics, stress, poverty, addictions and the overuse of pharmaceutical drugs. Whatever the cause a large percentage of young people right on into their senior years develop a lack of the proper Hydrochloric Acid (HCL) levels that are required in the stomach for healthy digestion. For many of the same reasons the other digestive juices also do not flow properly either. Review Chapter 3 Digestion. Another challenge with digestion regardless of age is that people frequently do not take the time to eat properly. To help the body improve digestion and extract the nutrients it needs applying good eating mechanics and guidelines are a must. First and foremost children and adults must both practice improving the chewing process. The following highlights give the important eating guidelines that make a big difference in lowering your gas, heartburn and other digestive symptoms and improve health significantly!

Highlights for a Healthy Digestive System
- Chew your food well into small particles before swallowing.
- Drink more water in-between meals, not during the meal and reserve iced drinks for a treat and not a ritual at meal times. Excessive water and iced drinks slow all digestive juices down and prevents digestion from working properly at mealtimes.
- Don't overeat at one meal. Only 2 – 3 cups of food fit nicely into an adult's stomach. More quantity than this reduces digestion and absorption and can bring upon symptoms of heartburn and pain. Remind yourself, "You Get to Eat Again!"

Hydrating your body daily, with drinking 6 – 8 glasses of good water helps to keep hunger under-control, fewer headaches and better energy. It also assists in helping out the Pancreas to release its *digestive enzymes* and *insulin* needed to control blood sugar. Water is required by all of the glands to function better besides being essential for life itself!

Relax at Meals

Relaxing during meals is important as well to allow for proper digestion. Do your best to sit down while eating and as often with the family as possible. To incorporate this time regularly may take reviewing your daily schedule. Scheduling our daily activities takes some practice to give you downtime however you and the family deserve it. Rule of thumb, "Don't overbook your life!"

Stress inhibits the digestive process. If you are upset or wound up, it is better to calm down before eating. Take a breath and once you've relaxed, do your best to enjoy your meal with some light conversation, reading (if by yourself), candlelight, music or light TV watching if you must. Remember this, we truly are what we eat yet only if we digest it and absorb the nutrients into the cells. Don't eat on the run and relax!

Supplements Help Digestion

Digestive complaints of gas, heartburn and bloating are not a disease in themselves yet are considered the most common class of symptoms in our society. Chapter 3 describes digestion in length including the relationship to gluten intolerance and the GIS inflammation. The entire GI tract requires attention because of its significance in the health of the body. Keep in mind that if you add up all the parts from the mouth to the rectum, the GI tract is the number one site of cancer above lung, colon, breast and prostate.

We need to give our digestive tract good nutritional support and experiment with the different basic digestive supplements defined in Chapter 8. For some of you this may be more of a preventative step to discourage disease from developing and for others it just might be what saves your life.

The word "Probiotics" refers to the friendly bacteria found in fermented foods and supplements and is often missing from our intestinal tract due to antibiotic use and or a poor diet. They are paramount to health and are required by infants to seniors. Targeting any bacterial or yeast overgrowth in the gut, Probiotics are used for the short-term to reduce nausea and gas right away and for long-term use to support a healthy active immune system. Remarkable in their ability research finds the friendly bacteria able to fight off infections, reduce the chance of H. Pylori bacteria, cancer and other debilitating disease development.

The basic herbs that also lend important support to digestion include; Aloe Vera, Chamomile, Ginger, Gentian, Mint and Slippery Elm. Each of these herbs has shown significance in addressing different factors of the digestive system to help get out of a crisis situation and support the body to heal. Aloe Vera when taken before a meal along with the appropriate GIS Diet Zone foods as tolerated supports the body to digest better and receive more needed rejuvenating nutrition. As pointed out in the TIPS section in Chapter 7 Organic baby foods have come to the rescue in severe eating crisis to give the body required nutrients and stabilize ones health back to eating normally along with Probiotics and Aloe Vera as tolerated.

Electrolytes Are Minerals the Body Requires for Life

You must replenish the electrolyte balance back into the body on a daily basis for energy and well-being especially if you experience loose stools. Foods that are more tolerated are tender lean meats and fish, vegetables and ripe bananas and cooking fruit like peeled apples and other choices with a little honey work very well. Minerals from vegetables (that include the electrolytes) include celery, carrots, squash and greens are generally well tolerated. A squeeze of lemon or lime in water or on certain foods like papaya fruit contain an abundance of electrolytes including; sodium, chloride, magnesium, calcium and potassium that naturally bring up the body's energy. The papaya fruit is loaded with vitamins and minerals and even enzymes that may be eaten with Greek yogurt (low in lactose) and with a little honey makes up a mini-meal. The papaya seeds are valuable and contain a concentration of enzymes that can be dried and ground like peppercorns onto your food that also helps with digestion.

Digestive Enzymes

Digestive enzymes can be a valuable help to digest foods in the short term yet their recommendation comes with a cautionary note. Only use digestive enzymes temporarily as needed. The body is designed to make its own digestive enzymes if you give it the correct nutrition and core nutrients it requires. The overuse of enzymes may actually create a digestive challenge mimicking Reflux in certain individuals. This appears to occur more often when enzymes are taken as a preventative supplement to give extra detoxification however they are expensive and by investing in the ECN's as defined in Chapter 8 the body receives more value long-term. The primary reason Reflux develops is that the liver is not working properly! I realize this explanation sounds odd at first, however as you review Chapter 3 Digestion and consider the bigger picture of health I believe you will begin to see the relationship. Proceed with taking enzymes using my rule of thumb in health - that if it works continue. Yet if you are not feeling any better and in fact feel worse at times stop using enzymes for a period of time accenting the rest of the GIS supplements.

Heartburn

Heartburn is regarded in health as a state of LOW Hydrochloric Acid (HCL) in the stomach. The symptom that is identified most commonly is a burning sensation in the chest yet this is due to improper acidity flow coming from other gastric juices not HCL that is essential. When a person is low in HCL the result is poor digestion of proteins and minerals. This incomplete digestion of these nutrients causes gas to build up in the GI tract creating pressure in the upper stomach causing pain in the chest. The secondary inflammation symptom of a burning sensation is due to other gastric juices flowing that do not help the digestive process. Both a quality Aloe Vera and the B-Complex are essential for the support of the body to produce proper HCL flow. Proper HCL allows an increase of mineral absorption from vegetables and protein from every source. The minerals the body is supposed to be absorbing are to assist in many facets including pH balancing of the body which further adjusts improper over-acidity in the GI tract. Heartburn is often misdiagnosed as Reflux yet there is approximately 20% of the population experiencing true Reflux symptoms. The original or full diagnosis of Reflux is called Gastro Esophageal Reflux Disease (GERD).

Reflux / GERD

Both conditions of Heartburn and Reflux can develop from advancing GIS however true Reflux is caused by an under-functioning liver. The liver is an important organ that is responsible for making bile. Bile is stored in the gallbladder and when a person ingests fats they depend on the bile flow to assist in their digestion. The Pancreas gland is also supposed to secrete Pancreatic Enzymes into the small intestine to first begin the fat digestion with lipase. Next and only if the bile is flowing from the gallbladder into the small intestine as designed, the bile will further help to digest fats in the small intestine.

At this stage in digestion the bile is supposed to perform a second job of alkalinizing the food content in the duodenum. The food coming from the stomach was supposed to be acidic. However, if not enough bile has been produced and mixed into the food content during digestion to then alkalinize it the food will stay very acidic causing over-acidity! This acidity affects the tissue in the stomach and can flow back up into the esophagus especially when the gastric sphincters are not closing properly. This condition of over-acidity may worsen and begin to cause inflammation and burning of the lining tissue. One of the actions required to reverse Reflux is to reduce any unnecessary drugs and at the same time start a good detoxification of the liver that will allow it to make healthy levels of bile in the future. Individuals must act responsibly working with a physician to reassess their medical requirement of any drug protocol. Following the GIS program will begin the detoxification to support the liver and glands, rebalance your pH and remedy Reflux in the future.

This process can be fast or take up to one year or longer depending on the individual's health state. Remember to not ingest capsules or gelatin and keep high acid foods and beverages low or out of the diet until symptoms improve!

Nutrition Highlights: Probiotics, Daily Greens, Alfalfa, Vitamin E Complex, B-Complex, EFA's – Flax and Cod Liver Oil, Vitamin A (fish oil), Aloe Vera, Chamomile, Catnip, Mint Tea, Cat's Claw, Sheep Sorrel, Licorice Tea, Slippery Elm and Digestive Enzymes (only as needed). Review the herbs in StomachPlus by *Aloe Life* in Chapter 8 to see why it has been so popular to support digestion in the body.

9. Diverticulitis & Abnormal Colon Conditions

Diverticula's are small, bulging pouches that form most often in the large intestine. They can also occur in the small intestine, stomach and even occasionally in the esophagus. Diverticulitis occurs when one or more of the pouches become inflamed or infected causing; pain in the abdomen, fever, nausea and even sometimes rectal bleeding.

Bowel habits often change from diarrhea to constipation in people living with Diverticula. The incidence has increased from a mere 10% of the population in the 1920's to 50% in the 1960's. It is commonly found presently in people age 40 and older yet occasionally it is observed in younger people in their 20's often living with obesity.

Medical personnel warn that this condition can become serious if infection sets in and a pouch breaks open exposing the abdomen to infection called *peritonitis*. Seek medical attention immediately with any acute symptoms of pain and or fever. GIS is a factor to developing diverticula's and the condition responds very favorably to the GIS health program. Review the slant board instructions in Chapter 12 which has been extremely beneficial to people living with Diverticulosis to attain better health.

Facts about Diverticulosis
- Research Sites Dehydration as the Cause.

- Commonly Diagnosed in People 40 yrs and above.
- The Symptoms are Associated with Gluten Intolerance and GIS.
- Low Level Infection in the Diverticula's Pouches Reduce Immune Function.
- Symptoms lessen with Probiotics, Aloe Vera, Fish Oil, Water and the GIS Diet.
- Practicing the Slant Board Exercise is Extraordinary Helpful.

The slant board allows the drainage of fluid inside the pouches. Once they drain an individual can feel more energy and develop an even stronger immune system. A client of mine living with episodes of Diverticulitis called and I suggested she experiment with the slant board. She used her collapsed ironing board placing two phone books under one end with the other end resting on the floor. She then carefully lay down on the ironing board with her feet up on the high side head down. After approximately 10 minutes with her head on the down side, she felt the need to go to the bathroom. She experienced a release of extra fluid in a bowel movement that had a very sour-like odor. This occurred several times during the first week of using the slant board as described in Chapter 12. After this experience, to her amazement she began to feel better in everyway. She didn't have the bloated feeling in her belly any longer. Her energy increased and a sense of well-being began to build in her that she had not experienced in many years. All we could surmise is that the fluid that came out of the pouches had held infection. Once her body no longer had to combat the infection the body was revived!

Dehydration appears to be a major factor leading to the development of the pouch like tissue sacks lining the colon found most commonly on the left side around the *sigmoid* portion. The AMA states a lack of roughage of food fiber in the diet is at fault. Make certain your intake of fiber is only from the gluten free sources of fruits, vegetables, beans and NOT from psyllium seed, flax husk or whole grains. Diverticulosis is a common condition experienced by many people. It requires a gluten free diet along with healthy water intake to avoid pain and to ward off any future spread of the condition. The highlighted supplements are critical including the addition of a quality Probiotics, Aloe Vera and a Fish Oil supplement that contains Vitamin A and D because infection and regeneration of the tissue requires these core nutrients.

Abnormal Colon

Abnormal Colon can be any condition that is outside the normal 23 feet of small and large intestine which may include a longer than normal large intestine called a "Redundant Colon". Other colon conditions include; "Encopresis" which is an enlarged rectum often experienced by children, "Fissures" and hemorrhoids. Hemorrhoids are very common among adults yet not discussed and can be extremely painful and problematic. Resections where portions of the colon have been removed are fairly common and ulcers (all types) within the GI tract effect many teens and adults. Lazy bowel, Leaky Gut, Spastic Bowel, entire bowel removal and strictures (that are the narrowing of areas in the bowel) are far too common. Why I mention these conditions is to validate that I understand that many individuals do live with these colon concerns. Secondly, I want to convey that each of these colon conditions listed respond excellently to the GIS Program following the diet and experimenting with the supplements.

An important medical tip I wish to share - that helped me take an even greater participation in knowing as much about a disease or condition as possible - came from dealing with my Mother's doctors. Even though we like to think our doctors know everything about our body from the tests they conduct - they often only have limited information. They make educated guesses about what is going on with the diagnostic tests that are available and the time they spend evaluating them. The chances are that you know more about your body and your colon from tracking your symptoms than your doctor does. Especially if you have been learning about the way the body works.

Patricia's Resection Lesson

After years of having different medical doctors follow my Mother's Diverticulitis condition, which by the way improved remarkably with the GIS program, she developed a break in the descending colon wall from old scarring. Food and stool was passing through the colon break being eliminated out of the body with urine. The testing could not pinpoint the area of the troubled colon so a surgical date was set after a year of searching. In an unhealthy person "Sepsis Poisoning" is all but a given because of the stool that passes through the abdomen before being eliminated.

I attribute my mother's use of Aloe Vera, Probiotics and a comprehensive GIS supplement protocol coupled with a healthy diet - to keeping her alive. She survived the surgery resection at 80 yrs. of age yet several surprises came to the doctor as he observed Patricia's large intestine from the inside. The surgeon shared with me he was shocked that the break was almost 2 inches long allowing for the high amount of discharge Mother had shared with him. He had not believed her account which was one of the frustrating comments he had made over the months.

The second big surprise was that her colon had actually folded over onto itself like a taco only God knows why. My question was, "Couldn't the doctor see that from the Ultrasound Tests?" He not only removed the scarred and leaking portion of her colon with the resection by taken out approximately 6 full inches, he also unfolded the colon. He repositioned the large intestine correctly in the abdomen into the traditional 7 shape - AMAZING! Mother went on to recover after a second follow-up surgery due to adhesions that developed in the abdomen and she is presently 86 years young requiring no pharmaceutical drug medication what-so-ever! The trade-off is that she eats healthy 95% of the time keeping sugar and caffeine almost out of the diet completely and takes about 6 – 7 supplements and a few liquids but in turn enjoys a relatively pain free quality life!

Nutrition Highlights: Probiotics, Aloe Vera, Fish oil containing Vitamin A and D and Filtered Water. See Immune System section for the full GIS supplement regimen.

10. Environmental Toxicity & Allergies

According to the Environmental Protection Agency (EPA), as of 2010, there are over 88,000 potentially harmful chemicals in our environment. The challenges they pose are complex to our world and the solution is to avoid them wherever you can and kick up your preventative health measures significantly. Many of the toxic compounds impact the health or proper development of children, adults and all living creatures. Research is becoming more consistent in connecting the massive amount of toxins we are bombarded with to the many current health challenges and diseases in our society. How did we get into such a toxic mess you may be asking yourself? I believe it has been either through selective legislation and or behind closed door agreements giving many manufacturers a go ahead to freely pollute. Why else would we now have such a toxic world that is in need of mega clean-up?

Toxic Substances Control Act of 1976

A gesture of protection came from the government in 1976 called the Toxic Substances Control Act (TSCA). There were 62,000 chemicals being used at that time with many lacking their safety tests. The travesty is that even with this deluge of chemicals; the EPA only banned or limited 5 "chemical classes" as of 2006. It is also astonishing that out of the 3,000 high volume manufactured chemicals made each year in the US, a whopping 93% of the chemicals are missing one or more of the six basic safety tests. Get ready for this last statistic, 46% of them had no testing in the files about their safety whatsoever!

It appears that companies are only fingered for wrong doing when blatant polluting brings awareness of their toxic crime. This was the case in the 2000 film called, *Erin Brockovich*. The town of Hinkley, California was having unprecedented birth defects and cancer in their community. After uncovering the toxicity source in the town's groundwater supply, which came from the electricity company PG & E, a multimillion dollar suit was won for the townspeople! This is just one of thou of cases dealing with communities living with the ravages of chei pollution. The current research is revealing just how badly the FDA has dropped the ball in policing industrial waste. Half the battle is learning the scope of the problem and then our country needs some innovation through Environmental Biochemical Recycling Processes to help save the environment!

Medical Research Confirms Chemical Toxicity is Linked to Disease!

Fortunately, we have some high integrity university researchers testing right along-side private laboratories. Both are proving how the environmental toxins relate to disease on the rise. For example, Mt. Sinai School of Medicine's study in 2003 found an average of 91 chemicals in their 9 volunteers, as they tested their blood and urine.

Of the 167 chemicals discovered, 94 are toxic to the brain or nervous system, 76 are carcinogenic and 79 are linked to birth defects. They stated that the volunteers tested do not work with chemicals on the job nor do they live close to any industrial facility. They represented the average body burden of an ordinary American citizen. The diseases directly related to these toxins in our environment include; Cancer, Alzheimer Disease, children's birth defects, learning disabilities, Allergies, Asthma and other lung diseases.

Many of the children's health issues of today are worsened by the toxins in their environment. Their bodies are smaller in size so even less toxins impact them more severely. Recently the EPA stated there has not been clean air in the US for over 25 years! It is especially important to monitor our children's environment and give them lots of health support to compensate for toxicity.

Consumer action groups and determined patriots have helped plow the path for the few laws that have gotten harder on chemicals and better labeling of products. Slowly, important regulations have improved and come about over the years including the banning of the dangerous chemicals; DDT, PCB's and Lead. However, we cannot relax too much because they are still very much in our environment. These and other chemicals like Dioxin and Arsenic have made their way into the food chain by way of water and soil contamination. This is why in today's world the demand is rising quickly for organically grown foods in all categories as well as the requirement to drink purified filtered water. Even in choosing Organically Grown everything these environmental toxins have permeated into them as well. You must live proactively to protect yourself and your family's health and take preventative supplements to give the extra DNA support.

Water Must Be Filtered to Be Safe!

Drinking tap water and heavily sprayed commercial foods is frankly like playing with a ticking time bomb. In 2005 the EWG watchdog group analyzed data from 40,000 utilities serving 231 million people in the US and found disturbing results. Besides the normal dangerous chlorine by products in all public drinking water today they unveiled 141 unregulated chemicals and 119 regulated ones in higher than desirable levels. The five top chemicals that they saw pose risk from cancer, reproductive challenges, impaired neurological function and even auto-immune disease included; Radon, Chlorine and Chlorine Byproducts, Trichloroethylene (TCE- a solvent used in industry), Prescription Drugs and Pesticides like Arsenic. Learning more about the grave challenges facing Americans and throughout the world in the water supply is motivational to act preventatively and drink purified water. Necessity is the mother of invention and you must make this a priority even if you have never thought it to be important before!

Prioritize Safe Water for YOU and your Family!

- Seeking affordable filtered and purified water for yourself and or family is the first step. It may be purchasing water from a purification machine at your local grocery store or other outlet. I chose this method when I first began drinking filtered water.
- Next I ordered distilled water for many years. This is 100% safe and takes the guess work out of purity. Then I graduated to choose a purification system from the jungle of home systems

that is no longer being manufactured. My home system that I have used for twenty years is a Sediment, Reverse Osmosis and Carbon Filter. I have recently decided to go back to drinking distilled water because of the increase in pollution including the addition of Fluoride which is a trace mineral by-product which holds unsafe side effect in larger amounts. Also, Ammonia Perchlorate (rocket fuel) has been found in half of the U.S. drinking water (along with other chemical spills) that polluted the public drinking water like the recent Chromium 6 spill which is a potential carcinogen.

The EPA is well aware of the "Toxic Soup" that permeates our lives with over 700 identified chemicals found in humans. The legal catch with the U.S. Toxicity Guidelines has been that they have "allowable limits" of contamination. Unfortunately research is costly and revealing therefore work has not been conducted to test the safety of multiple chemical impacts on children and adults. We do know that disease is on the rise such as cancers including Non-Hodgkin's Lymphoma for example. This type of cancer has increased three fold since 1950 and our society is experiencing many more childhood diseases that come from a reduction in immune function. In case you are one of the people living in the illusion of wondering where cancer comes from – look to the bowl of toxic soup we all partake in!

In the face of all the new research that is confirming the toxic facts we have the CDC that just completed an overview report. Hopefully the content will impact the CDC to make some hard decisions about who they will serve – big business or the citizens. We must encourage and support any legislation that is proposed in the future - to help create long-term solutions to pollution. Pardon my sarcasm – but don't hold your breath!

CDC Human Toxicity Study

It is clear from the massive amounts of pollutants we are absorbing into our bodies that the EPA has not been protecting the citizens thus far. The shocking truth is that on a daily basis each one of us may receive over one hundred chemical hits per day. It is easier to fathom this fact considering the toxins found on commercially grown apples in 36 samples contained up to 9 different pesticides, herbicides and some growers were using stabilizing chemicals as well! Several cancer causing chemicals were among them.

Four of the most common hazardous chemicals to avoid in our environment, in particular because they effect our ability to think, function at optimum levels and they also decrease immune function include; Mercury, Lead, Dioxins and PCB's. Other metals that also add to the arsenal of environmental toxins are Arsenic, Cadmium and Radon.

At last, fueled by public pressure, the CDC began conducting studies on toxicity. Testing that was recently completed in 2009, from the fourth CDC study called, *Analyze Toxins in Humans*, revealed that all 212 potential chemicals they tested for showed positive in the adults subjects. The CDC's study also revealed that 97% of the subjects had higher than expected levels of oxybenzone found in sunscreens and lip balms. The research has shown a relationship of this chemical to greater allergies, hormone disruption for men and women along with cell damage due to it increasing free radicals from the chemicals they create. Also, in a companion study, Oxybenzone was associated with a much higher incidence of low birth weight in infants whose mothers had the highest levels. Hopefully the findings of this research will put this chemical and others found to cause toxic symptoms on the do not use list. 700 sunscreen products contain this problematic ingredient. One stumbling block has been that the FDA has shelved the standards for sunscreens over the past 30 years. Citizen groups are ratcheting up the pressure on legislatures to honestly use the regulating guidelines to protect the consumer. What a novice idea!

Harmful chemicals and pollutants can be found in the water, air and food. Unfortunately, an individual's living environment to include personal care products of lotions, soaps, hair dyes, shampoos and household supplies can also be more dangerous than anyone wants to acknowledge. In fact 29 Personal Care Products have been isolated to contain harmful chemicals that absorb into the body. You need to understand that the body is like a sponge for every chemical that is applied to the skin along with ingesting them.

Even mainstream bubble soaps for children have been found to contain a newly discovered toxin by the name of Dioxane. This chemical which has no odor or color to speak of was exposed to the public somewhat recently by a study orchestrated by author and activist, David Steinman. Look for his book entitled, *Living Healthy in a Toxic World* and *Diet for a Poisoned Planet,* plus other books by Steinman who is also known as the Green Patriot. Dioxane is an important chemical to learn about because it has been directly linked to causing cancer in animals in even very small amounts.

Earth's Toxic Soup; Over 88,000 Toxic Chemicals Confirmed by the EPA

- Environment; Work, Home, Schools, Recreational Areas.
- Coatings; Paint, Sealers, Play Equipment, Processed Woods.
- Toys; Painted Toys & Children's Jewelry.
- Gardening Supplies; Weed Control, Pesticides.
- New Cars; Plastic Molded Parts, Rugs, Wiring.
- Household Cleaners & Appliances; Laundry Soaps, Dryer Sheets.
- Personal Care Products; Soaps, Laundry, Cleaning, Make Up, Hair Color, Shampoo & Rinse.
- Pots, Pans & Appliances; Non-Stick Coatings.
- Plastics & Chemicals in the Home; Paper Plates (chlorine by-products), Fast Food Leftovers (Don't reheat them in the Styrofoam containers.), Saran Wrap (Food should not touch the wrap and not all products are for use in the microwave!), Avoid Styrofoam with hot liquids.

- Dry Cleaning Chemicals & Fire Resistant Clothing and Furniture.
- Mercury; Fillings, Coal Burning, Vaccines, Large Fish Consumption.
- Commercial Foods (hundreds); Eat Organic Foods (as possible) including Baby food.
- Water & Beverages; Choose Filtered, Distilled, Organic Juices (as possible) and Baby Formulas.

Newborn Toxicity Study

A study, conducted by a steadfast consumer advocate group, has encouraged a ground breaking toxic review involving the innocent unborn child. In a 2004 study, conducted by the Environmental Working Group (EWG) in collaboration with the Common Wealth of Canada, 10 newborns from US hospitals had their umbilical cord blood tested for chemical toxicity. At one time it was hopeful that the fetus was protected from pollutants by some natural bio-filter system throughout the full gestational period. To everyone's regret this research put that hope to rest by discovering in the last weeks before the birth, the blood does carry chemical contamination straight away into the infant through the blood.

What these two laboratories found in this EWG study, were 287 different chemicals contaminating the newborns. The chemicals consisted of a variety of plastic compounds like PCB's, organic toxins of mercury, pesticides including DDT and Arsenic, coal burning chemicals, gasoline by-products like Lead, clothing flame resistant toxins, Teflon and even toxicity from fast food containers and garbage waste. We can all agree that this is a sad situation, brought about by the non-stop industrial revolution and runaway government.

My hope is through sharing these studies of the body burden of toxins in infants and adults that the public as a whole might begin to grasp the importance of avoiding and combating environmental toxins more than they do at present time. This work can motivate all of us to be more preventative in the choices we make each day to reduce toxins and arm the body with improved health to compensate for some of the unavoidable health damage (Ch. 8).

Chemical Toxicity of Newborns in the 2004 Study; Identified 287 Industrial Chemicals, Pollutants & Pesticides and classed each of their potential.

- 180 Found to Cause Cancer.
- 217 Found to Be Toxic to Brain Tissue and the Central Nervous System.
- 208 Found to Cause Birth Defects.

Mercury is in the Air, Water, Food and Our Teeth!

Mercury is one of nature's natural occurring metals on the planet. It becomes toxic when the body receives too much of it. Mercury is in the top four most deadly toxins and it is important to avoid it whenever possible. It is the second most harmful neurotoxin in the world with "Lead" taking first place. Mercury is found in coal. It spews into the atmosphere through coal burning electric plants. Coal burning unleashes tons of Mercury into the air every year. The US has over 600 coal-burning electric and industrial companies scattered about. In the northeast corner alone 5 tons of Mercury escapes into the atmosphere. Clean coal technology is a must in the world's future for the preservation of humans!

Once in the air it spreads uncontrollably across cities, farmlands and waterways, permeating into the food chain. It is this portal that the fish become contaminated in our rivers, streams and oceans. Some research states that there are also other forms of mercury toxicity originating from the ocean floor as well.

In our food supply people must curtail the amount of larger fish they eat because of the accumulation of mercury and other potential pollutants like PCB's and Dioxins both classed as probable carcinogens. Freshwater fish from rivers and lakes have also been fingered for having some responsibility to the higher cancer rates including breast cancer. One of many areas for example is around Lake Michigan where people have connected hot beds of higher cancer statistics to the local fish. In today's world I believe it would be the exception to find any fish that did not contain some contamination however, ocean fish do not contain the same potential of toxins found in some fresh water varieties due to the pollution coming from local city's manufacturing run-off into streams, rivers and lakes.

Dentistry has also been another source for mercury poisoning. Most people studying health are well aware that the traditional fillings, called *amalgams,* consist of a large percentage of mercury. Mercury is a very soft metal therefore during the chewing process, as you bite down on harder dense foods; it releases the soft mercury into the blood stream. More and more people are NOT getting the silver (mercury) amalgam fillings. If you have been considering the removal of them from your teeth it is important to do so by the correct method, to avoid more contamination. Also, with future dental work there are several other safer choices that include; composite or porcelain fillings. Dentists like to use the silver mercury fillings for children however I opted for the composite for my kids despite their recommendation concerning the amalgam (silver colored) mercury ones that worked out very well.

Symptoms of Mercury poisoning are similar to lead because both toxins kill nerve cells. The exception to mercury that experts in this field have shared is that it is difficult to get a positive reading on a blood test for mercury toxicity. The metal appears to lodge in the body and does not exit with any speed. Checking the blood does not reveal storage of toxins in the fat and body tissue. Chronic fatigue, failing immune function, mental illnesses and overall Central Nervous System irregularities that begin showing up following a mouth full of amalgams, seem to be the best litmus test.

One woman I met had over 25 silver fillings in her mouth and was unable to hold a job or have much of a life. She lived on government assistance through SSI monies. Only upon having her complete set of teeth removed did she begin the slow process of feeling better month by month. *Note:* It is important to work with a dentist that has been trained in proper removing of the amalgam fillings. In this woman's case the dental expert felt she would have experienced extreme toxicity if he removed so many fillings and suggested false teeth. Most people opt for removing the fillings gradually one by one with a trained dental expert or alerting the dentist that you are working with of the potential danger.

Mercury in My Youth

By age 13, I had 13 mercury fillings in my mouth. I received them over a three year period. I'm convinced that because of my full blown sugar addiction as a child that resulted in lots of dental caries requiring the fillings it impacted my learning ability as a youngster. Looking back with my perspective now, I can see how my learning capacity slowed way down over the following 10 years. I continued to experience many health challenges throughout my teens and young adulthood coming from both my sugar addiction, toxicity from Mercury and a budding gluten intolerance that my body had to endure.

Choosing to work in the health field and applying health has most definitely extended my life, I am most certain. My ability to learn has improved steadily over the years instead of going the other direction as with many of my peers. Applying the GIS program has allowed my body to detoxify and renew itself as I removed my mercury fillings one by one. I have optimized my body's capacity through including many different "Special Needs Supplements" over and above my everyday "Essential Core Nutrients" and have eaten the best I could. For certain by accenting the B-Complex, Fish Oil by *Nordic Naturals,* Aloe Vera, Daily Greens, NAC and Prevagen (Chapter 8) – has made a remarkable improvement in my ability to think more clearly and sharply and multi-task better than ever!

Mercury is such a harmful neurotoxin and we all get lots of it. Besides the dental fillings people receive it through vaccinations. It is used as a preservative in vaccines and you must request a non-mercury injection to avoid it in most injections. Also, be cautious to not eat too many larger fish products like tuna fish (sandwiches), swordfish or salmon, as good as it may taste or be for our hearts and brains. Small fish can be eaten more often like sardines, cod and even halibut from Alaskan waters or other safe areas. Sardines and other cold water fish are valuable to the body for Omega-3 Fatty Acids however you can also get the Omega 3's through properly distilled Fish Oil (Ch. 5 Highlight and 8) to reach an optimum level more safely. Remember to look for quality fish oil products that don't contain the mercury and other pollutants like *Nordic Naturals*.

Lead Poisoning Took Down the Roman Empire!

If you have studied Roman history you will remember that lead poisoning coming from the Roman vases and plates was speculated to have caused the fall of their empire! Lead is the number one destroyer of the human's Nervous System effecting proper brain function. High amounts can even be fatal! The amount of lead present in many children and adults bodies far exceeds the safe limit imposed by the FDA and the CDC. If our government was truly concerned with the citizen's well-being, testing for lead toxicity would be a requirement on every blood test from birth right up through to the senior years.

According to the Mayo Clinic our environment contains dangerous levels of lead especially in older homes that require more caution in daily living. This is because lead is found in higher amounts in the soil around older homes, schools, churches and other buildings. These older dwelling often still have leaded paints on the walls that cause paint dust that pollutes both the inside and outside environments. Extreme caution is advised in its removal. Also, water from lead pipes and or lead soldering material, children's jewelry and toys, cosmetics, candy contamination and miscellaneous other foodstuff especially imports may contain higher than safe lead content. Even a small amount of lead can seriously affect mental health and physical development of children. Older adults may be equally impacted yet have somewhat different symptoms. Some seniors may even have old lead amalgam fillings, used decades ago, in their teeth still causing them toxicity.

Higher Lead Toxicity Sources

- Older Schools, Offices & Homes; paint, soil, pipes, water.
- Toys, Jewelry & Paints; paint on jewelry and painted glasses, fishing weights.
- Cosmetics & Make-Up; color additives may contain the lead content.
- Industry & Fuels; making stained glass, manufacturing processes, industrial and cigarette smoke.
- Household Products; pottery, some China & Porcelain dishes, canned foods from imports (possibility, cleaners including rug cleaning chemicals.
- Candy & Foodstuff; chocolate candy and other, dairy, meats, vegetables and other.

The Mayo Clinic states that the detection of lead is not easy from just symptoms so if you think you or your family may have a toxicity issue seek professional guidance to be tested and get treatment called "Chelation". The blood test is simple for lead. It involves just a finger prick and according to the AMA guidelines, if the level of lead is above 10 mcg / dL or higher they suggest immediate treatment. Following the GIS Program including the detoxification supplements will help greatly with or without medical intervention.

Safety Tips for the Family

The Consumer Product Safety Commission joins the choir stating that people can easily be contaminated by up to 150 different chemicals in the environment that may increase the risk of allergies, birth defects, cancer, higher blood pressure, migraine headaches, hyperactivity as with ADD, ADHD and other psychological abnormalities. So often the chemicals in our homes are not obvious and come from the carpet and carpet cleaners, building materials used in the walls and flooring containing toxic glues, plastics and coatings that out-gas for many years. Make healthier choices whenever available. Airing out newer and even older homes, cars and offices is definitely a good practice to reduce toxic gases.

In this section I did not include all of the potential toxins that can be in the home that add to health challenges including molds and animal dander coming from insects and pets. Just keep in mind that there are many potential toxins found indoors that pollute the air of a home or office adding to the speculation that the air inside can be up to 5 times more toxic than the outdoors air!

Make Your Environment Safer by Eliminating Toxicity

- *Children's clothing and toys may be toxic;* Flame retardant pajamas come with potential toxicity risk so choose cotton and natural fibers that are safer for the whole family. When in doubt on painted jewelry and toys from China leave it out.
- *Dry cleaning chemicals are not the best choice for regular wear;* Any chemical we put on our body including soaps, lotions, shampoos, certain hair dyes and cosmetics can add health risks. Air-out any Dry Cleaning clothes outdoors or at least in the garage if possible before placing them in your bedroom.
- *Candles made from petroleum wax and certain wick materials can emit dangerous chemicals;* benzene, styrene, toluene and acetone. Purchase candles from a health food store or a reliable source that confirms that they are the most natural and safe. Air Refreshers may also contain very toxic chemicals depending on the particular product purchased.
- *Replace your non-stick pans with stainless or cast iron and glass for safety;* In fact the EPA states that non-stick pans are now rated the 2nd most harmful source of chemical toxicity for individuals, next to environmental chemicals. Recent ruling has classed Teflon as a carcinogenic chemical!

- *Wear gloves when handling certain electrical appliances, tools with moldable handles, wires that may contain coating with undesirable plastic toxic chemicals absorb directly into the skin;* Use protection when working with any known toxic material including a carbon filter mask and gloves.

- *Household cleaning solutions such as laundry detergents, anti-cling and dryer sheets, spotters or bathtub cleansers;* Mainstream cleaners may contain a plethora of mutagenic and cancer causing chemicals. Switch to organic cleaners and soaps from a more reliable safer source. Stop using any artificially scented cleaners, soaps or dryer sheets!

- *Garden Organically;* Weed killers and pesticides are poisonous to bugs and people. Plants in and around the home is a great way to help filter some of the toxins from the out gassing or chemicals and give off more oxygen people require for health. If you must use a toxic chemical use protection and clean up properly afterwards. Keep in mind that bare feet from children, adults and pets will absorb the poison residue (left from spraying or treatment) of chemicals directly into the body. Any toxicity in coatings on wooden play ground equipment and decks can be very toxic to the family.

- *Out Gassing of Toxins;* New or remodeled cars, offices and homes can have multiple toxic chemicals, a shocking 17 from new cars coming from the plastics, coatings and building materials also used in homes of today.

What is the Solution to Pollution?

Would they sell it if it wasn't safe? The answer is YES! I share this important information so you can understand when I say that avoiding toxic chemicals is a goal to looking, thinking and feeling your very best. People living in the 21st century are truly living in a toxic soup and hair analysis and blood tests are available to give that seal of confirmation.

My husband and I had the hair analysis performed for toxicity. It was a valuable exercise to confirm our own toxic chemical body burden. Testing helped to get our heads out of the sand and coming to grips with reality and was a giant motivator. Testing is not a requirement to get healthier yet if you are interested refer to the Reference for Hair Analysis home testing kit. If you are further curious about toxicity you may also wish to check out the website for California Proposition 65. It contains over eight pages of chemicals that made the list of known toxins found in California that are confirmed to interfere with proper metabolism or cause cancer and the list is mandated to be updated yearly. Let's keep getting healthier together by following the preventative steps making the wisest choices each day.

Steps to Avoid Environment Poisoning
- *Nutrition & Health*; Drinking good filtered water and include the best nutrition you have available accenting vegetables and food fiber. Review in Chapter 6 the Detoxification protocol that takes the body through a natural chelation and or removal of toxins as much as possible. Healthy fats, exercise and hot baths can speed up the detoxification process.
- *Increase Antioxidants;* Tuft's University has been measuring the amount of antioxidants it takes to reverse DNA damage resulting from toxicity within the body. The researchers advocate each of us to strive for 12,000 mg of ORAC daily. ORAC is defined as Oxygen Radical Absorbency Capacity or in other words the repair nutrients needed to allow the body to heal itself. Following the GIS Diet and Program will give abundant amounts of ORAC every day to help mend the damaged DNA and support detoxification. "Never enough Antioxidants!"
- *Create a Healthier Happier Living Space*; Open-up the windows or run the air circulation in the AC unit making certain to change the air filters with the seasons. Oxygen is very important for health. Plants in the home can assist with adding more oxygen

and also to offset chemical off-gassing to some extent. Spider plants have been touted to absorb air pollution. Clean the clutter and add some Green color. Color can affect our moods. Green is the color of life!

Nutrition Highlights: Aloe Vera, Daily Greens by *Aloe Life*, 2-3 cups of Vegetables and a couple of (organic) fruits (food fiber plus ORAC) daily, water, Minerals - Calcium, Magnesium & others, Vitamin C & Bioflavonoids, Antioxidants, NAC and Alpha Lipoic Acid.

11. Immune System Balance

All human beings are born with an immune system with varying degrees of function. Infants generally have a lower functioning immunity until they ingest the valuable "Colostrum" received in the first hours and days of nursing. Every woman needs to understand the great service they give their child through breastfeeding even for a short time if not longer like 12 to 18 months which is the average. Fortunately children and adults who were not nursed even for a short time, whatever the reason, can take a colostrum supplement (Ch. 8). Even though it is not exactly the same as from "Mothers Milk", research reveals it can enhance immunity at any age.

Immunity in the body can be categorized as coming from three main areas to include; Fluid Systems of the Blood and Lymph, Innate Immunity which we are born with and the Adaptive or Acquired Immunity. The value of learning more about the specific parts of the Immune System is to underline the importance of building a foundational network from nutrition. Once the Immune System is built it then requires stimulation and balance through exercise and a healthy lifestyle.

Immunity in the Body is Three-Fold

- *Fluid Systems*; Blood (made in Bone Marrow from Stem Cells) and Lymph circulate the Lymphocytes T & B cells. T- Cells are matured in the Thymus gland.

- *Innate Immunity* (genetically born with it and it operates within the Fluid Systems); Natural Killer (NK) Cells, Lysozyme Enzymes destroy gram positive bacteria found in the tears, saliva and nasal secretion. Healthy Friendly Flora Bacteria in the gut is part of this immunity working through lactic-acid pH protection and other pathways to ward off bad bacteria.
- *Acquired Immunity* (produced in the Bone Marrow and works within the Fluid System); Lymphocytes – White blood cells (WBC), T & B cells. T-Cells require balance to avoid auto-immune conditions and proper immune response. Macrophages stimulate the phagocytes so they can work together to destroy bad bacteria, viruses, fungus and other pathogens.

The Immune System elicits a response against an "Antigen". This is a substance that can be a virus, bacteria, fungus and even a sliver in your finger can bring upon a response. Immunity has a series of dual natures to help it recognize the difference of the body itself from a foreign invader. Research published in the September, 2001 issue of *Journal of Experimental Medicine*, underlines the importance of the Natural Killer cells (NK) to keep the Immune System in healthy balance. Since the AMA has reported up to 80 confirmed autoimmune diseases that affect many people's health, this work of balancing the immune system is very important.

Researchers from Brown University and McGill University, discovered by keeping the body making sufficient NK Cells, it directly regulates the T-Cell Immunity so valuable for both a healthy immune response and avoiding an over-response against the body's healthy tissue. This destructive autoimmune over-response is exactly what happens in the case of gluten intolerance. The researchers said keeping the NK cells around and functioning will help many conditions (besides GIS), from HIV and Cancer needing a robust Immune System of T-4 Lymphocytes to even keeping patients from rejecting organ transplants with high T-8's. The important lesson to take away from this work is that the body does not always manufacture these essential regulators of the immunity network. It takes supporting health to build a healthy NK supply.

Essentials of Building NK Cells and a Balanced Immune System

- Nutrition; Protein, Vitamin A Rich Foods, Essential Fatty Acids (EFA's), Vegetables (4-5 servings) & Fruits (1-2) high in Essential Core Nutrients and Antioxidants; A, C, E, B-Complex Plus Minerals and more.

- Supplements; Probiotics, Fish Oil - Vitamin A & D3, Vitamin E Complex, Aloe Vera, Pycnogenol and other Antioxidants to avoid DNA damage.

- Exercise; 30 - 45 minutes daily of Aerobic type, as tolerated, Rest and Good Sleep.

Vitamin A & Exercise Activates NK Cells

Stimulating the NK Cells for greater health was supported years ago through scientific research which indicated the need for higher levels of Vitamin A (found in vegetables, some fruits and fish) to keep the immunity strong. Researcher Dr. Ronald Watson a professor at the University of Arizona, College of Medicine found that enhanced immune response was noticeable at 30 mg equal to 50,000 IU of Vitamin A and above to increase the numbers of NK cells and activate lymphocytes.

Exercising for about 45 minutes that raises your heart rate around 75% over the resting rate has also proven to activate the NK response in the body. Exercise has been found to even help during chemotherapy for increasing not only the NK Cells but also the White Blood Cells (WBC's) thereby reducing Neutropenia that is common with lower immune function. Conversely, a marathon runner generally over-stresses the Immune System especially after running at top speed for 90 minutes or more. It may take hours or days to rebuild healthy immunity after such a strenuous workout!

Building a healthy immune system also requires quality foods such as Proteins from both vegetable and animal sources and Essential Fatty Acids found in seafood, fish oil, flax seed oil, greens, walnuts along with the other core nutrients required for cellular metabolism. Vaccinations are called "Active Artificial Immunity" and do provide some anti-viral support from activation yet in themselves they do not build any part of the Immune System. Injections of Gamma Globulin are given with a Hepatitis infection and a few other conditions and are referred to as Passive Immunity. Both of these are man-made creations to kick-up the body's immunity and are helpful yet extremely limited in their results. Investing in your health through nutrition which builds the Immune System is paramount to getting the most from your body for health protection.

Aloe Vera Research Proves Anti-Tumor Support

Natural supplements can be very beneficial and science is helping to bring this information to the attention of more people especially in regards to immunity support from Aloe Vera. Research has been repeatable showing the natural phytonutrients from the plant supports both Innate and Acquired Immunity. Aloe Vera stimulates the macrophages which increase the proper phagocytic response very similar to little Pac-men gobbling up microbial invaders in the blood stream. The anti-tumor activity from ingesting Aloe has most significantly come from the larger chains of polysaccharides or long chain sugars called Glycol-Proteins also called Acemannans. In both animal and human studies tumors regressed in just a matter of weeks depending on the quality of the Aloe Vera. Seeing a quality Aloe Vera at work supporting health on such a critical system as the immune system along with the core nutrients has been quite thrilling as a health educator. The scientific research reveals that to receive the immunomodulation response it must be dose dependent. Therefore, drinking a few ounces can soothe a troubled stomach or balance immunity and taking more 6-8 ounces (or tablets) revs up the Immune System to even bring about tumor reduction!

Vitamin E Significantly Raises Immune Response in Only One Month!

Tufts University has been a leader in the field of nutritional support of the body for healthy aging. During their 30 year longevity research study, they proved that by adding a Vitamin E supplement for as little as one month greatly enhanced the vitality of the immune system. Jeffrey Blumberg, head professor of Antioxidant research at Tufts shared during an interview that Vitamin E is not dangerous for an adult but in fact the body requires a regular higher quantity of it than can be delivered through diet alone. He went onto say that toxicity was not even observed with 7,000 IU much less a smaller amount. The conversation with Dr. Blumberg was in defense of the previous slanted media coverage, an obvious smear campaign against Vitamin E. He was in no way advocating the average person to take this mega amount however he strongly reassured the public that Vitamin E is safe to take and a valuable supplement. Just think about it for a minute, if Vitamin E truly posed a safety threat you know darn well that the FDA would have taken it off the market years ago!

Selenium Research has Revealed a 63% Lower Prostate Cancer Rate in Men

Minerals play a very key role in our immunity for both men and women yet we seldom hear about their importance. They are known as co-factors to metabolic pathways in the body including immunity. Selenium taken in the organic form from yeast has shown the best activity to raise the levels of Glutathione Peroxidase in the liver needed for detoxification. All people living in today's world can benefit from cleansing and detoxification of the body.

In a study conducted in China, researchers looked at the correlation of higher incidences of cancer in one village compared to another with low cancer rates comparing the levels of Selenium in the soil. The soil in the gardens that were depleted in Selenium had the increased cancer rate. Research has been very specific on the form of selenium used in each investigational study. The most remarkable outcome has come from the Selenium rich Nutritional Yeast taken in powder form or a 200 mcg tablet daily called "Selenium Yeast". The research has revealed a 63% reduction in the incidence of Prostate cancer in men from a 1996 study over a 10 year period with 974 men. Another study showed an over 50% decrease in all cancers with a group of over 8,000 people during the same time period 1996 compared to the controls not receiving Selenium Yeast. Selenium Yeast is one of the GIS daily recommended special needs supplements.

Another health enhancing compound found in nutritional yeast is called Beta-Glucan. Recently the research has been so compelling for extra immune support that scientists are considering the addition of Beta-Glucan to baby formulas.

The Value of Vitamin D is Not a Secret Anymore for Increased Immunity!

Healthy immune function requires all of the essential core nutrients including Vitamin D in sufficient amounts. Researchers have been doing their very best for the past decade to get the attention of the AMA in regards to the health importance of Vitamin D3. At last research facts were so compelling the AMA could no longer ignore the need to promote a supplement. Research on Vitamin D revealed that 50% of men and women with Osteoporosis did not have anywhere near the necessary amount of Vitamin D they required to absorb proper minerals including calcium to build healthy bones. Vitamin D3 is required not just for strong bones and teeth but the entire body's health hinges on having the correct quantity. Deficiency of Vitamin D is associated with many diseases to include; Failing Immune Function, Multiple Sclerosis (MS), Asthma, Digestive Issues, Bone Loss, Rickets, Inflammation, CVD, TB, Hypertension, Epilepsy, Parkinson's, Skin Conditions, Diabetes and even Depression.

PubMed which is the on-line service of the US National Library of Medicine has a total of 780 peer reviewed studies conducted over the past 10 years on Vitamin D3. They have been published in respected journals like the *New England Journal of Medicine* on the value of Vitamin D for adults and also studies on D3 include the infancy deficiencies. The AMA's past recommended daily allowance RDA has been a mere 400 IU daily, when in fact what biochemists are revealing is that humans may actually require up to 20,000 or more IU daily. Many doctors are not prescribing more than 5,000 IU per day just to be on the safe side because it is classed as a fat soluble vitamin however the test to check for healthy levels can be easily prescribed in the doctor's office.

The test to check for low blood levels of D3 is the 25-Hydroxy Vitamin D test. Many doctors are now routinely suggesting the test if you show any of the symptoms. Ask your physician to order a D3 test to uncover any shortcomings you may have. As I mentioned minerals are extremely important to reach optimum health and a good supply of Vitamin D and getting your digestion working well is critical to help absorb them all!

Why are People so Deficient in Vitamin D?

There appears to be several co-factors missing from the body with deficiencies that prevent the synthesis of Vitamin D to take place in the skin. Dark skin people absorb even less of the suns UV rays needed to make Vitamin D and often have the greatest deficiencies. Surprisingly, with the recent slew of testing being done it is revealing that even when people are getting a good 45 minutes of sunshine most days - they are still coming up deficient! My guess is, it could be that deficient individuals do not make enough of the good cholesterol in their bodies to begin with which requires a healthy liver and good nutrition, to metabolize Vitamin D.

Taking a good source of Vitamin D3 (Cholecalciferol) is important and my favorite is the natural products from fish oil that come with both the Vitamin D and if you choose also Vitamin A and the other Omega-3 fractions. Doctors are prescribing the D3 yet why not get Omega-3 Fatty Acids (that encourage production of good cholesterol HDL) along with the other healthy co-factors of EPA and DHA with the Vitamin D. Nordic Naturals is my number one choice in fish oils and they make several formulations to choose from. I take the Arctic-D at least 2-3 teaspoons daily to cover the nutritional bases. For special needs you may temporarily still require a higher prescription of a single Vitamin D3 however one focus you want to make certain of and that is to get some rays from the sun whenever possible.

Take Action to Build a Strong & Balanced Immune System!

Support your own immune system to work the way it was designed by taking ACTION - applying health and you will stay healthier and able to fight off invaders. As the American Cancer Society has proclaimed, the development of cancer is the end result of 10 – 20 years of neglect and abuse to the body. Genetic predisposition is only sixth on their list of why a person may develop the cancer disease!

A "Balanced Immune System" is the result when you make the healthier choices that allow auto-immune conditions to improve if not go into complete remission as many people have experienced. Review the Detoxification and Candida sections. Rest assured that the GIS Program will lead you along the right path as you choose health!

Nutrition Highlights: Protein, Vitamin A, Probiotics, EFA's – Flax and Fish Oil Vitamin A & D, Vitamin A (10,000 IU 1 – 3 times daily for 45 days as desired), Aloe Vera by *Aloe Life*, Antioxidants (a variety to reverse DNA damage) - 12, 000 ORAC, Vitamin E Complex 400 – 1200 IU., Nutritional Yeast (Selenium & Beta-Glucan) by *Solgar*, Zinc, NAC, Liquid Silver - Hydrosol Sovereign Silver, Multiple Vitamin & Mineral, Colostrum, Exercise, Water and Special Needs as desired (Ch. 8).

12. The Liver, Organs & Glandular Function

A group of organs also referred to as glands make up the Endocrine System of the body. They secrete hormones that are specialized to perform life supportive action throughout the metabolic pathways for health. The "Endocrine Hormones" regulate growth and development, tissue function and mood. Some organs are minimally important like the Spleen and the Gallbladder and can be removed without necessarily decreasing critical hormonal activity or threaten the life of a person. Other organs we cannot live without such as the Liver. It is highlighted in this section because of its enormous importance. In fact failing health can often be traced back to a lazy liver. The Thyroid and Parathyroid glands are very necessary however if they do become damaged or under-functioning modern medicine has made it possible to supply the body with similar hormones. Organs each have their individual purpose in the body and we want to make every effort to keep all of them. We also want them to function as well as possible and following the GIS Program gives that support.

What does the Liver Do in the Body?

- The liver is an important organ that preforms hundreds of actions and literally makes thousands of chemicals that allow metabolic processes to be successful all over the body every day.

- The liver is so important to the health and well being of the body some experts refer to it as a second brain.

- The liver plays a critical role in the digestive process and also helps to filter and disarm harmful toxins from the blood making potent antioxidants that even reverse cancer and DNA damage. It also makes cholesterol contributing to the manufacturing of hormones, the protection of cellular health and supporting metabolism of Vitamin D.

- The liver is a storehouse of nutrients including Vitamin A and glycogen when required for a quick energy source. When an emergency or shortage occurs as with hypoglycemia or during a famine or other physically stressful situations the release of stored nutrients is designed to be able to keep the brain thinking and the body alive.

- Another job of the liver supporting digestion is to process and synthesize amino acids, 22 different ones, from the eight essential amino acids called building blocks of proteins. The liver makes hundreds of protein compounds throughout the body which help to build the immune system, hormones, anti-bodies and all of the individual cells. Most fat soluble vitamins are also processed in the liver before traveling on to the cells for health support to include; Vitamin A (Beta-Carotene not the fish oil type), Vitamin E-Tocopherols, Vitamin K and Essential Fatty Acids (EFA's).

Hormones are needed for hundreds of different processes in the body including to wake us up, to go to sleep, experience happiness and to regulate our sex drive for men and women (estrogen, progestin and testosterone). It is no wonder that obese children and adults experience a high percentage of illnesses associated with a fatty liver. A fatty liver slows its metabolism way down and that causes it to malfunction which in turn affects the entire body.

What other factors cause the liver to go awry? In a very simplified explanation the liver becomes slow and ineffective with a reduction of the Nervous System as is the case with other glands being impacted by GIS. Also, constipation, poor and limited nutrition that includes the abuse from sugar, junk foods and alcohol result in more waste products and congestion in the liver slowing it down. Another challenge to the liver is when excess fat starts to accumulate on the body with obesity. Whenever the body is storing excess fat anywhere you can trust that the liver is getting bogged down with fat as well. The irony is that the liver is responsible for fat metabolism after the food contents are absorbed from the small intestine through the villi. When the liver does not work properly it cannot process fat or fat soluble Vitamins A, E, K, D and EFA's efficiently. This sets up a major shortfall because these nutrients are responsible to help build immunity and skin health two areas that suffer with a sluggish liver. Poor liver function indirectly affects every cell of the body negatively.

Abusing OTC and prescriptive medication is another reason for disruption of healthy liver function in the body. Once the body is not able to work properly from the damaging effects of the drugs and any other factors the result is Dermatitis and or other skin inflammation like Acne, Rosacea, Eczema and Psoriasis. Diseases such as Hepatitis, Lyme's Disease and Cirrhosis can also greatly damage proper liver function and require therapeutic supplements covered in Chapter 5 and 8. All rashes and skin condition are a result of food abuse including gluten inflammation, constipation and an unhealthy liver.

The body must have proper nutrition and a good functioning liver to build healthy lining cells in the GI tract and the outer surface of the skin. Healthy skin, anti-aging support and gut repair is totally reliant on a healthy liver!

Metabolic X Syndrome & Diabetes

Besides the Liver, the Pancreas and the Adrenal glands are two other organs also affected by GIS. The GIS inflammation can cause the Pancreas to reduced Insulin flow resulting in Diabetes. "Adrenal Exhaustion" coming from poor nutrition and stress coupled with the GIS inflammation further reduces glandular function. Continued stress creates high levels of the Cortisol hormone that lowers immunity while triggering fat storage, dizziness, skin conditions while increasing allergies and sleep disturbances. Together these under-functioning glands and low Liver function often result in "Metabolic X Syndrome" (MXS). This is a condition compiled of a cluster of symptoms. If you have three of the five symptoms doctors feel that you are developing this glandular shutdown called MXS which may lead to CVD and many other illnesses if no intervention is made.

Symptoms of Metabolic X Syndrome

- Fasting Blood Sugar (Glucose); 75 – 85 mg / dL Normal with 110-125 mg /dL a factor in MXS. The HA1C blood test out of range is also a symptom.
- High Triglycerides (Blood Sugar Fats); Normal 150 mg / dL, Abnormal above 200 mg / dL.
- Low HDL Cholesterol – Men below 40 mg /dL, Women below 50 mg /dL.
- High Blood Pressure – 135 / 85 and above.
- Obesity (Apple Shape) – Men greater than a 40 inch waist measurement, Women above a 35 inch waist.

The solution is to follow the GIS Program and kick up your daily exercise. Liver and glandular health is paramount for reversing MXS, weight loss, increasing healthy skin, reversing digestive conditions like Reflux or other digestive disturbances and more. Through perseverance you can reverse these symptoms and attain optimum health sometimes just within a couple of weeks. Follow the Detoxification and Cleansing guidelines along with the GIS Diet. This will allow the liver and the entire endocrine system to rebuild and function better. Review the Addiction section in this chapter as well. Doing the 2 day Gallbladder Flush may also be helpful (Ch. 12) and it is pretty easy for the value it brings.

Thyroid is Two Glands in One

Thyroid mal-functioning affects nearly all people of today. The actual gland is two separate parts referred to as a butterfly gland. The upper portion is the Thyroid and the bottom is called Para-Thyroid. What takes place within the imbalance is either an over-functioning of the gland seen with auto-immune disorders called Hyper-Thyroid (related to GIS) or an under-functioning as in Hypo-Thyroid associated more with poor nutrition and toxicity. Each part of the gland is critical for both the health of the body and the mind. Search out a physician or health professional experienced in Thyroid health if possible. Regardless as to the exact diagnosis (because they can fluctuate back and forth) nutrition is always important for renewal and medical intervention can be lifesaving at times.

When the Thyroid gland does not produce the required hormones the developing symptoms include; mood disorders, a challenge to regulate heat and weight, a variety of metabolic deficiencies, potential dizziness and even coma. Unregulated and high calcium levels in the blood may indicate that the Para-thyroid gland is out of balance. High Calcium due to the over production of Para-Thyroid hormone can bring on confusion, anxiety, depression, muscle and nerve pain and even a progressive walking disability resulting in immobility! With laboratory confirmation of high Calcium in the blood and or urine stop any Calcium supplement yet continue other minerals and supplements. It is also advisable to ask your doctor to run a Para-Thyroid hormone level. Surgery is often the only resort requiring the partial removal of the four glands. Rarely is it due to cancer however the potential is there so it is important to work with an experienced Endocrinologist. Post-surgery has shown remarkable improvement of symptoms in a relatively short period of time.

Adrenal Exhaustion is a Common Factor in Chronic Illnesses

The Adrenal Glands when healthy produce hormones that help to control the blood sugar balance, maintain proper muscle mass, support healthy energy both mentally and physically, increase immunity, reduce inflammatory conditions and allergies in the body. Most physicians do not acknowledge Adrenal Exhaustion as a medical diagnosis regardless of the symptoms. Some of the symptoms are a bit vague and might get mixed up with other conditions of the body including an under-functioning Thyroid gland. Often I have found that when one gland is not working efficiently that they all can require extra health support. The cause of depleting the tiny pair of Adrenal glands that sit on top of each kidney is generally the over use of stimulants, poor nutrition, excessive stress and or a traumatic incidence like a car accident or other tragedy.

Symptoms of Adrenal Exhaustion

- *Exhaustion;* Very tired at night yet unable to fall asleep. You may also wake up feeling tired even after a full night's sleep.
- *Digestive Symptoms;* Cravings for sweet foods alternating with salty foods can be almost an uncontrollable tendency (to give the body a quick pick-up) and the extra salt cravings come because the body requires potassium. Potassium is very nourishing to the Adrenal glands yet the taste buds get confused and try to quench the body's need with salt. Vegetables and fruits are what the body needs to get the potassium and also Vitamin C that nourishes the Adrenals.
- *Blood Pressure;* Running a very low blood pressure and at the same

time feeling cold a lot of the time is indicative of low Adrenal function. Dizziness upon getting up from a laying position is also low Adrenals.

- *Emotional Challenges;* A feeling of being overwhelmed by life is a common denominator.
- *Brain Fog;* The inability to concentrate or to think clearly and or having trouble remembering things that are obvious.

The good news once again is nutrition gives the body the building ingredients to rebuild the Adrenal glands highlighting protein, Vitamin C and Bioflavonoids, Vitamin E, B-Complex, Glandular and Herbal support. Ginseng stress formulas are very supportive to the Adrenal glands in teas and tincture form. When the Adrenal glands rebuild all the symptoms improve with more energy, feeling more optimistic about life, the skin becomes much healthier, sharper thinking and allergies improve too!

Nutrition Highlights: Vitamin E Complex 400 IU (1 – 3 x daily), Vitamin A – fish oil source best 10,000 IU (1 – 3 per day for 2 months), Multiple Vitamin & Mineral for Hypo-Thyroid and other glandular support as needed, B-Complex (and other separate ECN supplements to avoid Calcium with Hyper-Para-Thyroid (Review Chapter 8), Iodine (from seaweeds or liquid), EFA's, Vitamin C 1,000 – 3,000 mg, Aloe Vera and Glandular Supplements; Adrenal, Liver, Thyroid/Para-Thyroid for 3 months alternating and water is very critical to reduce any high Calcium levels down. Note: Surgery is 99% required with high Calcium due to Para-Thyroid and Stress Formula (to support Adrenal health) by *Herb-Pharm*.

13. Mental Health, Stress & Relaxation

Depression and mental health issues have become the number one health challenge of today. Mental illness affects 1 in 4 adults including seniors, teens and a growing percentage of children under the age of 13. Mental illness has barely gotten out of the closet in the past 100 years yet finally the door is opening. A handful of professionals working with mental health have been turning away from the limited and many times trap of the solo focus of prescription drug therapy and incorporating diet and supplements. The importance of the Body-Mind connection in regards to overall health can no longer be ignored (Ch. 5). I encourage each individual whether taking medication or not to begin a health regimen to support their mental wellness. The GIS Program leads the way.

Factors Influencing Mental Illness

- *Poor Nutrition*; Blood sugar, gluten intolerance, toxicity and heredity.
- *Stress;* Financial, working long hours, danger on the job, commuting, trauma, pain, relationships, environment, lack of relaxation & exercise.
- *Social & Peer Pressure*; Ethnic, Monetary and Social Standing prejudices. Longing to belong may lead a person into an addictive lifestyles and bad relationships.
- *Absence of Role Models & Family Support*; Fear of survival, lack of self-esteem, bullying, poor living conditions and trauma.
- *Negative Stinking Thinking*; Lack of Faith & Belief in GOOD, need for positive communication skills, forgiveness of self and others.
- *Bio-Chemical Imbalances of the Gut, Brain and Hormones*; Nutrition, GIS, Toxicity, Drug Use, Heredity, Exercise and a Need for Detoxification and Regular Sunshine Exposure.

The factors that account for the high numbers of people suffering with poor mental health have many subsets. In reviewing the factors that influence mental well-being I think many of you will relate to how each factor can mold and build up or wear down a person's mental attitude and character. Besides learned behavior our choices and actions are influenced by the biochemistry of our bodies. We often use the term chemical imbalance to describe people who act abnormal or in bizarre patterns – with the potential to harm themselves and or others. As the actor Robin Williams stated in a recent interview, "You cannot tell someone else to not be depressed or demand that they act normal. When you are in that frame of mind it is because you cannot escape it!" With chronic depression and psychosis the body's chemical balance must get chemically rebalanced.

Nutrition directly affects a person's chemical balance and can be used therapeutically to improve behavior and well-being regardless if the mood change is coming from a young woman's menses to a crazed Panic or Schizophrenic attack. Temporary and correctly prescribed drug prescriptions may be essential for some people, even life-saving at times. However, it does not authorize a free pass to ignore nutritional support. The fact is "Drugs" do not right the cause of the imbalance and further impact the nutritional stores of the body from use from both pharmaceutical drugs and or recreational type.

Excessive amounts of pharmaceutical drug chemicals must be metabolized and in doing so they have a tendency to run the body's nutritional stores dry. This can bring about more symptoms of poor health in the body. Even taking one drug may increase the body's requirements of the important core nutrients. A good example of this is blood pressure medication. The number one side effect from taking it is depression; therefore kick up your daily intake of B-Complex to compensate for this deficiency and it will greatly help to off-set depression.

Prozac prescribed as an anti-depressant and many other drugs categorized as "Anticholinergic" require super nutrition to compensate for their nutritional needs to metabolize them in the body! Over time this group of drugs can cause the entire Nervous System to under-function according to a Harvard Medical newsletter. The liver can become so overworked with drug use and a poor diet that it may begin to malfunction as discussed in number twelve of this chapter. *Caution:* Read the insert in all medications including any for mental health support because often the side effects can be much worse than the symptoms an individual may be living with.

Often people who suffer with mental health issues get into alcohol, food and drug abuse to medicate their feelings of inadequacy and discomfort. Drug treatment programs to stop abuse are helpful including the "12 Step Programs" but to be more successful individuals need to incorporate the GIS Program to address all the Mental Illness factors and it really works!

Thinking about mental health and chemical imbalances within the body, how many of you have ever considered gluten intolerance to be one of the factors? Move it up to the top of your list as it is discussed in Chapter 5 because GIS is tied closely to mental wellness. Eating gluten and gluten triggers develop symptoms that vary greatly from experiencing melancholy and sadness to Bipolar and Schizophrenic personalities.

Review the foods eaten by people experiencing chronic mental illness and you will often find that it consists of surgery carbohydrates, salted carbohydrate snacks and fried foods with limited quality un-denatured protein. Close to 100% of the time the diet is heavy on the GLUTEN foods that can even be the so called healthy whole grains my friends! The first step to follow is outlined in Chapter 7 suggesting to STOP ALL WHOLE GRAINS including oatmeal. Next make certain to eat 3 regular meals that include quality protein, eggs, meat or special dairy products or other suggestions (Ch. 7) along with vegetables and fruits in the diet daily. Don't dismay you can eat red potatoes and yams as desired on the diet – ha! The GIS Diet is heaven sent for all people to reach their mental and physical health goals!

The Serotonin Hormone Relaxes the Body Naturally

When you begin to connect the puzzle pieces of the Brain-Body connection by taking action in your own life you will learn that one of the most important hormones that helps the body relax is called "Serotonin". As you build healthier biochemistry in your gut through taking a good Probiotics every day and follow the GIS Diet the liver, digestive system and brain gets healthier and will begin to make natural

Serotonin - the feel good relaxant hormone - that so often is missing with chronic depression and other psychosis. To speed the process up a bit you can also add the supplement 5HTP discussed in Chapter 8 along with other brain supplements that are short cuts to brain wellness.

Daily exercise is also important for achieving mental health because it reduces the build-up of stress hormones including Cortisol levels especially doing fast pace aerobic walking, running or other activities. Review Cross-Crawl in Chapter 12 that everyone can do in the privacy of their own home, office or school or out in nature. Yoga stretching and deep breathing also allows the chemicals in the brain and body to find balance.

Monitoring the types of TV and media viewing is helpful as well to provide a more peaceful and fun living space allowing the body to relax. Listening to classical and melodious songs that promote peace in the body have been proven to increase pleasure hormones called Endorphins (as does exercise) and it stimulates amazing healing for every cell in the body. Research has shown that plants grow at an increased rate when classical music is played regularly and the opposite was observed with the electric synchronized music that actually stunted the plants growth!

Always seek healthy counseling or support with drug intervention therapy as needed. People are social creatures and thrive in a loving environment. A quick exercise that can dissipate anxious thoughts is drawing a heart in your mind or on paper and place your name or another person or event inside the heart. You can feel it right – like clouds clearing away allowing for a blue sky - relaxation surrounding the subject returns. Love is always healing – forgive yourself and others. Move towards healthier choices in all aspects of your life combining drug therapy as truly needed with health because people do have choices!

Nutrition Highlights: Aloe Vera, EFA's especially from Fish Oils, Protein, Chromium GTF, Zinc 30 – 50 mg, Calcium/Magnesium, 5HTP, Vitamin A, Vitamin B-Complex, Methyl B12 Sublingual-high dose or methyl B12 Injectable, Vitamin C - 2,000 mg, Protein, St. John's Wort, Kava Kava, Amino Acids – GABA, PS, L-Tyrosine and 5HTP. *Note:* Review Chapter

8 GIS Supplements which includes the brain supplements and only add one or two of these special needs supplement at a time to evaluate how well they complement your health program. An example might be the 5HTP and the GABA. A Multiple Vitamin & Mineral may be substituted for many of the individual vitamins and minerals as explained in Chapter 8 to keep the supplements to just 5 – 6 per day or as tolerated. If choosing only one supplement you may wish to begin with the Probiotics every day towards restoring the gut balance. Next the Aloe Vera and the fish oil may be combined together and in the future any liquids may also be combined into one health drink mix including a protein supplement with a little diluted juice to develop a very workable health regimen to feel your best. Remember that taking 6 – 10 supplements daily can ultimately fast track mental and physical health progress!

14. PH Balance of the Body

All metabolic processes of the body depend on pH balance therefore attaining pH balance in the body is of utmost importance. The body is constantly working to balance its own pH to maintain life and will actually rob minerals from the bone if the diet is deficient in order to succeed which may contribute to Osteoporosis and other deficiency symptoms.

Balancing pH of the body sounds ridiculous to most medical doctors unless they have been trained in complimentary nutritional medicine. When most physicians think about pH they consider their studies which highlight the pH of the blood. The pH of the blood is so critically important that even a slight variance in it for long can result in death. The body works diligently also using the kidneys and the liver to control the pH chemistry of the blood and body tissue without humans being aware of the process.

However, if the pH does go out of balance in the digestive tract it creates a long list of health challenges. The symptoms can be subtle and also more intense and painful including; heartburn, gas, burning in the throat and stomach, fatigue, parasites, fungal infections, bladder and Interstitial Cystitis, skin rashes and sensitivity, headaches, allergies, frequent colds, arthritic and joint pain, finger, bone and muscle pain, irritability, emotional outbursts, ringing in the ears, tired legs, ulcers, eye and vision conditions, hormone imbalance including hot flashes, Osteoporosis, chronic illnesses and even cancer.

PH Facts and Requirements of the Body

- Research reveals pH reactions control many if not all of the cellular functions of the body including the blood metabolism. Each fluid system of the body can be tested for pH to include the blood, urine, muscles and saliva.

- The pH scale ranges from the number 1 – 14 and can register test results of any fluid substance for Acidity or its Basic-Alkaline nature. Looking at the molecular chemistry of foods tells the pH reading from the content of Hydrogen, Oxygen (water H2O) and Minerals.

- On the pH scale the number 7 represents Neutral and below 7 going towards 2 measures Acidity. Above 7 gets more Basic called Alkaline. According to the University of Washington Science Center in Missouri, the healthy pH of human blood is 7.34. Water is an especially important factor in all pH balancing of the body and in turn affects the digestive systems pH as well along with the diet.

- The Kidneys and the Liver work hard to eliminate the high acidity in the body that comes from ingesting too many acid producing foods and beverages with a high consumption of; meat, alcohol, soda, sugar (junk foods) and a heavy grain diet (gluten). Alkaline mineral salts of potassium, calcium, magnesium and sodium bind and neutralize acids. The liver also assists by making LDL cholesterol that helps to bind and eliminate acidity. The kidneys in turn excrete the acid waste together with a functioning colon, lungs, skin and Lymphatic System.

- The pH of the GI tract is critical for optimum health because with pH balance it allows proper digestion and absorption of the foods people eat from the mouth, stomach and small intestine (see chart). Balancing the pH also avoids the over-acidity condition of Reflux and Esophageal Burning conditions.

- Testing the saliva and the urine ½ hour before meals or 2 hours after meals with pH paper is one way to confirm the GI tract status and then a person can work towards achieving a healthy pH. The saliva is fairly balanced if it reads slightly alkaline with a variance in testing of 6.5 pH to 7.5 tested anytime during the day. The urine's best pH goal is to test slightly acidic at 6.0 to 6.5 in the morning and perhaps a little more alkaline in the evening from 6.5 – 7.0 pH. It is far better for the urine to be a little more acidic 2 hours after a meal and the saliva test to show slightly more alkaline.

- Cancer patients that I have worked with have tested opposite on the pH scale having very acidic saliva and very alkaline urine which prevents the body from attaining health balance. Strive to adjust the pH balance of the GI tract through diet, supplements and a healthy lifestyle following the GIS Program.

The design of the body is to balance acidity on its own through the intake of eating a variety of nutrient dense foods from vegetables (including beans and low gluten grains) and fruit as tolerated. From these food groups and food supplements also come the essential core nutrients which the body requires to stay alive and also influence the body's pH. Each food that is eaten contains two pH readings. For an example take an orange. The orange contains its original pH of acidity before eating it. Once the food is digested - a ripe orange creates a more alkaline pH within the body tissue. This alkalinity of the orange affects the pH balance of the entire body; blood, muscles, cellular health and even the GI tract. Supplements will also impact the pH of the body therefor make certain you write an entry in your log or food diary to track when you add a particular supplement and how you feel taking it. If it causes you to feel over-acidic as Vitamin C does occasionally with people reduce the amount or discontinue the product perhaps using a buffered type lower in acidity.

Generally speaking, most protein foods like meat, beans or yogurt create an acidic pH in the body. On the other hand, most fruits and vegetables due to their high mineral content contribute alkalinity. Minerals, if digested properly, give the body the balancing pH along with water which is made from Hydrogen and Oxygen. Carnivores defined as people who eat animal meat, often run short on vegetables and fruits in their diets if they are not making the effort to get a plentiful supply. Conversely vegetarians who rely on beans, nuts and seeds, vegetables and grains may run short on protein or acidifying foods at times. Vegetarians can become too alkaline and be thrown out of pH balance resulting in reduced digestive capabilities, low immunity and other health challenges including auto-immune diseases.

Regardless of what you eat the goal is to strive for a ratio of 20% Acidic foods to 80% Alkaline. Keep in mind quality un-denatured protein is critical for making digestive enzymes for healthy digestion for every person. The 20/80 food ratio is similar to the diets of ancient societies that have survived over thousands of years like the famous Hunza people from the western Himalayas around North Pakistan to the Japanese culture. Both of these societies have produced a higher than average percentage of elders that live healthy lives into their nineties as well as the one hundred year mark eating meat and fish yet adding lots of vegetables coupled with a healthy lifestyle. The types of foods that give pH balance also contain an abundance of vitamins, minerals, phytonutrients like antioxidants, rich fibers and essential fatty acids needed to optimize health and wellness.

Optimum pH of the GI Tract

- Mouth > Alkaline
- Stomach > Acidic
- Small Intestine >Acidic > (then bile flow) Increases Alkalinity
- Large Intestine > Acidic

In Chapter 3 you can review the workings of the digestive tract and how it is supposed to function to retain a healthy pH balance. Unfortunately, situations do arise from infants to seniors that may throw the digestive process out of pH balance. What I have noticed that proceeds true Reflux or over-acidity includes; a person eating a poor (GIS) or mediocre diet, excessive stress and or a traumatic event like a car accident or having a virulent strain of the flu or infection (requiring multiple drugs including anti-biotics). Each of these factors can be a catalyst that consumes stored vital nutrients and shifts a person out of pH balance through over-whelming the kidneys and liver into higher than healthy levels of acidity. Some people are also born with a genetic impairment or birth defect that requires special needs as with Autism. Infants many times come into the world with a low functioning digestive system causing over-acidity, acute gastritis and bowel upset. They may even be more advanced lactose and gluten sensitive at birth requiring more help to balance the pH and optimize digestive juices. Review Chapter 9 Healthy Children for more explanations surrounding building a healthy child.

Toddlers, children, teens and many adults are often very picky about their food choices and sometimes evolve into limited mono-diets. The reduction in nutritional intake into the body (especially not eating enough vegetables) affects healthy pH leaving people vulnerable to more illnesses. Scientists have confirmed that as we age (due to many factors) the digestive juices have a tendency to slow down as well especially the production of Hydrochloric Acid (HCL). Adults and seniors must continue to support the body's health with nutrition if they are to increase the proper HCL and digestive juices required to utilize the food in the diet especially the mineral content in regards to pH and experience healthy aging. When the HCL levels are low in the stomach minerals and protein are not digested properly and health begins to decline.

What throws the pH out of balance? One factor that has only been slightly mentioned is the high pharmaceutical drug use by adults. Drugs disrupt the body's ability to properly digest and absorb food partially due to its increased requirement of the B-Complex. The B's are required to actually process the drug chemicals. Also, when the liver is overwhelmed with multiple drugs and obesity as discussed in the Liver, Organs & Glandular section it slows down the production of both bile and essential Low Density Lipid Cholesterol production. Bile is required to digest fats in the diet yet it also adjusts pH in the small intestine to be more alkaline. Cholesterol also binds to the acid wastes and assists in the removing of excess acid out of the body through the bowels.

Water is more important at regulating pH than given credit. The body when fully hydrated is 75% water and it is essential to maintain pH balance. Water most often has a neutral pH due to the two parts of Hydrogen and one part Oxygen – H2O. The Hydrogen and Oxygen matrix according to Dr. Robert Young, PhD, is the key factor in pH balance and it is the "Provider and the Protector of life" giving stability through all of its ability. Dr. Young's book, *The pH Miracle – Balance Your Diet, Reclaim Your Health* goes into detail of how eating the correct foods and supplements allow health to reverse disease.

Applying the GIS program and broadening the healthy dietary choices will give the emphasis of the alkalinizing nutrients (found in vegetables and supplements) for balancing the pH. Lowering meat and fish intake while increasing soups, stews and salads with a variety of vegetables including parsley, cilantro, cucumber, broccoli, asparagus, other greens, seaweeds and a rainbow of low starch vegetables all help because they are loaded with the alkalinizing minerals. Papaya and Mango fruit with a small amount of Ripe Banana and Organic Apples are also very alkalinizing. Adding a squeeze of Lemon or lime may further support the proper pH balancing unless inflammation in the GI tract as with Reflux is causing burning. Sipping on a little diluted Aloe Vera before meals (quantity as tolerated) may be extremely balancing to pH. It is not an accident that so many people living with cancer and other chronic illnesses do not have properly balanced pH of the GI tract. Review Candida, Reflux, Detoxification, Immunity and Exercise. Also, review the Liver & Gallbladder 2-Day Flush in Chapter

12 which is a short cut to be able to eat fats without so much heart burn and more.

Nutrition Highlights: Aloe Vera, Filtered Water 6 – 8 glasses (with added Trace Mineral drops), Minerals, B-Complex, Vitamin E Complex, Daily Greens, Chlorophyll, FiberMate by *Aloe Life*, Cucumbers, Parsley and Cilantro, Vegetables, Bentonite Clay (liquid), Probiotics, EFA's, Trace Minerals, Bee Pollen, Digestive Enzymes (as needed temporarily) Diluted Organic Apple Juice and other Vegetable Juices.

15. Physical, Mental & Spiritual Health Balance

In creating a healthier and happier life we can reflect on how a baby comes into the world with a relatively clean slate. All of the knowledge that a baby begins to learn about people, places and things are recorded into their remarkable computer like brains from day one. The good experiences are recorded right along with the hurtful and unfortunate ones and together all of life's experiences help to mold the person each of us become.

Our moral code of ethics and selection skills are guided and stimulated by our parental and peer role models coupled with our environment and our daily life experiences. This may sound like the entirety of what produces behavior that helps or hinders our lives yet there are a few more very important factors to include. These other factors contribute just as much if not more to who we become if not the foundation itself. These other factors include; dietary influence, mental stamina and fortitude along with spiritual substance and integrity. Our overall persona and how we live our lives from our beginnings are three fold; Body, Mind & Spiritual.

Body: The health of our physical body directly regulates our emotional well-being. When an infant receives the prenatal nutrition it requires as covered in Chapter 9 their sleep is sound and waking hours are more peaceful and enjoyable for both child and parent. As a child grows this emotional stability is an anchoring force that allows more effective learning during life and proper bonding to family members because of the focus a healthy body provides. Emotional health is dependent on good solid physical health at every age.

Physical health provides a growing child, teen and adult the opportunity to participate in life on every level; scholastic, athletic and creative endeavors for work and play. Many broken dreams and opportunities are missed as a result of an unhealthy body, addictions and disease.

Gluten and GIS may put a temporary roadblock in one's life yet when the roadblocks are removed once and for all the rebuilding of health to a higher level is totally possible. Allow the body to become the healthiest it can be and it will support a healthy mind and spiritual fulfillment as well!

Mind: Mental stamina and fortitude in life comes from one's ability to keep getting up even when you may fall down in life's emotional storms. The ability and success to develop this mode of action in life is fed from a desire to survive and awareness that actions give results. Friends, family and co-workers can help in this character development yet sometimes it is a very lonely road that leads us to succeed as we grab hold of every morsel of positivism along the way. Develop the "Can-Do Spirit!"

Spiritual Balance: It is my belief that faith and grace (being blessed when we do not deserve it) pulls us along and directs us as we each travel our spiritual path. Our spiritual longing of connection, love and understanding is one that is parallel to our physical life. As we seek the truth through developing our perfection of faith about our real spiritual self - it in turn strengthens belief in our goals giving us purpose while we are in the physical world. This realization allows us to let go of worry in the work we do and enjoy the people and experiences during our lives – Enjoy!

Both the mental self and the spiritual self are supported by a healthy physical body. In turn the body is uplifted to a higher level of optimum health and understanding of the Divine Design and Oneness with our Creator. This is truly why in seeking the highest optimum health and happiness in this life one must look towards all three areas for balance; Physical, Mental and Spiritual health. I encourage YOU to strive for balance and happiness will replace fear and worry - as we journey through life – and Breath!

16. Sleeping; Rest, Renewal & Detoxification

Healthy hormones are essential for healthy sleep. Besides detoxification, sleep is a time to rebuild the body and rest the mind. Interestingly the body is still at work on a very low level while asleep and because of this it continues to burn calories during sleep. The Circadian Rhythm and Healthy Hormones both dictate as to how sound of sleep a person gets during the night along with some other factors. Research reveals that too little sleep or the opposite with one sleeping too much during the day, either one, can take a toll on a healthy immune system and the overall feeling of wellness. Seven to eight hours of sleep is the average amount of sleep that most people require for health. Through detoxification of the liver and eating the GIS diet you will find better sleep awaits you in the future. The liver has a lot to do with proper hormone production of Serotonin and Melatonin function involved in reaching a deep sleep state. New research is also showing the gut and selective tissues throughout the body can manufacture Serotonin along with the brain keeping the body more relaxed 24/7 with renewal of the digestive tract taking Probiotics. Sufficient minerals and protein are also both needed in the daily diet to allow the body to make more of the Protein Compounds required in the brain such as GABA (see Ch. 8) that along with minerals allow people to relax and get sound sleep.

Certain environmental rituals, supplements, dietary and lifestyle choices like getting exercise during the day helps the body retire from the daylight hours more easily. It is interesting to find out how many people are not sleeping well yet are breaking many of the more common sense rituals or have not made the connection to important factors that will allow the necessary and rejuvenating sleep. I encourage you to experiment with covering the basics and judge for yourself how much easier it is getting some sleep!

Cover the Basics for Sleep

- Turn off lights in the house or bedroom at bedtime with only a small nightlight or flashlight as desired.
- Keep any stimulants from green tea, sodas, caffeine and or chocolate intake low during the day and do not consume them at all in the evening.
- Unwind with 30 minutes of exercise during the day at least and sometimes more for children and adults.
- Watch T.V. a Movie or the News earlier in the evening because of the potential for hearing about unpleasant events (that you have no control over that may be upsetting) or perhaps stimulate too much Adrenaline flow that wakes up the body from an exciting mystery.
- Writing in a daily log helps sort out life's challenges and clear the mind from unpleasant thoughts and pressure that sometimes replay as we turn out the lights.
- Take a warm shower or relaxing bath.
- Drink a cup of herb tea like Chamomile with honey before bed.
- Taking a supplement of Calcium, Magnesium and Zinc before bed is calming.
- Control blood sugar so you do not wake in the night hungry. Review Blood Sugar section.
- Prayer and meditation before bed is comforting and motivational.
- Foot massage that we give to ourselves can feel very good. Sweet dreams!

Nutritional Highlights: Protein, Calcium, Magnesium and Zinc (taken before bed), Melatonin and or 5HTP, Prevagen (daytime for adults), Herbs - Chamomile Tea, Catnip, Hops, St. John's, Valerian, Lavender

Bach Remedy (very soothing for relaxation anytime) and Mineral Cell Salts or Chamomile products (for infants, children and or adults).

17. Stimulants; Caffeine, Hot & Spicy Foods

A closer look into the world of stimulants reveals significant positive effects on the body both mentally and physically along with the opposite potential of depleting the body if used in excess. Caffeine and like substances found in herbs and foods including the coffee bean and the tea plant have been used since the beginning of civilizations.

The cocoa bean, which chocolate products are made from, contains a low percentage of caffeine and its use dates back to the 7th century Mayan civilization. In a 40 gram piece of chocolate (a 2 inch square) on average it contains 20 mg of caffeine or about 1/3 the amount of caffeine found in a medium cup of coffee. Coffee and tea is grown in many locations around the globe and is enjoyed by a variety of cultures on every continent. Most if not all of these stimulants also come with added health benefits of Phyto-nutrients and Antioxidants that enhance the body's health.

Spicy foods can have a more subtle stimulating energetic effect on the body and some like chilies can even support the improvement of one's circulation, digestion and healing capacity. It appears that each continent and population has become fond of different ways to enhance the effectiveness and enjoyment in their daily lives with stimulants and or spicy foods. To optimize our health on the GIS program an important guideline is to only use the amount of a stimulant or spice that adds joy or quality to life without creating any negative side effects!

Healthy Guidelines for Using Stimulants & Eating Spicy Foods

- Caffeine from Coffee, Tea or Chocolate and herbs can uplift one's Mood, Energy and through increasing the basal metabolism rate even support healthier Weight Loss.
- Always Lower Caffeine use from all sources if you experience Loose Stool or Nervousness and experiment with herbal teas or other beverages as desired.

- Chocolate contains added extra nutrients of high Oxygen Radical Absorbency Capacity (ORAC), Antioxidants of varying amounts (dark chocolate the highest) and Coffee also contains Antioxidants. Conversely Chocolate contains Anti-Nutrients (Review Ch. 6 Toxins) and also has high levels of Arginine (an amino acid) that can stimulate viral outbreaks (See Ch. 6 Viruses) and may actually contain higher Toxicity content of Lead than other candies and or foods.

- Black, Green, White or Herbal Tea is Best Tolerated (better than coffee) for GIS Zone 1, 2 and 3 and tea contains high Antioxidant value. Research shows it is best to not drink volumes of black tea at mealtimes because it lowers the absorption of Iron from the foods being eaten at the same time. Herbal teas would not have the same conflict with Iron.

- Hot & Spicy Foods Increase Circulation in the body but also increase Inflammation of skin conditions. Use with caution (including salsa) because this category is a GIS Trigger.

When people are experiencing advanced GIS symptoms in Zone 2 and in Zone 3 drinking tea seems to be a much better choice than coffee. Black, green and even the white tea varieties can give a varied selection. Coffee, as much as I enjoy this brew, it is from a bean. Therefore coffee tends to bring on more symptoms than drinking black or green tea with certain people putting them into a higher inflammatory cycle. All stimulants may also cause increased diarrhea so heed these suggestions and reduce the daily amount with loose stool.

Stimulants also act as a diarrheic and cause the loss of nutrition through frequent urination. This includes the loss of vitamins, minerals and proteins. As mentioned in reviewing the topic of Adrenal Exhaustion in the twelfth section excessive use of stimulants can lead to damaging the glandular health of the body resulting in grave circumstances. One to two portions daily of a stimulant seems to be a fairly acceptable range yet it always depends upon your body size and how you feel ultimately. Ask yourself how do you feel each day with your choices? If you feel nervous or anxious or find yourself in the bathroom excessively reduce the amount of caffeine or energy drinks you are consuming. Herbal teas are surprisingly satisfying and the many choices of flavors and combinations to experiment with for pleasure and even medicinal value are unlimited. I keep a half a dozen on hand so if I desire a warm beverage I can have a non-caffeinated choice. The herbs contain many different medicinal properties from Licorice that gives some extra energetic glandular support to Chamomile that is very relaxing!

My words of advice to the "Purist" and I use that expression with fondness because I have been one is, "Lighten up!" If a cup of coffee gives someone pleasure or eating a piece of chocolate, so be it. When choosing special treats and beverages search out quality in your choices and enjoy the indulgence. Even if that means to have an occasional French fry fling! Be prepared that it might bring on a bit of a surge to blood sugar from the deep frying oils – no big deal unless it triggers your addiction to fast foods. Oil and sugars are both a type of stimulant as reviewed in the blood sugar sections. Regrettably if junk foods are eaten in excess they can be very detrimental to one's health starting with blood sugar, blood pressure, weight gain and digestive symptoms. I indulge very rarely in fried foods or desserts because I enjoy living healthy and reaping the benefits. Review the recipe section to find tasty healthy choices for making home fries and desserts that you can enjoy 100% guilt free!

Hot and spicy foods do increase circulation in the body yet unfortunately they may also bring on inflammation for some folks not desired. Tomatoes in themselves can be extremely acidic and cause the pH to become overly acidic for many people. The positive side to hot peppers and ground black pepper is that they add delicious seasoning to foods and good health effects in the right amount. Herbalists have recorded many good therapeutic effects of these spices on the body from help with digestion and even the resolutions of stomach ulcers if used in small amounts. Their stimulation to the body's circulation may also help keep the Cardiovascular System a bit healthier and they certainly bring about warmth on a cold day.

However, caution is required especially for people in Zone 3 and also people living with Herpes Simplex Virus I or II. Review the Virus section. You may be able to use a small amount in certain dishes and condiments yet if you are living with advanced IBD or any major inflammatory auto-immune disease or condition like Rosacea, Psoriasis, Diabetes or Lupus keep the spices down until you are on the GIS diet for approximately 6 months or longer. The body does renew itself and once the liver begins to detoxify and the pH rebalances many people reverse skin conditions and can broaden their food choices once again. Making healthier choices can feel awkward at first yet the more we make the better decisions of what we eat and drink and begin to reap the rewards of feeling better it gets a lot easier – Cheers!

18. Sunshine, Fresh Air, Water & Exercise

People were made to spend their wakeful hours out-of-doors. Perhaps surprising to some, the sun's rays are important and have therapeutic affects on the body. It is almost easier to grasp the importance of breathing fresh air for oxygen, drinking water for hydration and the value of exercise than getting daily sunshine these days.

Growing Children & Adults Require the Basics
- Sunshine
- Fresh Air
- Clean Water
- Exercise

Sunshine, fresh air, water and exercise are each important for health and we must incorporate these health practices into our schedules targeting them on a regular basis. The facts are that with our busy modern world and some extenuating circumstances, people often spend very little time out of their homes, work and or vacation spots. The body rebels with bone loss, failing health, obesity and depression.

Sunshine: Regardless of a person's lifestyle the body requires sunshine for valuable health support including; promoting healthy Vitamin D3 development in the skin and other hormonal stimulation. D3 is a catalyst involved in mineral absorption, stimulating hormone production that influences our energy, immune function and even our mental attitude. To reach optimal health each infant, child and adult requires the health promoting rays of the sun at least 20 - 30 minutes daily.

Who hasn't walked into the sunlight and given a sigh of relief. The sun is life giving and people, just like in the plant kingdom, die without proper sunshine. Full spectrum lighting can be purchased during seasons that do not provide adequate sunshine. Fish oils that include Vitamin A and D (D3) along with the important Omega-3's are very helpful during the winter months or unnatural cave dwelling - ha! Death due to a lack of sunshine may not be diagnosed as such yet a weak and failing immune system and a crumbling skeletal structure with Osteoporosis is directly related to a lack of the suns rays. Just 30 minutes of sunshine can create up to 10,000 or more units of Vitamin D3 in our own bodies. Harvard Medical University recently stated that the Vitamin D deficiency, that is being diagnosed in young children through to seniors, is a "Pandemic Situation" and people must start getting more sunshine along with taking supplements of Vitamin D3! The sunshine Vitamin D3 is made in our skin from cholesterol and it helps the absorption of calcium and other minerals vital for keeping the immune system strong, bone health vital and is also essential to our mental well-being.

Seasonal Affected Disorder (SAD) which causes depression in many people during the winter months can be greatly decreased and even avoided with cod liver oil (fish oil) and perhaps part of this remedy is the proper levels of Vitamin D3 called Cholecalciferol. We need sunshine to be healthy so rethink how you can get at least 30 minutes of sunshine per day and or purchase a few full spectrum lights for your home!

Fresh Air: Learning the basics of health is not only giving the body the correct nutrition health demands but we also must meet the body's physical needs for fresh air. The blessed "Oxygen" cannot be taken for granted. Open up the windows and bring plants into your home because it is the plants that make the life promoting Oxygen humans and mammals alike are designed to breathe. Also, keeping plants around the outside of a home, business or apartment whenever possible will contribute to the life promoting valuable oxygen supply. Holding ones breath is a bad habit for many people. With proper nutrition fueling the Autonomic Nervous System which controls the breath, making a conscientious reminder to your body to breathe - in the nose and out the mouth regularly - will optimize your health.

A side benefit of proper oxygenation is the extra protection against an overgrowth of bad bacteria and viruses. That's absolutely correct that many potential enemies of the flesh, even cancer microbes, cannot survive in the body with proper oxygenation. Also, keep your refined sugar intake down for all the reasons including the fact that an excess of sugar will cheat the body of valuable oxygen. So give yourself the extra boost to the trillions of body cells that make up the body while even helping out your immune system and breathe!

Water: The body is approximately 65-75% water by content when fully hydrated. This underlines the great importance water plays in optimizing the health of your body. Water makes up a large percentage of the blood, hormones, muscles and skin mass and without a sufficient supply the entire metabolic process of the body falls short. In other words, fatigue, overeating, blood sugar abnormalities, constipation, low functioning immune system, increased inflammation and pain, headaches, increased allergies and other chronic illnesses symptoms will all increase if the body is dehydrated. The daily suggested intake is half your body weight in ounces per day to at least get in six 8 oz. glasses. The Mayo Clinic suggests that adult women drink at least two quarts per day and men three quarts minimum! Water of any quantity is best to drink in between your meals. It is essential for good digestion but it is NOT good to drink in any quantity or especially iced beverages during mealtimes. STOP ICE WATER AT MEALTIMES! Warm beverages do not interfere as much with digestive enzymes and hormone functions as does drinking iced drinks. If you must have iced drinks enjoy them without food on an empty stomach!

Exercise: We hear repeatedly about the importance of exercising from an early age right on through to the senior years. Moving the body with exercise is honoring the divine design of how the body was constructed. The legs are pumps for the Circulatory System. The faster the legs go it supports the heart to pump faster which circulates the blood up to the brain and extremities more effectively. The very important Lymph System depends upon daily exercise to keep the immunity and detoxification of the body at its peak. It is also involved in filtration of impurities and recycling the old blood cells out which allows the body to rejuvenate itself. Our entire body depends on daily exercise to allow the glands of the body to control the blood sugar as with Diabetes, process fat in our body for Weight Loss and Maintenance, keeps our liver healthy and allows cellular waste to be cleansed called Detoxification. Good liver health is needed to have healthy Biorhythms throughout life including Menopause for women and Andropause for men. Sustained exercise also decreases the build-up of high damaging levels of the stress hormones called Cortisol and Adrenalin another name for Epinephrine (a hormone neurotransmitter). Exercise also encourages the flow of the feel good pleasure hormones called Endorphins. Besides balancing our hormones exercise helps in "Toning our Muscles" to maintain a healthy muscular frame important as a biomarker for longevity. Exercising anywhere is terrific yet out-of-doors can be a daily adventure. It is also best to exercise before a meal to not slow down the digestive process. A leisurely stroll is not a challenge so keep in mind that a slow walk does not count as "Aerobic" exercise. My favorite side benefits of exercising out-of-doors when the weather allows is spending time in nature and intermingling with other people.

Aerobic Exercise Goals

- 35 minutes; 5 – 7 days per week or 60 minutes 3 times per week.
- Resting Pulse or Beats Per Minute (BPM); Average for Men 70 and Women 75.
- Heart Rate Goal: Maximum Aerobic Increase 85% or 155 - 160 BPM*.
- Combine Aerobic Exercise with; Weight Lifting, Isometrics, Stretching, Yoga & other Balancing exercises.
- *Caution:* Check with your physician before beginning a strenuous Aerobic workout.

Whether in a class situation, at home, a gymnasium, walking in a neighborhood or park getting regular exercise is critical to reaching your health goals. 35 minutes at least 5 times per week is an excellent amount of time or doubling up for 60 minutes 3 times per week.

Setting individual endurance goals for yourself is a great way to increase and master your cardiovascular requirements. Weight bearing exercise routines will get you in shape and keep you more physically fit, into your golden years. Even working out with light weights can be very beneficial. Incorporating some stretching into your routine will also keep more flexibility in your body and allow you to reduce arthritic pain in your joints as they may tend to become rigid with age. Diet of course also has a lot to do with maintaining flexibility as well. Discover an exercise that gets your heartbeat up and perspiring if possible to include; Dancing, Brisk Walking, Running, Playing a Group Sport, Sailing, Hiking, Gardening, Aerobic Routine, Lifting Weights, Yoga, Stretching and more. Swimming is a terrific aerobic exercise great for toning and bone density however for some people they just do not lose as much weight as when walking or running so you can mix it up. To have fun while you exercise is a great added bonus. As the late exercise Guru, Jack Lalanne put it, "I hate exercising that is why I get up at 4:30 am in the morning to get it out of the way?" Exercise is all about taking responsibility for your own health – Move it or you lose it!

19. Viruses; Herpes Simplex, Shingles and the Like

Thousands of viruses come into our living environment and some enter the body even without our conscious knowledge including; cold viruses, Influenza, Shingles and the Herpes Virus so common with GIS. The Herpes Simplex Virus Type I – HVSI causes cold sores on the lip and on the inside of the cheeks and other symptoms from the waste-up. The Herpes Simplex Virus Type II – HSVII is responsible for genital herpes and flare-ups from the waste-down. Both types respond very well to following the same GIS health program and are considered Secondary Triggers in the Gluten Inflammatory Syndrome (GIS).

Learning About the Viral Profile

All viruses are anaerobic or in other words they thrive without oxygen. Exercising to increase the body's oxygen level is a great preventative measure to keep viral activity lower in the body regardless of the particular virus of concern. You may have noticed that when people are fearful or stressed it is common to hold ones breath. So it takes retraining yourself to breathe frequently. Remind yourself to do deep breathing throughout the day especially during a pensive situation. Before long with practice breathing becomes much more automatic.

Nutrition also supports oxygenation by increasing high Magnesium rich foods and Vitamin C. Chapters 5, 7 and 8 review all co-factors required in oxygenation including the sections on Anemia. The Immune System is built from eating a nutrient dense diet as found in the GIS Program from adequate protein and core nutrients that combat microbial attack and keep viruses in a more dormant state.

The reported cases of HSV total approximately 20% of the population yet I find it much more common than anyone would like to think. HSV is highly contagious and before an actual ulcer blister appears there are cells on the surface area that can spread to other parts of our body or to other people. I will state in a question for the record, "Who doesn't carry the HSV virus?" I speculate the number of carriers of HSV to be more like 90% of the population. Young children can easily become infected through sharing food, drink and through all the affection within families and friends.

Both strains of the HSV virus type I and II can be stimulated into activity by many of the same factors to include; abrasion, temperature, a cold virus and Illness, nutritional imbalances and overall increased inflammation as in GIS. Once you learn that you can carry the HSV1 cold sore virus and not remember ever having had an eruption on your lip, your inner cheek skin or elsewhere - then perhaps you will give it a pause of consideration. I have found that most people actually do carry the dormant/semi-dormant virus that lives on the nerve cell pathways. If the conditions are right, up comes a painful lesion sore or other symptoms like a headache or sudden fatigue even without a tell-tale warning ulcer blister at all.

So what does being positive to the HSVI or II mean? The important lesson for people to learn especially if they are dealing with an advanced stage of inflammation with Herpes is to understand the link to other inflammation in the body. Herpes can be stimulated by inflammation from eating gluten or a combination of other triggers. The activated HSV can set off more inflammation and sensitivity within the Nervous System causing any or all symptoms including; headaches, fatigue, diarrhea, low blood sugar and even heightening more of the Gluten Inflammatory Syndrome effecting digestion.

Factors Influencing HSVI & HSVII Flare-Ups:
- Stress & Abrasion
- Deficiency of A, C, E & Zinc and other core nutrients.
- Colds & Illness
- Extreme Temperature Change
- pH Imbalance & Gluten Triggers
- High Arginine Foods (See List) and or Supplements (High Vitamin C is not good at times because of its acidity pH.)

Shingles is a Common Ailment with Seniors

Shingles is another virus that affects the quality of life and inflammation for thousands of people daily. The senior population is troubled most often because of a weakened Immune System allowing the Shingles to erupt. Shingles has the formal name of Herpes Zoster. It is a painful skin rash caused by the varicella zoster virus VZV. It is not related to the HSV (Herpes) but to the virus that causes Chicken Pox.

After a person has Chicken Pox the virus stays in the body as other viruses do in a dormant state. If trauma occurs or a drop in the Immune System from heavy stress, poor nutrition, a car accident, excessive drug dosing during a bout of flu or cancer it may appear. Shingles looks like a rash of blisters that scabs after 3 – 5 days. One in five people continue experiencing pain in the area that may persist even after the rash clears up. Shingles may further lead to other severe infections if health is not supported. The chronic Shingles complications may include; pneumonia, hearing problems, blindness, brain inflammation and even death. All viral conditions, as in Shingles, respond favorably to the GIS Program regardless of a person's age.

Viruses Regress with a Functioning Immune System and Key Supplements

The goal in health is to keep the viral load of the body as low as possible to protect the spread of any virus. To keep viruses in dormancy we must keep inflammation as low as possible from all sources in the body and the Immune System strong. Scientists have faulted the HSV to be a culprit in increased plaque build-up in the brain and may also add to other disease states including Mental Illness (see Chapter 5) as well. Taking preventative steps with HSV will give protection to all of the body's systems from further attack from any microbial and decrease the potential of HSV from spreading throughout the body. Following the GIS Diet and Program builds a stronger Immune System and allows the individual to feel healthier while living with any viral condition.

Supplements are helpful to reduce the viral load thereby reducing the symptoms greatly. To begin with eat more foods on the Higher

L-Lysine list and less of the L-Arginine foods. Research suggests the adult dose of L-Lysine when carrying the HSV to be approximately 1,000 – 3,000 mg daily with 8,000 mg being the upper limit. You may find that less is actually required when you take a couple of the other anti-viral supplements along with it. Good varied protein intake is essential along with vegetables and some fruits that contain the core nutrients for proper immunity and continue to always strive towards healthy digestion.

Nutrition Highlights: Protein 60-100 grams daily (variety), Aloe Vera (juice or tablet), L-Lysine and B12 sublingual, Red Marine Algae, Daily Greens, Liquid Hydrosol Silver (45 days, 5 tsp. daily), Monolaurine (3 months), Olive Leaf, Probiotics and N-Acetyl-Cysteine (NAC).

HSV Requires More L-Lysine and Less L-Arginine in the Diet

Higher in L-Lysine (eat as tolerated)
Lean Meats – fish, turkey, chicken.
Vegetables – All (eat less tomatoes).
Fruits – All (eat less citrus).
Dairy Products – All as tolerated.
Grains & Beans – Low gluten grains and beans as tolerated.

Higher in L-Arginine (eat sparingly)
Nuts & Seeds - Seeds are found in all foods yet more in Figs or
    Flaxseed so use with caution.
Coconut & Peanut Butter
Popcorn & High Corn
Wholegrains (including low gluten)
Garlic & Onions
Hot Spices & Salsa
Chocolate
Ice Cream (carrageenan thickener is a big trigger to HSV)
Beef (only once per week if desired)
Grapes

Berries

Avoid High Arginine Eggs

Avoid Supplements of Arginine

20. Finding Your Healthy Weight; Weight Loss & Weight Gain

Weight is influenced primarily by three factors; the calories we eat, the exercise expended in a day and very importantly how the body's metabolism functions including a person's "Gut Health". Making sure the Thyroid and other glands are working well (the best possible) provides a pivotal difference of how easy you gain or lose weight as well. Body temperature is an important gauge for checking the Thyroid Balance. The normal temperature goal to strive for is 98.6 under the tongue. Remember, improvement in health is the goal not necessarily perfection. It can take a person years to attain the 98.6 mark that will vary to a small amount normally throughout the month.

Factors for Attaining a Healthy Weight

- Calories
- Exercise
- Metabolism

As significant as each of these key factors are in gaining, losing and maintaining a healthy weight there is still one more critical factor. Can you guess what it is? If you said the MIND you are right!

Regardless of whether you are one of the 24 million Americans living with an eating disorder, a person having a difficult time keeping weight on due to an illness or unknown cause or one of the millions of adults and children finding themselves in obesity – attaining a HEALTHY WEIGHT takes a conscious mental decision. You must - DECIDE - to change your body for the better.

Review the contact information in the Reference section for the National Eating Disorders Organization or contact a local group for support as you desire. Once you have made the decision to improve your health and begin to strive towards a healthier weight many different support channels are available as needed. I suggest that you take the stops out and follow through to locate a good program or even a specific book to give you the success you are after. Support groups are available through the community schools, YMCA, medical health centers, church groups and even the 12 Step Programs. They can all give emotional support and review the healthy steps essential to reaching your success. A great teacher and author is Kat James because she herself struggled with weight loss for years that almost took her life. She is available through the website at www. informedbeauty.com. She dropped ten dress sizes but more importantly she reversed multiple diseases. Her teaching through transformational classes reveal the importance of getting the gut in the body healthy first through supplements and diet even before exercising begins. This unique weight loss focus enlightens the critical significance of balancing the body's biochemistry in the brain and the body that in turn allows a person to reach their weight goal with a lot less effort!

DECIDE – COMMIT – SUCEED!

The good news is once you begin to take action towards your health goal – COMMIT - and experience some success - it does get easier. You will not have to agonize in the same way as in the beginning when you first start to break routines, eat differently and exercise. Review Addictions in this Healthy Focus Factor chapter that talks about the fact that it can take 30 – 40 days to begin new habits and leave others behind that no longer serve us. It is OK so please give yourself permission to take care of your health needs as we often do for others yet not ourselves. You deserve it and I declare that GOD wants all of us well!

Learning new healthy self-talk is so critical to becoming a healthier person in body and mind - especially if you have experienced overcritical people in your life. You can write your own mission statement to help during this process and books are also available such as, *Self Parenting: The Complete Guide to Your Inner Conversations - Nurturing the (Inner Child)* by Pollard and *Love Is Letting Go of Fear* by Jampolsky one of my favorite books of all time.

My personal affirmation that I wrote at least ten times per day when I began making improvements in my life goes like this; "I am a RADIANT BEING Filled with LOVE and LIGHT". You are welcome to use this positive affirmation until you create one that resonates with your needs perhaps even better. Claim health for yourself and family. Be a VICTOR and not a VICTIM!

There is always work involved to reach any goal and discipline and a biological resetting of our body's biorhythms that must take place over a period of time – be patient. The taste buds re-educate themselves to enjoy natural flavors of fruits, vegetables and home cooking. Exercise can begin to call out to us when we miss a day because the body feels better getting the stress hormones reduced through a fast walk or work-out. You can also start feeling the pleasure hormones called Endorphins as they release into our blood stream however you gotta kick it up by increasing your aerobic workout to a faster time of at least 35 – 45 minutes as outlined in section eighteen!

You can begin to enjoy a new way of life eating to live with tasty foods (see the recipe section) and moving it from the top of the head to your toes and everything in-between. The frosting on the cake, sugar free and gluten free of course, is living this new life can truly get you out of depression and promote anti-aging with more vibrant youthful skin. That's right - your body, through following the GIS Program can actually reverse disease and grow younger in all of your biological markers! Pretty good perks if you ask me!

Weight Loss & Maintenance

Two out of three adults in America today are either overweight or obese according to the US Dept of Human Services, CDC, 2009. Fortunately the increase in adult weight appears to be slowing slightly with only a 1% gain from the last reporting period. Even though national attention has been focused on the importance for citizens to lose their unhealthy weight - not a single state was able to meet the 2010 Healthy People Target of dropping 15% of their weight.

Results from the 2007-2008 National Health and Nutrition Examination Survey (NHANES), using measured heights and weights, estimated 17% of children and adolescents ages 2-19 are obese. Obesity is defined as being significantly over a person's heaviest weight by 100 pounds. The measurement standard for the US has become the Body Mass Index (BMI) which is figured on the following formula and scale for interpreting; Underweight, Normal, Overweight or Obese.

BMI	Weight Status	BMI Calculation
Below 18.5	Underweight	[Weight (in pounds/divided by height (in inches) squared]
18.5 – 24.9	Normal	Times by 703 gives the BMI
25.0 – 29.9	Overweight	BMI 28.12 = 180 lbs. divided by (67 inches x 67 = 4489)
30.0 & Higher	Obese	(Example) 180 / 4489 = 0.04 x 703 give 28.12 BMI (shows math)

Symptoms Associated with Obesity+

- Difficulty Sleeping; Snoring, Sleep Apnea and more.
- Excessive Sweating; Feeling Hot Frequently.
- Pain in the Joints and throughout the body.
- Fatigue; Feeling Out of Breath with even Minor Exertion.
- Skin Rashes, Infections in Skin Folds and more.
- Depression; Mental Fatigue and Past Trauma Solace.

+ Mayo Clinic Symptoms

There are many other symptoms associated with obesity including more digestive issues and a greater health risk during any surgical procedure due to inadequate blood flow from impaired circulation. Circulation is one of the most important functions to maintain for a healthy body. It is essential to receive the needed nutrition into the cells and eliminate the waste products properly. Most often overweight and obese people eat too many calories and do not expend enough exercise which allows the pounds to creep up. However, as in MXS once the weight is to a certain level a person may become temporarily trapped in obesity until they address the biochemistry of their body. See Chapter 6 Addictions, Candida, Liver and Glandular Health and Detoxification.

"Normal Weight - Obesity"

A condition often develops when people are not eating properly called "Normal Weight - Obesity. I see this often with people who are not over-sized yet they obviously have a very low muscle mass to fat ratio. How the Mayo Clinic describes this imbalance of fat in the body is when a woman has more than 30% body fat and men with more than 20%. To measure body fat percentage, it takes a piece of equipment called a Bioimpedance. The device uses an electrical current to register the body composition. By measuring the rate at which the electricity moves through the body the machine can calculate your body fat percentage. Experts recommend the optimum body fat percentage for men to be 3 – 5% and women 8 – 12%. If you find that your body fat is high the next important step is to sincerely improve your dietary and lifestyle choices through following the GIS program. As you apply your program your body will become more efficient at fat burning for energy and you will also notice your body composition will change in texture (not spongy soft) and the return of muscle definition. Each of the support supplements help especially the Fish Oil (liquid) coupled with exercise. You can take your fish oil liquid by putting it into yogurt to disguise the flavor if need be or a delicious fruit juice or even Aloe Vera juice to prevent any burping. The important goal is to get your fat content measured and then take the next step to DECIDE – COMMIT and you will SUCCEED!

People are Surrounded with Calories & Gluten

There are more fast food outlets than grocery stores by far. Some folks have to travel quite a distance through traffic or countryside to food-shop just for the basics. Marketing has taken this into account with the placement of fast food restaurants, coffee shops and pizzerias! Once you DECIDE to get healthier and lose the weight one discipline that has worked well for others is to not eat any food that comes through a window. Just cutting sodas out of the diet and replacing them with water can drop lots of extra weight. Sugar is calories!

Fast Foods

The fast food corporations of today count on people's addictive nature. Sugar, fat, processed cheeses and breadstuff are all extremely addictive. The National Restaurant Association said in 2006, consumers bought $142 billion worth of fast foods. With all the romanticizing of dessert coffees, fast food outlets and pizza-man-i-a that has exploded over the last few decades this could even be a low figure!

The PMQ Pizza magazine wrote that people spent $36.3 billion dollars just on pizza alone in 2010 from the nearly 65,000 pizzerias in the US! Think about what it takes to make a pizza? Do you recognize the ingredients? Yes - they are the GIS Trigger foods. It is no wonder people feel so bloated after gorging on the tantalizing stuff. Keep in mind that pizza is one of the worst choices you can make in getting healthier. It is loaded with Gluten and Gluten Triggers that keep people in their obesity and crazy to boot (Review Chapter 5)!

The CDC also estimates that adults are eating an average of 14% more calories today than they did back in 1971 before the battle of the bulge began. Of course the calories that come with most of the fast foods have something to do with it. But more than mere calories is causing obesity. It has a lot to do with a major lack of proper nutrition and exercise from both adults and children plus there is the "inflammation" factor. Believe it or not GIS is a major reason why people keep gaining the extra pounds. The GIS heightens the inflammatory response that occurs in the body from eating the gluten in the pizza dough, sugar, fried foods, too much milk and processed cheeses lighting a fuse to destruction.

The inflammation affects the Central Nervous System needed for proper glandular support including; the Thyroid and Para-Thyroid, Pancreas, Adrenals and yes even the Liver. These are the glands you need working really well to lose and maintain healthy weight! Of course the empty calories also rob the body of B-Complex and other valuable core nutrients that feed into the chain reaction that puts on the pounds too.

Every person I have worked with to guide them along the GIS Program loses the unhealthy weight when they follow through! Read about weight loss in the testimony chapter from others that have taken the excess pounds off and kept them off by following the GIS Diet and Program.

Habits of People Who Reach and Maintain a Healthy Weight

- *Eat Regular Meals from the Mediterranean Diet (similar to the GIS Diet);* Lean Protein, Eggs (as tolerated) Vegetables, Fruits, Beans, Olive Oil and Low Alcohol Consumption.
- *Exercise Regularly;* 30 – 45 Minutes Daily of Aerobic Exercise to Increase the Heart Rate to approximately 70% higher than your normal beats per minute.
- *Keep a Log or Food Diary;* They Recorded the Calories from their Daily Foods. The Daily Calorie Goal is 2,000 for Women and 2,500 for Men.

Nutrition Highlights for Weight Loss: Multiple Vitamin & Mineral by *Aloe Life*, Probiotics by *Dr. Ohhira*, Fish Oil by *Nordic Naturals*, Aloe Vera, L-Lysine 1 - 3,000 mg (supports fat burning and viral), Nutritional Yeast 2-3 tsp., L-Carnitine HCL 500 mg 2 x daily (supports fat burning), Protein, Aloe Boost by *Aloe Life* (supports blood sugar - Nopal Cactus & Aloe, FF Amino Acids), Chromium GTF, Vitamin E Complex, Thyroid / Para-thyroid (as needed), Water, Love and Forgiveness plus any Special Needs Supplements (Ch. 8).

Weight Gain Requires Healthy Calories & Glandular Health Too!

There are people who struggle at the opposite end of the scale to keep weight on their body. As a clinician I have spent many clinic hours reviewing the foods for healthy weight gain and nutritional support for eating disorders. The fact of the matter is unless the weight loss is due to advanced bowel disease or another disease state, (review GIS Zone 3 diet in Chapter 7), being lean is a healthier body weight in most instances compared to obesity.

Sometimes having a lighter frame is due to people just not eating enough calories in their diet. Interestingly, people who eat less food have better absorption of the nutrients from the foods eaten. When people overeat at a meal, absorption of nutrients from the foods decrease significantly and they generally do not become satiated as desired. Avoid overeating with weight loss or weight gain and remember you get to eat again in another four hours or so. Putting calories on for the underweight person requires high caloric food sources accenting healthy fats and oils, natural sugars and including meat if possible; fish and all types of meat, nuts and seeds, butter, dairy products and beans as tolerated. Foods that are very helpful include; avocadoes, fruits, honey and olives, sesame and pumpkin butter, flax and fish oils keeping the focus on healthy calories.

Higher Calories are in Fats & Oils
- 9 calories in every gram of Fat or Oils.
- 4 calories in every gram of Carbohydrate or Protein.

The inability to gain healthy weight is caused by several different factors. GIS can cause nutrient deficiencies from poor absorption leading to a break-down in calorie metabolism and weight loss. The classic Diabetic is actually a very slim person who finds gaining weight to be extremely difficult! I know this fact may surprise some of you. It has only been in the last twenty years that the new Diabetic profile has emerged with overweight and obesity.

Proper glandular health is paramount to gain healthy weight by supporting; the Liver, Adrenals, Pancreas, Thyroid, Para-Thyroid and Hypothalamus in the brain. The nutrients that are most critical to build glandular health in the body are protein and the other essential core nutrients like Vitamin E. The Branch Chain Amino Acids are a specific combination of amino acids that are key building blocks of protein that allow for muscle and glandular construction. A variety of other health supplements are also available that contain essential Free Form Amino Acids that play an important support foundationally to the body to regain weight and health as well.

To gain weight - strive to add calories at every meal and snacks from nutrient dense foods not sugar and carbohydrate junk foods. Refined sugars can promote overgrowth of the yeast called Candida Albicans. Candida can be a major challenge of difficulty in weight gain and consuming junk food empty calories often just compound the challenge of gaining weight especially if Diabetes is present. As you begin to rebuild the body pushing calories to 2,500 – 3,000 every day - the best you can from natural sugars in fruits, vegetables, red potato, yams and seed butter (like Tahini), pumpkin seed butter and peanut butter (as tolerated), adding fish and meats, dairy (as tolerated) like yogurt, half & half, some cottage chesses and hard cheeses, you will begin to experience the weight gain.

Reasons for Unwanted Weight Loss

- Malabsorption – GIS; Candida, Detoxification, decreased Digestive Ability.
- Fewer Calories Eaten than Metabolized – Must Increase to 2,500 – 3,000 per day.
- Illness – Seek Diagnostic Test to Rule Out; Cancer, Pancreatitis, Diabetes, Muscular Dystrophy, Parasites or other.
- Eating Disorders.

Following the GIS program will address any digestive and malabsorption possibilities. Review the Digestive section in Chapter 6 to consider any possible GI parasite infections in the bowel. Being your own health detective using professionals when needed, will also include eliminating any advanced auto-immune diseases including Muscular Dystrophy and cancer that can all cause unwanted weight loss at any age.

The deciphering exercise is to add up the daily calorie intake to see if it is normal first. Next, after reaching the higher caloric intake for a couple of months make note to see if the weight continues to drop. Always seek professional support for evaluation and regular check-ups as needed. The last area to check for is any potential eating disorders that might be present coming from Bulimia to Anorexia Nervosa.

Each person receives 100% support from the GIS program since it addresses mental and physical health whatever your goal may be. GIS is so easily coupled with healthy counseling to reach your health goal. I find counseling to be such a finishing touch whether it is individual one-on-one counseling or in a group experience. After three sessions you can generally get a feeling as to whether or not you are getting positive results from the professional you are working with. You may end up speaking with 3 - 4 different counselors before you find a good match to benefit you and perhaps family members as desired. Take the stops out and in health always do what works!

Gaining Healthy Weight Benefits
- When you reach a healthy weight goal your body has the proper fat stores to protect and insulate all of its parts from weather, injury and wear and tear.
- The Face & Body is more attractive when healthy weight fat stores are on the body.
- Fat stored in the body can also be used for fuel to create needed energy if a person does not supply the body with enough calories for a day.
- Healthy weight allows you the energy and brain function to enjoy your work and play and avoid disease.
- People whose weight is normal on the BMI scale experience less osteoporosis and other disease.

Getting stuck on either side of a weight challenge, either underweight or overweight can be very frustrating along with being unhealthy. People in both camps require goals that are similar; to make healthier choices of the foods that are eaten, keep a diary of what you eat and take some healthy supplements to reach your goals faster while you follow the GIS Program.

The important step is to decide to change your current weight – DECIDE! Next step is to COMMIT to following the GIS Program for at least 3 month for the first evaluation period. And do yourself a favor by asking for a referral to connect with a professional for help as needed or desired. I believe in healthy counseling for men and women whenever possible to help remove roadblocks!

I encourage individuals to make the choice for health even if your friends, spouse or family will not join in. Do it for yourself and often health is contagious. SUCCESS will surely follow as you take ACTION to do your best - One Day at a Time!

Nutrition Highlights for Weight Gain: Protein, Multiple Vitamin & Mineral (or take ECN's separate Ch. 8), Fish Oil, Aloe Vera, Probiotics, Free Form Amino Acids or Branch Chain Amino Acids, Vitamin E Complex 400 – 800 IU, Butter, Olive Oil (2 tablespoons daily), Water, Love and Forgiveness and the delicious GIS Diet and Program.

CHAPTER 7

Healthy Living; GIS Program – Diets, Menus, Healthy TIPS & Tasty Recipes

"Crash - the noise came from an antique chair one of the few possessions I valued, broken against the closed front door! Married life was quickly turning out to be more turmoil than I anticipated with the honeymoon coming to a loud ending. Why did my husband think breaking my favorite chair was the only way he could get his opinion communicated to the family? Only years later did we understand that once we married I had begun feeding him a high gluten diet that was a catalyst for his manic depressant behavior. It was as though I had handed him a list of all of my buttons to push that really upset me. What a day and night difference once we began following the GIS Program in our family. We are healthier, happier and still married!"

— Karen, California

The Gluten Inflammatory Syndrome (GIS) Program guidelines are exactly that, "Guidelines." I guarantee that by experimenting with the suggestions of eating new foods, starting to live a healthier lifestyle and taking a few dietary supplements - Good Health Awaits You. It works for everyone not just a select few and you get to be the judge of just how well you can feel incorporating the GIS Program into your life.

Laboratory tests are totally optional to reflect and compare your progress "Scientifically". Some people need that type of validation before they will change their lifestyle yet it is not necessary. Chapter 4 reviews the available blood and stool tests, pros and cons that test for inflammatory markers. Keep in mind that testing is not a requirement to follow the GIS Program and start improving your health today. If you are experiencing symptoms described in Chapter 2, 3 and 5 then without a doubt you do have inflammation to some degree. Most people decide to pass on testing and be their own judge through observing their improvements. The GIS Diet is also a great "Preventative Health" program to stay healthy.

As suggested in the Healthy Focus Factors Chapter 6, keep a log of what you eat, supplements you take, lifestyle choices and how you are feeling both mentally and physically to record your progress. With a record of what you are doing each day you will find it very helpful to reduce the stress of trying to recall what your daily activities have been. You may find carrying a small notebook in your purse or briefcase works to make notes. It keeps track of your symptoms just in case you may need to make a few adjustments from time to time. If you have a negative reaction, simply review what you have been doing and focus on the diet without the supplement you just added.

Once your symptoms are stable begin to add other selections again. Review the Detoxification section in Ch. 6 to better understand that as you apply health the body goes through this very natural process of eliminating waste it has been storing. During this detoxification cleansing process you can experience flu like symptoms. Keep in mind the Detox symptoms are only temporary. Critical for detoxification is to keep the bowels moving each day to avoid unnecessary Detox symptoms of headaches, skin breakouts, achy joints and fuzzy thinking.

Successful Diet Protocols for Bowel Disease

- **Elemental Diet (ED)** – Good Results, Used in Advanced IBD Only, Medical Liquid Diet from a Physician. Many doctors do not mention this because of the high cost from insurance companies or out of pocket expense.

- **Haas Diet / Specific Carbohydrate Diet (SCD)** – Medium to Good Results, Foods Low in Gluten, No Refined Sugar or Cow's milk – Very Strict & Maintenance has been followed by many people over the last 10 years. Supplements not encouraged only due to the author not having work experience in this area.
- **GIS Renewal Diet (GISRD)** – Excellent Results, Foods Low in Gluten, Reduce Refined Sugar, Cow's Milk and all GIS Triggers, Zone 1, 2 & 3 are outlined in this chapter and is the most comprehensive for daily living. A complete supplemental program that speeds recovery through health and further supports the body's metabolic systems is outlined in Chapter 8.

Medical personnel will occasionally suggest the *Elemental Diet* with advanced Inflammatory Bowel Disease. This dietary protocol is successful by giving the digestive tract a total rest from inflammation. The formula is designed to give the body the basic foundational elements to fuel the body consisting of protein, fats and carbohydrates plus calories without bulk fibers or thickeners that are potential catalysts for bowel disease flare-ups. The upside is it does decrease the inflammation cycle that causes tissue damage and pain. The challenge with the elemental diet besides it being an added expense – unfortunately it's boring. To only consume a strict liquid supplement takes enjoyment out of eating and may disrupt normal social patterns. Eating is a very social activity and is meant to be a source of great pleasure besides sustaining life.

The Elemental Diet is designed to be used only temporarily during a crisis situation to ease advanced symptoms. It does not change the fact that gluten intolerance requires a life long restricted diet to be followed or inflammation will return causing problems once again.

The second diet regimen that has achieved a certain amount of success is called the *Haas Diet*. This dietary guideline has offered a more enjoyable diet from foods with similar goals as compared to the Elemental diet which is to lower inflammation and help to reduce bacterial and microbial growth in the bowel. The Haas Diet led into the development of the *Specific Carbohydrate Diet SCD* by Elaine Gottschall. The SCD outlines healthy guidelines avoiding most of the trouble producing foods and introduces nutrient dense foods and supports the rebuilding of the body. It has helped many people live a healthier less symptomatic life yet in itself has not addressed many of the challenges facing people with bowel disease to include the foods containing mold and other food intolerances.

The *GIS Renewal Diet* is easier to follow and more effective because it allows greater flexibility in less symptomatic people in Zone 1 & 2 Diets. This helps for compliance and enjoyment in eating while giving more solutions than the previous programs. The GIS Renewal Diet restricts more of the irritants in the Zone 3 Diet that may bring on a chain reaction of greater symptoms with advanced bowel disease. It also works even better to reduce tissue damage and heighten tissue renewal faster through advocating the use of important nutritional dietary supplements. The GIS program also incorporates the Healthy Focus Factors (Ch. 6) to be implemented in ones life over the months and years. Only when a person addresses these health topics on an individual basis will you experience the joy of attaining full optimal health success.

The **GIS Renewal Diet** is the most comprehensive program to date. Give yourself a 30 - 45 day trial on the diet that is most fitting to your symptoms. The second assessment time is 90 days. As you make notes of your improvements in a food diary or log it will track your success and areas needed to improve. Sticking to it for a full 3 months allows the body to rebuild the GI tract on a cellular level through making new lining cells. The GIS Diet provides three separate zone diets; Zone 1, Zone 2 and Zone 3.

GIS Diet Levels
- **Zone 1** – Maintenance Diet, Low Gluten for Low Symptoms.
- **Zone 2** – Restricted, Gluten Free and Low Gluten As Tolerated for Medium Symptoms.
- **Zone 3** – Advanced, Gluten Free (As Needed) for the Highest Symptoms.

Keep Your Sights on Success!

There can be high and low (emotional) days as you experiment with your diet and lifestyle. It is truly a life long journey not a fad diet. Perhaps the best attitude is one of adventure. The GIS Program can be an exciting new chapter in your life with some unknowns that cannot only save your life but also give you a lot of extra returns of reversing disease states. All illnesses relate to your bowel health in one way or another. By focusing on the health of the gut you can reach a level of health greater than you ever anticipated regardless of where you begin or your age.

Scientists have proven that the body can reverse disease through nutrition, improved digestion, metabolism and detoxification. Now you can prove it in your own home. Health reform begins in each person's kitchen and not in any legislation from government officials. However, you must make the effort and take action!

I am well aware of the fact that it is easier said than done when you are not feeling your best! *Caution:* Always review any diet, supplement or exercise protocol with your health professional to be appropriately cautious with existing medication you may be taking. However, do not let a doctor discourage you from getting healthier following the GIS Program.

With advanced bowel disease I suggest that you follow GIS Diet Zone 3. Your symptoms may resolve a little slower for some people and because of this I find it is better to add a new food or supplement at a slower pace. When a person experiences fewer bowel symptoms it is safe to experiment with the next Zone either GIS Diet Zone 2 or 1. If you begin in Zone 2 in general you may see benefits a little faster and add new food recommendations and supplements sooner. Remember intolerance to foods is only found with experimentation. Review the Healthy Tips section at your leisure. I think you will find the information helpful. Do your best each day and bless the rest while you set your sights to enjoy this adventure towards greater health!

Good Food Choices & Practices for All Zones (as tolerated)

- Lean Meats, Fish & Sea Foods, Raw Nuts & Seeds, Eggs, Butter & Cream.
- Cold Water Fish, Fish Oil and Flax Oil & Omega 3 Sources. *Avoid;* excessive fried foods, chips, confections and high Omega 6 oils (in fried and processed foods) while increasing Omega 3 oil content.
- Red Potatoes, Yams & Sweet Potatoes.
- Beans and Peas - Canned or frozen is approved, washed, soaked, slow cooked or sprouted is best.
- Vegetables and Fruits - Each zone diet allows slightly different choices.
- Low or Gluten Free Containing Carbohydrates – Low Gluten grains including; millet, quinoa, white rice, wild rice, sorghum, teff, brown rice (small amount if any), buckwheat, potato, tapioca, corn, white wheat flour, sprouted sifted wheat flour and rice flours (see Reference *Authentic Foods and all as tolerated*).
- 100% Sprouted Whole Grains - Reduce or avoid all "Grain Fibers".
- Fermented Milk Products – Pre-digested milk sugars found in yogurt, cow or goat's milk ferments (Ch. 1), sesame or other seed milk, nut or rice (white) milk (see recipe section).
- Sweeteners – Single sugars; fruit, fruit juice, honey, stevia, Agave or Xylitol.
- Increase Alkalinizing Foods - pH balancing is a goal and is achieved through improving digestion and including a variety of vegetables, fruits and supplements and drinking purified water (Ch. 8).
- Experiment with a variety of new Foods (Ch. 7) and Dietary Supplements (Ch. 8).
- Daily Hydrate with Quality Purified Water, Exercise and Get Sunshine Exposure and Rest!

GIS Dietary Triggers to Reduce or Avoid Review

1. **Regular Whole Grains** - Wheat, Oats, Barley, Rye, Brown Rice, Soy, Corn and all whole grains including Gluten Flour (unless 100% sprouted). When 100% sprouted the grains change - the protein molecule grows into a plant form which is not as inflammatory. *Avoid;* grains used in manufacturing certain products including; Certain Wine, Beer & Spirits, Condiments, Protein Powders & Drinks, Flour additives example; gluten flour or other grains added to white flour, Soy Sauce (wheat type), other grain binding ingredients in processed foods.

2. **Beans That Bloat** - Certain beans do cause more digestive symptoms than others. Beans must be properly prepared and slow cooked to reduce symptoms. Fewer symptoms come from Lentils, Adzuki and Pinto beans. Sprouting improves digestibility of all beans yet eat only as tolerated. *Avoid;* Soy and Soy products because they also contain Anti-Nutrients that can reduce Thyroid function critical for attaining healthy weight, heart and mental health.

3. **Cow's Milk & Some Softer Cheeses** - Cow's milk contain lactose sugars (disaccharides) that cause bowel symptoms. Milk protein may cause a secondary allergy reaction in some people congesting sinuses and adding to bowel distress. *Use caution with some;* Baby Formulas, Dessert Coffee's, Milk for Cereal, Soft Cheeses, Ice Cream and Desserts. Fermented dairy like special yogurt, cottage cheese and kefir contain low lactose sugars and may be eaten as tolerated. Recipe for homemade yogurt is in the recipe section that is best for high sensitivity Zone 2 and 3.

4. **Refined Sugar** – Table sugar is defined as sucrose a disaccharide sugar and is very inflammatory. Sugar examples; Candy, Cookies, Desserts, Drinks, Sodas, Condiments, dressings, soups, jelly, jams and regular catsup. Substitutes are primarily mono-saccharides and allowed in reasonable amounts including; Honey, Fruit, Fruit Juice, Fructose, Zylitol, Stevia and Agave Nectar Syrup.

Maple Syrup or Malt sugar is not to be used regularly because it is regarded as sucrose. Catsup made with honey is available in the health food stores.

5. **High Starchy Potatoes** – Many potatoes contain higher starch levels as in Russets. There are thousands of types of potatoes that contain amylase sugars that may cause symptoms in Zone 2 & 3. Allowed for all zones are the delicious low starch potatoes; Red Potato, Yams and Sweet Potato. Chew them really well to help digest the complex starch sugars.

6. **Wrong Thickeners** - A variety of thickeners cause symptoms in prepackaged gravies, sauces, coatings, drinks, other packaged foods, supplements, prescription medicines, OTC Medicines. *Caution:* Most processed foods including beverages found in the mass merchandized foods have either listed or *undisclosed thickeners* such as in mainstream; yogurts, cottage cheese, chocolate milk, whipping cream, dressing mixes, processed packaged foods, sausages, hotdogs, luncheon meats and soups. Common examples; Corn Starch, Guar Gum, Tapioca, Soy Lecithin, Textured Vegetable Protein, Gelatin and more. Avoid all in Zone 3 and reduce in Zone 2 until renewal occurs.

7. **Gelatin** - Foods, Sauces, Supplements and Pharmaceutical Drug packaging in Capsules and Pearls (animal and vegetable types). They all cause GIS symptoms. Alternative choices; tablets, powders or liquids. This is very significant!

8. **Molds** – Avoid aged and older foods in the store or refrigerator that naturally develop mold growth. The better choice is to buy foods as fresh as possible, peel fruits or cook to denature the molds. Zone 2 & 3 may also need to reduce or avoid; Leafy herbs, Cruciferol Vegetables, Berries, Nuts and for some people both Chicken and sometimes Turkey temporarily. Experiment and see if you can pinpoint any that cause nausea or another reaction. They may spark mold reactions at the beginning causing the extra nausea and as you detoxify you can begin to

add back one food at a time if they do not cause a reaction. See Chapter 6 Candida Albicans and Detoxification.

9. **Chemicals because of Sensitivity** – Zone 3 and at times Zone 2 may be reactive to chemicals that are added to foods for stabilizing, pesticides and mold inhibitors. Sources can be canned Tuna and other Fish, packaged meat and MSG added to foods plus "Commercially Grown"; fruit, veggies, grains and all foods. Best Choice to reduce reactions; "Organically Grown" as much as possible to include; meat, fruits, vegetables, grains, beans and some cheeses the best you can to avoid reactions.

10. **Rare Chemical Sensitivity to "Green Foods"** - Avoid with Zone 3 if you are experiencing advanced symptoms of chemical sensitivity for one to two months. Most people can eat greens and take green vegetable supplements yet not all people. Green foods can cause a health challenge because of a natural compound. This is called Phenol and it is a natural occurring chemical compound in green foods that cause the reaction. The *phenol reaction* is experienced as a chemical sensitivity and is very real. It can bring on fatigue, nausea and a general feeling of sickness, unlike the normal detoxification symptoms that will pass as the bowels move regularly. A phenol reaction will only improve by not eating greens and following the GIS program. It is more common in people that are dealing with multiple chemical allergies and drug reactions. Stop eating greens temporarily to see how you feel without them. After a month or two reintroduce the greens and judge for yourself how you react. This is most common in people who have undergone *formaldehyde poisoning* from processed woods or chemicals found in furniture, dry cleaning solutions and other unknown sources.

11. **High Omega 6 Ratio** – Most people need to increase their ratio of Omega-3 Fatty Acids to the Omega-6's in their diet. As reviewed in the Chapter 5 HIGHLIGHT the ideal ratio is now considered one part Omega 6's to one part Omega 3 or

1:1 once an individual achieves EFA balance. However, due to the excessively high intake of Omega-6 Fatty Acids in most people's diets, some testing show people are as high as 16:1 (Om 6:3's) and are experiencing more pain and other inflammatory symptoms because of this imbalance in their body. By increasing the Omega-3 Fatty Acids it lowers inflammation and pain in the body and increases health and the feeling of mental well-being. Sources of high Omega 6's includes; crackers, chips, fried foods, candy and high usage of vegetable oils in the diet. Even healthier foods can contain higher Omega-6's than 3's please review in the Highlight of Chapter 5. Many people also develop loose stool from fried foods coming from the imbalance in EFA's causing more symptoms of inflammation compounding the unhealthy gut. Omega 3's are found in fatty fish, fish oil, select seafood's, flax oil, leafy greens and other vegetables.

12. **Imbalances in the Body's Health Basics** - Review Chapter 6 Healthy Focus Factors to understand the impact on the body of; Dehydration, Viral Triggers, Emotional Highs – Anger, Stress, Exhaustion, a Sedentary Lifestyle, Trauma from Surgery and Accidents, Antibiotics, Medication, Constipation, Smoking and Addictions, Excessive Exercise, pH Balance, Allergies, Environmental Toxins and more.

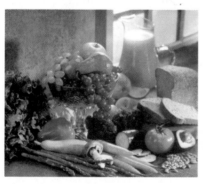

Diet - Choose the GIS Zone that best supports your body's needs.

For a variety of food choices you may wish to combine the food programs as desired and tolerated. The goal is to enjoy your meals and feel good after eating them!

GIS Zone 1 – *Maintenance & Low Symptoms*

Zone 1 is a maintenance diet with very little bowel distress or health challenges and has more variation in the diet. It still requires the avoidance of the GIS triggers to maintain health. It allows all animal proteins, most vegetables and fruits, specific nuts and seeds, fermented dairy products, hard chesses and the low gluten grains as tolerated. For vegetarians or raw foodists please see the Tips Section. Reduce or avoid all trigger categories in both the beverage and the food category 80% of the time. You can enjoy a 10 – 25 % "Food Flex" in Zone 1.

Keep non-sprouted white or whole grains (wheat included) very low in the diet if at all. Most beans, low gluten grains which include occasional brown and white rice, millet, quinoa, yams and red potato are tolerated best. Consider Zone 1 as a "Preventative and Maintenance Diet" for people with mild Irritable Bowel Syndrome (IBS) symptoms (review in Chapter 2) to encourage eating healthier and taking foundational supplements (Ch. 8).

Zone 1 is a maintenance program however some people may have occasional symptoms to include: heartburn, mild Reflux, bloating, slow regularity, maybe a bout of diarrhea or occasional food poisoning, nausea, melancholy or slight depression. Chew your foods well and begin the foundational core nutrients outlined in (A) of Chapter 8 Supplements at your own pace as soon as possible adding the Special Needs Supplements over a 30 - 90 day period. Chapter 6 and 8 give the extra guidelines for optional supplements as desired.

GIS Zone 2 - *Medium and Mixed High Symptoms*

Zone 2 experiences more symptoms of every type including frequent fast transit of loose stool with moderate to chronic constipation and bloating issues. This may include; emotional and mood changes, a variety of illnesses, diverticulitis, polyps, bowel narrowing, colitis, mild ulcerative colitis, hemorrhoids, chronic reflux, acute I.B.S., mild Celiac Sprue and occasional symptoms of Inflammatory Bowel Disease I.B.D. Behavior and mental psychosis as in A.D.D. / A.D.H.D., Bi-Polar and Manic-Depressive, O.C.D. (as reviewed in Chapter 2 & 5) fall into this category.

In Zone 2 some chemical sensitivity may be present along with malnutrition. Review the symptoms in Chapter 5. Chew your food well and begin the supplements one at a time (A) after being on the diet for at least (1) week. You may begin adding (B) and (C) Special Needs Supplements (SNS) as desired. Chapter 6 and 8 will give SNS (C) optional guidelines. Keeping a log of how you feel with each new additional supplement will be helpful and remember some symptoms can be due to detoxification and cleansing as you get healthier!

GIS Zone 3 – *Advanced Symptoms*

Zone 3 is newly diagnosed IBD or people who have been living with chronic bowel disorders with advanced symptoms as outlined in Chapter 2 and 5. Some of you may also be taking several daily and or periodic medications to control the GI symptoms or other maladies. As you experience your symptoms decreasing reduce your meds with your doctor's approval. Some doctors want to keep you on a medication even though you may no longer require them. In this case seek a second opinion from a pharmacist or a qualified health professional to help you make a smart decision to either discontinue a particular drug that is no longer needed or make another transitional choice because of your improved health.

Special Dietary Instructions

Chemical Sensitivity: A chemical sensitivity is often present with many people in advanced IBD. It is more important to buy organically grown foods as previously mentioned in this zone to reduce potential chemical reactions that add to digestive symptoms. Anemia is another major health risk with IBD due to blood loss. The concern in this zone is the potential of advancing malnutrition that can manifest to include lack of B12 along with other required core nutrients. This is why avoiding Gluten Triggers and selecting "Organic" foods whenever possible that contain higher levels of nutrients is highly suggested.

Quick Digestive Tips: Eating difficulties can be minimized by keeping a variety of soups, frozen foods, custom blender drink ingredients and even some organic baby foods on hand. These foods may serve as your main stay at times. Quick food reserves are especially valuable if you are having a lot of fatigue and other symptoms. Eating smaller meals more often every three hours is an important focus as to not over-tax the digestive system. Chew your food extremely well. This includes using the chewing motion with liquids to help the digestion process. Aloe Vera and Probiotics are both especially helpful to begin right away in this Zone. Foods that are nutritious and easy to digest are the primary focus in Zone 3. It is better to eat six smaller meals throughout the day. Three small meals and three nutritious snack meals work well. The menus and recipes are simplified for Zone 3 to avoid inflammation.

Stop Grains & Beans: Both Zone 2 & 3 need to reduce or eliminate beans and grains, at times entirely, until symptoms lessen. Yams and red potatoes are generally tolerated very well with a variety of very soft cooked fish or meat and steamed squash or other vegetable. It is necessary to avoid triggers in your diet that will delay healing of the bowel including 90% of all grains. Oatmeal is not on the GIS diet for a reason. *Unsprouted oats can be more inflammatory than wheat!*

Mold Triggers: Remember molds are GIS triggers. Avoid cruciferol vegetables like broccoli, cauliflower and cabbage in Zone 2 & 3, unless they are well cooked. Peeling your fruit and vegetables help to remove molds. Thoroughly cooking both vegetables and fruits kill any molds that may be lingering vs. raw foods. Because of the mold factor leave nuts and nut butters alone unless you feel well when eating a small amount. Seeds and seed butters seem to be much better tolerated as with sesame and pumpkin butter. You guessed it – seeds have less mold! After tackling the Candida challenge reviewed in Chapter 6, most people can go back to eating many foods they had avoided because it reduces the mold sensitivity.

Allergies: Fish is digested more easily than other animal proteins but it is not always tolerated from an allergy standpoint. Eggs, soy and whey powders may also be problematic for some people and OK for others. Careful consideration of protein powders and beverages are important and must be chosen carefully. Do not eat foods just because they taste good. Unfortunately, especially in Zone 3, it can prevent your body from healing and graduating into the Zone 2 Diet. Seasoning your food as tolerated is important for all people even if you are often blending foods into a soup or puree. Review the Seasonings section for Zone 1, 2 & 3.

Supplements: Begin the supplements (A) gradually within the first 2-3 weeks one at a time starting with a smaller than normal daily dose and increase as tolerated. Record the additions of supplements along with foods in your log making notes as to how you are feeling each day. This becomes very helpful to monitor how you are tolerating a new item even a new exercise, personal care or cleaning product. A fellow recently wrote up a testimony on-line that because he was using a mainstream laundry liquid that contained toxic chemicals he became very ill. The chemicals permeated his clothing so much so that when he realized the situation he went to an environmentally clean laundry solution and had to throw about $1,000 worth of clothing away. However, he began to recover as he plugged in health! As far as supplementing when you think about it, food supplements both herbal and core nutrients are just concentrated forms of foods and accelerate healing and renewal of the body ten fold. *Note:* **Make certain no gelatin capsules or pearls are being ingested in any zone diet especially Zone 3. Medications would be the only exceptions to this rule and do your best to replace any with a liquid or tablet.**

Nutrition is always the primary goal for repair and renewal with core nutrients regardless of the source being liquid, pureed or traditional in the food presentation. If you do have a reaction with a food or supplement stop it temporarily and then give it another trial in the future. Read the ingredients of all processed foods and review the Healthy TIPS section.

CAUTION: If it appears at any time on the GIS dietary program that you are having greater symptoms or continue to lose weight I recommend that you contact a medical doctor immediately. Remember you may request to use the Elemental Diet for a while which requires a prescription by your doctor. Be assertive! It can help to give you the nutritional boost you require and you may also take any of the GIS supplements as tolerated. I find the GIS Program works for everyone yet there may be ups and downs as you take the steps forward towards your healthier goal.

Protein

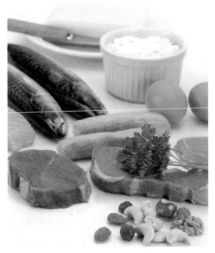

Choose 1 - 2 types of protein at every meal to receive nutritional variety. See TIPS Section for Vegetarian guidelines.

Protein is needed at each meal. High protein snacks are also important to support energy, stabilize blood sugar and body renewal. An example of a GIS snack would be an apple or banana with 1 ounce of hard cheese, 1 T. peanut butter or seed butter or ¼ cup of a healthy Trail Mix (see recipes). A small bowl of soup, fresh sliced deli meat (gluten free) or home cooked chicken, turkey or fish salad may also give variety to snacking with a few corn chips (or other sprouted cracker or chip) as tolerated. Daily protein needs may vary yet strive to get a healthy amount every day.

Daily Protein Requirements:		
Adult (21+): 60 – 100 g	Teen (16-20): 50 – 65 g	Senior (65+): 40 – 100 g
Infant (1-12 mos.): 14 g	Toddlers (1-6): 16 - 24 g	Children (7-15): 28 – 50 g

Why is protein so important? Protein starts with the letters - PRO. These letters are defined as "Number One" because of its great importance in the body. It is responsible for the major building and rebuilding structure of every cell. Trillions of cells make-up the tissue systems of the body for blood, skin, hair, nails, bone and nerve cells.

Also, proteins, which are made from smaller building blocks called Amino Acids, are responsible for constructing specialized protein compounds to include; Digestive Enzymes that process our foods, Antibodies that make up the Immune System and Hormones that control the body's growth and development. Many other "Specialized Proteins" are also made that we seldom hear much about yet are required for health. Sleep patterns, reducing water weight and even our emotional moods all require adequate quality protein. Protein is invaluable for life itself.

When children and adults are deficient they experience a break down in the overall health and metabolism of the body. A lack of protein brings about stunted growth patterns, fatigue, weight gain (especially water weight) and frequent illness. Make sure you include quality un-denatured proteins in the diet because it is essential for allowing the body to reach a healthy weight and heal itself. Excessively processed proteins and carbohydrates from sodas, junk foods, flours and pastas can weaken the glandular systems of the body allowing for poor protein metabolism and unhealthy weight gain as seen in the Metabolic X Syndrome (Ch. 6).

All of the nutrient dense foods including vegetables and fruits contain varying amounts of proteins yet vegetables also contain other valuable core and phyto-nutrients the body needs. Proteins from animals contain a greater quantity of protein in a smaller serving amount. However, meat lacks significant levels of vitamins, minerals and phyto-nutrients we receive from plants. For example (2) eggs, (¾ C.) cottage cheese, (6 oz) of meat from fish or poultry can each offer approximately 20 grams of protein. This is 1/3 of the average adult minimum daily requirement, in just one serving. Nuts and seeds (2 Tb) give us only 5 grams of protein. Beans for (1 C.) average protein count is about 10 grams. Each of these vegetable proteins contains less protein than meat per weight yet has more than common fruits and veggies. This is because seeds of a plant contain more concentrated and varied nutrition and meat is primarily only protein.

A Varied Diet of Both Vegetables & Meat Contain Protein, Fiber and a Lot More!

Each of these food groups contains important nutrition along with levels of protein to enhance the body's health. Humans require natural food fiber besides protein that also comes from beans, vegetables and fruits. Vegetables do contain the highest levels of essential core nutrients to include; vitamins, minerals, EFA's (however fish is the exception on EFA's), antioxidants and phyto-nutrients. The essential core nutrients work as co-factors along with protein to build the body and run its metabolic systems. The phyto-nutrients actually help to reverse oxidative tissue damage in the cells that if left unchecked brings about premature aging and disease.

In reaching for long term health I find it is truly valuable to have a combination of animal and plant protein in your daily diet. You do not have to eat meat to be healthy however you will have to work more diligently to maintain health in the body on the GIS program and throughout life without it. In Zone 1 & 2 strive to have a variety of protein from at least two food groups at each meal. Zone 3, it is best to simplify the meal and only choose one protein type per meal unless eating a vegetarian selection which requires two vegetable sources to complete the protein quality.

Protein Choices for Zone 1 & Zone 2

Meats: Chicken, Turkey, Beef, Buffalo, Lamb, Pork, Bacon, Wild Game, Sausages (GF), Hotdogs (GF).

Fish & Sea Foods: All types to include; Cod, Sardines, Bass, Tuna, Salmon, Snapper, Shrimp, Lobster, Clams, Halibut, Sole, Squid. *Caution:* Processed fish and sea foods may contain GIS triggers in the coatings, preservatives, seasonings and thickeners.

Legumes/Beans*: Lentils, Adzuki Beans, Split Pea, Pinto, Fava, Mung, Red, White, Black, Pinto, Garbanzo, Fresh Green Beans. *Note:* Avoid soy beans.

Sprouts*: Fresh Bean Sprouts, Seed Sprouts, Sprouted Grains and 100% sprouted breads and crackers.

Dairy*: Natural hard cheeses; Parmesan (fresh grated block type),

Cottage Cheese, Natural Yogurt, Half and Half, Whipped Cream, Goat Cheese, Goat Yogurt, Nut & Seed Milks, Rice Milk, Eggs and Butter.

Nuts & Seeds*: Cashew, Walnuts, and Blanched almonds, Peanut Butter, Coconut, Pumpkin Seeds, Sesame, Sunflower and Chia.

Breads & Crackers*: White Flour Tortillas, Corn Tortillas, Teff Tortillas, Corn Chips, White Rice Crackers, White Rice Cakes, 100% Sprouted Grain Bread Products, Homemade Bread & Crackers, White Water Crackers (GF) and some white bread(GF).

Cereals & Pasta*: Millet, Quinoa, White Rice, Basmati White Rice, Wild Rice, Buckwheat, Corn Grits, and Corn Pasta.

Flours*: Rice flour, White Pastry Flour, Nut & Seed Flour, Millet, Quinoa, Teff, Potato, Bean, Corn and Sorghum.

Vegetables*: Avocadoes, Broccoli, Leafy Greens, Yam or Sweet Potato, Red Potato.

* Complimenting Vegetarian protein meals requires two or more food groups at each meal.

Protein Choices for Zone 3

Meat, Fish & Sea Foods: May eat all same choices as in Zone 1 & 2 however proteins must be soft cooked and very tender fish and meat. Boiled chicken, chicken soup, fish of sole, tilapia, salmon, halibut and sardines are generally digested and tolerated very well.

Legumes/Beans*: Lentils, Adzuki and Green Peas are the best yet slow cook any beans to allow the beans to sprout before eating. Cook approximately 6-8 hours. Eat with caution. Some people must omit beans for 3 months or longer relying on fish or other meat, as tolerated while their symptoms improve. *Caution:* No soy products.

Sprouts* (fresh): The smaller seed and bean sprouts may be added to meals to give variety and nutrition. Excellent addition to soup, steamed vegetables, blender drinks, and salads as tolerated.

Dairy*: Natural yogurt and cottage cheese, some hard cheese, grated block type parmesan, half and half, butter, nondairy milk products, eggs and seed milks. Avoid Lactose sugar as much as possible found in dairy products. See TIPS Section. The Reference gives some brands containing less lactose. Recipe section includes homemade yogurt and other substitute recipes.

Nuts & Seeds*: Blanched almonds, peanuts, coconut, pumpkin, sesame, sunflower and chia. Some people wait to add any nuts for 3 months. Seeds as mentioned previously are best in Zone 3 and certified organic if possible to avoid added chemicals. Sesame and pumpkin seed butter is available in the market place or online. Peanut butter may also be eaten as tolerated. Delicious and nutritious nuts and seeds help to keep weight stable. Seeds either in ground form or butter may be used in a multiple of ways to enhance taste, variety, calories and nutrition of the daily diet. Eat nuts only if blanched and in small amounts as tolerated especially when having greater symptoms.

Crackers, Bread, Cereals, and Flours & Pasta*: Avoid until symptoms improve and weight is stabilized. Then you may begin cautiously with Zone 2 diet guidelines.

Vegetables*: Most vegetables can be included as tolerated including; Red Potato, Yams and Sweet Potato.

* Complimenting vegetarian protein meals requires two or more food groups at each meal. I highly recommend meat and fish be added as tolerated in Zone 3.

Note: Use caution when adding certain brands of fermented dairy products. Choose the products without thickeners. The unflavored and unsweetened Greek style yogurt is generally safer however many are being introduced to the market with irritating thickeners (read the ingredients carefully). By law manufacturers do not have to disclose all manufacturing aids they add to foods including certain thickeners in Dairy Products. See recipes for making yogurt and alternative milk recipes. Also, see Reference for approved brands of dairy. Milk substitutes may be used however it is best to rely on natural foods as tolerated (see TIPS). Cheeses are limited with extreme lactose intolerance in 99% of IBD. Cheddar and Swiss seem to be tolerated well, better than most other types.

Vegetables

Choose (4 – 5) servings of vegetables daily for adults to include a variety of different ones in your diet. Example: (1) cup steamed veggies plus (2-3) cups mixed salad or the equivalent would give you your targeted amount. Serving: ½ cup steamed is (1) serving and 3/4 cup raw is (1) serving.

Why have recent US polls revealed that only 25% of Americans eat the recommended daily amount of vegetables needed to be healthier? I believe the answer lies in a combination of reasons including; habit, ignorance, income and dislike. Each of these factors will keep people from enjoying and benefiting from the power packed nutrition found in vegetables. Vegetables fondly called "Veggies" are an important food source for human beings at any age from toddlers, teens, adults and seniors. The researchers who have studied the three most common diseases in our world – Heart Disease, Cancer and Diabetes, all agree that the science screams vegetables for prevention!

For people who are just beginning to eat more vegetables I understand that you may still have some mental blocks or a slim budget. Whatever might be standing in your way there is a wonderful option, a Daily Green Vegetable powder or tablet, supplement that is listed in the GIS supplements, Chapter 8. The daily cost can be less to take a vegetable supplement than buying fresh vegetables and you also have the convenience! Just follow the directions on the bottle and you start supporting your health with perfect compliance - fast, easy and very affordable as you do your best to incorporate veggies into the diet!

Daily Vegetable Requirements:
- Adults, Teens & Seniors (21+ yrs.): *4 – 5 Servings.* In addition you may take a Multiple Vitamin & Mineral or the equivalent in separate nutrients (Ch. 8).
- Toddlers -Young Children (1-3 yrs): *¼ C. cooked and introduce raw as tolerated in juice or veggies.* In addition give a Multiple Vitamin & Mineral supplement.
- Children (4 – 12 yrs.): *(1) full serving (1/2 C cooked or 1/2 C.*

raw) for every 4 years of age up to the adult amount. In addition give a Multiple Vitamin & Mineral supplement.

As a veteran vegetable lover who enjoys eating vegetables, I also include a daily vegetable green supplement plus a Multiple Vitamin and Mineral. I haven't always used a Multiple supplement preferring to take individual nutrients separately (see Ch. 8). For a long time I was also in the mind-set that I could achieve optimum health through eating the traditional way of salads and steamed veggies and occasional raw juices. When I finally added a daily greens supplement I was pleased and a bit surprised that I began to feel even better! Mind you this was over and above my normal good eating habits. That was many years ago and I wouldn't be without it today. It has been especially helpful when I was in a hurry to eat or couldn't make it to the market. Using a vegetable supplement really comes in handy especially if I am lacking vegetables. I can easily add an extra serving and maintain feeling my very best.

The body is never all grown up and we continue through life to require the valuable vitamins, minerals and phyto-nutrients abundant in veggies. Protein, as covered in the protein section, is also found in all vegetables although in smaller to medium amounts compared to fish, meat, nuts and seeds and dairy products.

Protein Value: Some veggies have more protein than others such as broccoli. Broccoli was appropriately listed in the protein section even though it is packed full of phyto-nutrients, vitamins and minerals being a vegetable. Broccoli contains 6 grams of protein in just (1) cup! It is twice the protein of leafy greens like chard or mustard greens. Broccoli is about the same as (¼) cup of cottage cheese (complete protein), (6) walnut halves, (1) tablespoon of peanut butter or (1) oz. of cooked Salmon (complete protein). See the TIPS Section that reviews the required caution to consider when choosing certain veggies. Most vegetables are allowed on the GIS program and significantly increase the health value of meals with variety, taste and nutritional content.

Organically Grown is the Best: Unfortunately commercial vegetables contain chemicals from pesticides and herbicides in varying amounts. Root vegetables require peeling besides a good washing to remove some of the outer residue. All of the vegetables including the organically grown type may also contain microscopic molds that may bring on more GIS symptoms as mentioned in previous sections. The other consideration in Zone 3 and perhaps Zone 2 for some people is an allergic response to green foods. However, don't let me catch you using this for an excuse not to eat your greens – Ha! See Chapter 6 Detoxification and Environmental Toxins. Choose as many organic foods as you can find and or that the budget will allow. Do your best and bless the rest is my motto!

Blood Thinners and Greens: An important warning concerning green foods is in order. Greens naturally contain an abundance of Vitamin K. If you are taking a blood thinner you must monitor the amount of green foods you eat on a daily basis. Vitamin K rich foods help to properly clot the blood and the medication is working to thin the blood. So you can see the challenge facing you. The doctor must be able to correctly prescribe the level of medication. Unless it is an absolute necessity as with some heart disease, get a second opinion as to the necessity of taking a blood thinner. Often a patient is prescribed the medication with a certain surgical procedure however does not have to continue it after the proper post-surgical period. When taking a blood thinner the general consensus is to eat the same amount of green foods every day and not change sporadically from one day to the next. Some doctors are writing a prescription for a blood thinner due to a heart murmur or irregular heartbeat. This is a situation that may be associated with GIS. See Ch. 5 Glossary of Conditions. Just by getting off the GIS Triggers the heart can beat regularly once again!

Each zone diet has individual parameters to help reduce the symptoms in the body while supporting renewal. Zone 1 can eat multiple veggies each meal as long as you follow the guidelines in the TIPS Section to avoid triggers. It is best to side on caution only adding one new veggie at a time in Zone 2 and 3 until you know how well your body will handle it. If you have no challenge eating many veggies at a time go for it!

Eat a Rainbow of Vegetables: The true family of vegetables includes; beans and peas called legumes, nuts and seeds, the potato family, the traditional vegetables and even the grains. Make sure to experiment with all of the vegetables including the dark leafy greens and the dark green lettuces. Iceberg lettuce can cause gas and irritation in the gut. Carrots, squash, broccoli, green beans and zucchini are all valuable to include as tolerated. Keep the high starch vegetables of peas, corn and rice lower in the diet. Potatoes are higher on the Glycemic Index scale yet they are OK to enjoy. Just make certain you start experimenting with a full variety of veggies to balance out the higher starch ones.

A fun vegetable food fact is that every color contains different nutrients. The goal is to eat from a rainbow of colors. One serving of vegetables is the equivalent to (3/4 -1) cup raw vegetables or (½) cup cooked vegetables. Fresh is best and taste superior - frozen is the second choice nutritionally and canned use sparingly with the exception of beans. Purchase "Certified Organic" and "Organically Grown" whenever your budget allows. Sometimes the cost difference is just pennies for a lot more nutritional value reducing environmental poisons and toxins in Organic. Gardening gives endless opportunities as well. The best buys are veggies in season and they are always tastier too!

Vegetables Zone 1 & 2

Choose (4 – 5) servings daily - including a variety of different vegetables in your diet. Example: (1) cup steamed veggies plus (2-3) cups mixed salad, raw or equivalent.

Leafy Greens: Dark Green Lettuce, Romaine, Bib, Green Leaf, Red Leaf, Arugula, Raw Spinach, Endive, Escarole, Dandelion Greens, Parsley, Sprouts, Cilantro, Watercress, Chard, Kale, Mustard Greens, Bok Choy, Beet Tops.

Root Vegetables: Carrots, Beets, Red Radish, Daikon Radish, Parsnips, Red Potato, Yam, Sweet Potato, Turnips, Rutabagas, Jicama, Scallions, Leeks, Onions.

Bush, Vine or Exotic: Asparagus, Artichoke (French Globe), Broccoli,

Cauliflower, Red & Green Cabbage, Chinese Cabbage, Brussels Sprouts, Eggplant, Mushrooms, Green, Red & Yellow Bell peppers, Okra, Acorn Squash, Summer Squash, Winter Squash, Crook Neck, Zucchini, Butternut, Pumpkin, Spaghetti Squash, Green Beans, Cucumber, Tomato (fruit as tolerated), Snap Peas, Chinese Peas, Celery.

Vegetable Zone 3

Choose only (1-2) different vegetables during the day to simplify the diet. Example: (1) cup of a steamed vegetable at two separate meals.

Leafy Greens: Dark Green Lettuce, Romaine, Bib, Green Leaf, Red Leaf, Arugula, Raw Spinach, Escarole, Dandelion Greens, Parsley, Cilantro, Watercress, Steamed Chard, Mustard Greens, Collard Greens, Bok Choy, Beet Tops.

Root Vegetables: Carrots, Yams, Sweet Potato, Red Potato, Turnips, Rutabagas, Jicama.

Bush, Vine & Exotic: Artichoke (French Globe), Asparagus, Cucumber (peeled and seeded as required), Okra, Green Beans, Acorn Squash, Summer Squash, Winter Squash, Crook Neck, Zucchini, Butternut, Pumpkin, Spaghetti Squash.

Note: Eat salad and raw vegetables only in moderation as tolerated after loose stools are no longer a challenge. All greens are excellent especially if you do not get nauseated or other symptoms upon eating greens. If symptoms result from eating greens avoid them for three months before trying them again. Concentrate on all the other colors of vegetables yellow, orange including as little green as possible. Add the vegetables listed in Zone 1 & 2 with caution as your symptoms decrease due to potential allergens of molds. Avoid tomato of any significant amount for the first 3 month period of the diet.

Fruit

Choose at least 2 servings of fruit per day or supplement with extra vitamins and minerals to receive the required ECN's. Fruit contains the important Vitamin C and Antioxidants and an abundance of other valuable nutrients.

Did you know that the early explorers and settlers became ill and sometimes died from a lack of a certain essential core nutrient found in fruit? If you guessed Scurvy you are correct and it is a deficiency disease I still see today! Scurvy was discovered to be due to a lack of Vitamin C and Bioflavonoids found naturally in fruits and some vegetables. Early explorers would travel with citrus to avoid the ravages of Scurvy including limes that resulted in the nick-name for sailors of "Limey"!

Modern day Scurvy symptoms can be seen today with many deficiency diseases including; arthritis, gum disease, bleeding gums, premature aging of the skin, a failing immune system and bone loss called Osteoporosis. Besides being a structural core nutrient Vitamin C works synergistically with iron, sulfur and protein to build blood reducing Anemia and is a natural anti-inflammatory agent responsible for other important functions in health.

US Recommended Daily Allowances	USRDA Minimum	Research Maximum* for Vitamin C
Adults, Children (4 yrs+), Teens & Seniors	60 mg	1,000 – 3,000 mg
Infants (11-12 months)	35 mg	60 – 100 mg
Toddlers (1-3 yrs)	40 mg	500 – 1,000 mg
Pregnancy & Lactating	60 mg	1,000 – 2,000 mg

*If diarrhea occurs reduce the daily amount.

Fruit is "Nature's Dessert" to humans and other creatures in the animal kingdom. Fruit contains higher levels of many vitamins when compared to the vegetable kingdom with only a few exceptions. Surprisingly, Vitamin C is high in citrus fruit yet it is topped in C content by bell peppers. Vitamins are practically non-existent in protein foods therefore fruits and vegetables play a very important role in health. They provide the required levels of Vitamin A, C, E plus other essential nutrients including minerals.

The word Vita means life! The body cannot make these important nutrients called vitamins from other compounds. This is why fruits and vegetables and/or to supplement is a must. Knowing this explains why more disease develops in people who rely heavily on high amounts of fast foods or mono diets that are higher in protein neglecting fruits and veggies.

Fruits are also an excellent source of minerals like potassium that is responsible for many healthy functions of the body. Known as a "Brain Food", Potassium is an electrolyte which supports metabolic function of the brain, reduces unwanted water weight, increases energy and helps to lower hypertension commonly known as blood pressure. Avocadoes, bananas along with most other fruits and vegetables contain potassium and other important minerals known as electrolytes essential for energy and stabilizing mood.

Flavonoids are also abundant in fruits like berries, citrus and some vegetables and are classified by researchers as extremely important phytonutrients. These compounds are in the top natural substances being researched today by Tuft's University in the U.S. and many other pioneering institutions abroad.

Humans benefit from eating fruit yet it is an acquired taste! Some of you may be saying, "That's for sure!" For fruit lovers it is hard to imagine that some people do not eat fruit. Yet many people have lost their desire for the natural sweet and flavorful taste of fruit. The over-the-top opulent multi-blended flavors of man-made desserts have made slaves of people's taste buds and it can be a challenge to break that addiction. Artificially engineered flavor systems in ice cream, candies, cookies and confections that combine natural and unnatural flavors of sugary, salty and carbo-fuel spiked ingredients - that you taste all at once can overwhelm the taste buds losing one's desire for fruit. The flavor and sugar addiction that develops in designer desserts may take a little time to let go of (Review Ch. 6 Addictions). It does indeed take a re-education of the taste buds to begin enjoying the natural treat of fruit and the natural flavors of wholesome foods again. I assure you that the change will take place like magic especially if you seek out delicious fruit. Search for mature fruits in season, organic if possible and enjoy the natural goodness - Guilt Free!

An exercise that can help in breaking the addiction of refined sugar is visualizing a symbol of cross bones on any refined sugar you may be tempted to eat! Yes this symbol of doom is a mind game that can help to break the addiction habit! Seeing refined sugar products as a potential poison is 100% truthful. Refined sugar both depletes the body of valuable nutrients in an effort to metabolize the empty calories and secondly sugar increases inflammation in the gut which is a factor in the GIS cycle. Entire books have been written on the evils of refined sugar and how the sugar trade has profited at the price of people's welfare since the beginning of civilizations. Refined sugar is highly addictive as all parents know who have given their youngsters the taste of refined sugar. Parents and adults I beg you to stop the refined sugar addiction and begin to enjoy one of the true healthy pleasures of this life – FRUIT!

Caution: Due to past abuse of sugar or poor sugar metabolism, as in Diabetes, Hypoglycemia or mood disorders many of you may need to add fruit sparingly for the first 3 month or so. Fill up more at mealtimes with other food groups including proteins, vegetables and allowable carbohydrates. Eat the fruits in season that are less sweet as with apples, berries, papaya and ripened bananas at first and avoid fruit juices. Remember water is good for the body!

Choices include; fresh, frozen, dried and canned sugar free fruit. It is OK to sweeten any fruit as needed with honey, fructose and or approved sweeteners. Fruit may be eaten raw or cooked according to your zone diet. Organic fruits are always best for all people especially children, people with allergies and advanced GIS symptoms as possible (see TIPS section for further suggestions).

Fruits Zone 1 & 2

Choose no more than (3 – 4) servings per day as tolerated. Example: (½ cup) of applesauce, melon or berries, (1) medium banana, (1) orange, pear or (2) Kiwis.

Tree: Apple, Avocado, Pear, Banana, Peach, Apricot, Nectarine, Orange, Tangerine, Grapefruit, Pineapple, Lemon, Lime, Cherries, Papaya, Mango and others.

Vines & Bushes: Blueberries, Strawberries, Boysenberries, Blackberries, Grapes and others.

Dried Fruits* & Exotics: Kiwis, Pomegranates, Mangoes, Papayas, Fresh Coconut and Dried*, Figs, Dates, Raisins and more.
*See Healthy TIPS section.

Fruits Zone 3

Choose (1 -2) servings per day as tolerated. You may need to cook and peel your fruits during this first phase for 1-3 months until diarrhea and or other symptoms resolve. Choose ripe and organic fruit when possible. Avoid berries that tend to grow molds very easily. Wait on adding citrus or tomato until symptoms resolve because of a possible pH imbalance. Review Chapter 6 pH section.

Tree*: Banana, Apples, Avocado, Pears, Mangos, Papaya, Peaches, Apricots, Nectarines, Cherries and other (best to peel and cook except with Avocados).

Vines & Bushes*: Avoid until symptoms decrease and then eat as Zone 2.

Dried Fruits*: Cooked to reconstitute dried prunes, raisins, apricots or other dried fruit in small amounts.
* See Healthy TIPS section.

Beverages

Water is the most important liquid that humans need to drink every day and people are dying from a lack of water in every town and city! It is true that most people as a whole are flat out not drinking the amount of water they need to support health in the body. The requirement for good pure water in the body is paramount to getting well and staying healthy! All of the body's vital organs and systems require water to function properly to include the brain, digestion, detoxification and renewal. Water is an absolute to reach and maintain a healthy weight for individuals. Some overweight people do drink sufficient amounts of water yet most kids and adults are drinking too much caffeinated soda, coffees, and alcoholic drinks that actually dehydrate the body.

Daily energy, healthy hormones and keeping the skin looking youthful at any age all require sufficient water. When feeling tired, hungry or depressed just have a couple of glasses of water and observe how much better you feel within the hour. A headache can vanish upon drinking a glass or two of aqua. Children require good quantities and it is the best liquid as they grow with a reasonable amount of milk or quality yogurt (eaten in-between their larger meals is best and as tolerated). *Note:* Supplement with a comprehensive "Mineral Supplement" when not giving your young children or teenagers dairy products.

Water is a Requirement for Life Itself!

- Daily requirement of water is Half the Body's Weight in Ounces. *Example:* 200 lbs. divided by 2 equals 100 oz divided by 32 suggests a little over 3 quarts of water.
- Water makes up 60 - 75% of the Body Weight When 100% Hydrated.
- Water Supports; Energy, Reduction of Headaches, Brain Health, Vital Organs, Hormone Production, Increased Digestive Juices, Youthful Skin & Sleep.

Enjoying a beverage is a "Mini Break" from life's mundane reality. People do not require any alternative beverages other than water but we enjoy them. As crucial as water is for every cell of the body choosing an alternative beverage has emerged as a social tradition and pastime. What would you like to drink? The choices are endless as you know so I encourage you to be selective and avoid sugar in its many forms including artificial sweeteners as much as possible. Long-term use of the artificial sweeteners may be hazardous to one's health. Review Chapter 6 Detoxification and Anti-Nutrients. Healthier beverages include; teas of many varieties, coffee, vegetable or fruit juices. Our beverage choices can lift our energy and spirits bringing enjoyment as we begin or end our daily rituals in life.

The goal on the GIS Program is to choose beverages that will complement one's health and not add to any bowel or GIS symptoms. People have many choices and pleasures in beverages however use caution within each of the zones. Alcoholic beverages are reviewed in the following section.

Juices can be fresh squeezed or blended, canned or frozen however use caution to avoid any hidden sugar and excessive salt. Organic is a better choice than commercial juices whenever possible. Also, only drink a small amount of fruit juice at one time to avoid overloading the body's sugar metabolism. A rule of thumb is to dilute your selection with water including an occasional mineral water with carbonation. *Note:* Carbonation is not a good choice for Zone 3 or anyone suffering with advanced digestive issues. Vegetable juices may be consumed in higher quantity (see recipe section for homemade blender juices). Food fiber plays such an important role in health and you kick up your daily intake through making home blended juice drinks that leave the fiber in the juice for Zone 1 and 2. Zone 3 may have better results with pasteurized apple or grape juice for the first 3 months due to the natural mold content of fresh juiced vegetables and fruits.

White, green and black teas are tolerated best in high symptom Zones 2 and 3 compared to coffee. Coffee is from a bean and for some people it may act as a slight trigger for inflammation. Other folks tend to tolerate it well on the GIS program in Zone 1 and Zone 2. Herb teas are generally tolerated by all zones yet it is suggested to avoid leafy green teas like comfrey and some of the mints if bowel symptoms are advanced. Chemically sensitivity people need to avoid leafy herbs because they naturally develop molds that cause allergy reactions. Do enjoy any of the teas and coffee in moderation as tolerated.

Avoid all caffeinated teas, coffee and sodas if stool is loose. Rule of thumb is to only drink (2) portions of caffeine daily to avoid excessive nutrient loss from its diarrheic property for most people. "Water Processed" decaffeination, is free of harmful chemicals and the best choice for daily use if it is available. Avoid milk solids and thickeners in beverages by carefully reading the ingredients on any instant coffee, tea or cocoa products. Review TIPS Section for further suggestions.

Beverages Zone 1 & 2

Water: Filtered, Distilled, Mineral, Carbonated*

Fruit Juice: Apple, Tomato, Grape, Prune, Orange, Grapefruit, Pineapple, Mixed Juices

Vegetable Juice: Any combination as tolerated – see recipes.

Teas: White, Green and Black Teas, Herb Teas, Mate, Homemade Hot Lemonade with honey+ and Cocoa*.

Coffee: Coffee, Espresso, Decaffeinated, Latte Espresso - black or with Half and Half.

Soft Drinks:* Diet Soda or Fruit Carbonated Soda.

* Occasionally + Approved Sweetener

Beverages Zone 3

Water: Filtered, Distilled, Mineral, Carbonated*

Fruit Juice: Apple, Grape, Prune, Other.

Vegetable Juice: Any combination as tolerated (if no loose stool is present) - see recipes.

Teas: White, Green and Black Teas, Select Herb Teas, Mate, Homemade Hot Lemonade with honey+ and Cocoa*.

Coffee: Regular* or Decaffeinated - black or with half and half.

Soft Drink:* Diet Soda or Fruit Carbonated Soda.

* Occasionally + Approved Sweetener

Alcoholic Beverages

Many people enjoy alcoholic beverages around the world. It can be a bit confusing at first as you begin to understand the parameters of the GIS Diet and become aware that most alcohol is made from whole grains. Whether or not a chosen drink will cause inflammation actually depends on the processing technique.

Beer is also made from grains. The beer making process leaves a large percentage of the grain food particulates in the finished product. The grain residue that is left unfortunately increases the amount of inflammation a beer drinker develops. This is why the regular consumption of traditionally made beer is not recommended on the GIS Program.

Malt beer is the worst choice to make. If a person enjoys an occasional regular beer it will not push that person into a GIS crisis. However, drinking a large amount of beer can definitely bring on detrimental GIS symptoms that may be interpreted as just a hangover. Review Chapter 5 to understand how people tend to self-medicate their mental imbalances because of the GIS inflammation. Regular drinking or choosing malt beer only perpetuates the symptoms of GIS – and the vicious cycle continues! Alternative gluten free beer is available for the determined soul. Ask at your local health food store or perhaps find a location through the internet for company brands sourced from several countries around the world.

Dry wine is permissible and it is better if it does not contain added sweeteners. Naturally aged wines are best and are allowed in Zone 1 & 2. However, use caution in Zone 3 because naturally aged wines may contain small amounts of mold adding to any allergy sensitivity. Many wines do contain sulfites to help retain their freshness and color. Sulfites are more commonly found in less expensive wines and can cause headaches and other physical maladies plus add to GIS symptoms.

Alcoholic Beverages Permissible for Zone 1, 2 & 3

Beer: Gluten Free or an occasional Beer.

Wine: Dry Wine, Semi-Sweet Wines or Champagne.

Liquor: Bourbon, Cider, Cognac, Gin, Rum, Scotch, Tequila, Vodka or Whiskey.

Fermented liquor spirits are not new to this world and are made from the fermenting of grains or potatoes. Most liquor is made through a distillation process which eventually removes the grain starters called mash, needed to make the alcohol. Not allowed on the GIS Diet are the rare products that add the mash back to the liquid as in Corn

Mash Whiskey. If consumed in moderation alcohol does not seem to undermine the health of the body. It is important however to avoid sweetened liquors. This section comes with a strong caution because we all live in such an addictive world that generally does not understand the definition of moderation. For many people MODERATION IS NOT EVEN A CHOICE!

Do not take this Alcohol section as a suggestion to use alcohol. In no way do I condone abuse of alcohol or even see the need for alcohol. I am blessed to have achieved a healthy happy life for myself alcohol and drug free. See Chapter 6 Addiction, to further understand that many people living with GIS use drugs and alcohol to self-medicate unnecessarily. In other words the alcohol and or drug use is a chosen lifestyle often to feel comfortable in one's own skin. Abuse of alcohol causes premature aging and is a factor in many diseases. It is my joy to share with you that as you get healthier on the GIS Program, you too can feel better than you ever thought possible and may choose to live without drugs and alcohol – Au Natural!

Desserts

Did you know that refined sugar consumption averages 200 lbs for every child and adult each year in the U.S.? Just think about what that means for a minute. For every person not consuming this horrendous amount of sugar, another person is eating twice the amount! The GIS trinity of inflammation is Refined Sugar, Lactose from Milk and Gluten from Grains. I suggest that you follow the guidelines in this section as if your life depends upon it because ultimately - it truly does!

Fruit is the focus for daily snacks and desserts on the GIS Program. Amazing dessert creations using fruit and natural ingredients are possible as you can review in the recipe section. Remember that there are varying degrees of inflammation for each family member. I suggest in the years ahead to follow the guidelines 80 – 90% of the time. At least if one strays a little and indulges for special occasions you will understand why you may be having certain GIS reactions. It has often been said, "I may not need the dessert but I want it!"

Natural sweets and allowable treats are great for the body. Every once in a while - a special dessert can be good for the soul called SPLURGE! At the beginning of getting healthier be as strict as your health dictates use discipline, especially on Zone 2 & 3 with higher and advanced symptoms. You can experiment and learn to be more selective having healthier choices when celebrating. I seldom choose a dessert when I go out to dinner any more. Yet when I do I thoroughly enjoy it having NO GUILT! Some people have found by volunteering to bring an alternative dessert to social gatherings helps them stay away from a dessert that is excessive. This exercise can also help others that may want a healthier choice!

Desserts Zone 1 & 2

Baked Goods (LG & GF): Fruit Bars, Pie, Cake, Cookies, Fruit Compote, Cheesecake and Custard are some of the basics. See Reference section for *Authentic Foods* gluten free dessert mixes.

Fruit Sundaes: Favorite Fruit in season with Yogurt or Whipped Cream topping. Add some toasted seeds or nuts (optional) on top of desserts or some coconut shreds. Ice Milk, Rice Cream, Fruit Sorbet, Frozen Bananas, Coconut Ice Cream, Applesauce with Whipped Cream, Yogurt Parfait, Puddings and more can be very tasty treats.

Blender Drinks: Smoothies & Frappes.

Snack Desserts: Trail Mix, Dried Fruit, Peanut Butter, Sesame Butter, Raw Nuts & Seeds, Select Dry Snacks, Cheese Slices and other non-bake snack creations are yummy.

LG Low Gluten & GF Gluten Free

Desserts Zone 3

Baked Goods: Baked Pears & Apples, Cooked Fruit Compote and Rice Custards are delicious.

Fruit Sundaes: Fruit Compote with Yogurt, Frozen Bananas, Apple-Yogurt Parfait.

Blender Drinks: Smoothies & Frappe

Snack Desserts: Dates, Sesame Butter, Peanut Butter, Raw Blanched Almonds, Raw Pumpkin Seeds, Cheese Slices.

Condiments

Nature provides people with a variety of foods that can satisfy the taste bud desires. A good example is the taste of sweet (Grapes), tart (Lemon Lime), salty (Celery) and pungent (Mustard Greens). Tasty foods come in all categories and are seasonal, best fully ripened and grown on good soil that facilitates the development of their full potential flavor and nutritional value. People have also been given a variety of natural herbs and condiments to enhance the natural flavor in foods. With practice you can create delicious flavor enhancement with your meats, beans and vegetables that will bring a lifetime of tasty enjoyment.

Top Seasonings Worldwide

- Salt
- Ground Pepper
- Cumin
- Garlic & Onions
- Ginger
- Oregano
- Rosemary
- Basil
- Thyme
- Peppers – All Types
- Lemon & Orange - Juice / Peel
- Curry Blend
- Bay Leaf
- Cinnamon & Clove
- Fermented; Fish & Soy Sauce and Vinegars

The GIS Program assists in the enjoyment of the foods we eat by cleansing our bodies and allowing the taste buds to fully experience the flavor potential. Often people do not taste the natural flavors from foods because of long term deficiencies of the mineral Zinc and the Candida fungal overgrowth. Once you replenish the Zinc stores your sense of smell and taste begins to return. This, along with improving the function of digestion in the body, will fan the desire to eat more natural foods especially as you learn to enhance the flavors of your foods with herbs and condiments. Start small and the combinations are endless.

Seasoning with your own condiment choices is not difficult once you learn the basics. Salt has been a basic flavor enhancer for foods since the early 14th century. Yet eating salt in excess is not healthy for the body and it overrides the other natural tastes that can be enjoyed! Too much salt can ruin an entire recipe! The same is true for excess of any one spice like pepper, catsup or even garlic. A small amount of tomato flavoring goes a long way. Garlic, onions, celery and peppers can all add taste expansion to any recipe and also bring with them extra health enhancing properties too.

Ground pepper and the spice cumin are two herbs that are in the top choices of worldwide popularity. You will learn how to use a variety of seasonings to flavor your foods creatively as you wish to increase the enjoyment of eating healthy foods regularly and in your own home. Thyme is a wonderful aromatic herb you may also wish to begin experimenting with. It compliments vegetables and meats from soups, to turkey patties, crab cakes and chicken dishes. Never enough Thyme!

Condiments Zone 1 & 2

Basic Seasonings: Salt, Pepper, Chili Powder, Cumin, Garlic, Onion, Bay Leaf (soups and sauces), Basil, Oregano, Thyme, Savory, Rosemary, Tomato.

Spicy Mild Hot: Cayenne Pepper, Hot Chili Sauces, Curry, Turmeric, Chili Flakes, Hot Mustard, Horse-radish, Ginger.

Pungent & Exotic Seasonings: Vinegar, Lemon / Lime, Fermented Vegetables, Cultured Yogurt, Sour Cream, Cream Cheese, Coconut Milk, Nut and Seed Milks, Mustard, Clove, Cinnamon, Nutmeg, Cardamom, Dill and Mint.

Broth Seasonings+: Chicken, Beef, Fish Sauce or Vegetable Broth, Miso Paste, Wheat Free Soy Sauce.

Thickeners: Xanthan Gum, Red Potato, Beans, Nut Flours, Low Gluten Flours.

Binders & Rising Agents: Eggs, Water Crackers, Low Gluten Flour, Baking Soda, Baking Powder and Dijon Mustard.

Sweeteners: Honey, Agave Syrup, Stevia, Zylitol, Fruit Concentrate, Fruit Juices, Raisins, Dates, Dried Fruit, Saccharin.

Fats & Oils: Butter, Coconut, Olive Oil, Sesame, Flaxseed and other (avoid margarine and hydrogenated fats and oils).

+ Best to use the canned or box broth seasonings containing less salt and binders.

Condiments Zone 3

Basic Seasonings: Salt, Pepper, Celery, Onion, Garlic and other as tolerated.

Spicy Hot Seasonings: Tomato and other as tolerated - use cautiously.

Pungent & Exotic Seasonings: As tolerated use cautiously.

Broth Seasonings+: Chicken, Beef, Fish Sauce or Vegetable Broth, Miso Paste, Wheat Free Soy Sauce.

Thickeners: Xanthan Gum, Red Potato and Beans.

Binders & Rising Agents: Eggs, Water Crackers, Low Gluten Flour, Baking Soda.

Sweeteners: Honey, Agave, Stevia, Xylitol, Fruit Concentrate, Fruit Juice, Dried Fruit, Saccharin.

Fats & Oils: Butter, Olive Oil, Coconut, Sesame and Flaxseed (avoid margarine and hydrogenated oils).

+ Best to use the canned or box broth seasonings containing less salt and binders.

Healthy GIS Menu Suggestions
Breakfast

Breakfast is defined as breaking the fast after a good night sleep.

Oftentimes people who have suffered digestive ailments skip breakfast due to experiencing negative side effects from cereals and breadstuff. Find foods that work for you even if they are not traditional choices. You may choose a light breakfast or a larger heavier meal for a day ahead that demands more physical activity. Keep in mind you can eat a healthy snack in a couple of hours as your hunger dictates. It is better to not overeat at any one meal and remind yourself you do get to eat again. Including a warm beverage at breakfast is very traditional or a glass of juice. The GIS Program suggests a tall glass of water upon rising to support cleansing of the body. You may wish to squeeze lemon or lime in the water for more astringent action and it tastes refreshing. After water then follow with a second beverage of choice. Common and enjoyable is to also include a fruit with your protein selection in the morning. *Note:* For Zone 3 it is best to have fruit alone or with a dairy choice like yogurt or a nut or seed butter as desired however not with a heavier meat meal. Review the TIPS Section to understand Food Combining.

Zone 1 & 2

Eggs – Poached, Scrambled, Fried, Omelet, Frittata, Smoothie or straight Protein Powder; whey (lactose free) or other type (See Chapter 8 Protein), Yogurt, Cottage Cheese , Nut & Seed butters, 100% Sprouted Bread, Lean Meats or Fish, Low Gluten Grain Cereal, GF Breakfast Bars, Miso Soup, Fruits, Vegetable Juices, GF Pancakes.

Zone 3

Eggs – Poached, Light Scrambled, Vegetable Broth Soup, Miso Soup (see recipes), Blender Drink, Cooked Fruits, Yogurt, Cottage Cheese, Sir Fry, Lean Meats, Fish.

Lunch

Lunch for the Mid-Day meal is called dinner by some people and is an extremely important meal to fuel the body. Striving to feel your best and maintain a healthy weight requires eating approximately every

4 – 5 hours. It can be a light meal yet we need 1/3 of the daily protein or approx. 20 grams of protein at each meal. Selecting half of the daily vegetables at lunch is also good unless you enjoy them for breakfast as some do in a Frittata or a vegetable juice (see recipes). Most common is to have vegetables with a protein at lunch. Ethnic foods to include; Mexican, Asian, Mid-Eastern and Chinese give a lot of variety to choose from. Simple but nutritious lunches, perhaps even some yummy leftovers are all great choices. Have you noticed bread sandwiches are not being talked about because on the GIS Diet bread is downplayed? 100% sprouted bread is not easy to come by yet some people are choosing white bread in this category even though it does contain some gluten flour these days. Wraps made with white flour tortillas or alternative flours like Teff are tolerated well by many people to replace traditional breads on the GIS Diet. See Reference section for alternative food product recommendations.

Zone 1 & 2

Lunch wraps with Chicken, Turkey, Fish, Beef or Veggie type, Special Sandwiches, Soups, Stews, Chili, Bean Dishes, Stir Fry, Lunch Salads, Ethnic Entrees, Fish Salad (Tuna, Salmon or Sardines), Raw Veggie Juices and Blender Juices, Fruit Salad with Cottage Cheese, Homemade or Greek Yogurt sides or dips.

Zone 3

Lettuce Wraps (Large Leaf - Dark Greens) with Meat or Veggie Filling, Soups, Stews, Beans-Lentils, Adzuki, Pea, Soft Salads, Stir Fry, Fish Salad (Tuna, Salmon and Sardines) and Chicken Spread. Raw Veggie Blender Drinks, Cottage Cheese, Yogurt and Fruit (Papaya, Mango or Applesauce) are good choices.

Dinner

Dinner can be a smaller meal if lunch has been larger for the day or visa-versa. You can decide what works best with your lifestyle and it can vary from one day to the next. The goal is to fuel the body with nutritious foods and make the meal as interesting and tasty – to find enjoyment during the dining hour. Preparing larger meals three times per week allows for some seconds to be enjoyed for a leftover dinner or a yummy lunch. Preparation can be simple or extravagant to match your food preparation ability, time and experience. In other words you do not have to be a gourmet cook to eat very healthy and prepare delicious foods. Practice, as with any skills, helps one to improve!

Zone 1 & 2

Enchilada Pie, Roasted Chicken, Spare Ribs, Lamb Stew, Turkey Patties, Fish, Chicken Vegetable Soup, Lentil Soup, Shrimp Stir Fry, Chili Con Carne, Sassy Salmon, Broiled Fish, Eggplant Casserole, Stuffed Bell Peppers, Tacos; Beef, Chicken or other, Shrimp Pad Thai (Stir Fry), Spaghetti, Dinner Salads and a quick Stir Fry.

Zone 3

Chicken and Vegetables, Fish; Sassy Salmon, Sole Portabella, Tilapia Parmesan and Asparagus, Chicken Red Potato - Vegetable Soup, Roasted Chicken with Yam Fries, Turkey Wild Rice Soup, Zucchini Bake, Egg Fried Rice, Spaghetti Squash with Italian Beef Sauce, Pumpkin or Squash Soup, Turkey or Fish Patties and Vegetables, Tender Beef Marinated with Green Bean Stir Fry.

Weekly GIS Shopping List

Purchase food basics that will last for 14 days or longer when possible including condiments, canned beans and frozen foods, onions, potatoes, eggs, meats, fish or other foods to freeze, breadstuff (gluten free – may freeze), olive oil and vinegar. Perishables need to be purchased more often shopping for at least 3 days of larger dinner meals each week. Some purchases will last longer and other categories will need to be replaced weekly as needed. In this way a person does not over buy and you can plan on having some frozen foods to help you get through your week until another trip to the market.

- Check the cupboards and refrigerator and make a shopping list.
- Shop for food basics every two weeks and perishables weekly for 3 – 4 lunch and dinner meals.

It helps to keep the routine if more than one adult in the family shares in the shopping. Older children can be helpful if you give them a few items to look for in the store. To prevent buying foods on impulse or missing important food items, make a shopping list before entering the store even if it is not complete. Generally this takes checking cupboards and refrigerator only about 5 – 7 minutes and it will lower stress and save you much more time and money once you are in the store. You will be able to resist over buying which will save you money and buying unnecessary items. See Reference for low gluten and gluten free food brands. Purchase food for both you and your family's particular zone diet.

Shopping List Zone 1 & 2

Key: (LG) Low Gluten, (GF) Gluten Free and (WF) Wheat Free.

Dry Goods – Water Crackers or (LG) Crackers, Grains including; Basmati White Rice & other types, Wild Rice, Millet (hulled), Quinoa, Puffed Grain Cereals (LG), White Unbleached Wheat Flour, Rice Flour, Rice or Corn Noodles, Beans; Lentils and others.

Frozen – Meal Entrees, English Muffins (LG), Flour Tortillas (LG), Corn Tortillas, Rice Bread, Frozen Vegetables-Peas, Seasonal Fruit, Bulk Raw Nuts & Seeds (freeze for storage).

Condiments – Olive Oil, Sesame Oil, Flax Oil, Sea Salt, Ground Pepper, Chili Powder, Cumin, Thyme, Bay Leaf, Oregano, Rosemary, Basil, Soy Sauce (WF), Fish Sauce, Balsamic Vinegar and others, Hot Sauce.

Canned Foods – Beans- Pinto, Lentil, Black, Kidney, Garbanzo, Stewed

Tomatoes, Tomato Paste, Black Olive, Red Peppers, Salmon, Sardines, Tuna, Sesame Tahini Butter, Peanut Butter.

Beverages – Filtered Water, Organic Apple Juice, Vegetable Juices, Herb Teas- Chamomile, Tea-Green, White, Black, Coffee, Diet Soft Drink, Fruit Carbonated Soda.

Dairy Products – Half n Half, Sour Cream, Cream Cheese, Yogurt Plain, Yogurt & Fruit, Hard Cheeses, Butter and Eggs.

Vegetables - Red Potatoes, Yams, Carrots, Celery, Bell Peppers, Onions, Garlic and Spinach (pre-washed), Radishes plus Seasonal Vegetables (3) Steaming Variety.

Fruits - Bananas, Apples, Kiwi, Seasonal Fruit, Lemon and Limes.

Bulk Items (as desired) - Raw Nuts & Seeds, Peanut Butter.

Meat & Seafood - Ground Turkey, Lamb, Beef, Chicken, Fish and Shrimp.

Deli Items – Sliced Low Sodium Turkey, Beef or Chicken (GF), Sliced Swiss, Provolone, Hard Cheese-Cheddar, Jack, Block Parmesan, Hummus Dip (Bean).

Snack Items – Fresh Fruit, Veggie Sticks and Dip, Corn Chips, Dried Fruit (sugar and sulfur free), Pop Corn, Cookies (LG), 100% Fruit Popsicles, Fudge Sickles Sugar Free, Cheeses, Meat Roll Ups, Dips, Dried Jerky, Trail Mix (GF).

Shopping List Zone 3

Dry Goods – Grains; Basmati White Rice and other types, Wild Rice, Rice and or Corn Noodles and Pasta (see Reference), Millet and Beans; Lentils and others.

Frozen – Meal Entrees, Vegetables, 100% Fruit Juice Popsicles as tolerated.

Condiments – Olive Oil, Sesame Oil, Flax Oil, Sea Salt, Ground Pepper, Chili Powder, Cumin, Thyme, Bay Leaf, Oregano, Rosemary, Basil, Soy Sauce (WF), Fish Sauce, Balsamic Vinegar.

Canned Foods – Lentils, Other Beans as tolerated, Caution with Tomato

& Soups, Black Olive, Red Peppers, Salmon, Sardines, Tuna, Sesame Tahini Butter, Peanut Butter.

Beverages – Filtered Water, Organic Apple juice, Herb Tea; Chamomile and others. Decaffeinated or Regular; Black Tea, Green Tea and or Coffee, Diet Soft Drink, Fruit Carbonated Soda.

Dairy Products - Half n Half, Sour Cream, Cream Cheese, Yogurt Plain, Yogurt & Fruit, Hard Cheeses, Butter and Eggs.

Vegetables - Red Potatoes, Yams, Carrots, Celery, Bell Peppers, Onions, Garlic, Spinach (Pre-washed), Radishes, Squash, Seasonal Vegetables (3) Steaming Variety.

Fruits - Bananas, Apples, Kiwis, Seasonal Fruits and (2) Lemon or Limes.

Bulk Items (as desired) - Raw Nuts & Seeds, Peanut & Seed Butter.

Meat & Seafood - Ground Turkey, Lamb, Beef, Chicken, Fish and Shrimp.

Deli Items - Sliced Low Sodium Turkey, Beef and Chicken (GF), Sliced Swiss, Provolone, Hard Cheese-Cheddar, Jack, Block Parmesan, Hummus Dip (Bean).

Snack Items - Stewed Fruits, Dried Fruit, Veggie Sticks and Dip, Custard, Deli Meat Roll-Ups, Soups and Homemade or Greek Style Yogurt.

Healthy TIPS

Cheeses Are Cart Blanc: Cheese can be a good protein source and a tasty snack. As convenient, nutritious and tasty as cheese is some cheeses are higher in lactose content and are best to limit or leave alone. As a food source cheese is also very concentrated and does contain higher saturated fat than may be expected. It is best to use control with cheese using it in moderation more as a topping on foods or a quick snack vs. making an entire meal of cheese. Some processed cheese products may also contain thickeners and sweeteners that trigger GIS symptoms. Regretfully, grated parmesan cheese is a good example of this and is used commonly as a food topping in the processed variety. Avoid the ready to use prepackaged grated parmesan cheese. Added milk solids are used in processing this product and they must be avoided. Choose the block parmesan variety to avoid the milk solids. When you freshly grate the cheese it has a stronger more flavorful taste anyway. It can easily be grated in advanced for a time saver and just keep it in a special container in the freezer for any prolonged storage. To avoid mold growth on any block cheeses don't contaminate the cheese with unclean hands and place it into a larger clean bag or container allowing the cheese to breath occasionally. Most cheeses can also be frozen to prevent spoilage and then thawed with only a slight change in the consistency. Dry Curd Cottage Cheese (DCCC) is a lactose free cheese that can be used in a number of different recipes for lactose intolerant people. The traditional cottage cheese contains varying percentages of lactose and thickeners that can be added without showing it on the label. See Reference for product brands and where to purchase DCCC. *Avoid or Reduce:* Cream cheese containing guar gum, excessive Feta Cheese, Gruyere, Gjetost, Mozzarella, Ricotta, Neufchatel, Primost, American and Processed cheeses including "Nacho" cheese and other processed cheese spreads. *Only Include the Softer Moist Cheeses Occasionally;* Gouda, Edam, Monterey Jack, Muenster, Limburger, Camembert, Brie, Stilton, Roquefort, Gorgonzola, Blue, Port du Salut, as tolerated. *May Include Dryer Aged Hard Cheeses Frequently;* Swiss, Cheddar (all types), Colby, Brick, Havarti, Asiago, Parmesan (hard block), Parmigiano Reggiano, Romano and the low lactose DCCC Cottage Cheese as tolerated.

Chocolate - The Good, the Bad & the Ugly: Chocolate has been defined as love and ecstasy for many people of today! The GIS Diet does not put it on the avoid list as some researchers have. Life is too short to not have some indulgences and enjoyment in diet and dessert selections. However, it is my responsibility to share the pros and cons and make the best suggestions to live within a healthy diet. Chocolate is best when consumed in its purest state as cocoa powder and then sweetened with honey or another approved sweetener. By adding some cream to sweetened cocoa you can have a delicious treat of hot or cold cocoa. Cocoa powder and making your own drinks or candies will help to avoid the refined sugar added to confections and also the bad hydrogenated fats. Review the recipe section for "Joy Balls" and "Chocolate Moose" which are really yummy! Unless you discover that you cannot even eat a small portion of chocolate because of allergies, a little once in a while can be a real treat and even good for you. Scientists have discovered cocoa contains very strong antioxidants within the dark chocolate specifically. Chocolate falls into the "Polyphenol Family" and the active ingredients are called Procyanidins and Epicatechins. Tuft's has shown that a cup of cocoa contains more ORAC than a glass of red wine to ward off free radicals that can damage healthy cells and cause premature aging! Before you get too carried away eating chocolate make a note that fruits and vegetables, which are a lot less caloric and come without sugar - are also abundant in antioxidants equal to chocolate and even greater! An occasional treat of chocolate is good for the soul unless you are in the process of breaking a major addiction to chocolate or sugar. The down side to chocolate is it contains some "Anti-Nutrients". Oxalates naturally found in cocoa, if consumed in larger amounts, can cause mineral loss in the body adding to Osteoporosis. Cocoa is also high in the amino acid Arginine which is a major trigger for the Herpes Simplex Virus (HSV). Another adverse nutrient in cocoa for some people is a natural chemical called Tyramine that sometimes triggers migraine headaches. With advanced symptoms of GIS as in Zone 3 it is best to put the Cocoa on the back burner at first. Carob powder made from the seeds of the Carob plant can be used in recipes in place of cocoa having a similar but milder taste than chocolate. The challenge in Carob product lies in that many products made today for drinks and confections come from the pods of the fruit not the seeds. On Zone 2 & 3 it is better not to take the chance with carob if you are having a lot of symptoms. The pods contain a potential trigger called locust which acts as a thickener. Be careful that you are making the correct selection of only the carob seed products following the GIS protocol. Locust gum is not an approved thickener. See Chapter 6 Addictions and Viruses for more about the HSV. See Recipes and References.

Condiments Are Crucial: Let's face it; foods require seasoning to enhance the flavors of our meals for pure flavor enjoyment yet be on your guard for hidden triggers in condiments. For instance regular ketchup may contain up to 40% refined sugar and ranks very high on the GIS Trigger list. The alternative is honey or Agave Nectar sweetened ketchup which is available in health food stores. Remember that pH can also be a factor in GIS so use ketchup sparingly. Tomato products are extremely high as an inflammatory food regardless of whether you may love the taste or not. It is best to use all tomato products in moderation - if at all. You can definitely use salt and pepper yet be warned to avoid starch, sugar and other triggers that are sometimes present in combination seasoning salts. MSG which stands for Mono-Sodium Glutamate is a flavor enhancer and still used in prepared Chinese foods, unless otherwise stated. MSG can bring on headaches, arthritis and increase inflammation causing disorientation in some individuals. Surprisingly, it is found naturally in fermented parmesan cheeses and is added to salad dressings, packaged sauces and occasionally other condiments. The important message is to read the food labels!

Cultured Milks Are Culturally Proven: Fermented cultured foods have been eaten throughout history and have been instrumental in keeping cultures alive. They are important to study and incorporate into the diet due to their support for improved digestion and immune function. Cultured milks are a valuable food category and include; yogurt (goat & cow), cottage cheese, buttermilk (keep low if at all), Kefir, Acidophilus Milk, Amazaki rice milk, sauerkraut, pickled vegetables and others. These foods are tolerated on the GIS Diet when regular cow's milk is not. Buttermilk is not to be consumed regularly yet may be eaten occasionally if it is an ingredient in dressings on Zone 1 and 2. It is also important to use only those products that are sweetened with honey, Agave or approved sweeteners. Remember the goal is to not ingest lactose (milk sugar), refined table sugar or any other disaccharide sugars. Use caution when adding fermented dairy products. If a product causes a negative reaction then you will know it contains a GIS trigger. This can occur frequently when you are still in an ultra-sensitive state of Zone 3. A fairly reliable choice is the Greek style yogurt, like *Nancy's* listed in the Reference section (available in the market). It is on the softer, more liquid side. Seek out the specialty dry curd cottage cheese without thickeners (see Reference). Unfortunately, mainstream manufacturers are allowed to add thickeners to dairy products and do not have to disclose all of the manufacturing aids present in dairy products on the label. Making your own cultured milk products is the best option and easier than you may think for some individuals. Mainstream "Milk Substitutes" may be used yet they do contain hydrogenated fats (Trans-fats) and so it is best to rely on natural foods as tolerated if you use them in any quantity. Best to avoid soy milk, and wait for 3-6 months after being on the diet before using coconut or almond milk. See Ch. 6 Detoxification and Recipes to make your own nut and seed milk.

Dried Fruit Can Be a Drag: Dried Fruit can be a great snack if your blood sugar is healthy (see Ch. 6 Blood Sugar). Look for unsulfured dried fruit not processed with sulfites that may cause symptoms of headaches and more. Sticky shiny dates and most banana chips have been processed with a refined sugar or a corn syrup coating. Avoid any gummy fruits and or supplements in the jelly bean form because they contain undesirable high levels of pectin and other thickeners not ideal for kids or adults. It is better to go with a liquid or chewable wafer children's supplement. Keep in mind that seasonal fresh fruit is always superior to dried fruits and some dried fruit can be contaminated with insects so always check carefully. It is suggested for fruits like prunes and figs to cook them for 3-5 minutes on a low simmer to make certain any contamination is pasteurized especially if one's immune system is on the low side. Organic raisins are available and preferred over commercial because grapes fall into the category of highly sprayed with pesticides that are dangerous for children and adults. Enjoy dried fruits but do limit yourself to the amount you eat in one setting. Too much fruit sugar can cause hypoglycemia reactions but a little is very enjoyable. Make sure you brush your teeth after eating dried fruit to avoid a plaque attack!

Fasting Can Fast Track Your Health: Fasting is going without food or limiting caloric intake for a period of time. Cultures have followed fasting protocols to give the body a rest and increase clarity of mind and spiritual insight for thousands of years. If you are not underweight a short fast of 1 – 3 days, is allowable. You must be monitored by a professional if you have any acute health challenges and are taking multiple medications. Of utmost importance is making certain you have proper intake of good water and your electrolytes are fully replenished. Both are essential for life. Fasting is not a requirement however some people find it a faster method of lowering inflammation especially if you continue to drink some vegetable broth or diluted fruit juice (adding lemon or lime) which gives electrolytes or fresh vegetable juices diluted with water. Getting the bowels to move before and during fasting is paramount for you to benefit from the fasting for renewal. See Detoxification in Ch. 6 and the Liver & Gallbladder 2-Day Flush, Enemas and Fasting in Chapter 12.

Anti-Nutrients Are Antagonists: Researchers studying cultural eating habits unveiled many secrets of fermenting foods by the Ancients. Besides fermented cultured dairy products eaten to receive the probiotic benefit, civilizations have also fermented grains, vegetables, beans, nuts and seeds to decrease the anti-nutrients in those foods. They found that the practice of sprouting and fermenting unlocks more of the nutrients needed by people by reducing the anti-nutrients that have been shown to significantly block absorption. Natural occurring "Anti-Nutrients" exist in the vegetable kingdom. These compounds, which include gluten, work as antagonists that block absorption of valuable minerals including phosphorous, calcium, magnesium, zinc and trace minerals. They also disrupt vitamin and protein absorption by creating inflammation in the digestive tract as reviewed in the first four chapters. This fact I share because it underscores the importance of choosing a varied diet that follows more of the Mediterranean Diet as in Greece and neighboring countries. Statistics show that these people are much healthier than the average American or Englishman. When you eat a variety of lean meats, fish, grains (LG, GF), red potatoes and cheeses (following GIS guidelines) with a large percentage of fruits and vegetables (including raw nuts and seeds) as tolerated, as suggested on the GIS Diet, you receive a better balance of nutrients, keeping the anti-nutrients lower including; Phytates, Oxalates, Tannins and Glutens. By including the cultured dairy products, sprouted and fermented grains and beans, as possible, it allows the body to reach a more optimum diet to build health. A few basic fermented recipes using dairy are included for the more advanced and braver student in the Recipe section that follows and look for fermented foods at your market place too!

Anti-Nutrients Naturally Occur in Foods

1. Phytates - Phytic acid is natural occurring in grains, beans, nuts and seeds and other vegetables. It is considered an anti-nutrient. Sometimes a food contains phytase an enzyme that counteracts the mal-absorption from the Phytic Acid. Fermenting bread by adding a culture which is a type of probiotics, as with a sour dough bread starter, can help reduce all anti-nutrients greatly in breads.

2. Oxalates - Oxalic acid is an anti-nutrient found more in certain green foods and it is activated by heat through cooking. Certain foods such as spinach, is better eaten raw to keep the oxalic acid from binding with other minerals in the foods and even potentially causing stone formation in the body. Chocolate contains oxalates and it is prudent to not overindulge. See Chocolate in TIPS.

3. Tannins – Tannic acid is found more in tea and chocolate and may cause a high acidity pH in the body causing primarily digestive disturbances.

4. Gluten – Gluten does fall into the anti-nutrient category and as explained in the GIS theory causes high inflammation and auto-immune reactions in the body leading to mal-absorption. Yet through proper 100% sprouting and avoiding the fiber in the grains as well, the damaging effects are lessened.

Fiber in Fruits & Veggies is the Healthiest Fiber: The U.S. government has made the recommendation or RDA for "Daily Fiber" intake of 30 grams a day for an adult. Unfortunately, the marketers have gotten ahold of this outrageous RDA and is brain-washing the consumers to think you must include the fortified whole grain cereals to be healthy. This is flat out not true! It is one of the reasons we are experiencing more gluten and inflammatory health challenges! The NIH and the other government agencies have not fully understood the challenge of gluten facing our nation and the world. Each adult and child does indeed require fiber from fresh fruits and vegetables and beans. The fiber in whole grains in its natural form causes great inflammation increasing GIS if eaten in larger quantities. DO NOT EAT HIGH FIBER CEREALS especially with IBS or IBD colon conditions. Following the GIS guidelines of a 50% raw diet, as tolerated, you will have more than sufficient fiber to assist in scrubbing the bowel from the fiber in apples, celery, carrots and beans. Fiber, both soluble (breaks down in the gut) and insoluble (remains intact), is good for regularity and can be instrumental to help reduce negative cholesterol called LDL. Low Density Lipid (LDL) cholesterol has been pegged as a culprit in plaque buildup in the arteries. Fiber does tend to keep the HDL, High Density Lipids or positive cholesterol higher and the LDL, also known as lousy (bad) cholesterol, lower because it encourages bulking of the stool and regularity. Regularity of the bowels rids the body of excess cholesterol so it cannot be reabsorbed. Also, regularity in turn allows the liver to function more effectively. Following the GIS protocol that includes daily intake of B-Complex and Fish Oil or Flax (increasing Om-3 Fatty Acids) from supplementing has been proven to decrease inflammation leading to plaque formation in regards to CVD.

Fish and Seafood Can Be Wild: Seafood is healthier if it is "Wild Caught" and fresh compared to "Farm Raised". A recent article in *Time* magazine, July 7, 2011 tells both sides of the fish story. Most consumers are unaware that the largest percentage of the farm raised seafood actually come from developing countries with poor unregulated standards. In the United States government's own study they state that farm raised sea foods have a wide variety of chemical contaminants (some cancer causing), added antibiotics and the potential for microbial contaminants from the weaker and sicker strains of fish! Because of the crowded aquarium like ponds that many are raised in, even in the U.S., they can even be contaminated by mosquitos carrying the West Nile Virus! Yes there is an upside that fish farms do bring to market more fish at better prices however it does come with some safety uncertainty that consumers must be made aware of especially for young children. The facts show certain types of farm raised fish eaten more often for their healthy Omega- 3 Fatty Acids like Salmon contain much lower content of the healthy fats because of the unnatural diet they are fed. Because they usually do not feed on the natural ocean sea life and river algae they do not develop the beautiful orange Salmon color and the farmers actually have to add fake coloring so the flesh resembles what nature has intended. Regardless, of either wild or farmed fish both types can have the addition of more chemicals added if they are frozen or canned to help maintain freshness. Some GIS Zone 2 & more 3 individuals may be chemically sensitive and if so it is best to eat certified organic meats and fresh wild caught fish purchased in the marketplace which generally contain no stabilizers applied. Frozen fish and canned seafood can usually be eaten by Zone 1 & some 2's if no chemical allergies are a problem. Ask your meat market clerks if they use stabilizers on their meats and seafood if you have allergies. Keeping a strong immune system can allow a person to eat miscellaneous fish at times yet ask for wild caught in restaurants to encourage their buyers to know that it is preferred! *Note:* Children and adults with a vulnerable immune system must be more diligent to avoid any food contaminants that may be coming from the food on the table especially if eating raw fish.

Food Combining Does a Body Good*: You must be kidding when you talk about one more consideration when choosing the daily diet? Let's not lose our sense of humor friends because truly learning about "Food Combining" is another discipline or choice to avoid more gas production from fermentation in your stomach. This is a valuable consideration for people that are extremely gassy or are in Zone 2 or 3. Some guidelines go so far as to say do not eat any starch vegetables like potato or rice with a heavier protein. Heavy fermentation in the stomach and in the GI tract occurs when one eats a concentrated protein like meat or fish at a meal and then follows it with a sweet dessert. Increased gas can even occur after the meal with the addition of fruit. However, when you add a sugary dessert or a very sweet fruit like a banana the gas build up can become very painful. The gas can start within minutes after poor food combining and for some escalate into painful and undesirable indigestion. The better your digestive system is working the less problematic fermentation has on the body. The ideal is to eat fruit alone or with dairy like yogurt or cheeses at a separate meal. A special dessert is best to be eaten 3-4 hours after a high protein meal however now that you know where the gassiness comes from you can decide when and where!

Keeping a Health Diary / Log Keeps You in the Driver Seat: If you develop symptoms from eating a particular food, beverage or supplement - record the reaction. If it is not a severe reaction do attempt to eat or include that item again in the future because the body renews itself and can possibly improve its tolerances. Zone 3 can evolve to Zone 2 and so on. Understanding the fact that all human beings are gluten intolerant for life yet it is a question to what degree - helps the daily prospective. Use your diary information to make remarks of any changes in your daily program, perhaps even to count your calorie intake with weight goals to include; diet, supplements, exercise, water intake, medications and how you are feeling each day. Your log can become a very good friend!

Foundational - Essential Core Nutrients (ECS) Are Foundational: For many if not all people following the GIS Program – the ECN's are 100% required to get the body going in the right direction for health! The suggested supplements in Chapter 8 will support your digestive system to do the work of improving digesting, reducing inflammation and supporting the natural detoxification action of the body through regularity and even slow down fast transit! Each ECN has hundreds and some have thousands of peer reviewed research articles to support their action in the body. As you add a supplement write it down and date on the lid or an entry into your Health Log. By making a note either daily or weekly as to how you are feeling you will see the reaction that the new product may bring. ECN's increase the entire metabolism of the body to work the way it was designed to be able to create health, wellness and youthfulness at any age much quicker!

Fungal Foods Are Ferociously Bad: Fungal conditions in the body, generally caused by Candida Albicans, create more symptoms upon eating certain foods and herbs. Eating garlic and feeling nauseous is a good example of what I am describing. What is needed is to detoxify the body - not keep reducing the types of food you can eat! Sugar is to be strictly avoided during the detoxification and check the recipes for alternatives. The advancement of fungal conditions in the body brings upon more GIS symptoms which create chemical sensitivities and allergies. Molds on foods can even become life threatening triggers for some. An allergy to some medicines like penicillin is also due to the overgrowth of fungus throughout the body. Eating turkey and chicken may even cause reactions such as nausea in some people with advanced Candida infection. Cruciferol veggies of broccoli, cauliflower, brussel sprouts and cabbage may cause similar symptoms including intestinal gas. Cooking foods does kill and denature the fungus or mold on most foods and proteins allowing more variety in the diet. Toxins on foods from sprays can also cause allergic reactions so experiment with more certified organic foods. Nuts, including peanuts, carry molds that may add to an allergic reaction including nausea. Molds can also develop a secondary toxin called Aflatoxin that can weaken the immune system in large amounts. Seeds have much less mold content and are included on the GIS Diet for all zones and nuts are to be eaten only as tolerated. See the Recipe for Blanching Almonds. Occasionally an individual who is in a heightened state of inflammation will react to seeds and some nuts until fungal growth is addressed. Anti-fungal herbs such as garlic and onions can both bring upon nausea and symptoms yet can help to detoxify if the bowels are moving well. When you get gas after eating certain foods or even taking the important Probiotics supplement, Aloe Vera or Daily Greens it can be due to the anti-fungal action of these products called "Die Off". Using anti-fungal supplements is a good idea yet temporary and sometimes uncomfortable reactions of flu-like symptoms, acne break outs, rashes and gas can occur especially with a history of constipation. Citrus is two-fold; first, it can act as an Antifungal causing die off and secondly it has an Acidic pH that may increase over-acidity adding to pain in the body, until the pH balance is regained. Absorbing minerals better with improved digestion will help to alkalinize the body for pH balance. Review Chapter 6 for pH Balancing, Candida and Detoxification. Zone 2 & 3 are best to keep low or avoid all grains with high symptoms of fungal infection.

Gardens Are Good: Gardens give back on many levels! Keep homegrown family gardens in mind for the future if you do not already garden. If you are not in a living space to start a garden project perhaps you can buy from a local farm or neighbor however don't stress over not gardening. Growing your own vegetables, fruits and herbs can add greatly to your health and give some extra financial savings to boot. Even a single pot or planter to grow herbs or a single tomato vine, fresh green beans or lettuce can be delicious and enjoyable. Gardening can be fun as well to connect us with the miracle of life itself and it can become a terrific stress reducer. The fun and enjoyment of sharing food with family and friends is really a treat yet not a requirement!

Grains & Beans Can Be Gaseous: Avoid soy, soy milk, gluten flour, whole grains not sprouted, regular Russet and other potatoes because they contain more starch than the approved red potato and yams. Many grains and beans are advertised as gluten free including the amaranth, quinoa, buckwheat, rice (all types), millet, triticale, bulgur, couscous (wheat) and spelt. Eat any grain with caution because many cause increased digestive symptoms. Oatmeal is a major GIS trigger grain discussed throughout the book. Popcorn and other corn products may also be a major allergy and trigger food for both children and adults. Simply said, any beans, grains or foods that give you symptoms from eating them avoid them for the first 3 – 6 months as you build up your gut health. Amaranth is not in the grass family like rice and has been problematic for many people. Quinoa, millet, teff and white rice are tolerated much better than other grains however the high Arginine in quinoa makes it difficult for many people living with HSV to enjoy it in any quantity or face a flare-up of their Herpes (see Ch. 6 Viruses). Because GIS symptoms are based on the amount of a trigger food eaten you may find that in the future you can enjoy some popcorn or a taco on a corn tortilla occasionally (at least no gluten flour) or a small amount of beans and not experience any noticeable symptoms. Less is best of a trigger! The good news is that the GIS supplements help to speed up the body's tolerance to a wider variety of foods and decrease inflammation to begin with if you do eat too much of a trigger food they can come to the rescue!

Green Foods Sometimes Get a Red Light: Zone 2 & 3 may include symptoms of heightened chemical allergies. This is generally due to an advanced state of inflammation brought upon by poor bowel health, Candida overgrowth and at times "Environmental Toxicity". Chemical sensitivity can cause reactions to many products and otherwise healthy foods including; drugs, cleaning products, molds – cruciferous vegetables requiring the peeling of most vegetables and fruits, green leafy herbs, berries and even a temporary sensitivity to all "Green Foods". It appears to be the molecular structure present in green foods called phenols. If symptoms increase upon eating green vegetables, green leafy herbs, green supplements these foods are to be avoided for approx. 6 months. See Ch. 6 and focus on detoxification and the anti-fungal regimen to reduce Candida. As the body renews itself individuals can introduce Greens back into the diet. Yes this is very odd but very factual!

Healing Takes Patience – Give the Body Time: The need to develop patience in life is important and that applies also to the body as it heals and reverses disease. Health educator Dr. Bernard Jensen stated that people heal from the inside out and from the present back through the past! Give yourself the time and permission to heal while following the GIS Program.

1. 30 days to rebuild healthier lining tissue in the GI Tract and decrease pain.

2. 45 days to let go of bad habits and reestablish healthier ones with support and the can do attitude – Decide, Commit & Succeed!

3. 90 days to greater improvement in the digestive function, increased skin health and energy.

4. 1 year to begin rebuilding the body's organs to function better experiencing remarkable energy improvement, reduction in major disease symptoms, better brain function, less depression, better fertility and libido plus sleeping better. Skin conditions will continue to improve with many experiencing 100% resolution.

5. 3 years for new tissue systems like a healthier Nervous System, Digestive System and balanced Immune/Auto-Immune System response and stabilizing glands for a healthier weight and more youthful skin.

6. 7 years to rebuild the human Skeletal System with less bone loss, less disease symptoms, greater brain function and overall greater quality of life!

Healthy and Fresh Fats & Oils are Essential for Life Itself: Essential Fatty Acids- EFA's called Omega-3 and 6's are needed for the Nervous System, brain functions and cellular health. How this translates into each person's life (Reviewed in Ch. 5.) is the necessity to increase the amount as needed if we are to maintain healthy body metabolism in preventing cardiovascular disease, maintaining a healthy weight, building needed hormones that run the systems of the body along with keeping GIS inflammation symptoms down. Researchers find that the lipids (fats) that people eat and how well they metabolize the fats can dictate how long a person lives. These healthy fats and oils are found in fresh vegetable oils like olive, flax, sesame and if at all possible a daily consumption of quality fish oil. These are all very important Omega- 3 food sources along with eating fresh raw nuts and seeds (as tolerated), eating fatty fish and green leafy vegetables. Using natural butter fat from butter not margarine is also a good idea because butter is a natural fat (as in other dairy products) which can be utilized for energy and add to protective fat stores. Children require natural fat that comes in full fat dairy products, fish and fresh raw nuts and seeds for healthy growth and development. Fat free is not for a growing body of an active child or for most adults either. If you must reduce your fat intake choose "Low Fat" dairy foods. *Very Important:* Adequate fat in the diet allows fat soluble vitamins to be absorbed properly. Rancidity of oils is another important topic. The word "Fresh" used in describing healthy oils is important because heated and aged oils cause peroxide by-products that are linked to faster aging and even cancer development. The unhealthy fats and oils to avoid include; heated oils from fried foods and margarine which contains hydrogenated oil also both are referred to as Trans-fats. Peanut Butter can also be from roasted peanuts yet AVOID HYDROGENATED peanut butter! Researchers find that consuming hydrogenated fats deplete our reserve of healthy fats and can add to aging of the body through its oxidation. Also, avoid the overconsumption of charbroiled or charcoal burned fats because the burning of fat and charcoal together make carcinogenic chemicals called PAH's, Polycyclic Aromatic Hydrocarbons on the food surface. The US Dept. of Health defines PAH's as a group of over 100 different harmful chemicals that are formed during the incomplete burning of coal, oil and gas, garbage, or other organic substances like tobacco or charbroiled meat. Fortunately, one study showed that by marinating meats before charbroiling - actually reduced the amount of toxic residual by over 50%. Enjoy your Bar-B-Qing safely!

Herbs - Friend or Foe: Molds acting as GIS triggers may be present in herbal combinations that will cause poor health symptoms. It is best to use fresh herbs, for example garlic and onions or dried single herbs vs. a combination of herbs to season foods or in a supplement, unless you are 100% convinced that they contain no starch base or other triggers. Herbs, especially the leafy green ones, may contain molds which may significantly add to allergy reactions. Curry may be one exception to the rule. However, avoid; beef and chicken bouillon, instant soup mixes, multiple herbs together in combination or in a Multiple Vitamin and

Mineral supplement especially for chemically sensitive people in Zone 3. See Recipes for making your own delicious broth!

Label Reading for All: Become a good label reader to spot any undesirable additives and triggers; avoiding gluten and other unhealthy factors like high sodium, sugars or Trans-fats (hydrogenated). Fresh and frozen foods have more nutritional value than canned foods. Be aware that the government does allow some thickeners that are GIS triggers to be added to dairy products and processed foods and they do not demand full disclosure of ingredients. Only use canned foods as a last resort to fresh or frozen. Dried foods can also be used with discretion yet sugar may be added to dried fruits as mentioned in other sections and especially if the fruit is unusually shiny and sticks together. Avoid sugar sweetened canned fruits as well. Some bulk or box grains may contain wheat starch used in the enrichment process like instant rice.

Milk Does A Body Good or Does It? The milk of mammals has been consumed as a food source since the beginning of domesticated animals back in early times. Animal milks are naturally very sweet to encourage the young to nurse. This sweetness comes from lactose sugar in the milk. When the enzyme called lactase, designed to break down the lactose, is in short supply the lactose sugar causes inflammation in the gut and people develop gas and other symptoms (Ch. 2 and 3.). The good news is when the disaccharide of lactose changes through the enzymatic process of fermentation as in the aging of cheese and yogurt it is digested much more easily without igniting the immune system which causes the GIS reactions. Most cultures use the local animals to make dairy products to include; cows, goats, water buffalo and even camels. Nature's intent is for the baby animal or child to consume its mother's milk during infancy and once teeth develop the child or animal is weaned from the milk. Nature has not intended for adults to continuing nursing. That sounds ridiculous but it is similar to the continuation of drinking another mammal's milk! Adults are designed to receive their required nutrition from green leafy vegetables and vegetable sources. Vegetables contain the required minerals and the other non-milk protein sources available in fish, meat, beans or nuts and seeds that the body needs. Adults do not need milk but people like it. The fermented milks and milk products that contain reduced lactose can be eaten by babies at about 6 months and also by children and adults as tolerated as per the GIS Diet. The fat or cream from milk is close to 100% lactose free and therefore butter, pure cream and even whipped cream and half n' half (1000 mg per 2 T of lactose) can be enjoyed on the program for Zone 1 and many on Zone 2. Caution is required in Zone 3 with commercial whipped cream because it does contain some lactose and refined sugar. Unfortunately, milk manufacturers have added several thickeners to the "Whipping Cream" causing potential digestive upset with mainstream commercial products. *Caution:* Avoid traditional prepared ice cream due to the milk, refined sugar and thickeners that are added containing high levels of lactose and GIS triggers. New varieties in alternative ice creams are now available like Coconut ice cream or to also enjoy an occasional Soy ice cream. 100% fruit sorbets are available as well which are delicious. For the innovative person you can even make your own frozen fruit blender desserts that are exquisite and avoids the carrageenan, guar gum and other triggers. Just add a little honey or approved sweeteners as desired as outlined in the Recipe section.

Milk Alternatives Are Delish: It is no wonder that people are having increased gluten intolerance with the "Soy Craze" that started over the last decade and swept the country. Besides soy beans being a GIS trigger food another challenge with soy is that the soy milk that most people drink is highly sweetened! Refined sugar is very inflammatory remember? I have counseled more people that were experiencing Reflux and digestive symptoms shortly after beginning to drink soy milk. After stopping the soymilk they felt immensely better. Pasteurized cow's milk has already been pinpointed as a primary GIS trigger. However you can make some delicious alternative milk that is approved on the GIS Diet. Tasty milk like beverages have developed over thousands of years from different cultures. Rice milk from Mexico and the Amazaki fermented rice milk originating in Japan are both delicious. In the market you also have the choice of almond milk on the Zone 1 and some 2 folks yet not the perfect solution by any means for many people because of the mold factor and the added sugar. If you use an approved sweetener like honey or Agave Nectar to sweeten your own recipe you have several selections you can make at home. The number one choice is sesame milk made with Tahini butter. After being on the GIS diet for 3 – 6 months you can experiment with cashew nut or blanched almond milk too. They both make delicious nut milks. You can use any of the alternative milks in a recipe calling for cow's milk. Coconut milk has also become very popular and can be used after the initial 3 months. Other foods or beverages that may contain hidden dairy triggers would be dessert coffees, instant coffee mixes, instant chocolate, processed foods for luncheon meats and sausages, sauces, dressings, soups made with milk solids, thickeners and desserts. Half n Half is tolerated by most people in the Zone 1 & 2 however Zone 3 may do better using the Lactaid milk substitutes or Sesame milk. As odd as it may sound using white beans, pinto or red potatoes as natural thickeners in recipes that call for milk work well and tastes good! Use Caution friends with drinking nut and seed milk if you have Herpes. Review Chapter 6 Viruses section.

ι *Plan Your Eating for the Outing:* Establishing the discipline of taking food with you when you leave your home is very important. Most of us carry water as we travel about and if you take a small cooler or lunch pack with a blue ice you will have the option to take food back home if you find foods you can eat on an outing. Give yourself permission to experiment with packing your own snacks and meals if you don't already do it - Enjoy!

ι *Quality of Food Matters:* Foods are grown with different growing methods including; commercial, certified organic, locally grown from farmers markets and homegrown. "Commercially" grown foods are the most common from the grocery stores and mass merchandizing outlets. More "Certified Organic" foods are becoming available in these stores so look for them and purchase organic whenever possible. The nutritional content can be much greater in certified organic besides being safer and the taste of the food can also be superior. Health food store markets carry more certified organic foods and you can now look for the USDA seal on many food products that confirm their organic status with a few exceptions*. Canned, bulk items, fresh produce, dairy and meats can all come in commercial or certified organic variety. Fresh locally grown foods can be found at farmers markets and many times at reduced prices fresher and tastier and sometimes without as much chemical sprays (if marked) than the commercially grown produce. Zone 2 and 3 may have greater reactions to the chemical herbicides, pesticides and stabilizing agents found on commercial foods. Toxicity from the chemicals can be catalyst for allergy reactions adding to GIS symptoms for everyone yet make certain you read in Chapter 6 under Environment Toxicity and Allergies to understand the full impact and health risk. Shockingly some experts expound that adults and children receive up to 68 toxic chemical exposures from the foods and environment every day. Start to make an effort purchasing a few organic food items to decrease the total amount of toxic pollution you receive each week like choosing organic apples and fruits and perhaps spinach, lettuce, peanut butter, dairy products and beans.

Some Certified Organic products are not able to use the USDA Organic Seal even though the contents are Certified Organic because of food grade preservatives contained in the ingredients therefore, read the ingredient panel on the back that fully discloses the fact of "Certified Organic" status.

Make A Regular Yearly Check Up A Priority: Seek professional support when needed! If you feel that your health is not progressing following the GIS Program (which I might add is rare) and you are experiencing increased symptoms get a check-up from your doctor right away. My rule of thumb is if symptoms flare-up then simplify the program focusing on the diet and detoxification. Most people tolerate the Probiotics and a little diluted Aloe Vera juice. I am a big advocate of taking the Probiotics supplement (see Ch. 8 and also in the Highlight of Ch. 2) and many medical doctors are beginning to also see the value. Secondly, review your diet sticking to the basics while eliminating processed foods and grains (corn or rice may be causing a challenge so only eat a red potato or yam for your starch temporarily). Many people are unaware of their chemical sensitivities so review that aspect. Yearly physicals are important to maintain preventative health along with keeping up with your oral hygiene. Also, check out your environment at home and work for possible toxicity. Seasonal molds can be a separate challenge needing attention so review Allergies in Chapter 6.

' ***Raw Foods Are "Rad"***: Raw Foodies are becoming more common in society today. However, living on only raw foods is a distortion, in my opinion, of how the body was designed to be nourished on this planet. Why I believe we are seeing more "Raw Foodists" is due to the GIS that absolutely bogs a body down. Think about it for a minute, a diet that alleviates a large percentage of inflammation through only eating raw and sprouted foods is understandably a better choice than the typical over processed sugar, wheat and junk food laden diet! Most people, including myself enjoy a variety of hot cooked foods combined with raw foods as tolerated. I also crave fish and meat with some dairy thrown in. In my opinion it is the best of both worlds to seek a 50% nutritious yet properly cooked food diet with 50% raw foods - following more of a Mediterranean diet which mimics the GIS Diet. Protein for the body whatever food sources it comes from is a must! The protein also needs to be absorbed into the blood stream to ultimately build a healthy body. Digestion is very critical with all diets. The bottom line with whatever foods you choose to nourish the body with - raw or cooked - vegetarian or carnivorous - each must provide the core nutrients the body requires to survive and thrive – Bon Appetit!

Refined & Synthesized Sugars Are Not Your Friend: Do your best to visualize a neon-light flashing that states, "Avoid refined sugar to reduce inflammation at all cost!" This one step of letting go of refined sugar will help you maintain health and your family's health to such a higher degree! The best alternative is to use honey, stevia, and fruit juice concentrates and the delicious new sweetener on the scene in moderation called Agave Nectar syrup. Sugar substitutes that are also safe include; Zylitol, 100% fructose, some dextrose and surprisingly saccharin that do not cause inflammation when used appropriately. Sweeteners to avoid include; *Splenda* trademarked Sucralose, Aspartame, High Fructose Corn Syrup (HFCS), 99% refined white sugar, brown sugar, molasses, maple syrup, malt sugar, sugar coated cereals and snacks, beverage drinks like canned cocoa and coffee, sweetened liquors, sweetened vinegars, sweetened jams, salad dressings (that contain a lot of sugar), canned fruits (with sugar) and beverages including fast food sodas, candies and confections. People who abuse sugar experience a variety of disease states including more allergies, bowel disease, bone loss, depression, mental illnesses and premature aging. Review Chapter 6 Addictions to get some motivation to leave it alone and reap the rewards of better health including finding a Healthy Weight outlined in Chapter 6. Giving it the 30-Day "Just Say No to Sugar Trial" can give you the edge on showing your body who is boss!

Soy Bean Surprise: Soybeans are not recommended on the GIS program as you have been reading. Many of you will gasp in disbelief at hearing this news and some of you will defiantly keep eating and drinking the soy milk for a while anyway. Soy has a lot of marks against it as a food regardless of all of the promotions from marketers. Yes - Tofu made from soy is a traditional food and I personally love it in dishes yet I rarely eat it anymore due to my own GIS.

1. Soy is a gluten trigger due to the carbohydrate protein compound that exudes in its jelly like thickener content. If not 100% sprouted, soy is highly problematic in the GIS.

2. Soy is high in Phytates an "Anti-Nutrient" and may prevent healthy Thyroid function keeping you from healthy weight loss and contributing to other health challenges in the body.

3. Soy is high in the natural Estrogen hormone, as other beans contain a smaller amount and in my opinion is contra-indicated for women and men who are at risk for hormone related cancers of the breast or prostate. Some researchers have even suggested that boys and men eating excessive soy products may become

effeminate keeping a higher pitched voice and developing female-like breast tissue.

Stick to Your Zones - No Cheating: With high symptoms you do not want to rush adding a lot of new foods. Zone 3 and even Zone 2 may want to avoid all grains and triggers until you are on the diet and lifestyle program for at least 3 months to lessen the GIS symptoms. You must make certain your bowels are moving daily and diarrhea is under control with advanced symptoms before adding low gluten grains for a trial. White rice, millet and quinoa seem to be the three grains that you can introduce 1 – 2 times per week along with sweet potato, yam and or red potato fairly soon.

Feeling poorly? I suggest you go back to the basics of your zone diet. There is nothing wrong with going without solid food and relying on light soup for a few days. Next add light foods perhaps squash and a tolerable protein of white fish or soft cooked chicken as an example. Organic baby food is another tip to keep on hand for rough days. Consult your physician as needed for the "Elemental Liquid Diet" if you are not able to tolerate food for more than a week or if other symptoms escalate stay in touch with your physician and other health professional supporters.

In following Zone 1 of the GIS Diet more preventatively because of low symptoms eating with flexibility doesn't appear to rock the boat. On a cellular level your body may be having some inflammation in the gut and in some rare individuals quite a bit. However, for most people, if it doesn't cause you to run to the bathroom, have gas or constipation, eating a sandwich with regular bread once a day is no big deal. If it is causing challenges then a lunch salad may be a better choice. You may also be able to partake in ice cream and other GIS trigger foods occasionally without any obvious mental or physical distress. Yet I do encourage you to stop abusing your body by eating an abundance of trigger foods. GIS is real and you who choose not to heed the warnings may end up with Diabetes, increased CVD or even Cancer if you do not already live with these diseases! Review Chapter 5 Glossary of Conditions to make a more in-depth inventory of your true health status. The Mediterranean Diet (MD) is very similar to the GIS Diet only it has more whole grains included in it! Researchers find that eating the MD the incidence of all diseases is reduced along with mortality! Recent findings in Spain showed an even greater improvement in all health markers when participants included a small handful of raw seeds and or nuts. In the GIS Diet it customizes to three categories of people and the degree of inflammation and illness in their bodies that they experience. It then makes recommendations (as tolerated) to keep the gluten grains lower along with the other GIS triggers making it the most effective diet for mankind!

Survive Restaurant Foods: Eating in restaurants demands "Assertiveness Training" to order successfully off the menu while adhering to the GIS Diet and enjoy your meal while eating it and afterwards. Remember it is OK to be polite and assertive at the same time - YOU are the customer. Fortunately with the evolving awareness about gluten intolerance in the restaurant world - you can say that you are on a special diet that forces you to ask for substitutions. Offer to pay a little more and most of the time I find a waiter is happy to comply with your wishes. You will enjoy your meal more and tipping is a great way to reward a business that truly works with its patrons! A last word when eating out, beware of added gluten flours to corn and flour tortillas and unfortunately even sour dough breads are resorting to adding extra gluten flour to avoid crumbling! Even breads in the marketplace that were once ideal for gluten intolerance have resorted to adding the additional gluten flour. This is why it is important to read labels. Rule of thumb is to avoid breadstuff when eating out and go for entrées, soups and salads. Many restaurants are now putting their menus on the Internet as well so you can check them out ahead of time for GIS prevention possibilities!

Thickeners - Pick Them Carefully or They Will Pick on You: Unfortunately our government allows some thickeners (including wheat flour) in products that are not disclosed to the public on the ingredient panel. Chocolate milk has thickeners as does yogurts, cottage cheese and some processed cheeses, roasted chickens, luncheon meats and other meats including sausages. Use caution when purchasing already cooked whole chickens or sliced deli meats where wheat and other seasonings are often injected into the meat to enhance the flavor. Look for the brand *Boarshead* Deli Meats and their other meats that are Gluten Free (GF). The GIS Diet approved thickeners to use in recipes include; eggs, Xanthan Gum powder, beans and red potatoes which are tolerated by most people. White pastry flour even though it is from wheat and tapioca flour contains the lowest percent of gluten triggers and is allowed in small amounts especially in Zone 1 diet and occasionally Zone 2. Most thickeners and grain ingredients are found in processed foods or are added in home food preparation. It is much better to switch over to non-trigger thickeners because you feel better. 9 out of 10 people feel better eating Gluten Free even if they do not consider themselves Gluten Intolerant! See Recipes that use the GIS approved thickeners. *Avoid*: guar gum, carrageenan, agar-agar, pectin (jams & jellies), amaranth, gluten flour, whole wheat flour (brownish in color), gelatin (all types) and starch (include the following as tolerated - tapioca, arrowroot, corn and sago).

ᴠ *Variety in Food Choices Count:* Variety is one of the most important habits people can develop in reaching an optimum diet at any age. By choosing different foods within each category of protein (meats, beans, dairy and nuts and seeds), carbohydrates (vegetables & fruits) and also fats and oils - it gives the body more of an "All you can eat buffet!" When people eat a mono diet or eat the same foods day after day it is very boring along with limiting the daily nutrition greatly! Busy or undisciplined people like to simplify their choices yet by doing so they cheat themselves in the long run with limiting their selections. Developing natural cravings for whole foods can become a guide to choose more variety in the diet. Researchers have compelling evidence to show that the cells actually signal the senses that give people a craving for a particular piece of fruit as when the body is requiring more Vitamin C! Continue to experiment with new and different foods broadening your choices to reach a higher level of enjoyment and health.

Vegetarians Beware: Eating a Vegetarian diet has lots of pluses yet it is important to pay attention to warning signs of possible nutritional deficiencies that may develop and GIS warnings as well. All humans must follow the biological rules that govern health including Vegetarians to live a full and long healthy life. People cannot make up their own rules and expect to live healthy! This is true especially if you are excluding all flesh foods, dairy products and eggs as in the Vegan Diet or are following a diet of just fruit or limited raw foods. Make certain whatever diet you are following that you give the body all the nutrition it truly requires by getting blood work and physical check-ups routinely.

To go without all flesh foods eliminating sea foods and meats (all types) is unusual in the history of the world. Auto-Immune diseases have been on the rise in the Vegetarian and Vegan community at an alarming rate. Philosophies can be very confusing with groups of people and the facts show that many of the foods that non-carnivores (non-meat) are eating fall into the GIS trigger classification with a high grain emphasis. Ancient indigenous people who have lived long lives have all eaten a collective diet including flesh foods, fish, fermented milk and other food ferments, dairy products, vegetables and fruits and a small amount of nuts and seeds. This has been successful for healthy aging and longevity for the Hunza's and the Japanese society that have the proof in their many Centenarians or healthy aging populations. It may surprise some of you (because there is a high incidence of disease in the US) that America is home to the greatest number of people living over 100 years of age than anywhere else in the world. The researchers think this is partly attributed to the long term care facilities but also because 100 years ago the US population was eating healthier with an emphasis on wholesome foods including fruits, vegetables and more fish in the diet. Japan has the second highest number of centenarians and researchers credit their long-life to diet and cleanliness. Historians wrote that some cultures would save the meat primarily for the men so they would have greater glandular health which as a matter of fact is essential to prolonging one's life. Men used to out-live women back in the ancient days. Yet to speak objectively going without all animal products is an odd and potentially dangerous practice especially if people have not been properly educated on the core foundational nutrient needs of the body and Anti-Nutrients. Foundational nutrients such as adequate protein must be included along with B12, not attainable in large enough amounts on a Vegan diet without supplementing. All 8-9 essential amino acids must be included from foods - in a window of 4-5 hours to make quality proteins in the body for Vegetarians. This is called "Complimenting Proteins" and is a requirement to be healthy. Animal protein is considered complete if not overcooked. Within the Gluten Inflammatory Syndrome I state that all people are gluten intolerant – it is just a question as to what degree? To be Vegetarian on the GIS Diet is not easy. It calls for eating a large percentage of fully sprouted foods not a diet based on just cooked beans and grains since those are the foods that can heighten destructive inflammation. To be a healthy Vegetarian or Vegan learn to sprout your foods if you have not incorporated sprouts already - complimented by fresh raw juices and the use of quality food supplements to compensate for any nutritional deficiencies you may experience and enjoy!

Veggies Are For All Zones: The CDC states that only 25% of Americans are eating adequate vegetables for health and that only about 10% are incorporating a healthy balanced diet! Join the health revolution before your health is pulled out from under you. I call that the "Rug Syndrome" when people keep eating just protein and junk foods WHAM – sickness shows up! People who get the sickest on the planet eat the least amount of vegetables. Eat fresh, frozen and very little from a can due to potential chemical triggers and over processing. Nutritional value plus flavor has been found to be superior in fresh and frozen vegetables. Children who are raised eating vegetables of all types grow up to enjoy the taste of vegetables. You can learn to like the taste of vegetables by slowly reintroducing them back into your diet on a regular basis. Many people that have not been eating sufficient veggies often like them better raw in salads and with dipping sauce - Delicious! Remember during your health transition you can take a vegetable supplement to compensate for the lack of intake (Ch. 8) and you just might continue it like I did because you find out how good you can truly feel! Eating vegetables and some fruits with a variety of protein sources will allow you to once again experience vibrant and youthful health!

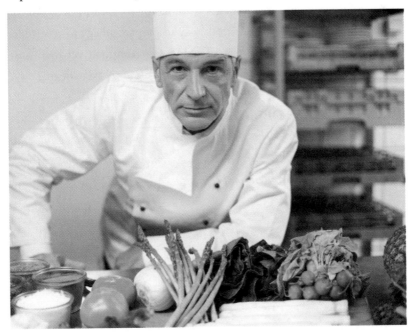

Healthy & Tasty Recipes

Zone 1, 2 & 3

Breakfast, lunch and dinner selections may be traditional choices, ethnic fun foods or whatever you and your stomach are in the mood for. The following recipe section gives ideas for each meal and some healthy dessert ideas that come with no guilt. A very important decision you will want to give consideration to whether you are eating out or dining at home - and that is the decision to include food selections that support health at least 80% of the time!

Eggs

Eggs are easy to prepare and give excellent nutrition for all ages. They are known as the perfect protein which all other proteins are compared to for nutritional value. Eggs can be part of any meal or snack and also used as a good binder for a casserole, muffins, sauce or dessert dish. Once digestion improves on the GIS Program most people find that they can digest egg protein very well. One egg gives approximately 8 grams of a complete protein and provides a good source of B12 if not overcooked. Poached eggs are the most nutritious way to prepare an egg to receive its optimum nutrition. Other styles of fixing eggs are good yet high heat destroys the B-Complex including B12 and protein to some degree.

POACHED EGGS - DELICIOSO!

Poached eggs are easy to make and are actually more successful than cooking soft boiled eggs that are awkward to remove from the shell at times. Both styles have similar nutritional content.

2	**fresh eggs**
1½	**cups raw spinach**
2 -3	**slices Portobello mushroom**
1	**sliced English muffin 100% sprouted (optional)**
	Butter
	Olive oil
3	**tablespoon white vinegar**
1	**teaspoon Soy Sauce - wheat free low sodium**
	Basil Leaf or Flakes
	Parsley
	Salt & Pepper
	Quick Hollandaise Sauce, Ranch Dressing or Mock Mayo

Mock Mayo Sauce

1	**cup Greek yogurt**
1	**tablespoon sour cream**
1½	**teaspoon mustard**
2	**teaspoons rice vinegar or lemon**
	Salt and pepper

Zone 3 – Omit Muffin and serve poached eggs over spinach leaves. Serve with Pan Fried Red Potatoes or fruit compote.

1. Easy to prepare; slice the muffin ready for toasting.
2. Clean spinach and mushroom slices and pat dry.
3. Next add olive oil to an 8 inch sauté pan turned to medium heat. Add mushroom slices and 1 tsp. soy sauce and slightly brown both sides and remove from pan onto plate.
4. In a second clean skillet add (1) inch of water, add vinegar and salt and bring to a boil. Reduce heat and add both eggs. Prepare eggs for water by breaking eggs one at a time into a small bowl and gently slide eggs into the water at a close angle. Let the eggs cook in boiling water until whites are set about 2 minutes. *Microwave Cooking:* Fill medium size custard cup halfway with water and (1) teaspoon vinegar. Next crack egg into water and heat at medium for 60 – 75 seconds covered with a napkin. Works nearly perfect every time for busy people.
5. Push toaster down while cooking eggs, butter toast and place on plate. Place half of the spinach on each muffin or on plate, place poached egg on muffin or on spinach (using slotted spoon), sauce as desired and top or dress the plate with slices of portabella and Basil Leaf.
6. Makes 2 servings add salt and pepper – Voila!

MOMMA MIA - FRITTATA

Pronounced Freet-TAH-tah it is an open faced omelet that originated in Italy. It takes on the shape of the pan it is cooked in with the ingredients mixed into the eggs before cooking. Frittatas can be made fried on top of the stove in a skillet or half fried and then baked in the oven.

4-6   eggs
2   cups vegetables; greens chard, kale, asparagus, zucchini, red or green bell pepper and more (best to precook)

½ -1   **small onion**

1   **clove garlic; fresh or ½-1 tsp. powdered**
       Olive oil
       Butter
       Salt & Pepper

2T.   **Herbs; parsley, thyme, basil, cayenne (hot), or other**

1   **cup precooked meat or fish as desired – salmon, chicken, turkey, etc.**

1   **cup grated Cheese; Swiss, cheddar, misc. or topped with 2 T of grated parmesan cheese**

½   **cup sour cream or cottage cheese (optional)**

1. Pick a large skillet 12 inches approx to cook on top of stove. Heat olive oil 1-2 T medium heat and sauté chopped or sliced onion until color changes. Add minced garlic and herbs toward the end to warm. If chard or kale is used make certain to wash first and pat dry, chop into medium pieces then add to the onion and herbs or add other precooked vegetables that have been cut into bit size pieces. Once warmed turn heat off.

2. In a separate large bowl beat eggs and add the cheese, meat, salt, pepper and the rest of the skillet contents and blend completely by hand.

3. Add 1 T olive oil back into skillet and turn heat to medium.

4. Add all ingredients back into hot skillet pan and cook approx 1 ½ minutes then turn heat to low and set timer for 12 minutes with a COVERED tight fitting lid. You may wish to cut the Frittata in half and carefully flip the frittata to brown on the top surface completing the cooking and avoiding any raw egg.

5. Alternative is to Oven Bake: Turn all blended ingredients into an oiled 2 quart casserole dish 9 x 2 x 11 inches and cook uncovered at 350 degrees preheated oven for 35 – 50 minutes or until set. Insert a toothpick or a knife into center and pull out. It is cooked if no egg or ingredients shows on the tester.

6. Approx 20 grams of protein in a 4 x 4 inch square.

7. Serve with fresh Grated Parmesan cheese & sliced basil leaf or parsley on top. Enjoy for breakfast, lunch or dinner. Just add a side of fruit, salad or soup to serve 6 – 8 people or have great leftovers!

SPICY BREAKFAST EGG BURRITO

This is a quick breakfast that tastes great and the varieties are endless with scrambled eggs. White flour of Teff tortillas (without gluten flour added) can be eaten on Zone 1 & 2. Zone3 enjoy your scrambled eggs with fried potatoes, no tortilla unless well tolerated.

2-4   eggs; scrambled in olive oil
1   tablespoon diced onion; scallions or any type (opt.)
2   slices cooked turkey or other bacon (Zone 1-2)
      or low sodium deli turkey or other meat (Zone 3)
2   tablespoons shredded cheese
2   white flour tortillas or corn tortillas heated on the side (opt.)
      Salsa (opt.)

Dry heat tortillas in a pan on top of the stove both sides as desired.

Butter and place on a plate. Place your eggs, meat and or shredded cheese and salsa, as desired, inside the tortilla and fold.

Makes 2 large burritos - Ole!

QUICHE

Great for Breakfast, Lunch or Dinner Quiche has many variations including;(a.) vegetables like zucchini, spinach, chard, onions, mushrooms, red sweet peppers (b.) meats like bacon, ham, chicken, turkey, sausage, seafood's and (c.) cheeses like Swiss, Jack, Parmesans, Cheddars and even Cottage cheese. Be creative and customize your Basic Quiche recipe to your own appetite.

Basic Quiche Crustless (GF)

10   eggs, beaten
½   cup butter
1   cup Cottage cheese, Nancy's brand or large curd
1   pound Jack cheese, shredded
½   cup GF flour, rice type or white flour as tolerated
1   teaspoon baking powder

1.   Melt the butter and place in a medium bowl. Beat eggs until fluffy and add them to the butter mixing together. Next add the rest of the ingredients and blend thoroughly.

2.   Add 1 cup of any other ingredients to the mix making certain they are cut into bite size pieces, vegetables, meats or seafood's and additional herbs. Blend well and pour into large 9 x 13 oiled baking dish uncovered.

3.   Bake in preheated oven at 350 degrees for 35 – 40 minutes until the top is lightly browned. This is good for Zone 3 without crust and little dairy.

4.   Serve with fresh grated parmesan cheese, steamed vegetables or a simple salad – Enjoy!

QUICHE LORRAINE

2 Flaky Pie crust, store-bought white crusts or homemade with rice flour by *Authentic Foods* listed in Reference or other

6   eggs, beaten
1   cup half and half
¾   cup vegetable and or meat/seafood's filling; spinach and mushroom
¼   teaspoon salt
¼   teaspoon ground white pepper
¼   teaspoon freshly grated nutmeg
1½   grated Gruyere or regular Swiss, may combine with Jack
2   tablespoons parsley, chopped

1. Preheat oven to 375 degrees. Fork stab each pie crust on the face before cooking empty for 5 - 6 minutes in oven to allow air to escape during prebaking. This also guarantees the crust to be thoroughly cooked and better tasting.

2. In a medium bowl place eggs and beat well then add half and half and herbs and blend well with a whisk. A second bowl will be holding the desired filling pre-cooked meat and partially steamed vegetables heated in the microwave or other.

3. Next take pie crust that have been precooked and fill each with half the cheese setting aside 2 tablespoons of cheese for the topping before cooking. Next take half of the filling and layer over the cheese on each pie. Lastly, divide the liquid egg mixture evenly between the two pies and top with 1 tablespoon of cheese on each pie plus some parsley as desired.

4. Bake on middle rack of oven until eggs are totally set approximately 35 – 40 minutes and pies take on a slightly golden color. Remove from oven and let cool on a wire rack for 15 minutes before serving. Serve with a simple salad – Enjoy!

Cereals

Box cereals may be eaten for breakfast and snacks (as tolerated) and provide some nutritional value but are not the best choice because they are highly processed using high heat that destroys a lot of the original nutrients. Corn, rice or millet cereals are the more common choices in ready to eat varieties for low gluten. Check out the oat-free Trail Mix recipe eaten more for a snack than a meal. Also, any grain can be soaked for 1 - 2 days allowing them to sprout (even oats) and then cooked for better digestion like the traditional Muesli eaten in European countries. For now the whole grain breakfast recipes of hot cereal, porridge, pancakes and muffins using the low gluten grains do give a lot of variety for kids and adults in Zone 1 & Zone 2!

HOT MILLET APPLE CINNAMON CEREAL

Hot cereal taste great on a chilly morning or anytime for that matter if you prepare it with some complementing toppings and spices. Remember oatmeal is not a recommended GIS food. Millet is an oatmeal alternative being considered a low gluten grain, in the grass family like buckwheat, originating in China, India and Japan and spreading into Asia, Africa and over into South America and the US.. Millet has a pleasant corn-rice flavor. It is very high in Iron with impressive levels of protein for a grain at almost 9 grams per one cup cooked. Millet is also referred to as an alkaline grain as is Buckwheat. All grains need to be complemented by another protein source at the same meal; yogurt, nuts or seeds, eggs, meat or beans will do just that. Millet can be enjoyed for breakfast, lunch or dinner meals. Cooking larger amounts of millet to enjoy for several days is a time saver. Serve it hot with butter at any meal or with stewed or fresh fruit and yogurt for breakfast - tastes delicious!

1   cup of Millet (hulled)
3   cups of water
1   apple; sliced
1   tablespoon butter
½   teaspoon cinnamon (opt. - may sprinkle separately on top)
1   teaspoon honey or Agave Nectar syrup

1. In a 2 quart medium sauce pan bring the water to a boil. Add millet and all other ingredients and cover with a tight fitting lid. Cook for 20 minutes on a medium to low heat simmer boil. Millet grains puff up expanding like rice to make approximately 4 cups of cooked millet.

2. Makes 3-4 Servings.

3. Serve as a breakfast cereal with yogurt, butter and 100% fruit preserves or seasonal fresh fruit – Enjoy!

POLENTA OR BOILED CORNMEAL

Polenta was originally eaten throughout Northern Italy, during the cold winter days as porridge. Multiple grains were used in the polenta porridge such as; millet, buckwheat, spelt, barley, chestnuts, chick-peas and broad beans. As corn became more plentiful the polenta made from corn meal became very popular and caught on throughout Italy. It traveled down through the south where it was once snubbed and began to be eaten as a side dish with vegetables, fish and meats. This cornmeal mush or corn cake as it is made can be included in the diet by most people on Zone 1 and 2, unless a person has known corn sensitivity. Zone 3 can sometimes enjoy corn!

Basic Polenta

6	cups water
2	teaspoons salt
1¾	cups yellow cornmeal
2-3	tablespoons butter

1. Bring water to a boil in a heavy sauce pan.
2. Add the salt and begin pouring the cornmeal into the boiling water as you stir with a whisk.
3. Makes 6 servings.
4. Reduce the heat to a slow boil as you stir often for about 15 minutes. Turn off the heat and stir in the butter - Enjoy!

Another alternative to eating it as porridge is to cool it and cut the polenta into strips. Then top it with cream cheese or sprinkled with fresh grated parmesan cheese and enjoy as finger bread.

COCONUT POLENTA CON MANGO

Make this delicious recipe that can be eaten as a breakfast or a dessert meal. A second alternative is to replace the coconut milk with 1 ½ cups water and ¼ cup of half n half omitting pepper and mango and serve it with other seasonal fruit such as papaya or pears – both delicious!

¾   cup Quick Cooking Polenta or regular corn meal

1   cup of coconut milk, unsweetened

½   cup water

2   ripe mangos, peeled into cubes

Salt

Cayenne pepper, opt.

1-2   tablespoons honey

1. Bring milk and water to a boil in a medium size pan.

2. In a second pan with butter sauté mango or other fruit (papaya, peach, apricot or pears) for 3 minutes then mix with honey, salt and pepper as desired.

3. Add polenta to boiling water and stir frequently for 5 – 7 minutes at a medium heat and then stir in ¾ of the fruit mixture. When done it should have a creamy texture.

4. Serve in bowls topped with a little more fruit and yogurt-enjoy! Makes 3 Servings.

GUILTLESS PANCAKES

Pancakes are a traditional breakfast food that can still be enjoyed by many people in Zone 1 & 2 Diets unless you flat out do not feel good eating any flours. Some people choose not to indulge because of lingering symptoms even though both millet and the white rice flours are the best gluten free grains in my opinion. White pastry flour even though it is from wheat is tolerated quite well by many people for pancakes occasionally or eaten out in a restaurant as per Chapter 1 states because it has the lowest content of irritants compared to any other type of wheat flour. Varying the spices and additions you can make pancakes for breakfast, lunch or dinner as a bread or dessert. Crepes which have a thinner consistency than a traditional pancake can also be enjoyed on the GIS Diet as you wish for a little more of a gourmet twist!

2   cup rice flour

2   eggs-beaten

¾   cup yogurt, Greek style or homemade

½   cup half n half or other

4   tablespoon honey

¼-½   cup water

1- 2   tablespoon Olive Oil

¼   tsp. Spices: cinnamon, clove and vanilla

2   tablespoon Butter, melted but not hot   as desired.

4   tsp Baking Powder

1   tsp. Salt

1. Every kitchen needs a skillet you can make pancakes on. Use a cast iron skillet, non stick or reliable pan that the cakes will not stick to.

2. Oil your skillet with vegetable oil.

3. Skillet is ready to cook your cakes when a drop of water easily evaporates off the surface.

4. In a large bowl place rice flour. Next blend wet ingredients with a fork and mix into flour. Adjust thickness of batter with water as needed to a medium thick yet fluid texture.

5. Add any fruit desired to batter at this point like cut up ripe bananas or apples.

6. Drop about 1/3 cup of pancake batter on hot skillet. A solid measuring cup works well.

7. Cook approx 2 minutes on each side until nicely browned. First side keep pan lid off and once flipped put a lid on to speed cooking throughout the pancakes. Usually done when they puff up.

8. Makes 8 – 9 medium pancakes.

Serve with fresh fruit or 100% fruit preserves, yogurt and peanut butter (as desired). A small amount of maple syrup (or better yet Agave Nectar) is permitted on Zone 1 & 2. Break apart your first batch to make certain egg has completely cooked - Enjoy!

MUFFINS ANYONE?

A basic muffin recipe can be altered according to your desires. I have used the following recipe with rice flours, cornmeal, cooked millet and other flours. Experiment with whatever low gluten and gluten free flours that you think will work for you and the family for Zones 1 & 2. Zone 3 is generally too sensitive for grains at this time. As the 100% GIS flourless flours are made available then more people will be able to enjoy bread products. I fix muffins every few months by purchasing (GF or LG) flours and mixes from "Authentic Foods" listed in the Reference section. Their products guarantee a delicious recipe!

2	cups flour (any LG or GF variety)
4	tablespoons honey or approved sweetener
1	tablespoon baking powder or equivalent (omit if already in the flour)
½	teaspoon salt
2	eggs, well beaten or other binder
¾	cup water
¼	cup half n half
¼	pound butter (½ cup), melted and cooled slightly

1. Preheat oven to 400 F degrees.
2. Sift together the dry ingredients.
3. Mix the eggs, milk and butter and add to dry ingredients.
4. Only beat the batter until smooth.
5. Scoop into buttered or oiled muffin pans or cups filling about 2/3.
6. Bake 20 minutes or until toothpick or knife blade pulls out clean upon checking.
7. Makes 12 – 16 muffins.

Variations: Add ¾ cup chopped cranberries or other dried fruit like dates or chopped nuts to dry ingredients. May drop honey and add ¾ cup of grated cheese to dry ingredients plus any herbs – Enjoy!

QUICK FRESH STRAWBERRY ENGLISH MUFFIN

1   **100% sprouted English muffin, cut and toasted**

2   **fresh strawberries, sliced**

1   **tablespoon peanut butter**

     Butter

- Spread butter and peanut butter evenly on muffin.
- Top with sliced strawberries – Enjoy!

SWEET POTATO CORNBREAD

1   **cup cornmeal, stoneground**

1   **cup GF Multi-flour (rice),** *Authentic Foods* **brand or other**

½   **teaspoon baking soda**

1   **teaspoon baking powder**

     Pinch of sea salt

¾ **cup sweet potato puree or pumpkin, cooked fresh or canned**

3   **eggs**

½   **cup olive oil**

4   **tablespoons honey or natural sweetener**

1   **teaspoon pure Vanilla extract**

½   **teaspoon cinnamon**

1   **teaspoon pumpkin pie spice**

1. Preheat the oven to 350 degrees. Grease the bottom of a 7 – 8 inch cake pan and dust it with flour. In a large mixing bowl, whisk the eggs and oil together. Add the sweet potato puree and mix together.

2. In a separate bowl mix together cornmeal, flour and other dry ingredients. Add the dry ingredients into the wet stirring by hand until it is smooth. Pour batter into pre-greased pan.

3. Bake on the center rack in oven for about 45 minutes or until the cornbread is firm to touch and a tooth pick or a sharp knife blade pulls out clean.

4. Recipe courtesy of Internet WebMD – Delicious!

CRANBERRY NUT BREAD

2	cups GF Flour, *Authentic Foods*, Classical Blend
1	cup sugar, Xylitol recommended
2	teaspoons baking powder
½	teaspoons baking soda
¾	teaspoons Xanthan Gum from *Authentic Foods*
1	teaspoon salt
¼	cup butter
½	cup plus 2 tablespoons Orange juice
¼	cup half and half
¼	cup water
2	eggs, slightly beaten
½	cup walnuts, shelled and chopped
2	cups fresh Cranberries, coarsely chopped
1	tablespoon freshly grated orange rind (organic)

1. Preheat oven to 350 degrees. Grease a 9 x 5 inch loaf pan and dust with flour.

2. Mix dry ingredients together and then slowly add butter until well blended. Next blend in orange juice and lastly add the rest of the ingredients mixing evenly into batter.

3. Pour batter into pan and bake for 55 – 60 minutes or until a knife inserted in the center pulls out clean. Remove bread from oven and let cool 10 minutes and then cool completely on rack. Wrap in plastic wrap and chill before cutting. Can be stored in the refrigerator for one week and in the freezer for 5 weeks. Serve with nut butter, sweet butter or Horizons cream cheese - Enjoy!

RED POTATO HASH BROWNS

Make plenty of this recipe to enjoy at breakfast and even another meal perhaps. Yams can be used with this recipe if you like however I find them more delectable at lunch or dinner for my own taste. Serve hash browns with eggs, meats or as a side at any meal.

6	medium red potatoes, cooked and cooled
2	tablespoons olive oil
1	tablespoon butter
1	medium onion, sliced or diced
1 - 2	cloves of garlic or garlic powder
	Salt & Pepper
	Parsley or Cilantro, chopped

1. Boil potatoes in a medium pan covered until tender 35 minutes, drain and cool.
2. Slice potatoes to the size you prefer either cubed, coin or moon shape.
3. Simmer onions in a large skillet with olive oil until caramelized, 10-15 minutes.
4. Makes 4 servings.
5. Add the sliced potatoes and brown about 3-4 minutes then turn add seasoning and butter. Enjoy!

BREAKFAST STIR FRY

A Stir Fry for breakfast can really give a refreshing taste break from the traditional eggs and cereal especially if you have issues with some breakfast foods. Any leftover meat, beans or eggs may be used for your main protein in the stir fry. Vegetables can vary to what you have on hand. Serve with noodles or white rice in Zone 1 and 2.

1	cup diced meat or 2 eggs (beaten for scrambling)
1 -1½	cups of vegetables; snow peas, red or green bell peppers,

broccoli, green onions or zucchini, tomato, red potato, chard, spinach

1 tablespoon onion, chopped

1 tablespoon cilantro or parsley

1 - 2   teaspoons herbs of choice; ginger, garlic, tarragon or other

1 - 3   teaspoons soy sauce, wheat free and low sodium

1   tablespoons water

1 - 3   cups cooked rice or soba noodles (optional)

1 - 3   teaspoons oil; sesame, olive or other

1. Heat 1 - 2 teaspoon(s) oil in a medium size skillet on medium heat.

2. Add onion, herbs and firmer vegetables like potato, zucchini or others first and sauté for 3 minutes turning then add cooked meat, water and other vegetables and cook for 2 minutes with lid.

3. If eggs are used instead of meat omit water and add another teaspoon of oil. Add to vegetables and cook using spatula to fluff eggs. Mix cooked eggs into vegetables well. Makes 2 or more servings.

4. Serve over precooked noodles or alone – Enjoy!

SAUSAGE STIR FRY

Review the ingredients on the package of any sausages you may be purchasing because sugar from corn syrup, milk solids and wheat or grain fillers are used in making most sausages. If in Zone 1 or 2 you may wish to enjoy a brand that is 90% (GF) or better like the Apple Gate by Sheldon's. Zone 3 may be able to enjoy this brand as well. Sheldon's also makes delicious turkey, chicken hotdogs and sausage patties that are gluten free too!

6   or more sausages, sliced

½   cup onions, diced (opt.)

4   cups greens; chard, kale, spinach, etc, chopped

1 - 2   teaspoons olive oil

1. Heat olive oil in medium size skillet on medium heat.
2. Add onions and sausages (pre-cooked boiling for 6 minutes) turning to brown on both sides 4 - 5 minutes total. Makes 3 servings.
3. Add greens (washed and cleaned) and cook with lid on pan for another minute or until tender. May serve with low lactose cottage cheese, cheddar cheese or alone and Enjoy!

HEARTY DAYBREAK MISO SOUP

Japanese have enjoyed this traditional soup for centuries. Miso is made from fermenting soybeans so it is warm and soothing without the potential irritation of eating soybeans.

Miso soup is thought to wake up the nervous system while providing valuable nutrients possibly B12, the body requires for health. Research also supports miso's protective action for people guarding them from radiation toxicity. This hearty vegetable miso soup may be enjoyed for breakfast, lunch or dinner. I love this soup served with Julienne cut radishes and hard boiled eggs!

½ - 1   cup onion, sliced longwise very thin
1 - 6   mushroom; portabella, shitake or other
1 - 2   zucchini, sliced or grated
1   cup carrots, sliced or grated
5 - 6   tablespoons miso soup; red miso is very medicinal (1 tsp miso = 340 mg. 14% DV of sodium)
2   quarts water
2 - 6   tablespoons cilantro

1. In a large 6 quart soup pot combine 2 quarts water and bring to a simmer.
2. Add vegetables except cilantro and cook covered about 10 – 15 minutes until tender.

3. Remove one cup of liquid to blend with the miso paste and then carefully add it back to the pot. Makes 3 or more servings.

4. Blend the cilantro into the warm soup a few minutes before serving and Enjoy!

Smoothies for Meals and Treats

Smoothies can be enjoyed for breakfast, lunch and dinner or a highly nutritious snack. Dessert Smoothies can also be a scrumptious treat in-between meals. Remember to "chew your drink" which allows the necessary flow of digestive juices into the stomach which is required for healthy digestion. Smoothies also provide a short cut, to consolidate powdered and liquid food supplements by adding them directly into the blender drink. There are lots of variations to choose from yet the most important step is to get started with a protein choice if used for a meal replacement. Most people do not get enough quality protein into their daily diet which is needed for health. Smoothies are a terrific way for both children and adults to hit their health target!

Choosing a Protein Powder

Blender drinks have been used for a quick nutritious meal by millions of people of all ages around the globe. Purchasing a protein powder may be a new experience for you yet it is a very smart step to incorporate one and it helps to achieve three nutritious meals daily whether mixed in a glass with juice and water or made in a blender with foods. Keep in mind that you want to buy or decide on a protein source to use right away so you can begin experimenting but it must agree with your particular digestive parameters.

The best choices for a protein supplement on the GIS Diet include; a 100% Whey Isolate low in lactose sugars yet some products are a combination blend of regular whey and can cause symptoms and digestive upset. Egg protein powder is also tolerated by many people (either whole egg, or egg white) and generally is a good choice if a person can eat eggs without GI distress. Sprouted brown rice, rice mixtures, yellow pea, hemp or another specialty protein supplement such as fish meal (if it doesn't sound too far out) works well for many in the Zone 2 and 3 Diets! I have reviewed this subject over the years and quite honestly with the high price of fish meal supplements (for humans mind you) and as tasty as some of the veggie or fruit blender drinks are in the juice section - an individual that is OK with fish such as sardines or precooked fish can add it directly into the blender plus the other ingredients in the recipe for an enjoyable drink. There is 14 grams of protein in just two sardines! *Caution:* If using other cooked fish for drinks make certain any bones are removed before adding to the blender.

Common Types of Protein Powders or Foods for Smoothie Drinks with GIS

- 100% Whey Isolate (Zone 1 can also use Whey Combination products and other sources as tolerated) – Zone 1 and 2.
- Egg Protein – Zone 1, 2 or 3.
- Sprouted Rice, Hemp, Pea or other Vegetable Powders – Zone 1 or 2.
- Fish Powder or Free Form Amino Acid Liquid (follow directions on bottle) – Zone 3, 2 or 1.
- Dietary Choices for the blender; beans combined with nut and seed butter, sardines or precooked fish (deboned), sprouts, yogurt or other – All Zones as tolerated.

Many people on Zone 1 and 2 can use several different types of protein powders except from soy, casein or "milk powder solids" variety. A good Homemade Yogurt or an acceptable Greek Style one that agrees with a person's digestion can also become a protein addition to the smoothie if other products create symptoms. Some of these protein powder choices are just asking for GIS trouble with certain people that have advanced symptoms in Zone 2 and 3.

Zone 3 does best taking the liquid amino acid supplements. If working through a GI upset or temporary crisis use the liquid amino acid supplements, a fish supplement (remember no gelatin) or a food protein* from several sources to include raw vegetable juices (see recipe for Blender Juices), plus relying on eating protein available in the diet and or occasionally from baby foods. The prescription for the Elemental Diet can also be requested if severe malnutrition is present obtained through a physician.

Some exceptions do exist for Zone 3 individuals using the sprouted pea, hemp or rice protein powders successfully (see Reference). Sometimes the straight whey isolate is also tolerated in Zone 2 along with Zone 1. To be honest it takes experimenting with two or three different products to see what works best and then at times you might need to change the source. Because a manufacturer is blending the ingredients with more than one protein in some of the products it can make experimenting a bit more challenging to find the one that agrees with your body the best. The rule of thumb is when confused always rely on the dietary choices and perhaps experiment with vegetable juices. *Note:* Ensure drinks are generally not well tolerated. They can add calories and some nutrition yet often they will increase GIS symptoms of the GI tract and even bring about mood disorders because of the ingredients (review Ch. 5)!

*May use ¾ cup of cooked beans and 1 tablespoon of seed butter like peanut, sesame or pumpkin seed butter (this makes a GF complete protein) for one serving or use another suggested protein following any recipe in this section. This may sound odd like using sardines yet it can taste delicious with the other ingredients added and it is very nutritious!

BANANA DATE SMOOTHIE

8	oz water
1	Scoop Protein Powder (16 grams protein approx.) - Example; Whey, egg, pea, other
1	ripe banana
3	pitted dates or other; apple, kiwis, blueberries or ½ cup other
¼ - ½	cup yogurt (optional) – Greek Style or 1 tablespoon nut

or seed butter; Sesame Tahini, Peanut Butter (as a milk substitute)

½   teaspoon vanilla extract

Supplements – greens, aloe, probiotics, multiple liquid or powder, fish oil or flax oil

1. Start with pouring water into blender making certain it is in full working order.
2. Add the rest of the ingredients for your creation.
3. Buzz to mix for about 2 minutes.
4. It is possible to make extra and keep in the refrigerator until desired.
5. If making for two people you can add a second scoop of protein powder and adjust the liquid and fruit as desired. Makes about 16 ounces of Smoothie-Enjoy!

FRUIT JUICE SMOOTHIE

8   oz water

1   scoop protein powder

½   cup of apple juice

1 - 2   seasonal fruits (for a blender)

Caution: Only include fruit and juices as blood sugar allows

1. Start with placing water into the blender or a large glass.
2. Add all ingredients and buzz in blender or mix rapidly with a fork if using only fruit juice and water. Smoothie is ready to drink and you may desire to include; a small handful of trail mix; cashews, pumpkin or sunflower seeds, a 100% sprouted English muffin or a piece of gluten free toast or homemade muffin.
3. May Add: Liquid or Powdered Supplements to this recipe – Enjoy!

VEGETABLE SMOOTHIE

8   ounces water

1   scoop protein powder, 16 grams

1½   teaspoons powdered vegetable supplement, Daily Greens or other

Optional; ½ ripe banana, apple, ½ cup of frozen berries

- Blend with fork or a blender when whole fruit is added - Enjoy!
- A time saver is to make several servings and store in a pitcher in the refrigerator especially when you use the blender.

HOMEMADE YOGURT

Let go of any reluctance to making your own yogurt because this recipe is very easy to make if you have the simple equipment and ingredients. To have success and make better yogurt than you can purchase from the health food store just takes some time and a little patience. By letting your yogurt stand for 24 hours you will be guaranteed to have the lactose sugar completely fermented from the good bacteria's action and you will generally not have bloating or other symptoms unless you are allergic to casein!

1   quart of milk

¼   cup of "Starter Yogurt" - quality commercial plain yogurt

1. Bring the milk to a simmering boil, stirring non-stop and then remove from heat.

2. Cover and cool down until it reaches the room temperature around 70 degrees. You can put it in the refrigerator to help it cool.

3. Next remove about ½ cup of cooled milk and stir in "Starter Yogurt". Store the rest of the store bought container for a future batch in the coldest part of the refrigerator.

4. Mix and stir the starter paste into the rest of the milk evenly.

5. Pour into a ceramic or heavy plastic container and cover.

6. Find the best place in your home to keep the yogurt mixture between (100 – 110F degrees) or (38-43C degrees) for the next 24 hours.

7. The heat source used during the fermentation process is critical; crock pot, warming tray, inside oven with a 60-watt bulb placed in oven then change it back after you are finished. *Caution:* Use a digital cooking thermometer or the type you take your body temperature with to make certain the heat is within the range for a full 24 hours.

8. When the 24 hours are complete store in clean containers in the refrigerator - Enjoy!

COTTAGE CHEESE OR YOGURT N' FRUIT

Purchase the products with the lowest content of lactose sugars and beware of GIS thickeners that may cause symptoms. Some Greek Style products are good (not all of them) and see the Reference section for better brands. In Zone 2 and 3 consider making your own yogurt or purchase more fully fermented products. See recipe for homemade yogurt (above) to insure the lactose content is the lowest for your body. Choose fruits like mango, papaya, peaches, apricot when they are available to reap the benefits of the high beta carotene content. Fresh berries and other seasonal fruits are great as well because they will be low in molds. See Tips section for more dietary recommendations.

¾ cup cottage cheese or yogurt

½ cup seasonal or stewed Fruit

EINSTEIN'S BREAKFAST

1 can of sardines; Crown Prince or another quality brand.

1 sliced fresh apple; Organic raw or applesauce.

½ cup Greek yogurt or Cottage Cheese, optional

1 100% sprouted English Muffin, buttered, optional

1. Open the can of sardines and drain. Place on a plate as desired with fruit.

2. Select organic apples from the market whenever possible due to commercial apples containing over nine potential toxins and a couple of these chemicals have been linked to cancer.

3. Many persons are also allergic to the stabilizers and toxins in the peel or commercial apples (microscopic molds), so peel if needed.

4. In one 6 oz. can you receive 28 grams of protein and with it the brain food of Omega 3's containing DHA and EPA - Enjoy!

5. Stuart Tomc's Power Breakfast.

Raw Vegetable Blender Juice Drink – Delicious!

Breakfast starts the day so why not have a power packed healthy head start with a blender juice drink? With only using a normal kitchen Oster blender you can make very successful and delicious blender drinks and it does not remove the desired fiber we all need. Of course purchasing a Vita-Mix or another specialized juice blender can reduce the fiber into smaller particulates yet they are a little pricey and heavy for some people to move about the kitchen. Regardless of which juicer you have it is fun to experiment making your own fresh vegetable juice recipes at home and less expensive than purchasing them! Keep fruit lower in the recipes because of the potential for very high glycemic (blood sugar) reactions to even fruit sugar fructose. Fruits also contain more natural molds that have the potential of increasing intestinal gas. Juicing is a great way to clean out the vegetable crisper and avoid vegetable casualties along with building a healthier body! *Caution:* If fast transit has been a challenge strain vegetable drinks until the bowels slow down. Mesh strainers are available in most food stores.

DELICIOUS BASIC JUICE

3	carrots
1	stalk celery

1 apple

2 radishes, ½ bell pepper or cucumber

2 cups water sieve if you desire.

  May add any herbs or seasoning of choice!

1. Scrub, peel and cut carrots into chunks.

2. With lid tightly placed on blender let it buzz for 2 – 3 minutes.

3. The fiber is desired yet strain through sieve if you desire.

DELUXE GREENS

1 bunch of greens; chard, kale, spinach

1 stalk celery

2-3 tablespoons parsley

⅓ cucumber

2 cups water

¼ cup fresh pineapple or (1) orange

LIVER DETOX

2 carrots

1 small beet

1 stalk celery

1 cup water

1-2 cloves of garlic, peeled

2 tablespoons cilantro, watercress or parsley

½ cup unsweetened cranberry juice

½ cup apple juice

1 ounce Aloe Vera juice

DIGESTIVE SOOTHER

2 cups cabbage; green or red

2 cups green lettuce

2 stalks celery

⅓ cucumber

2   tablespoons parsley

2   cups water

1   ounce Aloe Vera juice

ENERGIZER

1   bunch watercress, spinach or dark green lettuce

1   cup sprouts; mung, alfalfa, mixed sprouts

1   stalk celery

2   carrots

1   apple

2   cups water

ALKALIZING CHILLED AVOCADO CUCUMBER SOUP

½   medium cucumber, remove skin if not organic

1   small avocado, pitted and peeled

1   green onion, chopped

1   fresh garlic clove

2   tablespoons coriander (cilantro) or parsley, chopped

2   tablespoons fresh lemon juice

½   cup Greek yogurt or homemade

½   cup water

2   ice cubes

1. Detoxification of the body often demands one to achieve a better pH balance of acidity and alkalinity. This recipe along with vegetable juices helps greatly.
2. Mix all ingredients in blender until smooth, add salt and pepper and top with chopped coriander leaves – Enjoy!

Sandwiches

The bottom line is people of today want the convenience of sandwiches yet bread in most of its forms can be the enemy escalating GIS. Unless you have been fortunate to come across an acceptable bakery or bread product sold in your local store that is low enough on the scale of gluten to not cause symptoms – start experimenting with the alternatives.

The Webster dictionary tells us "the sandwich", was named after Earl of Sandwich and defines it as two or more slices of bread with a filling of meat, fish, cheese, peanut butter and jam, dating back in history to the 1ˢᵗ century B.C. People have been eating sandwiches for a long time so of course when you find out most bread may be the cause of your bloating and ill health it sets up a dilemma. The Tips section gives more detailed information about selecting breads, crackers and non-irritating foods. See the Resources for bread products and manufacturers for bread mixes and flour alternatives. Baking your own low gluten bread is an alternative for the daring and talented especially if you purchase a bread machine. The following recipes will give you the alternative choices people are using with Zone 1, 2 and 3 to keep their diets enjoyable and healthy!

Wrap It Up!

As previously mentioned many people in Zone 1 and 2 can eat white tortillas in moderation as long as the manufacturer has not fortified the blend with gluten flour as so many companies have done. To eat an occasional sprouted grain tortilla can also be tolerated by some however the bran can be problematic if eaten regularly for any zone. It is better for Zone 3 to experiment with the delicious "lettuce wraps" or "roll-ups" that follow in the recipes. They are very tasty and coupled with a cup of hot soup made fresh or from a can are extremely satisfying for the whole family and nutritious!

ITALIAN WRAP

2	**tortillas**
6	**slices deli turkey; or ½ cup or more of cooked turkey, chicken or salmon**
2	**slices of Provolone, Swiss or Feta cheese (1 oz.)**
1	**cup spinach or lettuce leaves**
6	**slices red bell pepper or ripe tomato**

Herbs; fresh or dry basil

2   tablespoons sour cream; may blend with ½ tsp of honey, mustard and lemon juice.

1. Heat or brown tortillas to desired doneness. Consider using a tortilla warming plate to brown both sides and place on a medium size serving plate for filling.
2. In a small bowl mix; sour cream, honey, mustard and lemon juice and place half on each cooked tortilla.
3. Arrange filling on tortilla with meat down first on half, next cheese, then vegetables on the other side; spinach, peppers or tomato then top with herbs of choice.
4. Serve open and each person may sprinkle grated parmesan as desired and black olives; fold it up - Enjoy!
5. May make ahead of time and take it to go. Just fold in a paper towel, saran and foil or placed in a reusable container to eat later.

BASIC LETTUCE WRAP

High in nutrition 100% gluten free (GF), lettuce wraps offer a great alternative to the bloat and fatigue that can follow eating bread sandwiches or fast foods. Depending on the filling and dressing you choose they can be neat or juicy but always delicious!

1   head lettuce; Bib or large leaf Green lettuce leaves.
½   pound of filling; sliced meat, cheese, fish salad, cooked filling Dressing; bottled salad dressing or homemade

Basic Dressing "Mock Mayo"
1   cup Yogurt
1   tablespoon sour cream
1½   teaspoon mustard
2   teaspoons vinegar or lemon juice
     Salt and pepper

1. Wash and prepare lettuce trimming as needed to provide a good leaf about the size of your open hand. Cut the rib end off of firm lettuce like Romaine so it will roll up.

2. Choose filling to give approximately 6 - 10 grams of protein in each lettuce wrap; 2 medium slices of turkey or other deli meats, ¼ cup (2 oz.) of Salmon or ground turkey. One slice of cheese (1 oz.) is about 4 grams of protein.

3. Medium appetite for lunch plan on two filled wraps for each adult. Larger appetite perhaps for a dinner meal, plan on three. If you are serving the lettuce wraps with a side soup, vegetables or a starch like yam, you will be very satisfied.

4. Lettuce wraps will travel with a blue ice or kept in the work refrigerator to keep chilled until eating. You may want to use a large cocktail toothpick or wrap in saran tucked into a handy reusable container - Enjoy!

THAI LETTUCE WRAP

1	large onion chopped
½	cup mushrooms chopped
1	cup water chestnuts (canned)
1	pound ground turkey
1	tablespoon soy sauce; low sodium gluten free Ground black pepper
2	cloves fresh garlic or 1 teaspoon powder
1	head of lettuce; Romaine, bib or other green type

Topping: ½ cup carrots shredded

Thai Peanut Sauce

1 ½	cups peanut butter
½	cup coconut milk
3	tablespoons water
3	tablespoons fresh lime juice
1-3	teaspoons soy sauce

1	tablespoon fish sauce, optional
1 - 3	teaspoons hot sauce, easy does it and optional
1	tablespoon minced fresh ginger root or 1 – 2 tsp powdered
1 - 3	cloves fresh garlic, minced
¼	cup fresh cilantro, chopped

1. Option: Peanut sauce can be purchased in your health food store. Read the ingredients to avoid GIS triggers.
2. Sautee the turkey meat first by adding a few drizzle of olive oil to a medium fry pan and cook on medium, cooking until browned on both sides then add soy sauce.
3. Next add some ground black pepper as desired and the vegetables – except carrots and simmer just a minute to wake them up. Do not overcook the vegetables.
4. Take cleaned lettuce leaves about the size of your open hand and patted dry and fill the center of each leaf with ¼ cup of filling. Place some carrots on top for crunch and presentation.
5. Makes 4 servings 2 per person. Add sauce as desired and Enjoy!

TURKEY CASHEW WRAP

4	oz cooked turkey, sliced
1	tortilla wrap, white or vegetable
1	medium Romaine lettuce leaf
1	oz. feta, cheddar or other cheese
8	fresh grape halves
4 - 6	cashew nuts, raw
	Red onion, as desired, half-moon strips
1	oz. creamy yogurt dressing

1. Heat wrap for 1 minute on medium heat fry pan until slightly browning.
2. Spread desired dressing either bottled or homemade (Creamy Sweet Yogurt Dressing is delicious on this wrap) and arrange

ingredients on one side closing over the top. Apply enough pressure to keep it closed – Enjoy!

Creamy Sweet Yogurt Dressing – Makes 1 Cup

1	**cup yogurt, Greek style or ½ cup sour cream and ½ cup yogurt for richer taste**
1	**tablespoon honey**
1	**tablespoon mustard**
1 - 3	**teaspoons lemon juice**
	Salt to taste

Pizza – GF

Why has PIZZA swept the country? It tastes good is the obvious answer yet tasting good and being good for children and adults are two separate topics. The GIS Program is about health education and keeping gluten triggers as low in the diet as possible for wellness. As explained in the previous chapters the once white flour used in pizza making is now being fortified with high gluten flour to give the finished products stability for a firmer more sturdy finished pizza.

Unfortunately that extra gluten flour is causing a lot more health challenges for people of all ages. Overeating in pizza can become a food disaster! Besides the gluten in the crust the body must cope with the high acidic tomato sauce, sugar in the sauce and the milk solids found in the less expensive dairy cheese products used in making most pizzas.

The solution is to eat thin crust pizza reducing the amount consumed, eat less pizza and another option is to make your own using a low gluten flour or gluten free (GF) from Authentic Foods or other alternative flours.

HOMEMADE PIZZA PIE

1	**box Pizza Dough Mix, www.AuthenticFoods.com, Zone 1 & 2**
1	**bottle Pizza Sauce**
¾	**cup toppings; precooked - chicken, turkey or seafood's, black olives, mushrooms, bell peppers, pineapple and other choices**

1   cup shredded Jack cheese and or white cheddar (softer cheeses are not the best choice)

2   teaspoons dried Italian herbs; basil, oregano, thyme, garlic, onion, parsley, other

    Parmesan cheese, grated fresh

1. Prepare and bake according to directions adding sauce, herbs, toppings and cheeses.
2. Variation: White Alfredo sauce can be made using half and half from a custom recipe – Enjoy!

TART PIE CRUST

1   package *Authentic Foods* or other LG / GF Pie Crust Mix

1   large egg yolk

2   tablespoon half and half or non-dairy substitute

4   oz. sweet butter, cut into small cubes

Tart Filling; may be a sweet filling with fruit or meat and or vegetable filling

Sweet Filling

3   white peaches, cut into ¼ - ½ inch wedges

¼   cup plus 2 tablespoons peach preserves

1. Preheat oven to 375 degrees. In a small bowl mix the egg yolk and cream then set aside. Use an electric beater cream the butter to smooth and gradually add in the tart mix. Add the egg mixture and beat at a low speed until the dough pulls away from the sides of the bowl. Add an extra tablespoon of cream if necessary. Remove the dough from the bowl and form it into two balls – to make bottom and top crust.
2. Refrigerate the dough for 30 minutes to (1) hour to ensure it will roll out more evenly.
3. Place the dough on a piece of wax paper that is taped down to a

larger counter so it won't move unless you have a "silpat" baking sheet. Flatten down your your hand and begin with a rolling pin starting from the center and rolling out with light even strokes. The goal is to form a 14 inch circle approximately ¼ inch thick. Repeat the process with the second ball of dough.

4. Place a tart pan in the center and flip it over on top of the pan covering the pan. Fit the dough down into the pan and trim the extra away on the edge.

5. Pour the filling into the tart pan and cover with the other 12 inch circle dough pinching the edges together with a fork motion around the entire edge making several cuts toward the center of the top dough.

6. Bake in the oven for approximately 35 – 40 minutes until golden brown. Remove from oven and let cool on rack for 15 – 20 minutes before cutting – Enjoy!

Salads

Men and women can enjoy a salad entree for lunch or dinner and they offer a good solutions to avoid digestive upset that may be experienced with sandwiches and other carbohydrate foods. Even though recipes are included to make your own dressings - store bought dressings work especially if you read the ingredients and find they are not loaded with GIS triggers. Add a cup of soup from a can or homemade to give the warmth element to any salad meal!

SPINACH SALAD

1½ - 2   cups fresh spinach leaves

¼   cup onion – preferably red for sweetness, thinly sliced

2   mushrooms; sliced medium

Salt & pepper to taste

Parmesan cheese, freshly grated as desired

Optional: celery, radishes, cooked turkey bacon, sliced hardboiled eggs. Cheese, cashews, walnuts, pears, apples, orange slices, can each give another yummy taste. Serve with cooked beans, fish, sardines, chicken or other meat for a larger meal.

Favorite dressings include; House Vinaigrette, Raspberry vinaigrette, Balsamic Olive Oil Vinaigrette.

1. Rinse and clean spinach and pat dry.
2. Red onions add a fabulous flavor.
3. Choosing at least 3 toppings adds color and compliments texture and taste.
4. Option: Heat dressing in microwave before serving to slightly wilt the salad as desired.
5. Makes 4 servings. – Enjoy!

Balsamic- Olive Oil Vinaigrette
¾   **cup olive oil**
¼   **cup balsamic or red wine vinegar**
⅛   **teaspoon freshly ground pepper**
¼   **teaspoon salt**
1   **clove garlic, freshly pressed**

Optional: sweeten by adding 2 teaspoons fruit preserves or honey. Herbs may be added as desired 1 - 2 teaspoons, mixed or blended to a good consistency. May wish to increase vinegar for more tartness.

1. Mix all ingredients in a dressing jar or blender.
2. Store in refrigerator to use in soups, salads and other recipes that need a zip!

RED CABBAGE SALAD
¾   **head of red cabbage, sliced thin against the grain for shorter strands**
1   **medium carrot, shredded medium**

½ bell pepper; yellow makes a beautiful color contrast

1 stalk celery, sliced

¼ cup oil; olive, flax, sesame, other

⅛ cup vinegar; rice, Red wine or other (may wish to increase vinegar for greater tartness)

½ teaspoon herbs of choice; thyme, savory or basil

1 teaspoon seeds; poppy seeds or anise

Salt & pepper to taste

Cabbage salad can be easily kept in the refrigerator to enjoy as a side dish for lunch or dinner. Lasts for a good 7 – 10 days. May top with sour cream as desired.

GREEK VEGETABLE SALAD

5 - 6 leaves of Romaine lettuce

1 large cucumber, chopped

2 large Roma tomatoes, other

10-12 black pitted olives; Kalamata or other

1 small red onion, quartered and sliced thinly

1 cup baby greens; variety

4 ounces Feta cheese, optional small cubed jack cheese

Salt & pepper

Vinaigrette Dressing

6 tablespoons olive oil

1 teaspoon each; garlic powder or 1 clove fresh dried oregano, basil.

1 teaspoon Dijon mustard

1 teaspoon lemon juice, fresh

1 cup red wine vinegar

1. Wash and pat dry lettuce and place in large bowl. Tear into medium pieces.

2. Combine the rest of the vegetables in a smaller bowl and add dressing allowing it to marinate.

3. May combine all ingredients shortly before serving or keep separated until ready to eat to maintain lettuce crispness - Enjoy!

QUINOA SUMMER SALAD

1	cup uncooked Quinoa
2	cups water or low sodium chicken broth
½	pound green beans, cooked and chopped diagonal
½	each red, orange and green pepper, chopped
1	tablespoon green onion, finely chopped

1. Bring 2 cups of liquid to a boil in a 1½ quart pan with lid and add uncooked Quinoa.

2. Cover and reduce heat to a simmer for 10-15 minutes until liquid is all absorbed and grain turns translucent and puffs up.

3. Mix all ingredients together in a large salad bowl and add dressing. May serve as a side dish or serve over lettuce leaves (as a salad). Best to compliment with a side of more protein; beans, meat or a handful of nuts and or seeds - Enjoy!

4. Recipe by Chef Pamela Croft

Olive Oil Dijon Dressing

¼	cup lemon juice
1-2	teaspoons lemon zest (grated skin of lemon)
2	teaspoons Dijon Mustard
1	clove garlic, minced
½	cup Olive oil

1. Place lemon juice, mustard and garlic in a medium bowl.

2. Drizzle the olive oil slowly into the bowl while whisking.

3. Add the lemon zest, salt and pepper and mix into salad.

TABOULI QUINOA SALAD

2   cups cooked Quinoa or other low gluten grain
1   cup parsley, chopped
2   green onions, thinly sliced
2   tablespoons mint, chopped
1   clove fresh garlic, minced
3   medium ripe tomatoes or 1 cup red sweet pepper, diced
½   teaspoon basil
½   cup lemon juice
¼   cup olive oil
    Salt and pepper
    Lettuce leaves, washed

1. Mix all ingredients in a large serving bowl. Allow to marinate in refrigerator for at least 1 hour before serving.
2. Serve on lettuce leaves with favorite entrée – Enjoy!

YUMMY KALE SALAD

1   bunch of kale, torn
1   cup cherry tomatoes or 1 large tomato or 1 sweet red pepper, diced
1   stalk celery, diced
1-2   avocadoes, chopped
¼   head of red cabbage, chopped
¼   purple onion, diced
    Variations: Reduce cabbage and or add 1 cup
    Romaine lettuce or spinach

Kale Salad Marinade
¼   cup olive or flax oil
1   clove fresh garlic, minced
1   lemon juiced or 3 tablespoons red wine vinegar
1   tablespoon Agave Nectar Syrup or honey

Pinch of sea salt and pepper

1. Remove stems from kale leaves and tear into bite size pieces.
2. Combine Kale with marinade.
3. Prepare tomato, avocado, cabbage and onions.
4. Stir into kale and toss well – Enjoy!

THAI MARINATED BEEF SALAD

½   **cup Lime juice**
¼   **cup fresh cilantro, chopped**
2   **tablespoons honey**
1-2 **tablespoons Thai fish sauce, does contain sugar and salt**
1-2 **tablespoons chili paste with garlic**
2   **garlic cloves, minced**
1   **(1 ½ pound) flank steak**
1½   **cups red onion, sliced in moon shapes**
1   **red bell pepper cut in strips or 4 plum tomatoes cut in wedges**
1   **large head of Romaine Lettuce, 6 cups torn**
1   **medium English cucumber, thinly sliced**
2   **tablespoons fresh mint, chopped (opt.)**

1. Combine first six ingredients in a bowl until thoroughly mixed.
2. Set half aside for topping the salads and the other half in a zip lock baggie with the steak for marinating for 10 minutes in the refrigerator turning once.
3. Spray grill or broiling pan with non-stick or lightly coat with vegetable oil heated to a medium heat.
4. Remove steak from bag tossing the remaining marinate.
5. Place on hot grill cooking 6 minutes on each side or to your desired degree of doneness.
6. Let stand for 5 minutes off the grill and slice diagonally in strips.

7. Sautee onions and bell peppers or tomatoes for just 3 minutes in a skillet with light oil.

8. Place onion mixture on lettuce leaves with cucumbers, place 3-4 ounces of steak on each salad top with a tablespoon of the reserved sauce, cilantro and mint leaves. May cook white Jasmine rice or rice noodles for a heartier meal. Serves 4 – 6 - Enjoy!

ORGANIC 3 BEAN SALAD

1	can each of **Organic Kidney, Garbanzo & Pinto beans**
1	can roasted green chilies, diced
¼	cup Italian parsley, chopped
2	stalks celery, thin sliced
2	or more green onions, thin sliced

Chili Dressing

½	cup olive oil
½	cup red wine vinegar
1	garlic clove, minced
1	teaspoon chili powder
1	teaspoon dried or fresh oregano
¼	teaspoon cumin
1	teaspoon salt
¼	teaspoon ground pepper

1. Mix together in a bowl and add to beans to marinate.
2. May serve alone as a side dish or over a bed of salad greens alongside a protein entre – Enjoy!

CLASSIC CHICKEN CAESAR

1	pound of cooked chicken, grilled or steamed
1	medium head Romaine lettuce, cleaned and torn
4-5	green onion tops, chopped

¼   cup crumbled Turkey bacon or fresh toasted Sunflower seeds, optional

1   cup croutons, made with rice bread or sourdough, occasionally

Creamy Caesar Dressing

½   cup olive oil

¼   cup sour cream, yogurt or mayonnaise

1   tablespoon Soy Sauce, wheat free low sodium

1   tablespoon white wine or rice wine vinegar

4   cloves fresh garlic, minced

¼   teaspoon ground black pepper

1-2 tablespoons Dijon Mustard

2   tablespoons Anchovy paste

½   cup fresh squeezed lemon juice

1   egg yolk

2   tablespoons Parmesan cheese

1   teaspoon salt, as desired

1. Mix all ingredients together in a deep bowl with a fork or metal whisk or blender.

2. Let the dressing stand a few minutes before blending it gently into the lettuce.

3. Serve alone or add cooked chicken on top sprinkled with grated cheese and croutons. Fresh bacon pieces may be available for each guest to serve as desired or toasted sunflower seeds are also good – Enjoy!

ORANGE-AVOCADO WITH TAHINI DRESSING

1   avocado, sliced

2   oranges, chopped

1   stalk celery, sliced

1   bell pepper, green, sliced

1   head dark green lettuce, torn

2   tablespoons cilantro or parsley

1. Prepare lettuce tearing into bite size pieces into a large bowl.

2. Toss the remainder of ingredients together in a smaller bowl with half the dressing then top the salad greens with some chopped cilantro or parsley.

3. Serve the remainder of dressing as a condiment as desired – Enjoy!

Tahini Yogurt Dressing

1   cup plain yogurt, Greek or homemade yogurt

¼   cup Tahini, sesame butter

1 - 2 tablespoons mustard

1   tablespoon lemon juice

1   teaspoon soy sauce, wheat free low sodium

½   teaspoon cumin powder (optional)

1. Combine all the ingredients into a blender or mix with a fork until smooth.

2. If omitting cumin may add 1 tablespoon of honey or agave nectar syrup.

3. Stays fresh for 7 – 10 days refrigerated and is delicious on meat, vegetables, wraps and salads.

4. Recipe by Cheryl Forberg, RD for the Biggest Loser TV show.

CUCUMBER-RADISH SALADETTE

1   cucumber, sliced and chopped

1   bunch radishes, Julian style

1   stalk celery, sliced

2   green onions, sliced thin

     Salt & pepper

House Vinaigrette

1	cup olive oil or flax oil
3	oz. Rice Vinegar
3	oz. Balsamic Vinegar
1	teaspoon thyme
1	clove fresh garlic, minced, optional
½	teaspoon each Salt and Pepper

1. Prepare by whisking together and put into refrigerator storage bowl to use on Saladette, future salads, marinate or steamed vegetables or soups.
2. Variations of Saladette is unlimited: tomato wedges and steamed vegetable leftovers work deliciously.
3. Serve in small ceramic 4 – 6 oz. bowls to accent a larger meal – Enjoy!

Soups

The original comfort food "Soup" is eaten and enjoyed around the world. Soups are calming to the digestive system and the mind. Steaming some vegetables like carrots in a soup, allow the trapped nutrient of beta carotene to escape the cellulose fibers. Soup variations are endless and an excellent way to utilize foods that are due to expire while also extending higher priced foods like asparagus, meats or shrimp. From Gumbo and Minestrone to Bean Soups and Chili making soups is a scrumptious tradition year-round!

MINESTRONE

1	onion, chopped
1-3	cloves of fresh garlic
2	stalks celery, chopped
1½	tablespoons olive oil
4	cups fresh tomatoes or a
6	oz. can of paste or 8 oz. sauce
3 - 8	cups vegetable broth or water

2   bay leaves

1   teaspoon oregano

2   teaspoons basil
     Pinch of fennel seeds (opt.)

2   cups or more of fresh chopped vegetables; Zucchini, carrot, red potato, green beans, Bell pepper, peas, cabbage, parsley, other greens or vegetables

1   cup cooked or canned beans; garbanzo, small White or kidney
     Salt & Ground Pepper to taste

1. Sautee the onion in the oil in a large 3-6 quart pot with a lid for about 3 minutes and add spices.

2. Add the rest of the ingredients making certain you have enough liquid to cover all the vegetables.

3. Bring the soup to a boil and simmer on a low boil for about 20 minutes. Taste and correct seasonings as desired. If you desire a thicker soup carefully puree a few cups of soup in a blender and return it to the pot. Garnish with a favorite parmesan cheese and parsley. If meat is desired add precooked meat during that last cooking period on a high boil to reach at least 176 degrees Fahrenheit.

4. Recipe makes about 10 cups and it is even more delicious the next day – Enjoy!

LENTIL MEDITERRANEAN

1   onion, chopped

2 - 3 tablespoons olive oil

2   carrots, diced

2   stalks celery, chopped

2   medium red potatoes, cubed

2   cloves garlic, minced

1½   teaspoon dried or fresh oregano

1	bay leaf
1½	teaspoon dried or fresh basil
1	(14 oz.) can tomatoes or 3 – 4 ripe fresh, cubed
1½-2	cups dry lentils
8	cups water or chicken broth
2	cups spinach or chard, thinly chopped
2	tablespoons Balsamic vinegar
	Salt and ground black pepper

1. Heat oil in a large pot with a lid over medium heat. Add onions, carrots, potatoes and celery. Cook for 3 minutes until onion is translucent.

2. Add lentils, herbs, water/chicken broth and tomatoes. Bring to boil and reduce to a simmer for at least one hour.

3. Variation: (a.) Drop the tomato, red potato, spinach, oregano and basil herbs. Then add 1 – 2 teaspoons cumin, 1 medium yam, peeled and cubed and 1 medium carrot. Mix in 1 tsp. red miso paste into each bowl and top it with cilantro and a little more Balsamic vinegar or (b.) drop tomatoes and chard for red and yellow bell peppers perhaps tender beef cubes 2 cups, 2 T. red chili sauce or catsup, 1 T. soy sauce, top with cilantro and ½ tsp. miso paste in each bowl. These flavors are finger licking good!

4. When ready to serve stir in spinach or chard and let stand about 5 minutes and add vinegar, salt and pepper to taste – Enjoy!

GREEK AVGOLEMONO (CHICKEN SOUP)

Many variations of Chicken soup come from countries around the globe including this delicious Greek traditional recipe. The unique sour-tartness compliments the chicken and egg taste. The recipe is actually easy to make once you learn the sequence and a wonderful way to use extra rice or chicken that you may have previously cooked.

2½   quarts (77 oz.) chicken broth

1-2   chicken breasts, cooked and torn into small pieces

2   cups cooked basmati rice

2   medium red potato, cubed and cooked or 3 tablespoons cornstarch, not for Zone 2 or 3 use potato only

3   egg yolks

1 - 2   whole lemons, juiced

Salt

1. Start with 2 ½ quarts of water and cook the chicken with the skin in the boiling water until tender at a low simmer-boil for approximately 20 minutes.

2. Remove chicken from the water and allow it to cool. Next remove the skin and discard. Shred chicken into medium to small pieces and place in refrigerator.

3. In a small 2 quart pan with lid cook 1 cup of rice by bringing 2 cups of the broth to a boil with the rice and then turn down to simmer 45 minutes not lifting the lid until finished.

4. Thickening the soup traditionally is done with corn starch however some people may be sensitive to corn and red potato works to thicken soup as well. Remove 10 ounces of broth in a bowl and slowly whisk with fork or whisk the cornstarch into cold liquid first and then blend into the soup to thicken. If using cooked red potato place in blender with broth and puree. Either thickener will work to thicken the remaining pot of soup.

5. The egg yolks are also added to a separated cup of the original cooled broth with a whisk or fork being careful to not have it too hot or it will cook the eggs prematurely. It should not look like scrambled eggs but a thickened yellow liquid.

6. Lastly, add the lemon juice to the large pot while whisking the egg yolk slurry. Add back the shredded chicken and rice and salt to taste. Garnish with some fresh chopped parsley and Enjoy!

CHICKEN POSOLE

2-3	cups cooked chicken, shredded
2 (	14 oz.) cans low sodium chicken broth
1	(14 oz.) can garbanzo beans
1	carrot, chopped
1	stalk celery
	small onion
¾	teaspoon cumin powder
¾	teaspoon thyme
½	teaspoon chili powder
1-2	cloves fresh garlic, minced
1	cup cilantro, chopped
	Water, to preferred soup consistency
½	teaspoon salt

1. In a 3 quart soup pan add oil and sauté onion for 2 minutes.
2. Add herbs, carrot and celery and cook for another 2 minutes.
3. Next add the chicken broth, beans and chicken and bring to boil turning down to a simmer for 10 minutes. Liquid totals approximately 5 cups from the chicken broth and water.
4. *Note:* If cooking chicken with the skin you can keep the broth and use it for your soup stock.
5. Serve with a sprinkle of green onion tops and a favorite grated cheese – Enjoy!

CREAM OF CHICKEN, WILD RICE AND ASPARAGUS SOUP

2	cups cooked chicken, shredded or diced
4-5	cups chicken broth, low sodium
1	cup wild rice blend, cooked
¼ - ½	cup of rice flour
½	cup half and half
1	bunch asparagus, spears cut in 1 inch pieces or 2 cups broccoli

2   tablespoons olive oil

1   onion, diced

2   stalks celery, sliced

½   bell pepper, red, chopped

1   teaspoon thyme

1   teaspoon curry, optional

Salt & pepper to taste

Parsley, chopped

Wild Rice Blend

¾   cup Basmati White Rice

¼   cup Wild Rice

2   cups water

1. Bring water to a boil in a 2 quart sauce pan and add rice. Cover with a tight fitting lid and cook on a constant low simmer boil for 45 minutes. Do not lift the lid. To avoid burning the rice cook on top of a "trivet" available in cooking stores. A rice cooker may be used if preferred.

2. Heat a 4 quart soup pot on medium heat. Add oil and onion sauté for 2 minutes.

3. Next add celery, red pepper, asparagus and herbs cooking for another 2 minutes and then add broth.

4. Mix the rice flour in ½ cup of room temperature water and whisk with fork to blend well. Bring soup up to a boil and slowly add the thickened flour to the soup whisking to avoid clumps. Turn heat down to a slow simmer for 3 minutes allowing the flour to cook and thicken.

5. Combine the chicken, rice and half and half seasoning with salt and pepper to taste. A tiny shake of hot sauce into each bowl excites the taste buds and a sprinkle of parsley for color – Enjoy!

BORSCHT BEET SOUP

1	bunch of beets and green tops, 4 medium, cleaned and diced
1	onion, chopped
2	tablespoon olive oil
5	cups water or broth
1-2	cloves fresh garlic, mined
2	carrots
2	stalks celery
2	medium red potatoes, diced
1	can tomatoes or 3 whole, diced (as tolerated)
½	head cabbage, sliced thinly and chopped
1	bay leaf
1	tablespoon honey
1½	teaspoon salt
¼	teaspoon pepper
	Lemon wedges and or top with sour cream

1. In a large pot with a lid sauté onion in the olive oil about 1 minute on medium heat.

2. Clean and peel beets and remove stems from the green tops and cut into large cubes. Red color will dissipate yet wear an apron. Add other vegetables, herbs, salt and pepper and bring water or broth to a boil.

3. Turn down the soup to a simmer and cook for 20 minutes until vegetables are tender.

4. Carefully not to capture the bay leaf place 2 – 3 cups of hot soup in a blender and puree. Safely return the blended soup to the pot and stir into soup.

5. Serve with lemon wedges and top with sour cream as desired – Enjoy!

6. Recipe from *Laurel's Kitchen* by Laurel Robertson.

PUMPKIN SQUASH SOUP

This is a soup that has great "Fall Flavor" and can also be enjoyed year round. Canned pumpkin or other dark orange squash like Butternut can be substituted.

2	pounds of cubed fresh pumpkin or 2 cans of pumpkin
2	carrots, chopped
2	onions, chopped
2	tablespoons olive oil
2	red potatoes, cubed
2 - 3	cups water
2	tablespoons honey
2	cups chicken broth
1	cup half and half or coconut milk
1	teaspoons each allspice and cinnamon
	Salt & Black pepper to taste

1. In a large 4 quart soup pan heat oil on medium and sauté onions for 2 minutes.
2. Add the rest of the ingredients except the cream and bring to a boil.
3. Simmer for approximately 20 minutes and add half and half or coconut milk.
4. For a creamy texture carefully blend 4 cups of the soup mixture in a blender and return to pan.
5. Variation of a heartier soup add 2 cans of cooked black beans, 14 oz. of tomatoes and drop the Allspice and Cinnamon and add 1 tablespoon curry powder and 1 teaspoon of Cumin spice. Both recipes are delicious.
6. Adjust seasoning and top each bowl upon serving with sour cream, fresh parsley or grated carrot – Enjoy!

TUSCAN WHITE BEAN

2	tablespoons olive oil
1	small onion
1	carrot, diced
1	stalk celery, sliced
1	red potato, diced
1	can (14 oz.) or fresh chicken broth
1	teaspoon sage
1-2	cloves fresh garlic, minced
1	cup water
1- 2	cans (15 oz. each) white beans, Cannellini or other
½	head of Escarole, Kale, Chard or Spinach (2 cups), thinly sliced
1	tablespoon of butter
	Salt & pepper

1. In a 4 quart pan with a lid add oil and sauté on medium heat; onion, carrot, celery and potato until slightly brown about 5 minutes.
2. Add the rest of the ingredients and simmer for 15 minutes stirring occasionally.
3. Variation in taste; just add an 8 oz. can of diced tomatoes or fresh tomatoes adding a richer color and taste. Just drop the sage and add 1 teaspoon of Oregano fresh or dried. When using fresh herbs add more to achieve flavor results.
4. Serve with Grilled Garlic Shrimp for a delicious treat.
5. Top with your favorite fresh grated parmesan cheese – Enjoy!

TURKEY CHILI - 30 MINUTES

2	tablespoons olive oil
1	small onion, chopped
1	pound ground turkey
1-2	cloves fresh garlic, minced

2   teaspoons salt

2   teaspoons chili powder

1   teaspoon dried oregano

2   tablespoons tomato paste or 1 T. each of tomato paste and
     Chipotle chili en adobo coarsely chopped

1   (14 oz.) can of whole peeled tomatoes with juice

1   (15 oz.) can of kidney beans, rinsed and drained if desired
     Topping: 1 – 2 Avocados, sliced
     Cilantro, chopped
     Sour Cream
     Shredded Jack cheese
     Corn Tortilla Chips

1. Heat the oil in a large skillet with high sides on medium heat
   and add the onion. Cook 1 minute and add ground turkey in
   clumps. Allow to brown and turn at least once.

2. Add the tomatoes and all spices and allow the chili to cook on a
   low simmer for approximately 10 -15 minutes.

3. Serve in bowls topped with your favorite garnish. Serves 4 -
   Enjoy!

WHITE BEAN CHICKEN CHILI

1½   cups dried white beans of choice or may use 6 cups of cooked
     canned beans reducing chicken stock to 2 – 3 cups as desired

5   cups of chicken stock

2   tablespoons butter

2   tablespoons olive oil

2   cloves fresh garlic, minced

1   onion, ¾ cups, diced

2   stalks celery, sliced

1   medium carrot, chopped

1½   cups green chilies, canned

1   pound of cooked chicken, chopped

1   tablespoons cumin powder

1   tablespoon oregano

1-2   teaspoons each salt and pepper

1   teaspoon chili powder

Pinch of red pepper flakes

½   bunch cilantro leaves, ¾ cups, chopped

1. If cooking beans from dried rinse well and cover with water in a large pot with lid for two hours. Drain water and add chicken broth.

2. Bring beans to a boil and turn down to simmer for about 2 ½ hours until tender.

3. While the beans are cooking take a medium skillet add olive oil, onions and chilies and sauté for 5 minutes.

4. Add chili mixture to the pot of beans along with the rest of the spices and chicken.

5. Lower the heat to a constant boil simmering the beans until done.

6. Top with favorite grated jack cheese or sour cream, cilantro as desired – Enjoy!

GUMBO CALIFORNIA STYLE

1 - 2   pounds of meat or seafood; chicken or shrimp

1   pound sausage, cut into ½ inch slices, (opt)

1   pound of okra, fresh or frozen, cut in sliced bite size pieces

1   large onion, thinly chopped

2   tablespoons olive oil

4   tablespoons rice flour, white flour or Instant Roux (opt.)

4   cups chicken broth, low sodium

1   bell pepper, green, diced

3   stalks celery, thinly sliced

2   cloves fresh garlic, mined

1   cup stewed tomatoes, diced

½   cup fresh parsley, chopped

2   bay leaves

1   teaspoon thyme

1   teaspoon savory

2   teaspoons File, ground Sassafras leaves

2   teaspoons soy sauce, wheat free low sodium

    Pinch of cayenne pepper

    Salt and pepper to taste

2   green onions, chopped

4   cups cooked rice

1. In a large 6 quart stainless pot with lid heat olive oil on medium heat and sauté the onion for 2 – 3 minutes called smothering the onions.

2. Add the meat to the onions and brown the outside to sear in the juices about 3 minutes each side lowering the heat to avoid burning the fat. Remove the meat temporarily.

3. In the pots drippings sprinkle flour evenly and brown flour stirring with a heat tempered long handled spoon for 3 minutes until bubbling is consistent then whisk in chicken broth bring to a simmer adding back the meat, herbs and vegetables to continue cooking approximately 1 hour.

4. Take the meat out and check the temperature. Correctly cooked if 178 degrees or hotter. Microwave meat if not hot enough. Remove meat from bone and shred or cut meat into 1 ½ to 2 inch pieces. Cut sausage into ½ inch slices.

5. Season broth to taste with more spices, salt, pepper and a little more hot sauce being careful not to over season. It is always better for the individual to personally season for each person's desire. Serve with rice into the bowl first and spoon gumbo around rice. Top with extra filet and chopped green onions and have hot sauce on the table ya'll – Enjoy!

EGGPLANT "LOUISIANA CAJUN" STYLE

1	eggplant, medium to large, peeled and diced
1	pound ground; turkey, beef or lamb, (optional)
1	cup onion, chopped
2½	cups bell pepper; green, red, yellow, chopped
1-3	cloves fresh garlic, minced
2-3	tablespoons olive oil
½	teaspoon thyme
½	teaspoon oregano
1	bay leaf
¾	cup water
2	teaspoons soy sauce, wheat free, low sodium
	Salt, pepper & hot sauce, as desired

1. Bring a medium size skillet up to a medium heat adding oil and sauté the onion for 3 minutes with the herbs.

2. Add ground meat and allow it to slightly brown turning for at least 6 minutes.

3. In a separate 1 ½ quart pan heat water and steam eggplant until tender, drain and add it to the cooked meat.

4. Add soy sauce and mix all ingredients turning the heat down to a simmer for approximately 10 minutes.

5. Variations may include omitting the water and adding a small amount of red wine to the mixture steaming the eggplant with the meat by placing a lid on the skillet. The dish may also be baked in the oven adding some stewed tomatoes, ½ cup of white cracker crumbs, 4 beaten eggs to the rest of the mixture topped with feta cheese and baked for 45 minutes at 375 degrees.

6. Serve any of the versions with rice or potatoes and a favorite grated cheese. Have hot sauce on the table for guests (as desired) and top with Cilantro – Ya'll Enjoy!

7. Recipe by Patricia Falk "Mom".

ENCHILADA PIE

1	tablespoon olive oil
1	onion, chopped
1	cup bell pepper, green or red
1	pound ground beef or turkey
3	cups cooked beans, black or pinto
2	teaspoons cumin powder and soy sauce
1	(14 – 15 oz.) can tomatoes, diced
1	clove fresh garlic, minced
1	can (4 oz.) green chilies
1	cup corn (optional), frozen or fresh
1	(8 oz.) can Enchilada Sauce, contains some GIS triggers (Zone 1) or alternative Green Sauce (Zone 2)
¾	cup black olives, pitted and sliced in half
12	tortillas, corn or white flour, no gluten added
8	oz. shredded cheese, Jack or Cheddar
	Sour cream and Cilantro, chopped topping

Alternative Enchilada Sauce

¼	cup olive oil
1	(8 oz.) can Green Chilies
½	teaspoon Xanthan powder
¼	teaspoon; onion, garlic, chili powder

Place all ingredients in blender and buzz at high speed until creamy and use in place of red enchilada sauce.

1. Oil a 3 quart glass baking dish, 13 x 9 inches, or another appropriate pan for baking.

2. Heat oil in a large skillet over medium heat and add onion for a couple of minutes. Next add the ground turkey and sauté 3 to 4 minutes browning it on both sides.

3. Add bell peppers, spices and beans and cook another 5 minutes turning twice with lid placed on it for the last minute of cooking.

4. Blend half of the Enchilada sauce into filling and place the other in a shallow cooking pan to heat for the tortillas.

5. With baking dish within easy reach of stove - place one tortilla at a time into pan to moisten with sauce and layer the bottom of the baking dish with 6 tortillas.

6. Blend half of the cheese into mixture and then turn it into the backing dish covering the tortillas. Moisten the rest of the tortillas placing them on top of the filling covering the contents as well as possible. This may call for cutting two tortillas in half in order to cover the top completely.

7. Turn onto the baking sheet and spread evenly.

8. Bake 35 – 45 minutes until it begins to brown – Enjoy!

Variation for Zone 3: Fix filling and serve as a casserole without tortillas.

1. Heat oven to 350 degrees.

2. Spread any leftover sauce over the pie and evenly sprinkle the rest of the shredded cheese.

3. Cover the baking dish with foil and bake for 10 – 12 minutes until contents bubbles. Remove foil and cool for another 2 – 10 minutes before cutting into 6 x 5 inch wedges.

4. Top with a heaping teaspoon of sour cream and chopped cilantro as desired - Enjoy!

MEXICAN FIESTA SKILLET

1	**pound ground turkey or beef**
1	**onion, chopped**
1 - 2	**tablespoons vegetable oil**
1	**clove fresh garlic, minced**
1	**large can (14.5 oz.) diced tomatoes (or 1 sweet red pepper, chopped and 2 oz. catsup, 2 tsp. soy sauce and ½ cup of water)**
1	**large can (15 oz.) black beans**

1   large can (15 oz.) whole kernel corn
1   cup sliced mushrooms
2   teaspoons chili powder
1   teaspoon cumin
½   teaspoon oregano (or 1 tablespoon fresh oregano)
2-3 shakes of hot sauce, optional

Topping;

4   oz. cheddar cheese, grated
¼   cup sour cream
¼   cup cilantro, chopped

1. In a large skillet brown meat, onion and garlic in oil at a medium heat turning for about 6 minutes.
2. Add the rest of the vegetables, herbs, hot sauce and beans then simmer for another 5 minutes with the lid on the pot.
3. Serve in bowls topped with cheese, sour cream and cilantro and corn chips – Enjoy!
4. Recipe by Kathy Cappasola.

TERIYAKI BEEF GREEN BEAN SHITAKE STIR FRY

1   pound lean steak, cut into thin slices or other meat preference
¼   cup Tamari soy sauce, wheat free low sodium
¼   cup rice vinegar or white wine
1   tablespoon honey
2   cloves fresh garlic, minced
2   tablespoons sesame, peanut or olive oil
2   teaspoons Xanthan Gum (Zone 2 & 3) thickener or corn starch (Zone 1)
1   small onion, red, thinly sliced
6   Shitake Mushrooms, sliced medium
2   cups fresh green beans, trimmed, cut diagonal into 2 inch pieces
1   red pepper, seeded and sliced

Pinch red pepper flakes

Salt and black pepper

Topping: toasted sesame seeds, cilantro or lime

Jasmine rice or other

1. Whisk Tamari, rice vinegar, honey and garlic in a large bowl. Add steak and toss to coat. Allow meat to marinate, in the refrigerator for at least 1- 3 hours.
2. Precook green beans in a medium pot with a lid with boiling water for 2 minutes.
3. Remove meat into a second small bowl and reserve marinade. Whisk the 2 teaspoons of Xanthan gum in marinade to be added after cooking the meat.
4. Heat 1 tablespoon of the oil in a heavy large wok or skillet over medium to high heat and add onion for 1 minute then meat for another 2 – 3 minutes.
5. Add mushrooms and peppers and cook another minute before adding the thickened marinade and cook for (1) last minute stirring. Return the precooked green beans into stir fry heating only not to over-cook.
6. Salt and pepper to taste, serve over rice or rice noodles, topping with toasted sesame seeds, cilantro or lime as desired – Enjoy!

PAD THAI STIR FRY

1	pound cooked chicken (bite size) or shrimp
1	small onion, chopped
1	tablespoon sesame or other oil
1	stalk celery, sliced
1 - 2	cloves fresh garlic, minced
½ - 1	teaspoons fresh grated (best) or powdered ginger
1	pound fresh snow peas or frozen peas
2	cups white Mung bean sprouts
	Cilantro, chopped

1. Heat a medium wok or skillet (with high sides) and add oil. Next add onion and herbs for 1 minute and then add the meat for 3 more minutes turning to evenly cook. Remove shrimp to not overcook yet other meat can stay in pan.
2. Add the celery, peas and bean sprouts for another 2 minutes with lid on pan until vegetables are slightly tender.
3. Variation: Make vegetarian by omitting meat. The Mung beans and peanut butter complement one another for a complete protein
4. Sir ½ cup of peanut sauce evenly into the stir fry and serve over rice or rice noodles as desired topping with extra sauce, crushed peanuts if desired and cilantro – Enjoy!

Thai Peanut Sauce

1½	cups peanut butter
½	cup coconut milk
3	tablespoons water
3	tablespoons fresh lime juice
1- 3	teaspoons soy sauce
1 - 3	teaspoons fish sauce (opt)
1 - 3	teaspoons hot sauce or sweet red chili sauce, (opt)
1	tablespoon minced fresh ginger root or 1 – 2 tsp. powdered, (opt)
1 - 3	cloves fresh garlic, minced
¼	cup fresh cilantro, chopped

1. Prepare sauce while cooking the meat or use bottled peanut sauce stating "gluten free" for best results.

BBQ CHICKEN OR BEEF

Slather it on chicken, turkey or beef after cooking the meat or use it as a condiment. It is a snap to make and keep it in the fridge. If you can't find the fire roasted tomatoes canned tomatoes or fresh tomatoes will work well however they won't have the Smokey flavor.

BBQ Sauce

2	tablespoons olive oil
1	tablespoon onion, diced
2-3	cloves of fresh garlic, minced
3	cups (28 oz.) tomatoes, fire toasted, finely chopped
1/2	cup fresh lime juice
½	cup Balsamic vinegar
½	cup Agave nectar syrup
2	tablespoons chili powder

1. Heat the oil in a 2 quart sauce pan over medium heat. Add the onion and sauté for 3 minutes until soft. Add the garlic and stir for a minute not allowing it to burn and then add the rest of the ingredients. Bring it to a low boil and simmer for 20 minutes. Cool and place in blender. Process until creamy smooth and transfer to a sturdy container perhaps glass, to store in the refrigerator. – Enjoy!

2. Recipe is found in *Positively Ageless* by Cheryl Forberg, RD of the Biggest Loser TV show.

CHICKEN MARSALA

4	chicken breast; boneless, skinless
4	tablespoons butter
4	tablespoons olive oil
¼	cup of rice flour
1	cup mushrooms, sliced
½	teaspoons oregano
½	teaspoons salt
¼	teaspoon black pepper
¼	cup of apple juice or cooking sherry

¼ - ½   cup Balsamic vinegar or Marsala wine

1. In a shallow dish mix flour, salt and pepper and oregano. Coat the chicken breast evenly with mixture.
2. In a large skillet with sides heat olive oil on medium heat. Place chicken in pan and lightly brown both sides for a time of about 7 - 10 minutes adding the mushrooms during the last minute.
3. Pour liquid into the pan and cover with a lid cooking on a slightly reduced heat for another 10 minutes turning once. Stir juices and check temperature of meat for doneness at least 178 degrees or more. Meat juice should run clear no pink color.
4. Serve as desired over rice, potatoes, pasta or vegetables – Enjoy!

PAN GRILLED GARLIC SHRIMP

1½	pounds of raw shrimp, cleaned
1 - 2	shallots or green onions, optional
2 - 3	cloves fresh garlic, minced
1	tablespoon capers, optional
2	tablespoons fresh grated parmesan cheese
2	tablespoons butter
2	tablespoons olive oil
4	lemon or lime wedges
½	cup Italian parsley, chopped
	Salt and pepper

1. Clean and devein shrimp cutting the back open discarding the black thread.
2. Medium to large skillet with high sides required with a lid. Heat oil and butter on medium heat.
3. Add onion and shrimp using tongs to turn after about 1 minute. Then add garlic and other herbs and capers as desired. Do not overcook shrimp it should turn white and still be tender to the bite!

4. Use care to not burn the garlic. It takes on a bitter taste so add after the shrimp has turned completely white from proper cooking. Squeeze ½ a lemon over shrimp as desired.

5. Take off heat to prevent over cooking. Sprinkle lightly with salt, pepper and the parmesan cheese and parsley as desired. Serve over GF pasta , on top of Tuscan White Bean Soup or on top a dinner salad – Enjoy!

SASSY SALMON STEAKS

This is absolutely the yummiest grilled salmon recipe! It has the hot, sweet and the spicy flavors yet not overpowering. Adjust the red pepper to your desired heat even though the recipe is fairly medium heat to begin with.

8	salmon steaks, (1) inch thick
⅓	cup avocado or olive oil
1	teaspoon sesame oil, toasted variety if possible
5	tablespoons soy sauce, wheat free low sodium or Braggs Liquid Aminos
4	tablespoons Balsamic vinegar
4	tablespoons Agave Nectar syrup
2	teaspoons brown sugar, optional
1½	teaspoons ginger powder
1	teaspoon crushed red pepper flakes (adjust to desired heat)
1	teaspoon salt
2	green onions, diced

1. Place Salmon steaks in a Zip-lock baggy. Mix the remaining ingredients in a medium bowl, whisk together then pour into baggy and let stand in the refrigerator for 8 hours or overnight.

2. Remove fish from liquid and place in broiler or on grilling surface when the heat source is ready or follow next step.

3. Take a large piece of Aluminum Foil and coat it with Avocado oil or butter. Coat the cooking racks with olive or Avocado oil

to avoid sticking as the fish cooks inside the foil. Wrap the steaks tightly in the foil before placing on the cooking rack.

4. Cook for 2 ½ minutes on each side on a medium heat. The fish is done when it flakes – Enjoy!

5. Recipe by Chef Tamara Renee.

LIME CHICKEN TACOS WITH MANGO SALSA

4	chicken breast; skinless and boneless
1	large lime, squeeze juice
4	cloves garlic, minced
1	tablespoon of olive oil

1. Combine all ingredients in a zip-lock baggy or bowl and marinate for at least 2 hours or overnight if possible.

2. Grill for excellent flavor or cook using another method as desired. Baking is also a good method of cooking chicken for this recipe or a crock-pot. Grilling needs to be on low to medium heat until meat is no longer pink and food thermometer reads at least 178 degrees or higher.

3. Serve with Mango Salsa – Enjoy!

4. Recipe by www.FoodFriendzee.com.

Mango Salsa

2	mangos, peeled and chopped (1 ½ - 2 cups)
3	ripe Roma tomatoes, chopped
1	sweet pepper, red or yellow, chopped
1	hot pepper of choice, Serrano, Chipotle
¼	fresh cilantro, chopped
2	green onion, sliced thinly
1	lime, juice only
⅛- ½	teaspoon Stevia sweetener, if mangos are not sweet
	Salt & pepper

1. Prepare, mix well and serve. Stores in the refrigerator for up to one week.

MAGGIE'S SALMON PATTIES

1	can of wild salmon, cleaned
1	cup spinach or chard, chopped
2	tablespoons pine nuts or walnuts, chopped
1	teaspoon olive oil
1	stalk celery, diced
1	tablespoon onion, diced
1	egg, beaten
2	oz. water cracker crumbs
1	tablespoon lemon juice
2	tablespoons of feta or cottage cheese
½	teaspoon dill and thyme
	Pinch of black pepper
1	teaspoon soy sauce, wheat free low sodium

1. Sauté nuts, onion and celery in a skillet for 2 minutes until nuts slightly golden then add greens for another minute to wilt. Let cool before adding to mix.
2. In a medium bowl put fish which has been cleaned of skin and any bones. Separate with a fork into pieces then add the rest of the ingredients mixing well. With hands pat into patty shape and place on a plate ready to pan fry.
3. Cook patties on a hot skillet with olive oil about 3 minutes browning each side. Then place the lid on the skillet for the last cooking of about 1 minute.
4. Serve with yogurt dressing and a cucumber salad of choice. Boiled red potatoes with butter and parsley are a great compliment. Some may even enjoy the added flavor of an organic catsup sweetened naturally – Enjoy!

GRILLED FISH TACOS

1 - 2	pounds of fish, grilling requires skin left on fish or pan fried
1 - 2	tablespoons vegetable oil, as needed
10	(7 inch) flour tortillas, white or Teff flour (see Reference)
	Hot sauce
3	limes cut in wedges
1	small head of cabbage, Napa best
4	medium tomatoes, sliced
	Butter
	Guacamole Sauce

Guacamole Sauce

2	Avocadoes, halved, pitted and peeled
¾	cup Greek yogurt
1	tablespoon sour cream
1 - 2	tablespoons red onion, minced
½	cup cilantro, chopped finely
5	tablespoons lime juice
	Salt and pepper

Jalapeno pepper, diced or a pinch of cayenne pepper
Mash avocadoes in a medium bowl until creamy. Next
blend in the yogurt, sour cream and other ingredients
as you desire.

1. If grilling fish start this meal with lighting the grill to get the coals and or heat to medium. Brush the fish with oil and season with small amount of salt and black pepper. Grill over moderate heat until fish is slightly charred on both sides about 10 minutes. Transfer the fish to a platter to pull off skin.

2. In a large bowl toss the cabbage with 2 tablespoons of oil and 2 tablespoons of lime juice, salt and pepper.

3. Heat tortillas on metal plate on grill or on the stove top and

swipe with butter. Corn tortillas may also be used in this recipe as desired.

4. Assemble tacos by placing a dollop of guacamole, 4 ounces of fish, a couple slices of tomatoes and a generous helping of cabbage. Serve with hot sauce lime wedges and black beans or other on the side – Enjoy!

SOLE PORTABELLA

4   sole filets, 4 – 6 ounces each

1   pound of Portabella mushroom caps, sliced

½   medium onion, chopped

2   tablespoons olive oil

1   clove garlic, minced, optional

2   tablespoons lemon or lime juice

1   tablespoon soy sauce, wheat free low sodium

1   tablespoon fresh dill or ¾ teaspoon dried or other herb of choice

Salt and pepper to taste

1. Heat 1 tablespoon of oil in large skillet with medium heat then sauté onion for about 30 seconds then add both soy sauce and lemon juice.

2. Add mushrooms into skillet cooking and turning them until they plump with juices about 5 minutes then add herbs for another minute and turn onto a plate.

3. In the same skillet put another tablespoon olive oil heating back to medium temperature, add butter and the filets. Sole cook very quickly in just a couple of minutes so do not overcook. Turn once carefully with thin spatula to avoid breaking fish.

4. Serve with mushrooms on top of filets and a sprinkle of fresh grated Parmesan Reggiano cheese and a Dill sprig – Enjoy!

BROILED TILAPIA PARMESAN

4	Tilapia filets, ¾ inch
¼	cup parmesan cheese
2	teaspoons butter
1	tablespoon plus 1 ½ teaspoon mayonnaise (as desired)
½	teaspoon garlic salt or 1 clove fresh garlic, minced
⅛	teaspoon garlic powder (opt.)
⅛	teaspoon celery powder
⅛	teaspoon black pepper
1	tablespoon fresh lemon juice
	Salt and pepper

1. Preheat broiler after covering with foil.
2. In a medium bowl mix together the cheese, softened butter, mayonnaise and lemon juice. Then add the herbs; celery, garlic, pepper and a pinch of pepper. Mix well and set aside.
3. Arrange filets on the broiler sheet a few inches from the flames and cook for approximately 2 minutes turn and cook the other side. Carefully remove from broiler and cover each filet with the parmesan mixture and put back into broiler for a 30 - 60 seconds more until golden brown on top and around the edges.
4. Serve with steamed broccoli and red potatoes or alongside a dinner salad – Enjoy!

CARIBBEAN GINGER TURKEY

2	pounds chicken turkey breast, skinned for cooking
¼	cup soy sauce
¼	cup dry sherry or balsamic vinegar
2	tablespoons apricot jam
½	teaspoon ginger powder or fresh grated (best)
½	cup water
3	tablespoons Agave Nectar syrup or honey
2	tablespoons vegetable oil

2   teaspoons lemon juice

1   clove fresh garlic, minced

1. With sharpened knife remove meat from the bone. Cut into strips 2 inches wide and place in bowl with marinade and refrigerate.
2. To make marinade combine all of the ingredients into the bowl whisking with a fork or whisk reserving 1 tablespoon of oil for the grill or pan for stovetop cooking.
3. Let marinate for 1 – 4 hours to infuse the flavors into the meat before cooking.
4. Heat oiled grill to medium heat. Remove meat from marinade reserving liquid for brushing and place on grill with tongs. Cook for 6 minutes approximately and brush marinade onto meat before turning to retain meat moisture. Cook another 5 – 6 minutes and check with food thermometer for doneness.
5. 178 degrees or higher for poultry and beef can be cooked to desired doneness.
6. Precooked meats can be enjoyed with the Caribbean Dip (see recipe).
7. Serve with white rice and Julianne cut steamed vegetables – Enjoy!

LAMB CURRY

3   pound boneless leg of lamb, cut into medium pieces

2   tablespoons olive oil

2   tablespoons soy sauce, wheat free low sodium

½   cup water

2   medium onions, chopped

4   tomatoes or 5 tablespoons catsup

2   cloves fresh garlic, minced

2   bay leaves

1-2   tablespoons fresh ginger, grated from root, less if powder
        used perhaps 2 tsp.

½   teaspoon cumin powder

¼   teaspoon cinnamon and coriander (cilantro) or fresh leaves

¼   teaspoon red cayenne pepper

½   teaspoon salt

1   cup fresh cilantro, chopped

1. In a large pot like a Dutch oven with a lid heat the oil on medium.
    Add the cut up lamb and brown on all side for about 5 minutes
    then set aside. Next add the onions and garlic and sauté for 2
    minutes then add back meat and all the rest of the ingredients
    except the chopped cilantro and bring to a constant simmer.

2. Cook for about 1 hour until tender. Serve with fresh cilantro,
    a dollop of sour cream, white rice and vegetables of choice.
    Applesauce or a fruit salad on the table would complement the
    flavors – Enjoy!

3. Recipe by Anne Louise Gittleman.

SPAGHETTI FOR EVERYONE

*What is the catch? Zone 2 & 3 can both have a big challenge with pasta
and two solutions are offered to give everyone a spaghetti night. Several types
of corn pasta have been formulated that seem to be well tolerated and not
cause GIS grief. Another yummy solution is to cook1 -2 spaghetti squashes.
When it is good it is scrumptious!*

1   pound ground meat, turkey, beef or chicken

1   large (or 2 small) spaghetti squash, organic if possible or 1
        pound of corn pasta or other as tolerated, *Authentic Foods* or
        other (De Boles Zone 1)

½   cup onion, chopped

1 - 2   tablespoons olive oil

1   large jar or can tomato sauce (or Pesto Sauce)

½   cup freshly grated parmesan cheese
Herbs of choice; fresh garlic, basil, oregano and anise
1   tablespoon honey, optional
Butter
Salt and pepper

1. In a medium skillet with high sides and a lid heat olive oil on medium. Sauté an onion about one minute then add meat and cook for about 6 minutes until browned.
2. Add herbs and sauce and bring to a simmer for about 10 minutes.
3. In a large pot with lid heat water for pasta and cook according to directions of pasta of choice, drain and return to pot adding 1 tablespoon of olive oil and butter and toss to prevent sticking.
4. If cooking Spaghetti Squash scrub well and then choose to bake in a traditional oven, steam on top of the stove (cutting the squash in half) or in a microwave oven. The microwave does work but make certain you safely slice poke holes (with a knife) for steam to escape into the squash before cooking for approximately 5 minutes then another 5 minutes, checking to see how easily a knife inserts. If needed cook for another 2 – 3 minutes.
5. The object of cooking with any of the methods is to cook the round squash until tender. Once the squash is cooked you cut it open if cooking whole and with a fork remove the inner pulp that is very fibrous like "Spaghetti".
6. Serve with butter and prepared sauce and toppings - Enjoy!

Basic Pesto
1   cup walnuts
½   cup pine nuts (opt.)
2   cups fresh basil
½   cup olive oil
2 - 3   cloves garlic

½   **teaspoon salt**
     Pepper

Chop all ingredients finely and gently simmer in a pan to infuse the flavors for approximately 5 minutes. Serve over pasta, vegetables or wraps – Enjoy!

JULIENNE ZUCCHINI VEGETABLES

Variation in the cutting style of a vegetable influences the presentation and enjoyment of vegetables. Combinations are endless and applying the Julienne cut (long square matchstick shape) transforms ordinary vegetables and gives them a new look and taste experience.

1   **small onion, cut in half-moon slices or 3 green onions, chopped**
1   **red bell pepper, sliced**
1   **yellow bell pepper, sliced**
1   **medium carrot, sliced medium diagonal**
2 -3 **zucchinis, cut Julienne style, 2 ½ inch pieces**
1   **tablespoon vegetable oil**
     Pinch of red pepper flakes, optional
½   **teaspoon savory, thyme or oregano, optional**
     Butter
     Salt and pepper

1. Heat large skillet with vegetable oil on medium and sauté onion for approximately 1 minute.
2. Recipe works well with any smaller squash or broccoli.
3. Add the rest of the ingredients turning every minute for 5 minutes then place lid on pan for the remaining minute until tender. Serve with any main course or as a starter with the Caribbean Dip or other dip or salad dressing – Enjoy!

OVEN ROASTED CAULIFLOWER

1	head cauliflower
2-4	tablespoons olive oil
1	teaspoon smoked paprika
	Salt & pepper to taste

1. Preheat oven to 375 degrees.
2. Line a large baking sheet with parchment paper or foil.
3. Prepare Cauliflower by removing the long stems and cutting it into 1 ¼ inch slices reserving the crumbles and placing them into a large bowl.
4. Drizzle with olive oil and season with smoked paprika and salt and pepper as desired.
5. Turn onto the baking sheet and spread evenly.
6. Bake 35 – 45 minutes until it begins to brown – Enjoy!

ROASTED MARINATED VEGETABLES

6 - 8	cups of vegetables to include; zucchini squash, yellow crook neck squash, red onions, baby carrots (cut in half), asparagus, eggplant, red and green bell peppers, others, cut in medium slices
¼ - ½	cup of olive oil
¾	cup Balsamic vinegar
1	tablespoon each; fresh oregano and basil
2½	teaspoons thyme
½	teaspoon salt
½	teaspoon pepper

1. Place cut vegetables in a large bowl and pour vinegar liberally over them. Decrease the vinegar with less vegetables and increase with more quantity.
2. Next sprinkle them with the herbs, including the salt and pepper tossing them well. Lightly coat with olive oil and toss once more.

3. Place vegetables on a baking sheet into a preheat 400 degree oven for approximately 15 – 20 minutes. Remove from oven to cool slightly and arrange on a serving platter. Delicious as a vegetable side to any main dish or starter – Enjoy!

SAUTÉED CHARD

1	**bunch Chard greens, chopped**
¼	**onion, chopped**
1-2	**teaspoons olive oil**
	Pinch of red pepper flakes, optional
2	**tablespoons chicken broth, optional**
1	**teaspoon soy sauce**

1. Wash and inspect each leaf cutting off any black spots from damage and chop.
2. Heat medium skillet with olive oil and sauté onion for 30 seconds then add the chard and red pepper flakes. If you like heat you can use a small pinch of red cayenne or hot sauce instead. Place lid on skillet and cook for 1 minute. Lift lid and add chicken broth and soy sauce and cook 1 more minute until tender.
3. Squeeze lemon or a little vinegar of choice before serving as a side vegetable – Enjoy!

BROCCOLI RED BELL PEPPER

1½	**pounds of broccoli, stock stripped, cut into 3 - 4 inch pieces**
1	**red sweet bell pepper, cut strips**
2	**stalk of celery, chopped medium**
1	**cup chicken broth**
½	**cup water**
1	**teaspoon favorite herb; savory, thyme or basil**
	Butter or olive oil

1. Clean broccoli and peel back outer fibrous covering of the stalks.

2. Place all vegetables in a 2 quart pan with a lid including chicken broth, herbs and butter or olive oil. Bring to a boil and turn down to a simmer for 5 minutes removing from heat when broccoli is fork tender. Stir to mix herbs and oil/butter thoroughly and drain.

3. Best served warm yet remove the lid if vegetables sit to avoid over cooking. Delicious by itself or with a squeeze of lemon or lime to accent any meal. Makes a great addition to salads when cold – Enjoy!

VEGETABLE TERRINE CASSEROLE

2	tablespoons olive oil
2	large Red potatoes, sliced ¼ inch (medium)
1	bell pepper, yellow or other, thinly sliced and chopped
1	onion, diced
1	clove fresh garlic
1	teaspoon thyme leaves
½	pound plum tomatoes, sliced medium
2	zucchinis, sliced diagonal medium
3	tablespoons fresh grated cheese, optional
3 - 4	slices of cheese, Provolone, optional
	Salt & pepper

1. Preheat oven to 350 degrees.

2. Coat a 9 inch baking dish with olive oil.

3. Spread potatoes evenly across the bottom, drizzle a little olive oil, salt and pepper placing cheese slices on top.

4. In a bowl mix the bell pepper, onion, thyme, salt and pepper and garlic and spread half the mixture over the potatoes.

5. Layer tomatoes and zucchini slices on top next and spread remaining pepper mix a drizzle of oil and grated cheese.

6. Cover baking dish with foil and bake for 45 minutes then uncover about 25 minutes until tender and glazed over.

7. Remove from stove and let stand for 10 minutes before serving hot or also good at room temperature - Enjoy!
8. Recipe by Chef Pamela Croft.

SCRUMPTIOUS YAM FRIES

5   **medium or 2 large yams, peeled, Julienne cut**
1   **tablespoon olive oil**
1   **teaspoon cumin**
     Salt and pepper

1. Clean and prepare the yam potatoes cutting them 4 inches long by ¼ x ¼ inch or wedges.
2. Toss with olive oil in bowl then spread across a cookie sheet in a single layer.
3. Bake in oven at 425 degrees for 25 minutes turning half way, salt and pepper – Enjoy!
4. Recipe by Kelly Cappasola.

ROSEMARY POTATO WEDGES

8 - 10   **medium red potatoes, cleaned cut into wedges**
1   **tablespoon olive oil**
1-2   **teaspoon fresh oregano**
1   **tablespoon fresh rosemary**
1 - 2   **cloves fresh garlic, minced**

1. Prepare potatoes quartering the smaller potatoes. Toss with olive oil and herbs then spread evenly single layered on cookie sheet.
2. Bake in oven at 425 degrees for 25 – 30 minutes turning once. The rustic flavor enhances any chicken or fish entres and delicious with a Greek yogurt dip of choice – Enjoy!
3. Recipe by Kelly Cappasola.

RED POTATO AU GRATIN

1½	pounds red potato, 5 – 6 medium, peeled and cut into ¼ inch-thick slices
⅓	cup butter, softened
½	cup Gruyere or other Swiss cheese, grated
1	cup half and half
½-1	teaspoon salt
½	teaspoon ground black pepper
⅛	teaspoon paprika

1. Preheat oven to 350 degrees F.
2. Butter a 1 ½ quart baking dish with about 1 tablespoon.
3. Arrange a layer of potatoes in the dish and sprinkle with cheese. Continue to layer using all potatoes and cheese.
4. In a small bowl whisk cream with salt and pepper and pour over the potatoes. Dot with the remaining butter and sprinkle with the paprika.
5. Bake for 60 – 75 minutes or until the potatoes are tender and golden brown on top. Let stand for 5 minutes out of the oven before serving and top with parsley – Enjoy!

VEGETABLE MILLET/QUINOA - PILAF

1	cup hulled Millet or Quinoa, low gluten grains
¼	cup each vegetable; onion, carrot, celery and bell pepper, diced small
1	clove fresh garlic, minced
1	teaspoon thyme or savory
1	teaspoon oregano
2	tablespoon butter
3	cups chicken broth, low sodium
1	teaspoon soy sauce, wheat free or Bragg Aminos
	Salt and pepper
	Pinch of cayenne, optional

1. In a 2 quart pan with tight fitting lid, bring to medium heat adding grain only and stir for about 2 -3 minutes until grain begins to brown.
2. Then add butter, onion, garlic and celery and sauté for another 1-2 minutes.
3. Add the rest of the vegetables, herbs, chicken broth with lid on the pot. Bring to a boil then turn down to a constant simmer for 20 minutes, not lifting lid.
4. Variation: white basmati rice (1 cup) requiring the broth decreased to (2 cups) and cooking time 45 minutes with lid on pan.
5. Serve as a side to any main course or lunch /dinner salad – Enjoy!

WILD RICE BLEND

¾   cup Basmati White Rice
¼   cup Wild Rice
2   cups water

1. Bring water to a boil in a 2 quart sauce pan and add rice. Cover with a tight fitting lid and cook on a constant simmer boil for 45 minutes. Do not lift lid and to avoid burning cook on top a "trivet" available in cooking store. Use a rice cooker if preferred.

ZUCCHINI PARMESAN DELIGHT

3   Zucchinis, grated
1   small onion, chopped
1   teaspoon favorite herb; thyme, savory, basil
1   tablespoons olive oil
1-2   teaspoons butter
Topping: Fresh grated Parmesan or Jack Cheese

1. Delight your taste buds with this easy side dish. In medium

skillet heat oil and add onion and cook for 1 -2 minutes until translucent.

2. Add the zucchinis and sauté for 1 minutes with herb seasoning, butter, pinch of salt and pepper place lid on skillet and let steam in own juices another minute and it is ready to serve with a sprinkle of favorite cheese or alone – Enjoy!

CAULIFLOWER MASHED "POTATOES" (Potato Free)

1	head cauliflower cut in wedges
1	tablespoon olive oil
1- 3	tablespoons butter
4	tablespoons Half and half (opt.)
	Salt and pepper
	Parsley, chopped

Steam cauliflower in 2 quart pan with lid in boiling water, 2 inches in bottom of pan for 15 minutes until tender to fork test. Drain water and put in food processor or blender with oil, butter and half and half until smooth. Return to pan until serving keeping warm.

Serve in place of mashed potatoes seasoning with salt, pepper and a sprinkle of chives or parsley for taste and color – Enjoy!

Recipe by Loni Pickle.

PESTO STUFFED MUSHROOMS

14 - 16	button mushroom, cleaned and steamed
	Stuffing:
1	cup walnuts
½	cup pine nuts
2	cups fresh basil
½	cup olive oil
2 - 3	cloves garlic
½	teaspoon salt
	Pepper

1. Clean mushrooms of outer debris gently using a mushroom brush if possible and cut any bad spots off. Do not submerge in water. Next take a small knife and remove the center stump and then using a teaspoon clean the remaining inside surface as needed.

2. Place mushroom caps top side down on a baking pan appropriate for the broiler.

3. Blend all stuffing ingredients in a food processor or blender until smooth.

4. Scoop 1 heaping teaspoon of stuffing into each mushroom.

5. Variation includes placing mushroom in a dehydrator for 5-6 hours that blends the flavors and changes the texture to an enjoyable raw food taste treat or conventional cooking methods below.

6. Place in broiler for 5 – 6 minutes until bubbling occurs on tops and slightly toasted.

7. Variation for raw stuffed mushrooms: Place filled mushroom in a dehydrator for 5-6 hours that allows the blending of the flavors and changes the texture to an enjoyable raw food taste treat.

8. Crab stuffed mushrooms are also a favorite for many using; 1 cup crab meat, ½ cup white water cracker crumbs, ½ cup cream cheese, ½ cup chopped parsley, 1 – 2 chopped green onions, 1 clove minced garlic and 4 tablespoons parmesan cheese. Mix all together, stuff mushrooms generously, spray with olive oil or brush with melted butter and bake for 20 minutes in a 375 degree oven until slightly brown on top – Enjoy!

Dips, Spreads & Dressings

Experiment with making the following recipes to find out what you enjoy with complimenting; meats, vegetables and even fruits. A rule in food preparation is to use less of an ingredient that you may not be familiar with until you taste test. You can always add more but you cannot take away from a recipe. Yes you can purchase premade dips, spreads and dressings yet unfortunately many of them contain GIS triggers. Once you have the basic ingredients you can make your own wonderful delicious creations!

SALMON PATE

1	can of salmon, wild caught
1	can sardines boneless skinless
¾	cup cottage cheese (opt.)
¼	cup sour cream or plain yogurt (opt.)
1	tablespoon mustard, use personal favorite
½	stalk celery, diced
1	tablespoon onion, diced
1	clove fresh garlic, minced (opt.)
¼ - ½	teaspoon dill, optional
	Pepper
	Parsley or cilantro

1. Carefully open cans, drain and discard the skin of the salmon as desired.
2. Place all ingredients in a medium bowl and mash together with a fork.
3. Variations include using leftover fish, black olives and hot sauce.
4. Serve with white water crackers, wraps, corn chips or salads – Enjoy!
5. Recipe by Terry Koch.

TUNA SPREAD

1	(8 oz.) can of tuna or salmon or fresh cooked fish
2	tablespoons of olive oil
1	tablespoon of red wine vinegar
1	teaspoon Italian seasoning containing; oregano, basil, thyme, fennel, garlic
	Salt and pepper

1. Open cans of fish and place in a medium bowl or use leftover cooked fish. Discard any undesirable skin and add all of the herbs of choice and mix well with a fork. Ready to eat on a salad, wrap or as an entree for lunch or dinner – Enjoy!

CHICKEN SALAD SPREAD

2	**cups cooked chicken, diced**
1	**stalk celery, diced**
8	**black olives, pitted, sliced**
1	**green onion, optional, thinly sliced**
½	**teaspoon dill or thyme**
½	**cup Greek yogurt**
2	**tablespoons sour cream**
1	**heaping teaspoon Dijon mustard**
	Salt and pepper to taste

Variation: Use seedless grapes cut in half and omit olives.

Mix with a fork in a medium bowl – Enjoy!

WHITE BEAN SPREAD

2	**cups cooked white beans**
2	**tablespoons olive oil**
1 - 2	**cloves fresh garlic or (1) T. onion, minced**
2	**teaspoons fresh rosemary, minced**
	Salt and pepper
	Italian parsley, chopped

1. Heat oil in a 10 inch skillet on medium adding garlic and rosemary for 1 minute sauté being careful not to burn the herbs. Add beans and mash them as they heat with wooden spoon or potato masher. Cook together to a loose consistency about 5 – 6 minutes. Remove from heat and let cool and transfer to serving bowl or refrigerator container to use as a dip with vegetable, chips or on wraps – Enjoy!

HUMMUS DIP – (garlic-sesame free)

1½	cups cooked garbanzo beans, canned
¼	cup olive oil
¼	teaspoon toasted sesame oil
1 - 2	tablespoons fresh lemon juice (1 large lemon)
½	teaspoon cumin
2	tablespoons water to desired consistency
½	teaspoons salt

1. Place all ingredients in a food processor or blender until creamy.
2. Best combined with another protein source to complete protein; cheese slices, nuts and seeds or meat.
3. Serve with vegetables, chips or on wraps. Great for kids – Enjoy!
4. Recipe by Loree Wilstermann.

TAHINI YOGURT DRESSING

1	cup plain yogurt, Greek or homemade
¼	cup Tahini, sesame butter
2	tablespoons mustard
1	tablespoon lemon juice
1	teaspoon soy sauce, wheat free low sodium
½	teaspoon cumin powder (optional)

1. Combine all the ingredients into a blender or with a fork and mix until smooth.
2. Variation: Omit cumin and add 1 tablespoon of honey or Agave nectar syrup.
3. May be kept for a couple of weeks refrigerated and is delicious on meat, vegetables, wraps and salads!

QUICK MISO-TAHINI DRESSING

4	tablespoons olive oil
8	tablespoons water

1   lemon or lime, juiced

1   tablespoon Sesame Tahini, butter

1½   teaspoon Miso Paste, Red or other

1   small fresh garlic clove, minced

     Blend with fork until creamy – Enjoy!

TRADITIONAL HUMMUS SPREAD

1   cup cooked Garbanzo beans, canned

⅓   cup water

3 - 4 tablespoons fresh lemon juice

3   tablespoons Tahini, sesame butter

1   clove fresh garlic, minced

1   tablespoon olive oil

⅛   teaspoon salt

     Paprika, optional

     Parsley, chopped

1. Mix all ingredients in a food processor or blender until creamy. Sprinkle the top of the serving bowl with paprika and parsley. Serve with vegetables, meats and or chips. Great for a mayonnaise replacement in wraps – Enjoy!

HOT & SPICY MUSTARD VEGGIE DIP

1   cup cottage cheese or Greek yogurt

1   heaping tablespoon sour cream

1   tablespoon Dijon or Spicy Mustard

     Pinch of Cayenne pepper, hot or hot sauce

1   tablespoon honey, optional

¼   teaspoon onion powder

¼   teaspoon garlic powder

¼   teaspoon celery powder

1   tablespoon fresh parsley, chopped

1. Place all ingredients in a food processor or blender until creamy.
2. Store in a refrigerator container and use for potato oven fries, raw or cooked vegetables, chips, salads, meats or wraps – Enjoy!

SPINACH DIP

3	cups spinach, frozen defrosted (10 oz. box), chopped
1	cup sour cream
1	cup Greek yogurt
1	tablespoon honey
2	tablespoons olive oil
¼	cup green onions, thinly sliced
3	tablespoons red bell pepper, diced
1	can water chestnuts, diced
½	teaspoon each; dill and celery salt
¼	teaspoon black pepper

1. Mix all ingredients in a large bowl and let stand in the refrigerator for at least 3 hours before serving to allow the flavors to blend.
2. Serve with crackers, chips, veggies and on salads – Enjoy!

GUACAMOLE DIP

2	Avocadoes, halved, pitted and peeled
¾	cup Greek yogurt
1	tablespoon sour cream
1 - 2	tablespoons red onion, minced
½	cup cilantro, chopped finely
5	tablespoons lime juice
	Salt and pepper
	Jalapeno pepper, diced or a pinch of cayenne pepper

1. Mash avocadoes in a medium bowl until creamy.
2. Next blend in the yogurt, sour cream and other ingredients as desired and watch it disappear – Enjoy!

SWEET CARIBBEAN GINGER DIP

1	cup Greek Yogurt
1	tablespoon sour cream
1	tablespoon Agave Nectar syrup
⅓	cup apple juice
1	tablespoon olive oil
1	clove fresh garlic, minced
1 - 3	teaspoons fresh grated ginger or ½ tsp. ginger powder
	Sea Salt

1. Mix all ingredients in a medium size bowl with a fork or whisk.
2. Serve with cooked or raw vegetables, cooked meats or even on a fruit salad – Enjoy!

THAI PEANUT SAUCE

1½	cups peanut butter
½	cup coconut milk
3	tablespoons water
3	tablespoons fresh lime juice
1-3	teaspoons soy sauce
1	tablespoon fish sauce (opt)
1 - 3	teaspoons hot sauce or sweet red chili sauce, (opt)
1	tablespoon minced fresh ginger root or 1 – 2 tsp. powdered, (opt)
1 - 3	cloves fresh garlic, minced
¼	cup fresh cilantro, chopped

1. Mix all in a bowl with a whisk, food processor or blender – Enjoy!

BBQ SAUCE

2	tablespoons olive oil
1	tablespoon onion, diced

2-3   cloves of fresh garlic, minced

3   cups (28 oz.) tomatoes, fire toasted, finely chopped

½   cup fresh lime juice

½   cup Balsamic vinegar

½   cup Agave nectar syrup

2   tablespoons chili powder

1. Heat the oil in a 2 quart sauce pan over medium heat. Add the onion and sauté for 3 minutes until soft. Add the garlic and stir for a minute not allowing it to burn and then add the rest of the ingredients. Bring it to a low boil and simmer for 20 minutes. Cool and place in blender. Process until creamy smooth and transfer to a sturdy container perhaps glass, to store in the refrigerator for up to 2 – 3 weeks – Enjoy!

2. Recipe is found in *Positively Ageless* by Cheryl Forberg, RD of the Biggest Loser TV show.

MANGO SALSA

2   mangos, peeled and chopped

2   ripe Roma tomatoes, chopped

1   sweet pepper, red or yellow, chopped

1   hot pepper of choice, Serrano, Chipotle or other

2   green onion, sliced thinly

1   lime, juice only

⅛- ½   teaspoon Stevia sweetener, if mangos not sweet

Mix together in a large serving bowl and serve as desired - Enjoy!

HOUSE VINAIGRETTE

½   cup olive oil

½   cup flax oil

3   oz. Rice Vinegar

3   oz. Balsamic Vinegar

1   teaspoon thyme

1   clove fresh garlic, minced, optional

½   teaspoon each Salt and pepper

Mix with a whisk until blended well and store in the refrigerator.

ITALIAN VINAIGRETTE

6   tablespoons olive oil

1½   cups red wine vinegar

½   teaspoon each; lemon juice, Dijon mustard, garlic powder, dried oregano and basil

      Salt and pepper

      Mix with a whisk until it is blended well.

CREAMY CAESAR DRESSING

½   cup olive oil

¼   cup sour cream or yogurt

1   tablespoon Soy Sauce, wheat free low sodium

1   tablespoon white wine or rice wine vinegar

4   cloves fresh garlic, minced

¼   teaspoon ground black pepper

1- 2 tablespoons Dijon Mustard

2   tablespoons Anchovy paste

½   cup fresh squeezed lemon juice

1   egg yolk

2   tablespoons Parmesan cheese

1   teaspoon salt, as desired

      Black pepper

CHILI DRESSING

½   cup olive oil

½   cup red wine vinegar

1   garlic clove, minced

1   teaspoon chili powder

1   teaspoon dried or fresh oregano

¼   teaspoon cumin

1   teaspoon salt

¼   teaspoon ground pepper

BASIC "MOCK MAYO" DRESSING

1   cup Yogurt

1   tablespoon sour cream

1½   teaspoon mustard

2   teaspoons vinegar or lemon juice

1   teaspoon honey

Salt and pepper

Oil Free – Egg Free

CREAMY SWEET YOGURT DRESSING

1   cup yogurt, Greek style or ½ cup sour cream and ½ cup yogurt for richer taste

1   tablespoon honey, optional

1   tablespoon mustard

1 - 3   teaspoons lemon juice

Salt and pepper to taste

SEASON SALT

6   tablespoons Sea salt

½   teaspoon dried thyme

½   teaspoon dried marjoram

½   teaspoon garlic powder

2 ¼   teaspoons paprika

¼   teaspoon curry powder

1   teaspoon dried mustard

¼   teaspoon onion powder

⅛   teaspoon dill-weed

½   teaspoon celery salt

Recipe makes about 4 ounces of seasoning.

Desserts

Nutritious desserts are enjoyable and are also important on the GIS program for renewal of the body. These dessert ideas are delicious however use self-control on the quantity of any recipe because the natural sugars in fruits can still be a challenge for the body to process. Many people even not having a diagnosis of Diabetes can still be living with "tricky blood sugar" that effects health. This is true for children as well as adults so I suggest smaller portions in dessert cups even for the "Big Kids" the adults. Cakes, cookies and pies can all be made with LG and GF flours and alternative sweeteners yet I have chosen to include mostly "nutrient dense" dessert choices that add to the rejuvenation of the body while tasting scrumptious - Enjoy!

TROPICAL KIWI PAPAYA FRUIT SALAD

3	Kiwis, peeled, medium slices
2	bananas, ripe, medium sliced
2	Apples, chopped
2	cups Papaya, ripe, peeled, cubed (or Strawberries)
	Lime wedges

Quality fruit organically grown when possible will taste better and be better for the whole family. Preparing a fresh fruit salad for the family gives a special treat with no guilt attached and it contains nutritious building blocks for health.

Small fruit cups accompanying a lunch or dinner is a great dessert treat enhancing the flavors of the meal. Of course it can also be served in-between meals with yogurt, cottage cheese or slices of sharp cheddar as a mini-meal. Including a small handful of raw nuts and seeds or cheese helps to stabilize the blood sugar. However, for some people eating fruit with a meal is the best time so the protein can balance the glycemic sugar response (See Ch. 6 Healthy Focus).

Easy to fix fruit salads just require some time to shop, clean and peel any spoiled spots from the fruit. If it is to last for a few days prepare it in a refrigerator container. Combinations are endless and having children to help makes a fruit salad a fun activity. Younger children can help cut the bananas and soft fruits while older children can learn to handle a knife with supervision.

Combine all ingredients gently folding together and squeezing a couple of lime wedges or the juice of an orange over the fruit salad helps to retain the color and freshness. In general it tastes better to keep oranges to eat all by themselves. Organic grapes are also a real treat in themselves like melons.

Adding just a few ripe strawberries or other fruits in season on the plate of a traditional meal offers a yummy surprise – Enjoy!

CHOCOLATE AVOCADO MOUSSE

4	ripe avocadoes, peeled, pitted and mashed
¾	cup honey
1	tablespoon pure vanilla
1	cup cocoa powder

1. Blend in a food processor or blender until smooth and creamy. Serve in a dessert dish approximately ½ cup with squirt of whip cream and strawberry or other fruit slices. This is a truly decadent dessert – Enjoy!

FIGS RICOTTA, PISTACHIOS AND HONEY

8	dried figs
¼	cup unsalted pistachios or blanched almonds
¼	cup part-skim ricotta cheese (Zone 1) or Greek Yogurt (Zone 2 & 3)
1	tablespoon honey
	Salt to taste

1. Toast nuts in a dry skillet for 3 – 5 minutes until fragrant stirring frequently. Set aside to cool then chop finely.

2. Cut figs in half crosswise and place the fig pieces on a serving dish, cut side up.

3. Mix the honey and salt into the cheese or yogurt.

4. Make an indention with a spoon or your finger into the fig. Then place ½ teaspoon of the ricotta or yogurt filling on each fig and sprinkle with toasted nuts – Enjoy!

PEANUT SESAME DATE JOY BALLS

1	**cup peanut butter**
¼	**cup honey**
¼	**cup sesame Tahini butter**
1	**cup dates, pitted, chopped into small pieces**
1	**tablespoon pure Vanilla extract**
1	**cup puffed rice cereal**
	Coating; either shredded coconut or
	Cocoa powder, ¾ cup

1. This recipe is very easy to make however patience is required and some muscle to stir and blend the ingredients. It can be made with almond or cashew butter as desired and tolerated.

2. Mix all ingredients except the coating together well. A wooden spoon works fairly well. Next roll into bite-size balls in your palm and then roll through the coating of choice laying the balls flat.

3. Joy Balls can be stored in the refrigerator for months - Enjoy!

CASHEW DATE DELIGHTS

4	**Medjool dates**
2	**tablespoons cream cheese, Horizons Brand**
8	**whole cashew nuts, raw or freshly toasted**

1. Quick treat to make - just slice open the dates and remove pits and place on a serving tray. Next whip cream cheese with fork

or spoon and scoop 1 teaspoon into cavity. Place a half or whole cashew or blanched almond into the cream cheese

2. Variation is omitting the cheese and add one teaspoon of nut butter directly into opened date – Enjoy!

BLANCHED ALMONDS

1   cup raw almonds, with the brown skin - organic if possible

1. In a medium saucepan bring 6 cups of water to a boil then carefully slide the almonds into the water.

2. Boil on a simmer for approximately 6 minutes to make certain the skins softens.

3. Drain and as the nuts cool you can fairly easily slip the outer skin off like squeezing a grape out of its skin motion.

4. Pat almonds dry and store in the refrigerator for up to one week or freeze for an extended amount of time. The blanched almonds do not have the same allergic response for people due to molds that can grow on the skin.

5. Toasted almonds can be made by putting 2 teaspoons of oil in a frying skillet and stir constantly while they take on a golden color. Lightly salt as desired.

6. Another great use is making almond milk very easily!

ALMOND MILK

1   cup of blanched almonds
4   cups filtered water
1   tablespoon Agave nectar syrup or honey
2   teaspoons pure Vanilla extract

1. Place almonds in a blender or food processor on high. Add the other ingredients and blend well. May use as a milk replacement for a beverage and baking. Almond milk is not the best for an

addition to coffee or tea. Half and half (dairy) is used in hot beverages by many people on the GIS Diet.

2. Variation: Use sesame Tahini butter or cashew butter or nuts in place of almonds.

3. Stores in the refrigerator for 7 – 10 days and tastes delicious – Enjoy!

CANDIED NUTS

1	**cup of coarsely chopped nuts; pecans, cashews, walnuts or blanched almonds**
2	**tablespoons natural sweetener; Agave Nectar syrup or honey**
2	**teaspoons butter**
¼	**teaspoon salt**
1	**teaspoon herbs; oregano, thyme, basil and rosemary combined (opt.)**

1. Heat oven to 325 degrees and use a non-stick baking sheet or foil covered.

2. Combine in a small sauce pan on low heat; butter, honey and seasonings. Add the chopped nuts of choice and mix well. Turn out onto baking sheet as evenly as possible and place in oven for approximately 12 minutes turning every (4) minutes to achieve a golden brown. Clumping of some nuts is expected.

3. Great for sprinkling on a salads, wrap or grain dish. Store in an airtight container for one week - Enjoy!

4. Recipe by Cheryl Forberg, RD, Nutritionist for the Biggest Loser NBC's TV show.

GF TRAIL MIX

2	**cup Rice Chex**
1	**cup raw nuts and seeds, as tolerated like cashews, blanched almonds (thoroughly dry), sunflower seeds or other**

1   cup dried fruit, as tolerated like papaya, organic raisins or other cut in small pieces

1.   Mix together and keep in an airtight container in a cool cupboard. Don't refrigerate. Add other GF dry ingredients as desired. Fresh for approximately 2 weeks – Enjoy!

BASIC CHEESECAKE WITH GF GRAHAM CRACKER CRUST

13   Graham crackers, crushed, (regular crust for Zone 1 - GF cookies if possible)
2   tablespoons butter, melted
4   (8 oz.) packages of cream cheese, Horizons brand or other approved
1½   cups granulated Xylitol sugar
¾   cups half and half
4   eggs
1   cup sour cream, Horizons
1   tablespoon pure Vanilla extract
1   tablespoon Xanthan gum

1.   Preheat oven to 350 degrees. Grease a 9 inch spring-form pan.
2.   In a medium bowl mix graham crackers and butter and press into only the bottom of the pan.
3.   In a large bowl mix cream cheese and sugar until smooth. Blend in half and half and one egg at a time just enough to incorporate it. Then blend in sour cream, vanilla and Xanthan gum. Pour filling into pan.
4.   Bake for 1 hour then turn heat off and let cool in oven for 5 – 6 hours. Lastly, put the cheese cake into the refrigerator until you are ready to cut cake.
5.   Variations for Zone 2 & 3: Gluten Free (GF) Ginger snap cookies or other for crust available under the Trader Joe's brand or use the nut crust from *Authentic Foods* (see Reference).

Fruit Sorbets, Fruit Ice & Frappes!

Fruit Ice Sorbet is the easiest and most refreshing frozen dessert to make at home and it is great for lactose intolerant families. For most flavors all it takes is a fresh fruit puree, a little lemon juice, sweetening and the time to make a colorful and yummy tasting Sorbet. Fruit Ice and Frappes invite endless creations to enjoy for the whole family especially during the summer months!

Sorbets

Tips include using ripe fruit, organic when possible and trimmed of any blemishes. Refined Sorbets require; a pound of fruit, ¾ cup of sugar (Xylitol sugar is best), lemon juice and egg whites to give it an extra firmness. Adding ripe bananas to any recipe will give a smoother and creamier texture and taste. Also, using an ice cream freezer will make a smoother Sorbet. Berries should be strained after the puree is made unless a hand food mill is used. To learn more about making this luscious dessert just Google the *New York Times* article "Fresh Fruit Puree" - tips for making Sorbets.

FRUIT ICE

3	ounces frozen orange juice
1	cup ice cubes

1. Place in food processor or blender turning off to push down ice cubes until thoroughly crushed. Serve immediately or refreeze in ice cube trays.
2. Flavor variations: apple, lemonade, pineapple and fruit punch.
3. Look for sugar free or reduced sugar frozen juices.

Frappes

The following recipes are for quick sorbets called "Frappes" made in a blender. Frappe is French for a "chilled" drink. Mind you that using a blender even if it is advertised for making iced desserts may result in premature breakage vs. blending softer foods. Blend on high and always turn off the blender before adding more ingredients to blend. Serve immediately or refreeze in an ice cube tray. Both Fruit Ice and Frappes are great for busy people. Be creative and make your own tasty Frappe recipes - Enjoy!

BERRY BANANA YOGURT FRAPPE

1	cup berries; strawberry, blueberries, other
1	banana, ripe, peeled, frozen
1	cup Greek yogurt or Almond Milk (dairy free)
2	ice cubes
1	tablespoon honey
¼	teaspoon pure vanilla extract
	May garnish with whip cream and a few berries.

MELON FRAPPE

2	cups watermelon or cantaloupe
3-5	ice cubes
2	tablespoons frozen concentrated lemonade

APPLE CINNAMON HIBISCUS FRAPPE

3-5	Hibiscus ice cubes
2	medium organic apples, cut into wedges
½	teaspoon cinnamon
1	tablespoon honey

Variation: 1 small banana, optional
1. Make Hibiscus herb tea and freeze in ice cube tray then blend – refreshing!

CHOCOLATE PEAR EXTRAORDINAIRE

2	pears, ripe, cut in half
2	tablespoons cocoa powder, Ghirardelli unsweetened

1   **tablespoon honey or other approved sweetener**

1   **teaspoon pure Vanilla extract**

5   **ice cubes**

May garnish with whip cream and mint leaf.

BANANA SPLIT FRAPPE

2   **bananas, ripe, peeled, frozen**

1   **cup strawberries, organic**

1   **tablespoon Cocoa powder**

¾   **cups Greek Yogurt**

3   **ice cubes**

GIS Supplement Program; Shortcuts to Health

"Living with advanced Rheumatoid (Sclerotic) Arthritis pain was taking over my entire life. I woke up with pain and went to bed with pain. Even though I was only in my 40's I could no longer handle a full time job. The medication doctors gave me helped at first but gradually the four prescriptions I took weren't controlling my pain. As time went along I began gaining more and more weight and felt badly not just in my joints but all over.

One day I happened upon a health show called the Forever Young Radio Show and it seemed as if it just might be an answer to prayer. I started listening regularly and followed the health suggestions first focusing on my diet. As hard as it was I got off sugar. That seemed to help quite a bit. Next I began eating more of a gluten free diet with lots of vegetables, fish and lean meats and that helped reduce my pain even more. I was encouraged and asked myself, "What do I have to lose to perhaps feel even better?" So I got on the suggested supplements called the essential core nutrients, one at a time, plus I began to drink the Aloe Life Aloe Vera juice that was talked about. Wow - the supplements and Aloe acted like a catalyst in my body!

At about three months I started feeling more like myself

again and began to lose some weight. I kicked up my walking and began to feel even better. Applying health was honestly reducing my pain and I couldn't believe it! At the six month marker I started reducing the pharmaceutical drugs I had been on for many years one by one. My doctors were shocked and said my arthritis was a progressive disease that I would have for the rest of my life. I tried to tell them that I had switched to natural anti-inflammatory herbs and supplements yet they scolded me - saying I could find myself in worse shape if I got off my medications.

I was afraid and went extremely slow yet I knew deep in my heart that I was doing the right thing and was feeling better for it with less pain and more energy. Now after five years of supporting my body to heal - I am only taking one medication for pain as needed but off all the heavy drugs including Prednisone. Also, people who have known me are shocked to see how good I look and feel. My hope and prayer for anyone reading this personal testimony is to give it one year to get healthier. I was one of the most reluctant people because I had worked in the medical field in research most of my life. It took a lot for me to change my eating habits and swallow around seven or eight supplements a day yet I never want to be without them or my Aloe Life juice again!"

— *Anne, Wisconsin*

Why is it important to eat well and take vitamins?

Eating a healthy diet is the number one objective for health along with drinking water and getting some form of exercise, sunshine and fresh air daily. As important as these basics are for survival - statistics show that only about 25% of the population are eating the foods they require to be healthy. Research is hinting that only about 10% of the populace is living a healthy lifestyle which is also a shocking statistic! Because of these facts and the other factors challenging people in modern life

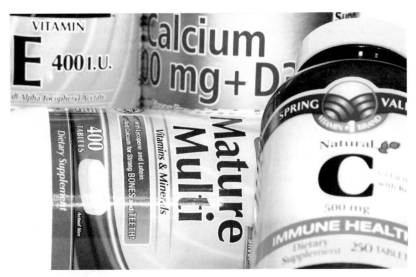

most experts, including more and more physicians, recommend taking at least a Multiple Vitamin and Mineral to offset any possible nutritional deficiencies an individual may be experiencing. Taking supplements will provide some of the required nutrients the body needs to help decrease and avoid malnutrition in the body and in doing so can be considered the best "Health Insurance" a person can collect on every day!

The catch with supplements is that to have effective supplementing requires using "quality products" and the "correct potency" to reach one's health success. Many products especially if they are just a "One per Day" cannot even come close to supporting the nutritional requirements that an adult truly requires for health even when someone is eating fairly well.

A good example of underlining the importance of supplementing with a higher potency supplement is in the case of Vitamin E. Jeffrey Blumberg, head scientist of Tuft's University Antioxidant Research, stated in an interview that as a general rule people are very deficient in Vitamin E. He elaborated that the RDI (Recommended Daily Intake) level is extremely conservative at approxi mately 20 IU per day for adults. He went on to say that because Vitamin E is an Essential Core Nutrient (ECN), required to protect and support the body's metabolism in hundreds of processes including immunity, higher levels of perhaps

400 – 1200 IU's are very beneficial. He explained that taking higher amounts even into the thousands of IU's daily is extremely safe, contrary to select reports that came out in the past decade. Tuft's research on aging found that by increasing Vitamin E to higher potencies in adults significantly increased the Immune System's function in only 30 days!

When supplementing it is critical to shop for quality supplements and the potency your lifestyle demands. There can be a sharp difference in the higher quality brands of products on the market today. Some brands of vitamins are very poor being made only from synthetic chemical isolates that can be purchased extremely inexpensively. Also, people today require the higher potencies to compensate for the environment and lifestyle stresses instead of the low potency referred to as "Minimum Levels". Do not be fooled to think that all supplements are the same. This is why many people take each of the nutrients separately to receive the potency, quality and the best type of a particular nutrient for their body's needs. Many people start with a comprehensive Multiple and add to this a few of the recommended individual ECN supplements as in the GIS guideline recommendations.

An advantage of taking individual supplements is that it gives more control of any minor allergy like reaction one might experience vs. taking a complete Multiple Vitamin & Mineral supplement that may contain up to 15 – 20 different nutrients in just one serving. This is the case with the B-Complex for some people as mentioned in Chapter 5. Often when an individual has a history of multiple allergies the best approach is to take nutritional yeast powder vs. a B-Complex of higher potency. Yet the higher potency B-Complex in the 25 – 50 mg. taken 1 – 3 times daily is a great amount for people not being hypersensitive for them to feel their very best. Most people do tolerate a higher potency B-Complex as explained in detail later in this chapter. As similar as people are we each have individual differences and needs especially when you factor in the GIS.

Higher quality natural Multiples are available with higher potency that will require more tablets per day. Some choices even formulate with the lower potency of the B-Complex from yeast for sensitive people. Reading the ingredients and descriptions on a bottle can help you decide if a product appears to meet your particular needs. Contrary to the belief that yeast base supplement are problematic most people tolerate yeast extremely well - benefiting from its natural occurring nutrients. Products that state they are from food extracts or state food based may cost a little more yet for many people they tolerate them much better and they receive more nourishment for the body. When you find a Multiple that gives a good range, then adding a few single nutrients such as extra Vitamin C and perhaps extra Vitamin E and even B-Complex (as tolerated) to your regimen may give you the optimum potency for your individual needs. Liquid, chewable or powdered Multiples are extremely low potency but a good place to start for some people in the advanced Zone 3 and high symptoms Zone 2 providing better absorption.

A person generally gets what they pay for in supplements as with quality foods. When it comes to your health you want to budget for quality supplements to get the health insurance you are investing in. A good Multiple may require 4 – 6 tablets per day taken with meals as directed. Remember to avoid gelatin. For budget restraints you can take half doses of quality supplements and they will last longer but you will still be getting the quality the body can better utilize.

Keep in mind that higher potency of some nutrients is often required to rebuild the body and to reach optimum health especially to compensate for deficiencies in the body during times of stress, illness, pregnancy, post-surgery, toxicity and mal-absorption and should be coupled with eating the best diet possible. As the body gets healthier then you can cut back on the quantity of the supplements and stay on more of a maintenance protocol as desired and outlined in this chapter.

Supplementing Supports
- Overall Body Metabolism that requires 92 nutrients for wellness.
- Daily Health Insurance providing missing nutrients due to mal-absorption linked directly to disease development.

- Optimum Health for regeneration of damaged cells including DNA damage, decreasing inflammation and improving immune function along with fat and sugar metabolism required for longevity.

One fact that experts agree upon is that the body requires nutrition to be healthy! The human body can be viewed as one big chemical laboratory with ongoing chemical reactions called "Metabolism" taking place from head to foot. The body was designed to fuel all of the metabolic systems in the body with nutrition sourced from foods. The metabolic systems support; Growth & Development, Tissue Healing, Immune Function, Thinking, Sleep and Energy. Many people have not felt well their entire lives and when they begin to give the body optimal foundational nutrition from the ECN's which supports; Digestion, Circulation, Detoxification and Renewal with a few select Special Needs Supplements (SNS) - they truly begin to reverse disease and pre-mature aging in the body!

Essential Core Nutrients (ECN)

The body makes energy from fuel sources that come from proteins, carbohydrates, fats and oils found in food and food supplements. Water is also required for the thousands of metabolic processes in the body to work properly and to help create energy. Water can be viewed as a type of lubricant in the body containing its own chemistry made from hydrogen and oxygen.

Besides giving fuel for energy the food sources contain other important factors for health called "Essential Core Nutrients (ECN)" that includes; Vitamins, Minerals, Amino Acids and Essential Fatty Acids that the body requires to function properly. Without the ECN's the body begins to run very poorly and sometimes creates symptoms of headache, fatigue, skin conditions, mental illness and multiple diseases. If the body is deficient of these crucial ECN's long enough it begins to actually die.

Current research estimates the human body requires "91" nutrients essential to maintain health which includes; 60 Minerals, 16 Vitamins, 12 Amino Acids and 2 - 3 Essential Fatty Acids. In addition it also requires the valuable Probiotics Micro-flora to support the health and metabolism of the intestines and tissue groups. Probiotics was first placed in the Special Needs Supplement category and because it has become such a daily necessity due to the overuse of antibiotics and processed foods in modern day I have now classed it with the ECN's. This brings the grand total of individual nutrients required by the body to "92".

Special Needs Supplements (SNS)

SNS are not required to support the basic metabolic function of the body for life. They are however extremely valuable and can add to the quality of life and longevity by increasing; Digestion, Circulation, Detoxification and Renewal. Sourced from unique Super Foods, Phytonutrients, Isolated Nutrients including Amino Acids and Herbs the SNS's give extra added health support. Glandular supplements such as liver and adrenal extracts are also considered valuable SNS's however I have chosen not to heavily emphasize them in this chapter because the most important focus for renewal comes from the ECN's. Homeopathic and Bach Remedies are two other very valuable types of supplements in support of emotional and physical well-being yet they work on a different premise than foundationally rebuilding the body. Each modality has the potential to reverse damage and imbalances in the body helping it to run more efficiently than left on its own without intervention. Volumes of good scientific peer reviewed studies support a large percentage of the SNS's for applications in the human body. Yet it has been the traditional use of herbs over thousands of years on this planet that has maintained their credence for health value attracting new users to the already great numbers of people supporting health with herbal therapy.

Super Foods are growing in numbers and are available in many supplements. Several of them are highlighted in this section being extremely valuable to include; Daily Green Vegetable powders and tablets, Alfalfa, Fruit Concentrates (alone or in formulas), Bee Pollen and Propolis, Fermented Foods as with the Probiotics, Nutritional Brewer's Yeast, Protein Powders, Seaweeds and more.

Phytonutrients is a broad name given to a class of SNS that include "Antioxidants" that are chemical compounds naturally occurring in plants. The value of adding antioxidants which also include the action of certain vitamins, has been proven in research to slow aging, reduce cancer risk, improve CVD and reduce the occurrence of other disease development. Green Tea, Resveratrol (an extract from several plants including grapes), Zeaxanthin (carotenoid from Kale and Spinach), Lutein (extract from edible flowers) and Astaxanthin (isolated from sea algae) are some extraordinary examples. "Flavonoids" also called polyphenols, is another class of phytonutrients containing both anti-viral and antioxidant properties and are present in many vegetables and fruits that people commonly eat. Quercetin has been found to be an important flavonoid. It's beneficial properties are currently being studied in great depth at prestigious universities, to include Tuft's, and is found naturally in foods including; sweet bell peppers, citrus, red and green onions and berries. Foods can contain many different SNS's yet when they are taken in higher potency as in a supplemental form they can work even more therapeutically without negative side effects 99.999% of the time. *Note:* "phyto" means "plant" so other than an occasional drug interaction they are not harmful. An example of an interaction is when chemotherapy is being given doctors will sometimes state they prefer the patient to not take certain antioxidants or phytonutrients that would prevent the drugs from destroying the bad cells. Once the treatment has stopped then the importance to increase the SNS's and the ECN's are critical to rebuild and boost the immune system and other tissues of the body. Keep in mind any small side effects from supplements overall are miniscule when taken as directed and they do not cause death. Review the health risks of some common OTC products and pharmaceutical drugs for a good perspective of risk vs. benefit.

Isolated Nutrients & Amino Acids are another subgroup in the

SNS's. There are many single super hero isolated nutrients including Liquid Silver that acts as an antimicrobial, Colostrum that supports immunity, Enzymes and Hydrochloric Acid that gives support to digestion through steps in the renewal process. The CoQ10 Ubiquinone Enzyme is a heavily researched nutrient that for over twenty years has improved and transformed cardiovascular support for the body along with fish oils. Researchers have clarified one of its major pathways of action that explains why it gives such tremendous inclusive health support. Repeatable studies have shown CoQ10 is needed in the "ATP Cycle" of every cell for generating energy efficiently which in turn optimizes all cellular function in the body. Taking CoQ10 in high enough doses 30 – 200 mg often stops the painful Myocardial Infarction by encouraging more oxygen to reach the heart muscle and it is great for any neuromuscular conditions like Parkinson's and a lot more.

The Amino Acid category is fascinating in the SNS's because when these building blocks of protein occur naturally in foods each 22 amino acids compete for absorption and the body utilizes each one on more of a maintenance level in the body. However, when an isolated single amino acid is taken apart from food the therapeutic action can impact the body in life saving ways as is the case with NAC. N-Acetyl-Cysteine (NAC) works in several remarkable ways including to stimulate the production of the antioxidant called Glutathione. NAC is a precursor to the body manufacturing Glutathione and is less expensive than taken Glutathione itself. People make this antioxidant naturally in the liver when it is healthy along with others including Super Oxide Dismutase (S.O.D.). These enzymes are called the Phase II Enzymes and research has found them to reduce cancer development and more. Glutathione helps with Mercury toxicity and other detoxification applications including anti-viral action. An example of NAC's true capacity was in an article written years ago when I was still working clinically with AIDS. The physician I was working with at the time handed me the *American Medical Journal* and there was an article that stated NAC stopped the HIV virus from multiplying. I had already been using NAC with our patients and he was quite taken by the documentation!

Herbs also fall into the SNS category. Thousands of different safe herbs dot the planet like gifts from God. History has revealed Garlic, Aloe Vera, Ginseng, Licorice and culinary herbs like Oregano, Parsley and Mint help with everyday ailments of indigestion, arthritis and keeping the immune system active to ward off colds - besides complimenting the flavor of foods. Research has also confirmed the therapeutic applications of taking these herbs including a quality Aloe Vera for example to stimulate the important Phase II Enzyme production in the liver. These naturally made enzymes are found to be one of the healthy longevity markers for people reaching 100 years of age. Herbs really work with rare side effects and that is why their use has continued throughout the ages. *Note:* Responsible companies such as Herb-Pharm do not formulate products using herbs that have any side effects for any concern with children or adults.

Supplements and Herbs Have a Long History

Health supplements have been used in the U.S. and other developed countries close to one hundred years. The use of herbs and some of the other Special Needs Supplements go back to ancient times. Aloe Vera's recorded use dates back over 3,000 years ago to the Egyptians. Fermented milk products which yield the "Probiotics", date back over 50,000 years and they are regularly eaten all over the world on every continent today. Archeologists came upon the herb Ginkgo Biloba as they excavated ancient ruins dating back over 5,000 years ago in China. Ginkgo Biloba is one of the oldest living tree species identified to have been growing over 300 million years ago and each individual tree can live to be 1000 years old. Both the leaves and the fruit are used medicinally and it is a very popular herb used today.

Ginkgo Biloba

Recently Western researchers have been studying Ginkgo Biloba as a treatment for senility, hardening of the arteries and oxygen deprivation. More than 34 human studies on Ginkgo have been published since 1975 showing a variety of health support for the body to include; increasing the body's production of the energy through "Adenosine Triphosphate" commonly called ATP. This activity has been shown to boost the brains energy metabolism of glucose and increase electrical activity.

Scientists also discovered Ginkgo contains high antioxidants of Vitamin C, Carotenoids and the highly studied Flavonoid compounds collectively known as "Ginkgolides" that have revealed the most remarkable actions to scientists. They act specifically to dilate the smallest segment of the circulatory system, the micro-capillaries, which have a widespread effect in the organs especially the brain. Ginkgo extracts effectively increase blood circulation and increase oxygen to the brain tissues. Its powerful antioxidants prevent platelet aggregation inside arterial walls, keeping them more flexible and decrease the formation of arteriosclerotic plaque.

Ginkgo's ability to improve blood flow has been shown in numerous studies with the elderly; leading German researchers to use it as a treatment for Atherosclerotic Peripheral Vascular Disease (AVD). A common symptom with AVD is experiencing severe pain felt in the legs when attempting to walk even short distances referred to as intermittent claudication. The German doctors found the patients receiving the Ginkgo had less pain and could walk much further. The extracts are considered safe from side effects although taking very large doses may lead to diarrhea, nausea, vomiting, headaches and perhaps a slight elevation in blood pressure. Always begin any herb with a single dose and then increase as directions are given and as desired.

The U.S. government conducted a study in 2006 on the use of Complimentary Natural Medicine. It revealed that approximately 33 million Americans use some form of natural therapy to stay healthy. Of the people polled Aloe Vera was the most popular herb to incorporate into their lives out of hundreds of herbs available and Ginkgo rated in the top ten. There are many valuable herbs to experiment with and are available in herbal teas to herbal tinctures. Herbal handbooks can also be purchased that will give the health highlights for use and any caution with a particular herb. Rest assured side effects are extremely low on the scale.

Any Toxicity Concerns ingesting ECN's & SNS's?

Toxicity is not a worry when taking most ECN's and SNS's, including herbs, if you follow the directions on the bottle and do a little homework before selecting a product. If you are taking pharmaceutical medications ask your doctor if there are any herbs or supplements that conflict with your drug protocol and ask for the documentation to support their comments. Aloe Vera has no bad side effects other than having a slight blood thinning property and loosening the stool for some people. These are positive benefits supporting healthy elimination and Cardiovascular Disease prevention. Aloe like Vitamin E naturally decreases excessive platelet aggregation or unhealthy blood clotting. Also, with so many people having slow elimination Aloe's cathartic help for regularity is generally welcomed like drinking a little prune juice. Just add it slowly if your bowels are loose to begin with and remember it helps to detox the body (Ch. 6 Detoxification). Because of the five anti-inflammatory agents present in Aloe Vera (if it is not over filtered) it gradually balances the bowels peristalsis action. Many doctors unfortunately still follow the rule that if they are personally not informed about a supplement they give thumbs down. You must become your own health advocate working with your doctor and pharmacist to find better, safer and lasting health!

CDC: Reports Half of US Adults Are Now Taking Supplements

A recent survey sponsored by the U.S. government Center of Disease Control (CDC) in 2011 revealed an increase in adults taking a Multiple Vitamin and Mineral and other supplements approaching 50% of the population. It appeared from the questionnaire that those taking the supplements were the people with a higher education, higher income and people who eat a more nutritious diet in the first place. A spokesperson from the National Institute of Health remarked, "It's almost like the people who need supplements the most are not the ones taking them!"

Education is so critical to understand the value of taking supplements because many factors in our lives today increase the need over and above what we can receive from diet alone. Unfortunately, over the past century it has increasingly become impossible for people living in today's world to receive the nutrition the body requires and reach optimum health without taking a few supplements. Many factors increase the need for supplementing even if people make an effort to "Eat Right" including the GIS challenge. It is imperative to eat the best you can and then kick up your nutrition whenever possible through choosing certified organic foods or growing your own vegetables. However, not all people have the time, talent or financial investment to do this and that is where supplementing can save the day!

Modern Life Demands Supplementing for Health

What increases the need for supplementing in today's world is a combination of factors. Two areas that are the most important to consider and rarely talked about is first the heavy pollution in the environment discussed in Chapter 6 that leads to toxicity and the genetic damage to the body. The second factor is the depletion of the top-soil that the food today is grown in. Statistics show that the soils from over farming and modern commercial farming methods are down 85% in nutrients from just 20 years ago. A world conference on farming in Brazil fingered the U.S. to be the most deficient in soil minerals with only 20% remaining from just 100 years ago. The fact is that if the nutrients are not in the soil they will not be in the food! Also, once the food is grown it must be transported to the market place and this is sometimes hundreds and even thousands of miles away which can further reduce the nutrient content from heat exposure and oxidation. Processing the foods is yet another factor that sometimes contributes harmful chemicals and often over processing denatures (destroys) the food value. When you add the poor food choices, pharmaceutical drug toxicity and addictions that so many people of every age are living with you can begin to see why kids and adults require greater nutrition. Chronic illnesses and bowel health conditions as discussed in previous chapters undoubtedly top the scales of reasons for increasing nutrition from foods and supplements for renewal. A rule of thumb is that it is much better to have a little more nutrition in the body than not enough. Lastly, yet very relevant, is the over stressed lives that people lead including both positive and negative stress. Stress-loads impact individuals' in their personal life and in one's professional work environment that increases the body's nutritional requirements. A big catalyst to the increasing daily stress of many developed countries is from the cultural evolution of families today that often demands both parents to work. This change in the core family dynamics has increased the stress on the entire family unit calling for more stress supplements in every category. Humans today must live defensively and preventatively by improving health to survive and even better to thrive and that calls for supplements!

Factors that Increase the Need for Supplements

- Pollution & Toxicity of the Environment
- Commercial Farming, Transportation & Processing of Foods
- Poor Food Choices & Omissions (Eating Mono-Diets)
- Pharmaceutical Drug Interaction & Food Addictions
- Chronic Illness & Reduced Bowel and Digestive Health
- Excessive Stress from Personal, Work & Cultural Evolution Impacting Individuals and Families

Research Supports Living a Healthy Lifestyle for Longevity & Wellness

The ongoing research for over 30 years by Tuft's University has pinpointed what it takes for healthy aging. Coinciding with Tuft's work has been the largest study on longevity and aging recently completed by the Boston Medical University (BMU) and together they identified the factors that are required by the body for healthy aging and longevity with or without bowel disease. Surprisingly, the research found genetics only played a 25% factor in the length of one's life. The environmental and social factors held a whopping 75% responsibility for people reaching their eighties, nineties and even one hundred years of age called Centenarians.

BMU & Tuft's University Factors for Healthy Aging

- Eat Nutrient Dense Foods & Supplement
- Good Digestion is Critical especially Hydrochloric Acid in the Stomach
- Reduction in Pharmaceutical Drugs to Avoid Interference with ECN Absorption
- Maintain Healthy Lipid (fats) and Glucose (sugar) Metabolism
- Don't Smoke and or Drink Alcohol - Only Modestly (if any)
- Healthy Liver Enzymes (Antioxidants) - Present in Blood Samples
- Functioning Immune System Markers
- Exercise Regularly & Practiced Weight Resistance Exercises
- Stayed Socially Active (Fun), Learned to Handle Stress and Set Goals!

Thousands of repeatable research studies have been conducted on health, disease and the connection to nutrition in the past 30 years. Check out the research yourself on the internet by going to PubMed and putting in the subject or nutrient you wish to study. People are no longer being brain washed to the fact that aging is uncontrollable and disease is inevitable. The human body does not have pharmaceutical drug deficiencies yet it does develop many nutritional ones. Purchasing a more in-depth supplement book is recommended to enhance this chapter however it is not required for health success. Follow the suggested GIS Program including the diet and supplements the best you can on a daily basis - will allow you to reap the benefits that others who follow it enjoy!

Food, Supplement & Health Diary / Log			
Date Started	**Food, Supplement or Activity**	**Date Stopped**	**Result**

GIS Supplement Program for ECN's & SNS's

Essential Core Nutrients ECN   GIS Supplement Program

Zone 1:

A. Maintenance Daily for Optimum Health (follow as tolerated)

1. Multiple Vitamin & Mineral (tablet, chewable or take each nutrient separately – Iron free if required). Add a B-Complex of 25 – 50 mg if Multiple is low.

2. Probiotics (dairy free - powdered, liquid or chewable - chew out of gels or pull apart from capsule)

3. Fish Oil (including Vitamin A & D for maximizing nutrients, 1 – 3,000 mg and or other Omega-3 sources – liquids are most convenient or chew out of gels)

4. Vitamin C with Bioflavonoids 500 mg – 3,000 mg (chewable, powdered, tablet)

5. Vitamin E, 400 IU (mixed complex, take the amount as needed – chew soft gels open)

6. Daily Greens Supplement (as tolerated - see definition in regards to blood thinner prescriptions)

7. Aloe Vera – Whole Leaf Concentrate juice, tablet or other (1 - 3 times per day)

8. Minerals, Calcium, Magnesium & Zinc (liquid or tablet, test for Calcium level in blood work) *Note:* Zinc may be taken separately if not in the selected mineral supplement and check personal blood levels for Calcium. Also important is to include a source for Trace Minerals.

9. Antioxidants (a variety)

10. Other Special Needs Supplements SNS (as needed and desired review Ch. 6)

Zone 2:

A. **Beginning Daily** *(A gradual process of introducing supplements is important to lessen detox symptoms. Suggested supplements are grouped and listed in sequence order. Begin with group A, follow with B and so forth. Work down the list adding (1) new supplement every 2 – 4 weeks.)*

1. Multiple Vitamin & Mineral (tableted, chewable or liquid - Iron Free if required or take separate nutrients)

2. Probiotics (dairy free - powdered, liquid or chewable - chew out of gels or pull apart from capsule)

B. **Additional ECN** *(Add one at a time as tolerated.)*.

1. Vitamin B-Complex, 25 – 50 mg. (1 – 3 times daily) or Nutritional Yeast (1) teaspoon (increase to 2 -3 tsp.)

2. Vitamin B12 – Methyl Sublingual 200 mcg (1 – 3 times daily)
3. Vitamin E, 400 IU (mixed complex, take the amount as needed - chew soft gels open)

C. **Core SNS** *(Begin this group with A. above as tolerated.)*
1. Aloe Vera – Whole Leaf Concentrate, juice, tablet or other (1 – 3 times daily before meals is best)
2. Fish Oil (including Vitamin A & D, 1 – 3, 000 mg or other Omega-3 source – liquid is most convenient or chew out of gels)

D. **Additional ECN**
1. Vitamin C with Bioflavonoids 500 mg – 3,000 mg, (chewable, powdered or tablet)
2. Calcium 1200 mg, Magnesium 600 mg, Zinc 30 – 60 mg (tablet, liquid or powder - check blood level of Calcium) *Note:* Zinc may be taken separately if not in the selected mineral supplement. Include a source for Trace Minerals also very important.

E. **Additional SNS**
1. Daily Greens (powder or tablet, as tolerated and or see definition in regards to blood thinner prescription)
2. Antioxidants (a variety)
3. Other SNS (slowly add as needed and desired see Ch. 6)

Zone 3:
A. **Beginning Daily** *(A gradual process of introducing supplements is important to lessen detox symptoms. Suggested supplements are grouped and listed in sequence order. Begin with group A, follow with B and so forth. Work down the list adding (1) new supplement every 2 – 4 weeks.)*
1. Liquid or Chewable Multiple Vitamin & Mineral (Iron Free if required or take separate nutrients – see Multiple Vitamin & Mineral description)

2. Probiotics (dairy free - powdered, liquid or chewable - dairy free, chew out of gels or pull apart)

B. *Additional ECN*
1. Liquid B-Complex with B12
2. B12 Methyl Sublingual (may require injections)
3. Nutritional Yeast, start with 1/4 - 1/2 teaspoon and increase to 1 – 3 tsp.

C. *Core SNS* (*Begin this group with A. above as tolerated one at a time.*)
1. Aloe Vera – Whole Leaf Concentrate, juice, tablet or other (1 – 3 times daily before Meals and diluted with water as desired)
2. Fish Oil - Re-esterification Triglycerides (rTG) form (1 - 3 teaspoons, containing the Vitamin A & D or use other Omega-3 sources as tolerated – liquid is best or chew out of gels)

D. *Additional ECN*
1. Vitamin C with Bioflavonoids, 500 – 3,000 mg (chewable or powdered - reduce with loose stool as needed)
2. Liquid or Chewable Calcium 1200 mg, Magnesium 600 mg, Zinc 30 – 60 mg (as desired and tolerated, check personal Calcium blood levels) *Note:* Zinc can be taken separately if not in the selected mineral supplement. Include a source for Trace Minerals also important.

E. *Additional SNS*
1. Daily Greens (powder or tablet, as tolerated and or see definition in regards to blood thinner prescription)
2. Vitamin E 400 IU (mixed complex and chew soft gels)
3. Antioxidants (a variety)
4. Other SNS (slowly add as needed and desired see Ch. 6)

Multiple Vitamin & Mineral

Taking a Multiple Vitamin & Mineral supplement is a convenient way to boost your nutrition. If you choose a more comprehensive product make certain you take it daily even if you may not get all of your other supplements in because of running behind or just do not feel well or are not motivated. This happens occasionally in my life and then I make certain I catch up with my other supplements later in the day or the following day making the extra effort to follow the complete program.

If a reaction does occur from taking the Multiple Vitamin & Mineral product with a developing rash or nausea please consider that your body just may be having a cleansing symptom as mentioned in Chapter 6 Detoxification & Cleansing. If it is a true allergy reaction it may be coming from existing molds that can be present naturally on certain leafy herbs used for herbal support or from the high B-Complex level as previously mentioned (see B-Complex). Allergies often show symptoms of bloating and gas in the intestines and if it doesn't pass stop the Multiple and take each supplement separately.

Safety of Supplements

The safety of taking supplements is a familiar theme in the media yet the research confirms that the overall safety if you follow the directions on products is excellent. You will also want to know the basic facts about your own body's needs through confirming with your doctor that no interactions exist (if taking life supporting pharmaceuticals drugs like blood thinners) and a little testing (of blood) as is suggested in this chapter. If you have never tested for malnutrition of core nutrients you may also wish to have this completed through a laboratory blood test to show if any poor absorption issues are present (review Ch. 4 Testing).

For your peace of mind there was a mandatory reporting bill voted into law not too long ago so that if any customers experience a reaction to a supplement or cosmetic requiring hospitalization or urgent care the notified company must promptly report the incidence to the US government. The outcome of this Mandatory Reporting Bill has been as health experts predicted with only rare reported incidences! Compare this to the adverse reactions of medical mistakes that resulted in over 100,000 deaths per year calling for Congress to pass a law in 2005 for more competent medical care! The fact of the matter is supplements are not dangerous! It is also important to dispel the notion that our government does not have control over the supplement industry. This is absolutely false because the federal government has 100% authority to control all supplements according to the DSHEA Law passed in 1994.

To review the safety of vitamins there are about 16 that are considered essential to optimize health counting each one separately. Vitamins come in both water and fat solubility yet only Vitamin A and sometimes D (especially with people taking the higher levels recently in the fish oil type) may be potentially toxic to an unborn or nursing child. When a person is or is not supplementing they can request through a health provider (Physician, Chiropractor or Acupuncturist) a blood test to show the levels of certain nutrients (in the blood and or plasma) in particular for Vitamin A or D. Running higher on beta carotene is never a challenge as some physicians have occasionally alarmed good vegetable eaters that turn a little golden orange from the vegetable pigment.

There are 60 minerals more commonly isolated in our foods and you want to make certain to not get too much unabsorbed Calcium and/or Iron. With supplementing people are often encouraged to take higher potencies (definitely above the low RDA's) to achieve a more therapeutic result in the body for renewal support. Yet don't think that just because you are having bone loss for example you need to take extraordinarily high amounts of Calcium. In this situation the challenge often lies in the body not digesting and absorbing properly and through testing the blood it will show if these minerals are getting dangerously high. So please understand the importance of NOT exceeding healthy safety limits on minerals. Minerals are essential to health and we need them to support the vital processes of the body. By blending the suggested supplements to receive the macro and micro (trace) minerals you will receive a Smorgasbord of them to support the body's health needs.

Many people do not digest and absorb minerals very well especially when first starting the GIS Program. Because of this fact minerals can be stored in the body's tissues as with Calcium that can cause bone spurs, kidney stones and sometimes dangerous circulating high calcium. This can come about from a poor functioning Thyroid – Parathyroid gland and the levels of Calcium need to be checked from time to time right along with general blood work ordered by a health provider. Iron has become a mineral that can build up in the body (from poor absorption) and cause headaches and left unchecked even death if it becomes too high in the body tissue. Iron has been commonly included in Multiple Vitamins and Minerals however because of declining absorption there is a growing number of people with high Iron and therefore more products are being made Iron Free. The following example is to give guidance in shopping for a Multiple Vitamin and Mineral product.

Multiple Vitamin & Mineral Potency: The following formula is an example of a supplement best taken by sensitive individuals and other supplements can then be added to reach the target potency. In addition to this Multiple an individual may add an extra Vitamin C, E, B-Complex, EFA's and Probiotics. Some people may also add an extra supplement of minerals as needed at bedtime of Calcium, Magnesium and Zinc and Trace Minerals. The SNS are added in addition to these core supplements by following your Zone recommendation to include; Aloe Vera and other products.

Nutrient	Potency	% Daily Value
Vitamin A (beta-carotene)	5,000 IU	100%
Vitamin C (calcium ascorbate)	200 mg	333%
Vitamin D3 (Cholecalciferol)	400IU	100%
Vitamin E (d-alpha succinate & mixed Tocopherols / Tocorinols)	100IU	333%
Vitamin B1 (Thiamin HCL)	1.5 mg	100%
Vitamin B2 (Riboflavin)	1.7 mg	100%
Vitamin B3 (Niacin)	20 mg	100%

Vitamin B6 (Pyridoxine HCL)	2 mg	100%
Folic Acid	400 mcg	100%
Vitamin B12 (Cyanocobalamin)	200 mcg	333%
Vitamin B5 (Calcium Pantothenate)	10 mg	100%
Calcium (Citrate, Glycinate)	350 mg	35%
Magnesium (Citrate, Glycinate)	350 mg	38%
Zinc (Citrate)	10 mg	67%
Selenium (from yeast)	100 mcg	143%
Chromium GTF	200 mcg	167%
Inositol	90 mg	t
Choline (bitartrate)	50 mg	t
Free Form Amino Acids Complex	200 mg	t
Trace Minerals (if available)		
Aloe Vera (if available)		
Alfalfa (if available)		

Measuring Weight and Oils of Supplements

Trace minerals are measured in micrograms or mcg. A review of measurements is 1000 mcg equals (1) mg and 1000 mg equal (1) gram. At times you might see the decimal equivalents yet most manufacturers still use the micrograms for trace minerals and IU International Units to measure fat soluble vitamins instead of milligrams (mg). If converting these measurements is ever in question a review on the internet or in a complete nutritional book or with a pharmacist will help to further explain the exchange.

Probiotics Micro Flora

Probiotics also known as the "Good Bacteria" has earned placement in the ECN category because of its required support for digestive health and body wellness (reviewed in-depth in the Highlights of Chapter 2). Foods that contain the friendly bacteria micro flora are fermented foods such as yogurt and sauerkraut yet they do not have the needed potency and variety of beneficial organisms that can be found in the Probiotic supplements. There are many Probiotic products on the market to choose from and this is why I offer my recommendations. Many have value however a few are truly superior. Rotating with a few different products will allow you to reap all the benefits available from the friendly bacteria category. *Dr. Ohhira's* Probiotics, soft gel caps - dairy free - do not require refrigeration and are easy to travel with and chewable for kids and adults. This product holds exceptional quality and value that is not found in other products and is based on fermented foods made solely by the Dr. Ohhira's company. One major attribute to this selection is the success of the good bacteria to colonize more efficiently in the gut. This 12 strain formula also contains the powerful and unique complimenting TH10 strain that has shown viability against the H. Pylori bad bacteria and drug resistant staph along with combating other bacterium associated with food poisoning so common with digestive ailments. The *Jarrow Formulas* Company distributes several good Probiotic products for infants and adults however are not food based or 100% stable without refrigeration. Their line includes a daily adult probiotics called JarroDolphilus and FemDolphilus that has been very effective for support of chronic yeast infections. Their line contains good potency, quality and nearly 100% dairy free. The *Flora* Company also distributes another line of quality probiotics made similarly containing a full range of good bacteria for all ages that are a notch above many other products.

Experiment with Probiotics to find the one for you and your family to feel your best by taking it regularly. Be aware that as the good bacteria creates a healthier "Immune Response" in the digestive tract through its Lactic Acid pH destruction of bad bacteria it causes pathogenic yeast "Die-off" which results in microbial debris waste. This waste can create symptoms of intestinal gas, body rashes and temporary flu like symptoms requiring detoxification to complete the cycle for renewal. Review Chapter 6 on the steps to take for healthy detoxification.

The benefits of using a quality Probiotics daily is the reduction of nausea, stomach pain, better regularity, healthier skin (long-term), increased immunity, energy and wellness. Follow the directions given for each product however many individuals take a larger loading dose amount 3 – 4 times what a package states and then reduce it back to a maintenance daily amount stated on the package. Experiencing loose stool is a normal die off reaction. Remember by taking a Probiotics daily instead of only during a crisis or after antibiotics will give you the best health results!

Vitamin B-Complex

B-Complex is known as the "Happy Vitamin." It is highlighted in Chapter 3 and 5 because of the critical support it gives to the entire body and brain's metabolic function. Being a core nutrient required for proper digestion it is listed as "A" in the ECN supplement list. A Multiple Vitamin & Mineral always includes the B-Complex in varying amounts and or you can take the B-Complex separately to reach a higher level. Absorption is very important so follow the zone suggestions for B's and other nutrients to receive the designated health support for your GIS Zone 1, 2 or 3. Tableted is generally tolerated well in Zone 1 and by many in Zone 2. Impaired digestion may require a chewable or a liquid B-Complex supplement to allow absorption for Zone 3. *Note:* If you notice any whole tablets or foods coming through the stool undigested rely on only chewable, powdered and or liquid supplements while your body goes through renewal to improve its digestive ability.

A sublingual form is also available for B12 which is to be placed under the tongue and allowed to slowly absorb. It may take up to 3 – 5 minutes to absorb in this manner. B12 is sometimes needed in the injectable form to increase absorption however this must be prescribed by a licensed professional. A deficiency of B12 is not correctly diagnosed from the common B12 blood test. Symptoms described in Chapter 3 and 5 are a more reliable consideration that tells you if a B12 deficiency is present. The result of receiving B12 injections will give the final endorsement of whether the body was in tremendous need by the results taking it for 60 – 90 days regularly of less fatigue, pain and confusion and improvement in body wellness. B-Complex is very seldom given in an injection form yet a liquid B-Complex and or the Nutritional Yeast is a good alternative. *Note:* Make certain to also review Magnesium deficiency and how neuromuscular and walking challenges may develop with not enough Magnesium to Calcium ratio.

Nutritional Yeast is a very good source for B-Complex and it also falls into the category of a *Super Food* only keep in mind that the potency is very low. B-Complex is not absorbed well especially with advanced GIS decreasing intestinal ability. Two other reasons absorption can be impaired is the overgrowth of Candida Albicans a fungal condition and also toxicity in the body both discussed in Chapter 6. Toxicity from the environment can block the pathway to utilize certain nutrients efficiently in the body including B-Complex. With this situation it appears that only low potency is tolerated. The symptom of intolerance with B is nausea upon taking higher potency as with 25 – 50 mg potency. Normally a higher potency B helps nausea that comes from either poor digestion and or pregnancy. *Note:* If you develop nausea while taking a Multiple, stop taking it and take each nutrient separately and replace the Nutritional Yeast for the B-Complex source in your program.

Eating carbohydrates increase the need for B-Complex and most people feel their best taking 50 mg 1 – 3 times daily with meals. Experiment with your own body's optimum level. Keep in mind it is a water soluble vitamin and does not cause any imbalance unless people take large amounts of the separate B's like 500 mg of B6. This practice had become very popular years ago for reducing water weight. This is not a good idea and can bring about nerve damage. Energy is a fabulous result of taking B-Complex so it is suggested not to take them late even at dinner time for some people having a challenge sleeping.

Niacin is one of the family members in the B-Complex called B3. *Note:* Occasionally a person taking larger amounts of B-Complex will experience the vascular dilation affect coming from the Niacin fraction. Please do not be overly alarmed. This reaction in the body is NOT dangerous and will occasionally take place when taking the Nutritional Yeast as well. Symptoms of a "Niacin Flush" include a sense of warmth to hot flushing on the face, joints and buttocks. Itching can follow for about 10 minutes or so. Just drink a glass of water and stay out of the sun until it passes. There is no need to go to the emergency room as many people have done over the years not understanding the reaction. It seems to occur when a person has been especially stressed. A feeling of relaxation is experienced once the flushing is gone which I find very enjoyable.

Taking a separate Niacin supplement of 25 – 50 mg is almost assured to bring on this flush. As long as a person takes a supplement of 50 mg of B-Complex with the Niacin it doesn't appear to create any imbalances within the body. Some people have found that by taking Niacin it reduced their high HDL cholesterol level by supporting better liver function even though one study did not show it to be remarkable at all. To maintain mental health, reduce hyperactivity, support all digestive processes, skin health and reduce chronic illness B-Complex is a must. Leafy greens, vegetables, beans, nuts and seeds, fish and some meats and dairy all contain a variety of B Vitamins yet remember that cooking foods destroys this water soluble vitamin complex and the body requires more than the RDA to feel it's very best!

B12

Vitamin B12 (Cobalamin) is essential for life itself. Even a slight deficiency for a prolonged amount of time can potentially cause permanent damage to the brain and Nervous System. Review Chapter 3 and 5 for symptoms of B12 deficiency. The only reliable food sources are from animals even though some people say a small amount may be found in the food ferment called miso paste. Authors have written entire books on the value of B12 and the B-Complex for wellness of the human body. Pain in the body is associated with deficiencies along with improper functioning of the Nervous System in the body. Mental health hinges on a good supply of B12. Seek out a medical professional that understands your needs of reversing B12 deficiency in the body when any symptoms are suspected and don't hesitate to take a B12 supplement.

The daily amount of either sublingual or injection type B12 is 200 mcg 1 – 3 times per day as required. If B12 is not supplied into the tissue early enough damage will occur adding to mental illness and even death. 1,000 mcg of methyl B12 by injection has been found to be effective as needed per the prescribing physician to help reverse chronic deficiency. Experiment with the type of B12 that gives you the best results including making B12 dietary choices. The top B12 foods include; yolk of eggs, beef and other red meat, fish, crab, lobster, octopus, mussels, oysters, clams, caviar (fish eggs) and dairy products.

Experimenting with the supplements available in the health food store is a good start to see if your body will absorb and respond to them however don't wait too long if they are not doing the job. The nerve damage that takes place from poor absorption and or lack of B12 due to deficiency can be irreversible! The missing Intrinsic Factor as written about in Chapter 3 that is required to absorb B12 can be the challenge even if Pernicious Anemia is not diagnosed. Interestingly, the Bioavailability Study with Aloe Vera at the University of Davis in California showed a sharp increase in absorption of B12 when taken with a quality Aloe Vera juice. B12 is water soluble and when taken in large doses, does not seem to throw the body's chemistry off especially if a person is also taking a B-Complex in larger amounts like 50 – 100 mg and or Nutritional Yeast. You must do your diligent best if the oral products do not work to experiment with B12 injections to bring back body function. You will know if you begin to absorb the B12 better by the results you receive with the injection type including; decreased pain in the limbs and allowing the person to walk, think and reverse the deficiencies. Also, study Magnesium to rule out this potential imbalance. Keep in mind that both B12 and Magnesium may be deficient at the same time. Tuft's University made the statement in their aging study that just taking one pharmaceutical drug can bring about several deficiencies of core nutrients including the B-Complex (that includes B12). It is easier to be happy when your body is getting its optimum amount of B's!

Nutritional Brewer's Yeast (NBY)

Nutritional Brewer's Yeast (Saccharomyces Cerevisiae) is considered both a good B- Complex supplement in the ECN class regardless of its low potency and also a "Super Food" in the SNS class. It is produced from beet molasses not a by-product of beer manufacturing. After the completion of fermentation which makes the Nutritional Yeast it is collected and dried to preserve the nutrients including; protein (18 amino acids), vitamins (7 of the B Vitamins), minerals (8 including Iron, Magnesium, Zinc, Selenium, Chromium, Copper, Manganese and Potassium) and special nutrients like Choline which is very good for the liver. It also contains RNA and DNA which is believed to enhance longevity. Nutritional Brewer's Yeast (NBY) is great for children and adults, very economical and a popular addition when stirred into juices and "Smoothie Drinks". Adding NBY to foods gives a rich slightly Smokey-like BBQ taste to cereals, popcorn (as tolerated), salads, stews, soups and gravies.

It is best to start with only ¼ - ½ of a teaspoon and work up to the desired amount to avoid extra intestinal gas. Also, it is good to add it right before serving the food as to not over heat the yeast which destroys some of its health value. Health experts have encouraged daily use of the yeast for just about any ailment. It is not the same as Baker's Yeast because it is not a live yeast therefore it does not contribute to Candida Yeast Infections as is talked about in Chapter 6. The health value is unmatched by including NBY in a health protocol for children, adults and even pets!

Vitamin C & Bioflavonoids

Known as the beauty vitamin this valuable core nutrient complex is plentiful in fruits and most vegetables. One of the foods containing the highest amount of Vitamin C is sweet bell peppers registering 70 mg in ½ cup. This is twice the amount found in oranges containing only 35 mg in ½ cup however citrus has been a very popular source over the years. Kiwis, melons, papaya, lemon and limes are all great fruit sources for C. Vitamin C supplements are sourced from different foods and are also made synthetically as in ascorbic acid. Corn has been a relatively inexpensive source to manufacture Vitamin C (ascorbic acid) from yet because of ascorbic acid's high acidity and a source of allergies for some people palm (Vitamin C) was used to make hypo-allergenic Vitamin C products. During manufacturing it is often blended with minerals including sodium, potassium, magnesium and calcium to make Vitamin C Ascorbates that are lower in acidity and tolerated better by most people with a sensitive GI tract. Calcium Ascorbate or Magnesium Ascorbate are more commonly formulated into products yet always consider that whichever mineral they use it contributes up to 100 mg at times with every dose of Vitamin C. Ester Vitamin C is yet another process to make Calcium-Ascorbate (Vitamin C) that contains a few other natural chemicals that some chemists and researchers promote as a superior quality providing up to four times the absorption of other types of Vitamin C. Even though this category of Vitamin C has an onslaught of different products the good news is it's much easier these days to choose a product that gives you the potency you are looking for in the type of Vitamin C that agrees with your stomach.

Vitamin C is rapidly metabolized under stress, pollution and smoking therefor it must be supplied on a daily basis. Vitamin C is found with a variety of bioflavonoids in foods that research has shown work together with C in the body for health support. They support collagen structure along with hundreds of other jobs and processes. Vitamin C is responsible as a co-factor nutrient as in the case of Iron absorption. Every cell, tissue complex and the glands in the body are dependent on the Vitamin C Complex. Human's literally fall apart one cell at a time without enough of it causing pain in the joints, anemia, shortness of breath, poor digestion, broken and split hair ends, poor lactation, premature aging, bleeding gums, poor dental health and a low functioning immune system. Good mental health, reduction in allergies, protection against heavy metal pollution and the ability to produce energy are all dependent on the proper intake above the minimum RDA of Vitamin C and Bioflavonoids.

People regularly take anywhere from 500 mg to 5,000 mg per day without side effects. When taking larger amounts getting into more than your body can utilize at one time symptoms include gas and or loose stool. Reduce the amount or spread it out over the day if diarrhea is experienced. Since it is a water soluble vitamin it is destroyed by heat. Consuming diuretics like coffee and alcohol will flush it out of the body. To receive greater value from absorption of Vitamin C take it with a quality Aloe Vera juice. Research has confirmed almost twice the absorption resulted in a timed release action in the study participants through testing the adults plasma levels. Vitamin C is energizing so take it earlier in the day if you are not a sound sleeper. Although physicians sometimes caution people about possible side effects of kidney stones the science shows that it adjusts acidity helping the digestive process of improving calcium and minerals being less apt to make kidney stones! The RDA Recommended Daily Allowance also known as RDI Recommended Daily Intake (established to prevent disease) has been set at only 45 – 95 mg per day and this is not sufficient for children and adults in the present day who are exposed to environmental toxicity and massive oxidative stress in daily life!

Bioflavonoids

Bioflavonoids sometimes referred to as Vitamin P are found together with Vitamin C in foods and work as partners supporting healthy collagen in the body. Hesperin, Hesperidin, Eriodictyol, Rutin, Citrin and Flavones as in Quercetin are all considered bioflavonoids. There are ten times the amount of bioflavonoids in fruits and vegetables when eaten in their whole form instead of filtered juices. It is found in the peeling of many fruits and vegetables like the white fibrous covering of an orange and also in the color portion of foods. Collagen is essential for health and anti-aging support and is the substance likened to glue that connects each individual cell together.

Research has shown bioflavonoids contain; anti-inflammatory, anti-allergic, anti-viral and even anti-cancer properties. 1,000 – 2,000 mg of bioflavonoids daily has been significant in reversing varicose veins. Quercetin has been found helpful in chronic viral conditions like Herpes and in Cancer protocols. Bioflavonoids function with Vitamin C to promote healthy blood vessels, anti-bacterial action, improve circulation, lower LDL cholesterol, treat and prevent cataracts, act as antihistamines reducing swelling in tissue and support overall healing in the body. Choose supplements that contain bioflavonoids especially Quercetin if possible and food sources including; onions, broccoli, peppers, apples, cherries and berries like raspberries, leafy greens and a variety of beans.

Vitamin A

Vitamin A is a fat-soluble nutrient found in nature in two different forms and is generally much underappreciated for the importance it plays in health. The first type of "A" is commonly known as beta-carotene and sourced from dark green, orange and yellow vegetables and fruits. The second type is from animal products especially rich is fish oil containing the Cod Liver Oil. Statistics show that people consume about equal amounts of the beta-carotene from vegetables called "Provitamin A" and the animal source called "Performed Vitamin A" available from fish, milk, cheese, butter and egg yolks. Essential for proper growth and repair of the body Vitamin A is a building nutrient and works along with protein and co-factors to build all of the lining cells in the intestinal tract and skin throughout the body keeping it functional, soft and youthful. It helps protect the mucous membranes of the nose, sinuses, lungs, eyelids, mouth, throat, stomach and intestines. The soft tissue of the kidneys, bladder and sex organs also demand Vitamin A for protection. Vitamin A is also required in the process of gastric digestive juices being properly secreted into the stomach and many other important metabolic functions to include; building strong bones and teeth, building rich blood, reproduction, healthy immunity and developing good eyesight.

It is essential for reducing and fighting infection in the body. Researchers believe that Vitamin A has the ability to counteract Cancer development in the body and keeps the Thymus gland from shrinking.

When animals were injected with a tumor virus and then given Vitamin A their tumors diminished and their Thymus gland regained normal size.

The requirement of Vitamin A is great in the body especially the more a person uses their eyes and also when eating higher amounts of protein from milk and meat. Algae supplements are a good source of beta-carotene for Vegetarians. The challenge however when only getting vegetarian sources is that it must be converted to usable Vitamin A in the liver. If the liver is lazy having impaired function from a fatty liver due to high sugar and carbohydrates, alcohol abuse, a high intake of pharmaceutical drugs or liver disease proper conversion does not take place. Fat soluble deficiencies of A, E, K and EFA's can occur from the inability to digest and absorb them properly in the body. Researchers have found in particular that Diabetics are unable to properly convert vegetable sources of Vitamin A. Mind you this mal-absorption can even happen with people attempting to eat properly. The remedy is to include fish oil that contains Vitamin A not requiring conversion. It is readily absorbed into the body within the same day of consuming it!

The dosage of Vitamin A according to the RDI is more of a minimum suggestion for children and adults so make absolutely certain to keep excellent food sources for the family and or increase the daily supplemental amount. Children's RDI is 20 IU and adults 5,000 IU. Using a quality fish oil supplement is very helpful to guarantee that children and adults receive a sufficient supply of Vitamin A and the valuable Vitamin D can also be found together with Vitamin A in a fish oil supplement.

Just one teaspoon or more, as needed, of the *Nordic Naturals Children's DHA* or the *Arctic* for adults (which can be given to children) is significant in Vitamin A content. Children can require as much as 1,000 IU and adults 25,000 IU's of "A" daily at times. Toxicity of Vitamin A is rare because the body uses it up so quickly. It only may occur when taking extremely high amounts for a prolonged period of time of the animal source because excess is stored in the liver. The vegetarian sources do not store in the liver therefore they do not have any potential for toxicity, only some temporary color changes to the pigment of the skin

(100% safe) may be witnessed. The symptoms of toxicity cannot be missed from a rational adult to include; nausea and cramps in the body that do not go away. Do not confuse these symptoms with bowel disease. More symptoms of toxicity may include the cessation of menstruation, vomiting, diarrhea, sores form on the skin, excessive flakey itchy skin, headaches, weight loss, itchy eyes and pain in the calves. By reducing or stopping the fish oil the body is allowed to use the stored nutrients and the excess symptoms resolve. If not taking any fish oil the above symptoms are also from a deficiency of Vitamin A. As you fill the body's deficiencies through following the GIS suggested protocol the symptoms clear and only if taking high levels as mentioned would one experience any toxicity so do not be uneasy about supplementing.

Food sources of Pro-vitamin A and hundreds of other carotenoids have been isolated from vegetable and fruit sources including carrots which led researchers to name the nutrient beta-carotene. Green leafy greens are even higher in beta-carotene than carrots which include beet greens, spinach and kale. Of the 500 carotenoids isolated from nature 50 of them need the full conversion to be utilized in the body including Lutein known to prevent Cataracts and Glaucoma found in broccoli, Brussels sprouts and cabbage. As the body gets healthier by following the GIS Program it goes through a natural detoxification. This cleansing will support renewal of the liver and allow better utilization of all the forms of Vitamin A more efficiently helping to reach optimal health. Do your part by eating a variety of foods in your diet of both types of Vitamin A along with supplementing.

Vitamin D

Vitamin D is called the sunshine vitamin. It must be manufactured through a special process of converting healthy cholesterol located directly under the skin to D3. The conversion occurs when the ultraviolet rays of the sun connects with the cholesterol. This is a good example of why cholesterol is required in the body. Cholesterol is utilized in several other important functions as well including; a component in the structure of each cells outer membrane, a building component for bile required for fat digestion and also making hormones that regulate the body.

Just 20 minutes of good sunshine daily has generated up to 20,000 IU of Vitamin D. This is a significantly higher level than the RDI suggests for children and adults of only 400 IU's each day. In fact, current research has now proven that most people are not generating adequate amounts of D3 known as Cholecalciferol. People living in the northern climates have always had a challenge with deficiency during winter and cloudier weather. New research reveals that even people receiving enough sunshine are still not producing the essential levels of D3 their bodies require. This may be traced back to a poor diet, an unhealthy liver and an overuse of sunscreen which blocks the UV rays from making contact on the skin.

D3 is critical to help absorb all minerals. This includes Calcium and Magnesium to avoid bone loss, support for mental health, to maintain good muscle action, proper growth, healing of wounds and even a healthy immune system. Vitamin D is essential in hundreds of metabolic processes of the body including sleep.

Many individuals are supplementing anywhere from 1,000 – 15,000 IU daily and sometimes more to rebuild the D3 back to a healthy level. The lab test needed to monitor D3 is called the Vitamin D, 25 – Hydroxy test with the reference range from 30 – 80. Although D3 is a fat soluble vitamin it doesn't appear to hold as much concern for overdosing as thought in previous years. The best natural supplement for D3 is a Cod Liver Oil which must state the amount on the bottle. Manufacturers have made D3 in capsules and tablets as well. Food sources include fortified milk (as tolerated), whole eggs including the egg yolk, beef or chicken liver or fish liver. Toxicity is possible so be cautious to keep D3 supplements away from small children and if using infant drops dose very carefully. The excessive warning about toxicity is being reevaluated yet be responsible with your D3 supplements – Don't guess - TEST.

Nordic Naturals has been making the finest fish oil products with several already containing the valuable D3. Now with the discovery of a more widespread deficiency within the population in the last few years they have increased some of the products to meet the needs of people including a primary D3 supplement. Children and adults both require sufficient D3, Omega-3 Fatty Acids and Vitamin A. If you have been living with any chronic health issues I suggest you get tested and or start taking a good D3 supplement regularly like the *Nordic* Arctic D liquid.

Research has been impressive on Vitamin A and D. Hundreds of recent research papers can be accessed through PubMed on the internet and other resources. One that was conducted years ago by Dr. C. J. Reich reported the following study in *Prevention* magazine in 1972. A total of 5,000 cases suffering from bronchial dermatitis, bronchial asthma and or chronic rhinitis were treated with Vitamin A and D plus a Calcium/ Magnesium supplement. The result was 75% of all symptoms were alleviated including 1,000 of the patients suffering with Asthma.

Vitamin E

Vitamin E is composed of a family group of compounds referred to as Tocopherols and Tocorinols. The different fractions of each group are referred to as alpha, beta, gamma and delta and together can be referred to as Mixed Tocopherols and Tocorinols. The reason the fraction "d-alpha Tocopherol" is seen most often in Vitamin E supplements by itself or in the largest percentage in a formula is because the body appears to require a larger amount of this fraction for metabolic health. In recent studies scientists have isolated all eight fractions and are slowly discovering the different responsibilities they each hold. For instance the gamma-Tocopherol supports more anti-inflammatory action in the body for reduction of arthritic pain. A few other Vitamin E fractions have been isolated that are not mentioned yet the eight listed are identified most frequently.

Ideally it is good to include all of the Vitamin E fractions with a higher proportion of d-alpha Tocopherol in a given supplement of approximately 400 IU minimum or as desired. All of the family components of "E" are found together in food sources to include; raw nuts and seeds, grains, beans and leafy green vegetables. Supplements of Vitamin E come in both natural and synthetic. The (d l)-alpha Tocopherol is the synthetic form or manmade version. It does offer some value yet experiments show it is only half the potency of a natural supplement which is designated with the letter (d) without the (l). Natural Vitamin E is a fat soluble vitamin, like A, D, K and Essential Fatty Acids yet comes in a dry powder form or the oil form. If you tend to burp oils or have tricky blood sugar it is best to use the dry form when first supplementing. Because oil soluble supplements may cause a surge in your blood sugar bringing about light-headedness and moodiness it is always best to take your supplements with foods to avoid this from occurring. Keep in mind that the natural Vitamin E Complex may contain more of the other fractions naturally occurring together that have yet to be identified and even though a bit more expensive the inclusion of the complex is ideal for reaching optimum health.

As fat digestion improves through the GIS Program people begin to digest oil soluble supplements and fatty foods better. Adding a little Aloe Vera to your program as soon as possible will help to increase absorption much more quickly. The Bioavailability Human Studies on Aloe Vera showed a 300% better absorption of Vitamin E into plasma vs. the controls not drinking a quality Aloe Vera.

RDI levels for Vitamin E are low at only 4 – 5 IU for infants with 50 IU upper limit, 10 IU for toddlers upper limit 100 IU, 30 IU for children up to 10 years of age with the upper limit of 300 IU and 17 IU for adults with upper limit as tolerated. The ridiculously low level of the RDI for Vitamin E will help a little however the research has proven it to be almost criminal to only encourage such a miniscule amount! In cases of adult illness some doctors have suggested to take up to 400 – 2,000 IU daily with excellent results. The average amount that an adult takes is 400 IU daily. During the winter I will often increase my personal intake to 800 IU to include a larger amount of the Vitamin E Complex. People who smoke or work with toxic chemicals or consume more fats and oils from junk foods and even taking higher levels of fish oils require more Vitamin E. Vitamin E is an important antioxidant that prevents cellular damage that comes from rancidity of oils and oxidation in the body. Oxidative damage is very destructive in the body causing premature aging, blood clots and cancer. Vitamin E is a protector of the body's DNA and also an anti-thrombin helping blood flow through the veins for improved circulation. Remember Tuft's research found Vitamin E taken in higher amounts than RDI improved immune function in only one month!

Vitamin E also plays an important role in respiration and breathing because it maintains healthy red blood cells that carry oxygen throughout the body preserving the longevity of every cell including nerve cells. This is one big reason "E" has been in the "Anti-Aging" category of nutrients. Vitamin E increases energy and relieves muscle cramping adding stamina and endurance to the body. Athletes require even higher amounts over and above normal adult activity and exercise. "E" protects the body against pollution as does Vitamin C and is more effective when taken with the mineral Selenium. People with Sickle Cell Anemia, the Rosacea skin condition, nerve disorders and failing health all require improved absorption of Vitamin E through digestive support and liver detoxification that will improve Vitamin E metabolism (see Ch. 6 Detoxification). Vitamin E is required by all the glands to function properly and is essential to off-set Electrical Magnetic Fields (EMF's) and low dose radiation people receive coming from cell phones, microwaves and TV's. Fertility is reliant on good levels of Vitamin E (see Ch. 9 Healthy Children). Vitamin E even works as a type of diuretic ridding the body of unhealthy water retention for people living with Cardiovascular Disease along with taking the mineral Potassium in a supplement and or accenting dietary sources.

Vitamin E is considered a fat soluble vitamin however toxicity is not considered a threat. Even larger amounts do not seem to cause an imbalance for most people yet there are a few guidelines to be cautioned about. For people with a history of Cardiovascular Disease start Vitamin E only using half doses for 3 – 4 weeks. This allows the body to adjust to working properly. If starting with too high of an amount like 400 – 800

IU, it can raise blood pressure causing slight hypertension response in a small number of people. If you begin with only 100 IU to 200 IU daily or just take a 400 IU a couple times per week (2 per week), you will find the body adjusts and studies show it actually assists the body to lower blood pressure in the long run by its therapeutic support to the body's circulation. *Note:* Always consult your physician about supplements when taking medications that are life supporting. Also, check with a pharmacist or get a second opinion from a professional to confirm that the advice you are receiving from your physician is accurate.

Selenium

Selenium is a trace mineral that is best sourced from nutritional yeast. Trace minerals mean that they are only required in small amounts yet are critical in the body to include; selenium, chromium, vanadium, molybdenum, manganese, zinc, iron, iodine, copper, cobalt, boron and silica. Over 150 other trace minerals have been isolated in the body yet their importance still remains undocumented. Selenium does come in inorganic sodium selenite and the preferred organic selenium is isolated from yeast. Research has confirmed that the selenium from yeast is effective in giving the body support as an antioxidant and supporting proper immune function. Studies show this essential mineral is needed in minute amounts yet is imperative for prevention of many diseases including; cancer, arteriosclerosis, stroke, cirrhosis of the liver, arthritis, emphysema, radiation and other chemical poisoning. Many other conditions also relate to the lack of selenium including; diminished vision, nerve disorders, mental impairment, growth retardation, Muscular Dystrophy, Leukemia, cancer of the; colon, breast, ovary, prostate, lungs, bladder and skin. Vitamin A and E are also found to be lacking with skin cancer. Selenium is essential for healthy reproduction (with Vitamin E) and supports good Thyroid health as well. Studies in Australia have even pointed to a lack of selenium being at fault with the crib death known as SIDS.

Foods containing selenium include; Nutritional (Brewer's) Yeast, organ and muscle meats, fish and shellfish, grains, Brazil nuts, broccoli, cabbage, cucumbers, radishes, garlic, onions and dairy products. Impressive results showed selenium (yeast type) to be supportive in preventing Prostate cancer in a very large study in the 80's. It works effectively with Vitamin E as a valuable antioxidant preventing DNA damage which may be part of the pathway reducing all cancer risk and contributing to anti-aging results as well. *Note:* With existing hormone sensitive cancers in breast and prostate primarily reduce the amount of Vitamin E to small amounts as what might be in a Multiple until remission is attained. Higher amounts of Vitamin E encourage hormone production.

Selenium RDI for infants is 10 mcg, 6 months to toddlers 15 mcg, children 1 – 6 years 20 mcg, 7 – 10 years 30 mcg, 11 – 14 years 40 mcg, 15 – 18 years 50 mcg, 19 and above 70 mcg for daily use. A good diet eating a variety of nutritionally dense foods may contain 35 – 60 mcg of selenium however experts suggest an additional 100 – 200 mcg may be the best for optimum health support for adults. High amounts of selenium exceeding 600 mcg daily may potentially become toxic. Choosing the natural type from yeast is least likely to ever cause any toxicity because it is low potency. Higher than 200 mcg daily of selenium needs to be sanctioned from a doctor or health professional. Toxic symptoms that are very rare are loss of hair and teeth plus the finger nails may become weakened and black. The body would exude a strong garlic odor, lethargy and paralysis. I think that will keep the irresponsible person from thinking that if a little helps more is better. Be responsible when you supplement with trace minerals and using a yeast form will serve as a safe guarantee.

Chromium

Chromium is an essential trace mineral often in short supply in the body. It is required for efficient carbohydrate metabolism necessary to sustain good energy. Chromium stimulates the enzymes involved in glucose metabolism. Glucose is the fuel for mental and physical growth and development in the body and without enough chromium a person will experience fatigue and moodiness.

Chromium is also a necessary co-factor for synthesis of fatty acids, cholesterol and to support the valuable RNA required by our chromosomes. Organic chromium is used in formulating a high quality product called GTF Glucose Tolerance Factor that includes Niacin, a B vitamin and Amino Acids. This GTF formula of chromium greatly supports Insulin metabolism which works in regulating glucose (sugar) in the blood helping all people feel their best especially those with borderline or full blown Diabetes. Chromium has become a popular nutrient added to weight loss protocols and is one of the few single nutrients tested that increased the lives of animals for longevity. The body appears to require higher levels of chromium after receiving a glucose IV and during a viral attack as with a cold or a Herpes Simplex Viral flare-up. A viral headache can develop from a drop in blood sugar and is often prevented in this situation by taking chromium. Chromium is also involved in the health of the Nervous System and building muscle. Mental health is dependent on healthy blood sugar therefore including the GTF chromium for conditions like hyperactivity to Schizophrenia is highly suggested. A comprehensive Multiple will sometimes include the GTF chromium. Besides improving mental clarity it can help slow down the in-between meal snacking and getting up during the night to eat. It is an important addition to a weight maintenance and health program.

Even though 200 mcg is the average amount to take for an adult you may feel you're best taking it 2 – 3 times per day with certain conditions. A medical review in 2004 of chromium showed no toxicity risk of any type even from chromium yeast GTF or the Chromium Picolinate type unless people exceeded 1200 mcg. A study with the Nutrition 21 Picolinate Chromium resulted in a 25% decrease in hunger, a 25% reduction in food intake and a reduction in craving of high fat foods! Taking mega doses irresponsibly is a rare occurrence above the high threshold of 1200 mcg yet has led to side effects for people including;

nausea, dizziness, headaches, sleep disturbances, loss of appetite, frequent urination, nosebleeds and unexplained bruising.

Iodine

Iodine is a valuable trace mineral that supports the healthy metabolism of the Thyroid gland. The Thyroid gland converts the iodine into iodide. Then the largest percentage of iodide is utilized to make the important Thyroxin hormone. Thyroxin regulates energy, heat, allows for the burning of excess body fat, growth and development, supports mental health, speech, healthy hair, nails, skin and good tooth development. A portion of the digestive metabolism of the body is also regulated by this hormone to properly metabolize protein and carbohydrates and help with the conversion of Vitamin A in the liver. Some researchers have also connected a poor functioning Thyroid gland to Cardiovascular Disease and weight loss can come to a complete standstill if the Thyroid gland is under-functioning. Deficiencies of iodine are extremely common without a single report of toxicity ever being linked to taking iodine supplements.

Besides a lack of the trace mineral iodine in people's diets chemical toxicity coming from the environment is another reason for an under-functioning Thyroid gland. Government officials have recently confirmed that the ground water in the US was contaminated over the last decade or so from the chemical Perchlorate used in rocket fuel and it decreases the proper functioning of the Thyroid gland. Scientists have revealed that this chemical collects in the fat of the Thyroid gland similar to the nuclear power pollution called iodine isotope causing a reduction in the glands ability to work efficiently. Good sources of iodine come from both plant and animal to include; dark colored seaweeds, kelp, fish and sea foods, garlic, lima beans, sesame seeds, spinach, chard, squash, beet and turnip greens. However, keep in mind that the soils must contain the trace minerals for the food sources to have them. Fortified salt can also contain a portion of an individual's iodine requirements yet use salt with caution to not consume more than 2,000 mg of sodium each day. The

RDA suggested the amount of iodine to be 150 mcg for adults and 70 mcg for children increasing to age 17.

Eating too much of certain foods containing Anti-Nutrients discussed in Chapter 6 can create deficiencies of iodine including; cabbage, peanuts, Brussels sprouts, soybeans and cooked spinach. Women who do not receive enough iodine, at least 200 mcg during pregnancy, risk giving birth to an infant with physical and mental impairments. Also, a deficiency can lead to the development of a goiter on the upper throat area causing a puffiness that may disguise itself as fat yet the area is firm to the touch. A reduction in the Thyroxin hormone will bring about obesity, sluggishness, depression, mental slowness, racing heart and pulse, dry skin, brittle hair and nails, tremors, nervousness and irritability. If you suspect you have a low functioning Thyroid seek out a doctor that is trained in both Thyroid and Para-Thyroid imbalances because both are important glands of the Thyroid and secrete two separate hormones that effect body function. Make certain you are including good sources of iodine while following the GIS Program for body renewal. Review Chapter 6 Finding Your Healthy Weight to understand the other factors important in weight maintenance.

Silicon (Vegetable Silica)

Trace minerals in our environment and in the human body number over 150. Scientists have found some to be labeled essential because of the importance they perform in daily metabolic processes like iodine, chromium and selenium. Silicon has not yet been given this title however it is found in all cells of the body and begins to decline with age. It has been found to be a building component alongside calcium, magnesium and other trace minerals for healthy skin, strong and flexible bones, teeth and finger nails. It appears to be responsible for more flexibility in the tissue structure which leads people to speculate it can be very helpful to prevent injury and premature aging of the body. Silicon appears to be preventative in the hardening of the arteries condition called Arteriosclerosis and flaky dermatitis skin conditions. Interestingly some researchers speculate that the body may actually manufacture any needed calcium from excess stores of silicon in the body. Years from now more research may reveal the exact pathway silicon works in the body. Until then individuals eating an abundance of organically grown foods that contain more trace minerals will receive on an average 200 mcg of silicon daily. Silicon can also be added to ones protocol in a liquid form very easily and sometimes found in special formulas for bone health. It is often used as natural vegetable filler in high quality supplements. Food sources include; plant fibers (to include the corn silk), brown and wild rice, organic bell peppers, beets, beans, 100% sprouted whole grains and sea foods.

Iron

Iron is a misunderstood essential trace mineral required for energy and vitality yet can also become toxic due to poor absorption. Iron is required for oxygen transport and cellular respiration. It resides inside the Red Blood Cell (RBC) being part of a biomolecule called "Hemoglobin" that binds the oxygen and also gives blood its red color. Red Blood cells do not have a nucleus. Oxygenation works by the RBC's picking up the oxygen from the lungs and then it is squeezed out of the RBC's when the cells travel through the tiny capillaries. Iron must be supplied to the body and be properly absorbed to prevent "Anemia" and also to avoid toxicity build-up in the body.

There have been 400 different types of Anemia identified besides the one caused by iron deficiency. To prevent Anemia the body must have a sufficient supply of folic acid, B12 and protein along with iron sourced from supplements and or the diet and be able to absorb the nutrients. Unbeknownst to most people drinking black tea during meals can reduce the amount of iron absorption up to 75%! Deficiency symptoms of iron are fatigue, weakness, dizziness and headaches. Besides eating good foods sources of iron like beans, greens, raisins and dates, persons must also have sufficient co-factors that include Vitamin C to utilize the iron supply. It is also recommended to not take iron at the same time as calcium. Taking an Iron Free Multiple in the morning that includes calcium leaves the dinner hour available for an iron supplement so as to not compete for absorption. Other options could be taking iron at a mid-morning or afternoon snack as needed.

Good digestion is also a factor to optimizing iron and other minerals from our foods and supplements. By adding Aloe Vera and or another digestive enzyme that includes HCL at meals is important to support digestion especially if you have gotten a high iron count on a laboratory blood test and or have been living with poor health.

Toxicity from excess iron in the body is becoming more and more common. Symptoms of excess or unabsorbed iron includes; abdominal pain and a rise in LDL cholesterol and occasionally has been linked to cancer growth. Another challenge with iron supplements for many is developing constipation. The best absorbable type of iron supplement in a tablet is the Fumerate or Sulfate form. For many people their favorite type of iron comes from food derivatives and one very popular product is called Floradix Iron and Herbs made by the company *Flora*. It is a delicious liquid and absorbed very well with no constipating side effects.

The RDA for adults is approximately 12 - 24 mg and for children 10 - 12 mg increasing with age. Loss of iron is very small on a daily basis unless you are a woman experiencing her menses or having advanced bowel disease symptoms discussed in Chapter 2. A simple blood test can confirm the level of iron and any Anemia that may be present requiring supplementation. Therefore, taking an Iron Free Multiple Vitamin and Mineral product may be the best choice for adults and to include a separate iron supplement only as needed at dinner or snack time (temporarily) to feel your best!

Zinc

Sense of smell and taste are both regulated by zinc and it also plays an important role in fighting infection, tissue healing and general support for a healthy immune system. Adequate levels of zinc are also needed to have healthy skin including; acne, psoriasis, eczema and even diaper rash.

Found in every cell of the body zinc is required for healing of cellular tissue, cellular growth and healthy hormone function. Stunted growth has been attributed to a zinc deficiency. It also works as a co-factor for absorption of vitamins including the B-Complex and others. Over 2,000 enzymatic reactions in the body require zinc for success including DNA synthesis and Insulin metabolism. Unfortunately the toxic metal cadmium often in our environment competes with zinc for absorption into the small intestine. Detoxification is required to allow the body to better absorb the zinc. See Chapter 6 Detoxification. Both stress and environmental toxicity along with an unhealthy lifestyle will increase the daily requirement for zinc. Fast transit from loose stool and also excessive fiber from grains containing Phytic Acid in the diet can also reduce absorption of zinc and other minerals. Good food sources include; seafood, Pumpkin seeds (raw), Nutritional Brewer's Yeast, beans, peas, meat and 100% sprouted grains. Nutritionally dense foods grown in certified organic fields will yield higher levels of trace minerals including zinc compared to commercially grown foods.

The RDI for adults is approximately 12 mg – 30 mg. Children's RDI is about 10 mg and then the requirement increases to age 17 years of age and then to the adult dose. Zinc is relatively nontoxic however high amounts greater than 60 mg daily are not advised. Adequate levels of zinc are required for proper Vitamin A and Vitamin K absorption paramount for good bowel health. When zinc is increased in the diet more Vitamin A is also required. Vitamin A is needed in generous amounts and is used up quickly in the body especially when individuals use their vision for reading and detail work. Good digestion is important for the absorption of all minerals including zinc which is available in liquid form as well as tablets.

Magnesium

Magnesium is in the class of "Macro-Minerals" which encompasses; magnesium, calcium, chloride, phosphorus, potassium, sodium and sulfur. The macro-minerals are required in larger amounts than the trace minerals in the body. Magnesium is a critically important mineral required in over 300 metabolic reactions that is often under supplied. Why this occurs appears three-fold; a lack of eating the correct food sources, poor absorption of minerals in general and a high demand in the body for magnesium. Good food sources for magnesium include; fruits, vegetables (leafy greens), raw nuts and seeds and yogurt. Specifically, figs, apples, bananas, oranges, avocado, peaches, apricots, raisins, almonds, potatoes, leafy greens including raw spinach, lentils, lima beans and garlic are magnesium rich. Proper digestion and absorption of magnesium requires a healthy flow of HCL in the stomach and researchers report that most people do not absorb sufficient amounts. Review Chapter 3 Digestion.

Detoxification is one important job of magnesium which is unknown to many people. The requirement of magnesium in the body increases greatly to properly manage waste removal through the channels of elimination when ill. All chronic disease especially having more of the opportunistic Candida Albicans fungus as in Fibromyalgia and Chronic Fatigue Syndrome require higher levels of absorbable magnesium. Also, if calcium levels become higher in the blood the need for magnesium increases whether it is from drinking too much milk, cheese or ice cream or an imbalance in the Thyroid gland or other challenges.

Magnesium helps to calm anxiety, nervousness and irritability. In fact Dr. Daniel Amen, M.D. says that it improves the brains pleasure centers so much that it in turn seems to reduce food cravings. Magnesium also plays an important role in energy production, reversing muscle weakness paired with other core nutrients and helps reduce hyperactivity. Muscles in the colon rely on magnesium for proper peristalsis of the colon along with B-Complex. Many people help their chronic constipation by adding an extra Magnesium Citrate supplement.

Another area of the body that relies on magnesium is the electrical impulses throughout the cells that regulate metabolism called neurotransmitters. They must have magnesium to function efficiently which in turn supports healthy brain function and reduces depression as well.

All muscles rely on efficient magnesium to function properly reducing spasms including the heart muscle. Some heart attacks are actually attributed to not enough magnesium for the heart muscle to keep working and it just stops! A rapid heartbeat and seizures may sometimes be attributed to a magnesium deficiency. Magnesium is required for proper digestion by its activation of enzymes needed for protein and carbohydrate metabolism. It is also a structural mineral with 70% of the body's stores located in the bones and soft tissue along with calcium and trace minerals.

Adults are recommended to consume approximately 400 – 1000 mg daily as needed however it is difficult to digest and you may wish to supplement with the slightly more expensive forms of Citrate or Glycinate. A laboratory test may indicate a deficiency (if you specify to check for magnesium) or by being your own health detective you can recognize a magnesium deficiency symptom and take action to supplement with an extra amount. If the symptom clears you know your hunch was correct. Magnesium is best taken with calcium either equal or half the amount daily. If levels of calcium become high (checking through a blood test) then stop taking calcium and only take magnesium to help balance out the calcium in the body. The kidneys are very efficient in ridding the body of excess magnesium therefore toxicity is not a challenge. Magnesium Glycinate can loosen the stool if needed and is often used as a natural laxative for some individuals yet do not exceed the higher level. Follow the other GIS guidelines for regularity reviewed in Chapter 6 and 12. If you experience diarrhea switch the type of magnesium to the Citrate type. Combination mineral formulas are available on the market that group several minerals together as with calcium, magnesium and zinc. This is a very popular way to supplement for both men and women or you may find that a Multiple Vitamin & Mineral also contains higher levels as well. Add up the potency of any products you are taking to stay within the ranges as desired and make the best food choices!

Calcium

Calcium is the most abundant mineral in the body. It is required during gestation for the developing fetus, for a growing baby and throughout a person's entire life including the senior years. It is one of the 15 required minerals for the body which includes both macro and basic trace minerals. 99% of the body's calcium is needed for structural building including strong bones and teeth and the other 1% helps support important processes including nerve transmission, the clotting process, healing of tissue, muscle growth and function. Calcium is also a catalyst for the hormone called Secretin which aids in the digestive process by encouraging Bicarbonate to be released into the digestive tract calming acidity. Calcium maintains proper pH balance of the blood along with magnesium. The body will actually rob calcium from the bones when sufficient levels of calcium are not in the blood to support its metabolism.

Calcium and magnesium are also natural tranquilizers, supporting sound sleep and are both sourced abundantly from many vegetables like carrots and it is especially high in leafy greens, nuts and seeds, beans and dairy products. Drinking soda pop causes malabsorption of calcium due to the high content of phosphorus and sugar in the ingredients. Purchase only natural sodas (not containing phosphorus) and or drink diluted fruit juice as desired to avoid high phosphorus. Calcium levels are best maintained at 3 parts of Calcium to 1 part Phosphorus. Eating too much meat and or sugar can tip the scales of this 3:1 ratio which is important to maintain to prevent bone loss. Calcium must be taken in balance with Magnesium, 2:1 as found in nature or 1:1 seems to also work well at times for some individuals as needed. The best types of calcium for absorption are supplements containing Gluconate, Lactate, Glycinate and or Citrate forms. Interestingly, many vegetables contain the 2 parts Calcium to 1 part Magnesium ratio!

Excessive amounts of calcium can throw off absorption of other minerals including both zinc and iron. High circulating calcium that is not being utilized can interfere with the nervous and muscular functions of the body causing mental confusion, constipation and neuromuscular problems. It is important to periodically request a blood test for calcium and other minerals like iron to prevent advanced toxicity. *Note:* It is the Para-Thyroid gland that is responsible for maintaining proper mineral balance in the body. If calcium tests abnormally high in the blood or the urine make an appointment with an Endocrinologist for either surgery or drug treatment as appropriate. Also, review Chapter 6 for Detoxification and Glandular support to help improve Thyroid health.

Calcium is very inefficiently absorbed. As little as 20 – 30% of calcium is utilized from foods and or supplements. To be properly utilized all minerals require healthy amounts of hydrochloric Acid (HCL) to flow into the stomach. Review Chapter 3 Digestion. With calcium it is also important to have the needed co-factors present such as Vitamin D, magnesium, phosphorus, A, C, E and trace minerals to be well absorbed, build bone and support body metabolism.

When calcium metabolism is not running according to design bone loss called Osteoporosis and other developmental deficiencies arise such as Rickets that occurs in children. Rickets can be observed in children and adults with the bowing of their legs. This condition accentuates the partnership of Vitamin D and calcium. Low back pain is a common symptom of calcium deficiency as is nervousness, insomnia, slow healing, muscle cramping and bone loss. The excessive consumption of diuretics including caffeine can cause mineral and vitamin loss through the urine. When avoiding milk with lactose intolerance and milk allergies it is imperative to supplement with a calcium and mineral supplement and ideally add a vegetable supplement (that includes greens as tolerated) as well. This will guarantee the proper calcium requirements for both children and adults. Adults and children (over 4 years of age) require an average of 1000 mg of calcium to 750 mg of magnesium. Toddlers need less about 800 mg of calcium, 200 - 400 mg magnesium daily. Remember to monitor mineral levels in the blood work and perhaps even get a hair analysis with multiple health issues. See Resources for a laboratory referral. *Note:* Men require calcium in the range of 800 – 1000 mg daily coupled with magnesium, Premenopausal women up to 1500 mg at times but not always and Postmenopausal women sometimes require up to 2,500 mg. *Caution:* Higher levels of minerals including calcium need to be monitored in the blood through routine blood work.

Potassium

Potassium is in the macro-mineral category and is called the "Brain Mineral". It also falls into the class of primary electrolytes along with sodium, chloride, calcium and magnesium. Potassium becomes undersupplied when people are not eating enough fruits and vegetables. Also, taking certain medications, eating an excess of sodium in the diet and the loss of body fluids through perspiration, loose stool and vomiting can deplete or imbalance the body's supply of potassium. Especially using hypertensive drugs for high blood pressure or heart disease can increase the need three fold because of the diuretic action they often have. A prudent physician will also give a prescription for a potassium supplement with these particular medications. Most fruits and vegetables including; Bananas, apples, papaya, broccoli, bell peppers, cucumbers, radishes, parsley and culinary herbs are all great sources of potassium. Potassium is relatively non-existent in meat, bread and dairy products. Supplying the needed potassium helps support normal regularity, energy, glucose metabolism, a regular heart rate, good blood pressure, good muscle action and brain power.

The RDA is 2,000 mg for age 10 years old through adulthood and 1,000 mg for toddlers increasing the amount through age 17. High sodium intake and caffeine use can cause an imbalance of electrolytes and a deficiency. Eating sugar can also upset the ability of the body to absorb minerals including Potassium. People eating poorly and not supplementing, to compensate for potassium deficiencies risk kidney damage, insomnia, nervous disorders, constipation, slow and irregular heartbeat and muscle damage. Potassium regulates daily enzymatic reactions and it has the important job of lowering blood pressure by balancing intracellular fluids including the sodium levels of the body. Potassium's action creates a diuretic response decreasing depression, increasing brain power and energy. Potassium is primarily found in the intracellular fluids and is essentially responsible for the transfer of nutrients into every cell and eliminating waste, both absolutely essential for cellular health. From infants to seniors all people require this valuable mineral!

Special Needs Supplements   GIS Supplement Program

N-Acetyl Cysteine (NAC)

An Antioxidant and Glutathione Precursor – NAC may be viewed as a natural "Garbage Collector" of the body. Waste products and oxidation are created naturally in the body and also from chemical poisoning coming from a person's diet and the environment. If the waste is not neutralized from antioxidants it damages the DNA of cells. Research now confirms that DNA damage precedes the development of cancer and premature aging. NAC is an isolated amino acid which acts as a chelator of toxic heavy metals and also stimulates the Phase II enzyme Glutathione which is required to stop viral replication for example in HIV, HSV, cold and flu and more. 600 mg of NAC daily for adults 1 – 3 times daily is the general recommendation. Include it for 1 – 3 months in a detoxification regimen or to kick up the support of your body's immunity for colds to cancer.

NAC is great for any lymphatic congestion, fibrocystic breast lumps, Rheumatoid Arthritis and more. Side effects are minimal with taking NAC however it is wise to supplement with more trace minerals while taking NAC because of its chelation properties. NAC also encourages an increase in stomach acidity which for 90% of the population is beneficial. If an over-acid stomach develops reduce the amount and make certain you are taking it during meals instead of on an empty stomach. It has such extensive detoxification action that on rare occasions it has brought on the elimination of kidney stones requiring medical supervision at times. Review Chapter 5 protocols to understand the great health support NAC provides for many conditions of the body.

L-Lysine

L-Lysine called Lysine for short is an essential amino acid that cannot be synthesized by the human body. Sources of higher levels of Lysine include; beans especially kidney, black, white, green snap beans, poultry, pork and lamb. Other sources lower in content include dairy products, sardines, cod fish, eggs, Spirulina and Nutritional Brewer's Yeast. Lysine is important to support healthy collagen production in the body that includes; skin, hair, nails, teeth, bones, cartilage and tendons. Osteoporosis requires an increase in Lysine along with addressing mineral deficiencies and metabolism including; Vitamin D, Thyroid health and strength training exercises. Lysine is also a partner with Methionine another essential amino acid for the production of Carnitine. Carnitine is a nutrient responsible for fatty acid metabolism known as a "Fat Burner" significant for energy, weight loss and lowering the more negative cholesterol called LDL.

People eating a varied diet receive adequate amounts of Lysine however athletes, vegans, people living with poor digestive health or individuals living with Herpes Simplex Virus (HSV) require two to three times the normal 1,000 mg daily recommendation for an adult. Children over the age of two require approximately 10 mg for every pound of body weight. All amino acids are heat sensitive and over cooking foods destroys the value of most nutrients including Lysine. A deficiency of Lysine can cause fatigue, nausea, dizziness, and headaches, loss of appetite, irritability, slow growth, anemia and reproductive disorders. *Note:* Upon experiencing a Herpes outbreak the suggested amount is 3,000 – 9,000 mg spread out over the day. A maintenance amount is 1,000 – 3,000 mg per day as needed. Arginine another essential amino acid must be balanced with Lysine to prevent a flare-up of Herpes Simplex Virus (HSV). Arginine is found in high amount in nuts, seeds, chocolate and ice cream. Review Chapter 6 Viruses for a more complete list of foods to include and reduce. Recent research has suggested Lysine may even be a deterrent to cancer. Do not take large amounts if pregnant because of a lack of information on fetal development. Review with your doctor if you have any kidney or liver disease before taking Lysine. High amounts may be linked to gallstones. If living with fatigue and other viral symptoms experiment with Lysine for at least 6 weeks to see how much better you may feel!

CoQ10 – Ubiquinone Enzyme

The CoQ10 Enzyme was identified in 1957 by researchers at the University of Wisconsin. It is a natural occurring nutrient found in every cell of the body required in the energy cycle of ATP. 97% of all the body's energy is dependent upon the efficiency of ATP. CoQ10 is especially valuable for the larger organs including the heart, liver and kidneys yet it also provides immense support for dental health.

Through providing energy for cells CoQ10 also optimizes oxygenation of the body and has become a supplement of choice for people living with heart disease or CVD prevention. It can decrease pain felt by many patients in the heart because of its ability to increase the tissue oxygen levels. CoQ10's action also appears to work as an antioxidant protecting cells from oxidation and death especially in the oxidation of fats. Taking this supplement preferably in tablets or chewable wafers you will experience why it is called the Ubiquinone Enzyme meaning it is everywhere in the body and helps everything!

Naturally made in the liver researchers have found it is still invaluable to take some extra CoQ10 every day. The average amount that people supplement with is 100 mg of CoQ10 however more has helped to off-set the side effects of long-term "Statin Drugs". It has such a comprehensive effect for the entire body with remarkable applications for the neurological support of Parkinson's, CVD, Diabetes, Cancer, Chronic Fatigue Syndrome, Skin Health, UV exposure damage and Anti-Aging action. The CoQ10 Enzyme is found naturally in foods and plants to include; fish, meats, parsley, avocado, peanuts, garlic and a small amount in most other vegetables especially when eaten raw. Side effects only include slight gastrointestinal upset at mega-doses above 1200 mg daily. Researchers have had subjects taking as much as 3600 mg with no undesirable side effects other than slight bowel distress. As important as this enzyme appears to be in attaining optimum health it is still unclear whether the body makes the largest percentage found in the cells and or if it is reliant on the dietary intake of CoQ10. Daily intake is approximated at 6 mg from eating a varied diet but keep in mind that cooking destroys about 30% of it. Supplemental therapeutic amounts vary from 50 mg to 200 mg and at times up to 1200 mg and above.

Digestive Enzymes

Digestive enzymes are critical to the health of the body. Chapter 3 describes the Digestive System and each individual digestive juice and enzyme needed by the body on a daily basis. The body must either make them as designed or an individual must ingest a digestive enzyme supplement to allow the body to digest food properly.

Three Major Steps to Supply the Body with Required Nutrition

- *Eating* the correct foods and or food supplements.
- *Digesting* them properly throughout the GI tract.
- *Absorbing* the digested nutrients into the cells to provide the fuel and metabolic support for cellular function.

Animal sourced "Pancreatin" digestive enzymes are the closest to the human digestive enzymes especially porcine derived from pigs. Vegetarian Enzymes are also available and if they work that is all that matters. Both types contain Protease, Lipase and Amylase to help digest protein, fats and carbohydrates from food and supplements. Unfortunately they generally are in capsule form. Look for a comprehensive product in a tablet or weigh the benefit-to-taste-to-bloating side effect of swallowing the gelatin capsule. You can pull the capsules apart and mix the powder into juice or a food (tastes a bit yucky) for example applesauce or other food which can cover the taste. You will know if the Digestive Enzymes are helping your digestion when you do not bloat or they lower other symptoms you may have experienced after mealtimes.

Many enzyme supplements line the shelves of the health food stores today however health in the body was not designed to require enzymes. Aloe Vera is suggested to take before you experiment with enzymes because it can encourage the proper flow of all of the digestive juices and enzymes in the body naturally including the valuable HCL within the first 6 weeks. I have found that many people do not require expensive enzymes at all to reach their greatest health potential! Occasionally, a full spectrum enzyme product such as the *EMZYMEDICA* - Digest Gold is recommended for post-surgery, cancer or other chronic illnesses. However, by focusing and including the supplements on the GIS Program it gives the body the rebuilding materials for renewal of the organs that make your own digestive enzymes and ultimately the optimum health results!

The primary ingredients for a digestive supplement includes; Pancreatic Enzymes, Hydrochloric Acid and Bile which is needed for extra fat digestion. Several combination products are formulated that contain all three and that may be the best type of a transitional supplement to take during meals if it gives more relief from bloating. Many people come to the GIS Program taking an enzyme product yet I always suggest that as they get onto the diet and supplements that they experiment stopping the enzymes because their body starts making their own once again. In health and supplementing the bottom line is to do what works!

Papaya Tablets

Papaya fruit or tablets contain "Papain" a very strong Pepsin enzyme. This enzyme helps to digest protein foods primarily decreasing gas and bloating. The unripe Papaya fruit contains more of the Papain however eating Papaya does appear to help the digestive process even as it ripens. Some health products contain the Green Papaya extract giving extra added digestive benefit. Papain is known as a protease or "Proteolytic" enzyme that will also help digest carbohydrates and fats to some extent along with proteins. Follow the directions for use on each product for best results and note that it does not replace your other foundational supplements.

Aloe Vera

Aloe Vera is an ancient herb needed in modern day to support human health foundationally beginning with digestion! Highlighted in Chapter 4 because of its great health support on many important levels begin taking Aloe Vera as soon as possible on your GIS Program even if it is only just a fraction of the suggested amount. It is a health shortcut to speed your overall health results. It works best if you purchase a quality product containing all of the active ingredients that support; the Soothing and Balancing of Digestion, Skin Renewal and Faster Resolution of most Wounds, Balanced Immunity, Fighting Infection, Reduce Symptoms of Allergies and Increase Cleansing & Detoxification for children and adults.

When taken with other herbs and nutrients Aloe Vera carries them deeper into the cells for faster results as documented in bioavailability studies. Aloe Vera is the Number #1 choice in herbs whether for topical applications for the skin or internal support for body wellness. The quality of each product varies greatly therefore if at all possible start with the most therapeutic Aloe Vera made from the whole plant and concentrated still containing the yellow sap. Unmatched in potency and quality look for a quality product at your local health food store stating no water or sulfites added! Any product that contains even a small amount of Aloe Vera will help a little yet be aware that a few products have been tested on the market in the mass merchandizing channels to contain little Aloe in the bottle whatsoever! A good Aloe Vera delivers what the ancients experienced taking Aloe Vera - Better Health! Taking it daily you will soon discover why Aloe Vera was known as - The Plant of Immortality! *Note:* If you experience loose stool upon using Aloe Vera decrease the amount to a very small amount, water it down and gradually increase as tolerated. Some people misinterpret the detoxification symptoms and think they are having a bad reaction to a stronger Aloe product. Review Chapter 6 Detoxification to understand the process of cleansing. YOU do not want to miss the opportunity received that only taking a quality Aloe Vera can deliver for kids and adults!

L-Glutamine

Isolated amino acids like L-Glutamine work very therapeutically when taken in a higher potency away from other foods on an empty stomach. However, a few small side effects from some of the amino acids including L-Glutamine have led me to suggest for many people to take them with foods and they still are found to be effective. L-Glutamine called Glutamine is best taken with meals for this reason. It has been studied extensively over the past decade and is found to be supportive during treatment of many ailments including; serious illnesses that cause weight loss, injury, burns, wounds or trauma requiring healing of the body. Individuals going through treatment for Cancer have found relief to ease side effects from chemotherapy with taking Glutamine. HIV individuals that are experiencing muscle wasting have used upwards of 30 – 40 grams daily with very good benefits. Glutamine is also used by body builders and other athletes to enhance muscle recovery after a big work-out.

Research has shown that Glutamine enhances the production of human growth hormone HGH stimulated by the anterior Pituitary gland. It has become popular to use it with digestive illness recovery to support the bodies healing ability in the gut even though one must begin using a very small amount and work up gradually to your desired daily dose. *Caution:* With advanced bowel disease some patients have reported intense pain upon using Glutamine. If allergic to MSG you may also show allergic symptoms to Glutamine because it converts to Glutamate during digestion. Also, people taking anti-convulsive drugs are warned not to take Glutamine because it affects brain chemistry that may be conflicting. No other side effects of any significance have been reported other than the above pain reference. Follow directions and mix powdered

Glutamine in water, gargle then swallow. This nutrient is NOT part of the regular GIS protocol however depending on your health goals you may wish to experiment with it.

Lecithin Granules – Inositol & Choline

Lecithin is a phospholipid needed by every cell in the human body. It contains partially dietary fat, the fatty acid Linolenic Acid (Omega-3) and Choline. A healthy liver produces similar compounds to lecithin and we can enrich these amounts by taking lecithin supplements. It is concentrated and used in the cell membrane possessing both fat and water solubility allowing nutrients to enter and leave the cell as needed like a "Gate Keeper". A strong cell membrane provides immunity protection from anti-microbial attack including viruses. Lecithin is a good source of Choline a B-Vitamin Co-Factor located in the compound Phosphatidylcholine. It is a valuable precursor to Acetylcholine a neurotransmitter required for an efficient functioning Nervous System and supports memory. Lecithin like compounds makes up 2/3 of the outer covering of the nerves and is called a myelin sheath. Lecithin is especially important along with B-Complex to help the body reverse Carpal Tunnel Syndrome. Lecithin is vital for a healthy brain and a growing fetus, infants, children and adults. Researchers state that the brain consists of 30% Omega-3 Fatty Acids (sourced from lecithin, fish oil and other Essential Fatty Acids) and Lecithin truly enhances one's brain function.

Lecithin's constituents are critical in successful reproduction along with other core nutrients. It also has "Emulsifying Characteristics" in the body for redistribution of fat stores. Because of this action it is used in weight loss programs and also in manufacturing salad dressings to keep the ingredients in solution. Lecithin contributes to Bile production needed to break down fat in the digestive tract (see Chapter 3) and it appears to work on cholesterol deposits helping in both weight loss and heart health programs. Studies have shown lecithin to lower LDL and raise HDL for a healthier cholesterol ratio. This action appears to be why it assists the heart, gallbladder, kidneys and liver to cleanse and detoxifying. Because of its fatty acid profile Lecithin also helps in absorption of fat soluble vitamins including; Vitamin A, E, K and D. Inositol is also a component in Lecithin and appears to give additional support to the Nervous System and protection to cholesterol from rancidity especially the LDL type. Lecithin is a valuable addition to any neuromuscular, brain, CVD and chronic illness program. Store in a cool dry area and use in a reasonable time period to avoid rancidity. Found naturally in foods like beans and is available in several supplemental forms including powder and granules suitable for mixing into juice, foods or blender drinks.

Red Pepper – Cayenne

Cayenne Pepper, generally used in its powder granule form comes from red hot chili peppers. Cayenne not only adds flavor to foods it can give great health support! It originated in Cayenne, French Guiana and now is farmed the world over. Many civilizations claim to have used Red (hot) Pepper as a staple including the Hunzas, Mayans and Aztecs. The nutritional value of the Red Pepper includes high levels of Vitamin C and flavonoids, beta- carotene and other antioxidants plus the highly researched Capsaicin. Science has observed Capsaicin has killed Prostate Cancer cells in preliminary research and it also seems to lower pain in the body. Cayenne Pepper is used by health enthusiasts including herbalist because of its many health benefits including; improvement to circulation and heart health, improved new tissue growth (research completed with frostbite), reversed hemorrhoids and even encouraged faster renewal of the stomach and intestinal lining due to ulcers. Other benefits reported include; raising red blood cell counts and increasing body temperature, lowering cholesterol and triglycerides, anti-parasitic, increased anti-microbial action destroying toxins in the blood and as mentioned it speeds the healing of stomach ulcers. *Note:* The heat from the Red Pepper may prevent its use by many people. Fortunately Aloe Vera is another traditional herb indicated as a remedy for ulcer resolution. *Important:* Use only a small amount of Red Pepper in daily foods before considering supplementing in larger amounts. Mind you Cayenne Red Pepper can be hotter upon elimination than the spicy heat you taste at mealtimes!

Seaweed

Seaweed is a vegetable that grows in the ocean. There are many varieties including Nori and Kelp which are both extremely rich in minerals. Kelp is one of the best sources for iodine and an abundance of other trace minerals. It is high in the Vitamin B-Complex, D, E, K, along with calcium and magnesium. Kelp contains a higher amount of natural sodium and because of this it is sometimes used for a salt substitute. It can be used in soups, salads, sushi or stir-fry's. Nori is so pleasant tasting it can be munched on as a snack food. Kelp and other sea greens may also be found in a single or a combination supplement giving extra daily nutritional value. The iodine in seaweeds provides special nutritional protection from nuclear pollution by protecting the Thyroid gland from Isotope Iodine.

Daily Greens (Vegetable)

Green Vegetables, including the leafy ones, are packed full of vitamins, minerals, proteins, chlorophyll, Essential Fatty Acids (Omega-3's) and phytonutrients from A-Z. Greens add to pH balancing of the body which requires minerals to alkalinize the sometimes over-acidic body tissue. Vegetarian individuals who do not eat animal proteins or cooked foods are known as "Raw Foodist." They provide their body's dietary requirements eating a large percentage from the category of Greens. To solely support the body with only greens and other vegetables (hopefully with an added supplement of B12) is a good example of the terrific food value vegetables hold.

The challenge with keeping a quantity of fresh Greens in one's house is that they are highly perishable and spoil within days and weeks of harvesting. Some people grow their own in gardens and or sprout beans, seeds and grains and allow the sprouts to make Chlorophyll to have a fresh supply of tiny vegetables. Greens and vegetables can demand a high price at the store when purchasing them especially if buying "Certified Organic". It is really no wonder that people are not eating the quantity of quality vegetables. Many people just can't afford them yet there is another alternative and that is to purchase supplements of vegetables "Daily Greens" in a carefully processed dried form as with the Daily Greens Formula that I take.

Most people eat a combination of foods including fish and meats, grains, beans and potatoes with varying amounts of vegetables both cooked and raw. The heat during cooking destroys a lot of the vitamin value of vegetables and proteins especially when excessive heat is used. Minerals are a bit more stable with heat. With 75% of Americans eating less than the recommended 7 – 11 servings of vegetables daily the overall health value of adding a vegetable supplement is tremendous.

Children and adults require a variety of vegetables to include the dark green, orange and yellow ones along with all the other colors of the rainbow to experience true health. There are a lot of Green supplements to choose from yet for just pennies a day the best buy and best formula of greens in my opinion is Daily Greens Formula. The powder or tablets contain Certified Organic Greens equal to 2 servings of green vegetables in each heaping teaspoon without the high price and it taste good!

Fortify a childs diet with just (1/2) teaspoon mixed in juice, yogurt, salad dressing or a blender drink. An adult daily serving is at least (1 – 1½) teaspoons or 2 tablets. Highlights include; support for the body's blood sugar (both high and low) and seems to settle down hyperactivity in children and adults. The formula is also geared to support a healthy weight through the addition of minerals, vitamins, proteins, Essential Fatty Acids that decrease the snacking tendency while supporting energy, cleansing and detoxification. Research has proven that Folic Acid abundant in all Greens is required for a healthy pregnancy, good growth and development of children and adults and a robust immune system. Shop around and you will see why it is easy to promote the Daily Greens Formula!

Alfalfa

The use of Alfalfa as a "Super Food" goes back thousands of years to ancient times. The Alfalfa roots can penetrate hundreds of feet into the soil absorbing more trace minerals and other nutrients than any other green vegetable. The name itself means "All Father - Father"! Alfalfa is a tiny seed and a health rule in nutrition is the smaller the seed the more nutrition there will be in the food that grows from it. Alfalfa grass is a powerhouse of nutrients including; many vitamins including beta-carotene, B-Complex, C, E, K, Chlorophyll and contains both macro and trace minerals. Minerals are seriously missing in today's population and this is why Alfalfa alone or in combination with other foods and herbs helps reverse so many ailments people suffer with from arthritis to a failing immune system. Alfalfa has a long history of use in Europe, China, and India and around the Mediterranean for indigestion, arthritis, bladder problems (diarrhetic), high cholesterol, allergies, rhinitis and hay fever, irregular menstruation and constipation. See Reference to locate companies that make great Alfalfa formulas to assist in gentle but effective cleansing of the bowel for children and adults heightening the success of the GIS Program by supporting healthy regularity without glutinous fibers – Psyllium Free!

Bovine Colostrum (BC)

Bovine Colostrum is richer in certain factors that tend to help the immune system than the whey isolate extracted from milk. BC contains high levels of immunoglobulins, growth factors, cytokines and nucleosides. It also contains oligosaccharides, antimicrobials and immune-regulating factors great for people who were never nursed or were weaned at a young age. The highlights of BC include; Immune System Support, Increased Athletic Performance, Improvement with Gastrointestinal Disorders such as diarrhea, especially with a history of heavy antibiotic use. One study following the support of BC was completed with a team of cyclists showing no difference on normal training between the participants using 10 grams of Bovine Colostrum or the regular Whey Protein Powder after the 8th week test point. However, once the study participants went into high training for 5 days after the initial 2 months there was a marked difference between the groups. The BC group experienced far less fatigue and performed at an exceptionally higher level of competition when compared to the performance of the group not taking the BC.

Bee Pollen & Propolis

Bee Pollen is gathered from plants by honey bees. It contains all 8 essential amino acids, Vitamins A, D, E, K, C and Bioflavonoids. It is also especially high in the B-Complex including Pantothenic Acid (B5) and Niacin (B3). Bee Pollen is extremely beneficial to the Adrenal Glands which often become weak due to constant stress, poor diet and excessive caffeine use. Skin conditions, allergies, fatigue, inability to concentrate and cope with stress are some of the symptoms associated with Adrenal Exhaustion. Bee Pollen has also been used traditionally as an Anti-Aging food and energizer. Many athletes have used Bee Pollen and Propolis both to improve their performance. Look for individual Bee Pollen and Propolis products to perk up the Adrenal glands or formulas containing them.

Bee Propolis is also found in the bee hive containing similar nutrition to pollen yet holds some unique and significant concentration of nutrients including "Flavonoids" especially important for boosting up ones immunity. This category of Phytonutrients is fast becoming the most scientifically studied category because of the powerful health action support it gives to the body achieved only through Antioxidant Action. In addition the Propolis holds significant Anti-Microbial properties which help prevent microorganisms from entering the hive. In the human studies researchers found Propolis very helpful for the immune system with its Anti-Bacteria properties as well giving support against dangerous gram positive bacterial strains including upper respiratory bacteria. Anti-fungal action is also significant with Propolis as well making it another great natural product that has many applications of use.

Chamomile, Peppermint, Catnip & Slippery Elm

Stomach herbs are important to keep in your herbal medicine chest including; herb teas, herbal liquid tinctures, liquid formulas or tableted herbal supplements. *Chamomile* is an all-time favorite for calming not only the stomach but the entire body and mind. It contains anti-inflammatory and anti-spasmodic properties and also stimulates renewal of lining cells in the intestinal tract. When applied topically on the skin as in lotions it helps to regenerate new cells quicker for anti-aging support. Applications include; digestion, colic, anxiety, insomnia, canker sores, conjunctivitis of the eye, Crohn's disease, diarrhea, Eczema, Gingivitis, hemorrhoids, menstrual disorders, migraines, IBS, Peptic Ulcers, Ulcerative Colitis and topically for all skin conditions. *Caution:* Persons with acute ragweed allergies may have an allergic reaction to the teas or tableted Chamomile. The Chamomile tincture is more hypo-allergenic. Chamomile also contains Coumarin a natural blood thinner which is an important consideration for people taking blood thinners or experiencing bleeding disorders. This property is a plus for helping the blood to naturally keep the platelets from becoming too sticky which contributes to CVD. Relax in the evening with a nice hot cup of Chamomile tea and see how much better you sleep!

Peppermint expels gas and calms a nervous stomach. In 2007 researchers showed 75% of the IBS patients taking peppermint oil for 4 weeks had major reduction in digestive symptoms compared to a placebo. In 2011 scientists tracked the pathway Peppermint works as an anti-pain herb through the TRPM8 channel. This study also confirmed that it relaxes the Gastro-Esophageal sphincter thus promoting belching. Because of the tendency to be a bit irritating when concentrated in the oil form researchers recommend using the entire plant which gives the therapeutic results without side effects. Peppermint also displayed protective action against the effects of radiation for cancer patients.

Catnip is in the mint family of herbs. It generally comes as a surprise that it can be used internally by people and that it helps digestion so much. Folk medicine claims it to contain disinfectant and sedative qualities making Catnip tea great for an upset stomach. The natural Tannins and Nepelactone active ingredients hold even more applications for respiratory infections as with asthma and bronchitis, lowering a fever, a decongestant and even warding off colds and flu. Catnip is a great herb for both children and adults to relieve colic and gas, nausea, ease headaches, menstrual cramps, general pain, arthritic soreness, sore throats, cough and croup, sinuses, ease allergies, restlessness (hyperactivity) and wonderful to induce restful sleep.

Slippery Elm is another impressive stomach herb that is indicated for GERD, gastritis, Crohn's disease and diarrhea. Slippery Elm also supports easing a sore throat and cough and is especially helpful for skin renewal of the intestinal tract. Throat lozenges are available and many good digestive and renewal formulas contain Slippery Elm.

Each of the Stomach Herbs is available to take separately or they can also be found in combination formulas. See Reference section to find more information for excellent herbal formulas in teas and tinctures.

American Ginseng, Cats Claw & Essiac Formula

Ginseng to an herbalist is synonymous with Long Life. It grows around the globe having different species however the American Ginseng root that was used traditionally by the American Indians is found by herbalist to be the most versatile classed as an "Adaptogenic Herb" for both men and women. The roots are light tan in color with gnarly roots that look human-like appearing to have arms and legs. Ginseng is packed with nutritional components along with phytonutrients called "Ginsenosides" that support glandular health including the Immune System. Research has proven American Ginseng to boost immunity perhaps one of the pathways is through its Antioxidant activity. It also exhibits anti-inflammatory properties and has been used successfully with many chronic illnesses including; Diabetes and Cancer. Often people will reach for Ginseng to ward off Colds and Flu and to assist with Adrenal Exhaustion supporting strength in the glands enhancing mental clarity and physical stamina. *Caution:* Ginseng is not for individuals already diagnosed with high blood pressure. Its stimulating qualities may increase blood pressure to higher levels in hypertensive people. Also, avoid Ginseng with hormone sensitive Breast and Prostate cancer because it appears to increase hormone levels. For all other individuals heightening hormones including ones libido is healthy.

The *Cat's Claw* herb is a climbing vine plant from South America receiving its name from the small thorns at the base of its leaves. The indigenous people refer to it as "The Sacred Herb of the Rain Forest". It became well known in America after the outbreak of the HIV virus. The active ingredients in Cat's Claw give support to the immune system, digestion and CVD. The main active ingredients in Cat's Claw include; Tannins, several phytonutrients and a major alkaloid called Rhynchophylline. The alkaloid elicits anti-hypertensive effects. This may reduce blood pressure and the risk of stroke and heart attack. Researchers have observed Cat's Claw constituents to support anti-inflammatory and antioxidant protection. Application for Cat's Claw includes support for symptoms of Crohn's Disease, Gastric Ulcers, Immunity, Parasites, Colitis, Gastritis, Diverticulitis and Leaky Gut Syndrome.

The original *"Essiac Herbs"* included four herbs; Burdock Root, Sheep Sorrel including the plant and root, Slippery Elm and Turkey Rhubarb. In 1920 Rene Caisse (Essiac spelled backwards) a Canadian nurse, experimented with herbs and nutrition with terminally ill patients suffering with Cancer and Diabetes. To her amazement all of her patients experienced benefit and some went into remission with their illnesses even in late stage cancers! Her legacy is bringing to light the value of herbs in the human experience and an alternative for people struggling for survival. Forty different Essiac Formulas have been developed from her original four herbal combinations. Each individual herb is available or in combination formulas. Quality and potency is important to experience the true therapeutic action that herbs provide for the body!

Licorice, DGL & Fennel

Licorice known as "Sweet Root" is in the Long Life herbal category along with Ginseng, Garlic, Gotu Kola and Aloe Vera. It is naturally sweet being 50 times sweeter than refined sugar. True Licorice is definitely not the same as the synthetic candy flavoring that contains no therapeutic value. Licorice has been used in both the East and the West in numerous health protocols from the common cold to liver disease. It contains elements that soothe and coat the mucus membranes of the intestinal tract and help as a decongestant ridding the body of excess mucus and phlegm from the respiratory tract. One of the active ingredients in whole Licorice called Glycyrrhiza can have side effects of increasing blood pressure and can bring about headaches and increase hypertension. Because of a special processing that removes this ingredient it allows the beneficial properties of Licorice to be available in support of peptic ulcers, cancer sores and GERD called "De-Glycyrrhized Licorice – DGL". Whole licorice, licorice tea and herbal formulas are valuable to support the body to perk up energy, glandular health, decrease cough and respiratory challenges especially with Asthma conditions. *Note:* Beware of gluten triggers in Licorice candies that can bring upon symptoms of GIS.

Fennel is in the Celery family and shares some key components with Licorice and is very soothing to the digestive tract. The use of Fennel goes back into ancient China. The Fennel root has been enjoyed as a food and the Fennel seeds as a supplement. The uses include; relief of gas and bloating, soothing an upset stomach, clearing mucus and congestion, conjunctivitis, stimulating appetite and increasing the flow of breast milk. Fennel is an anti-spasmodic, diuretic encouraging urine flow, expectorant and stimulant. It has been especially wonderful for supporting cancer patients while going through chemotherapy and radiation to reduce nausea and calm the body. It is also used for relief from upper respiratory conditions including bronchitis and Asthma symptoms. A traditional use is cutting the leaves or adding a tincture to boiling water and carefully inhaling the steam to soothe the breathing channels. Available as a single herb or in combination as found with other stomach herbal formulas.

Milk Thistle

Liver health is essential to maintain overall body health and Milk Thistle supports a healthy liver. It has relieved symptoms in many conditions involving the liver to include; cirrhosis, jaundice, hepatitis and gallbladder disorders. Other applications that research mentions include; lowering cholesterol LDL, support of Type 2 Diabetes, slowing the growth of cancer cells in breast tissue, cervical and prostate cancers. Silymarin is the highlighted active ingredient isolated from Milk Thistle. It is a powerful herb providing anti-inflammatory and antioxidant support to the body. It appears to stimulate proper estrogen levels so women who are staying away from increased estrogen may not want to take Milk Thistle. Another potential side effect is only a slight allergy if ragweed is a challenge. Milk Thistle is recommended to use in tincture form or tablet alone or in combination with other liver support herbs.

Brain Power: Prevagen, Phosphatidylserine (PS), L-Tyrosine & GABA

Brain support is critical to maintain ones "Brain Power" to be productive, engaging and to enjoy life to ones fullest in today's world. Dementia and advanced dementia called Alzheimer's disease (AD) and Mental Illness is on the rise due to poor diets, stressful lifestyles along with chemical and EMF pollution. AD is the seventh leading cause of death in the U.S. and experts predict it will quadruple in the next few decades! Brain supplements really work to support the body and it is just a matter of experimenting to find the best product for your needs blended with the GIS Program.

Prevagen is a one of a kind supplement that supports brain function significantly over and above the essential core nutrients by themselves coupled with a healthy lifestyle. The active ingredient in Prevagen is a specialized protein first isolated in a species of jellyfish called Apoaequorin. It works in the body and brain as a "Calcium Regulator" preventing nerve cells from premature death by up to 50%. The research at the University of Wisconsin has been impressive to show improvement in cognitive ability up to 80% in some instances. In just weeks Prevagen was able to improve advanced dementia to a mere common forgetfulness in some people. Besides supporting a healthier brain, sharper mind and protecting memory it allows for better multitasking, word recall, reading in general and even better sleep for many adults!

Phosphatidylserine (PS) is a single isolated amino acid involved in stimulating the brain to function sharply and seeming to lessen depression. It is found in all living foods including beans and when taken as a supplement in concentrate it improves cognitive function perhaps by supporting the Nervous System and enhancing the neurotransmitters in the brain as stated by the researchers. It has been written that the FDA admitted the success of PS research appearing to increase ones cognitive and memory function. The Mayo Clinic suggests however that a physician should be consulted with the use of PS although most doctors are not informed about the benefits of PS. To simply say there may be a conflict with medications and not give a reason for their warning is not a responsible reply when so many people require help with dementia. *Note:* The PS raw material is extracted from cow brains unless another source has been found to be effective. *Note:* The manufacturing of other single amino acids are derived from a micro-organism that is similar to a fermenting yeast healthy bacterial agent and not from animal tissue as with this particular nutrient.

L-Tyrosine and GABA are two other significant isolated amino acids critical for a healthy brain. *Tyrosine* is found in many protein containing foods such as meat, dairy products, fish, beans and grains. The benefits include; support of neurotransmitters L-Dopa and Dopamine, Norepinephrine and Epinephrine which supports mood and emotions. Deficiency of Tyrosine can bring about feelings of sadness, anxiousness, irritability and even depression. The body must have enough Tyrosine to feel satiated upon eating and prevent over eating. Chronic stress, junk foods with excess of sugar, caffeine and or alcohol depletes the body's stores of Tyrosine. Benefits of taking it include feeling more calmness, increased proper energy and enhanced libido. It may also improve the symptoms of Parkinson's disease, dementia and Alzheimer's disease. Consult your physician for any conflict with other mood enhancing pharmaceutical medications.

GABA is another isolated amino acid and has been reported to work very similar to the antianxiety drugs and anticonvulsive medication. GABA functions as a neurotransmitter in the brain and appears to stabilize the nerve cells encouraging a calming effect for people that experience irritability, short fuse temper and anxiety regardless of the origin. Dr. Daniel Amen, MD, in his book *Change Your Brain Change Your Body*, recommends adults to take from 100 – 1,500 mg daily and children 50 – 750 mg in addition to the core nutrients available in a Multiple Vitamin & Mineral (as tolerated) and Fish Oils.

Natural Tranquilizers: 5HTP (Serotonin Precursor), Kava Kava, St. John's Wort, Valerian & Melatonin

Depression and mental wellness is dependent on an individual's overall health status of the body which includes hormones. The expression that someone - living with mental illness has a "Chemical Imbalance" is primarily referring to the imbalance of hormones. The body makes over 50 hormones that regulate physical and mental well-being. Mental Health is discussed in length in Chapter 5 and how it relates to GIS.

The Special Needs Supplements (SNS) reviewed in this section have helped thousands of individuals through temporary and prolonged periods of mental imbalance and feeling uptight. These SNS along with other herbs, amino acids, supplements and lifestyle changes offer natural alternatives to pharmaceutical drug protocols. When a drug of choice works for mental health terrific yet I still suggest that a person follows the GIS Program to reap all of the renewal benefits it supports for mind and body. Once a person has followed the diet and supplements (as tolerated) for at least six months to one year then making alteration to any drug protocol under the strict guidance of a medical advisor is a possibility. Always consider any risk vs. the benefit of a drug protocol. Some SNS may be taken with pharmaceutical drugs and some may conflict. I suggest you

do your preliminary homework by talking with your attending physician about adding a natural substance. Do more in-depth study on the SNS you are considering. The ECN are not conflicting because they are just concentrated food supplements. With the SNS you can call the manufacturer of a certain product and also research on PubMed to find studies and or other people who have had similar experiences of use with a particular SNS. IMPORTANT: This is not a recommendation to stop your Pharmaceutical Drugs! *Note:* It may interest you that some blood pressure medicine has the side effect of depression.
You must make that important decision with a trained medical professional. Following the GIS Program will support the body for both mental and physical health and then experiment with SNS as tolerated and as desired.

5HTP is an intermediate form of L-Tryptophan easier for the body to absorb. Tryptophan is an essential amino acid the body cannot make therefore it is required in the diet. Tryptophan is essential to make a hormone called Serotonin in the gut and the brain. Tryptophan must be metabolized in the liver to make Serotonin and if the liver is under-functioning it cannot promote Serotonin to be manufactured. Serotonin is a necessary feel-good hormone that allows the muscles of the body to relax from the brain down throughout all the muscles of the body. A sluggish liver, a poor diet and low absorption of Tryptophan due to competition of other amino acids during digestion all appear to reduce the production of Serotonin. Good food sources of L-Tryptophan are found in protein rich foods including; turkey, chicken, dairy products, beans, nuts and seeds, eggs and 100% sprouted grains. Low levels of Serotonin symptoms include; depression, obesity, carbohydrate cravings, insomnia, narcolepsy, sleep apnea, migraine and tension headaches, pre-menstrual syndrome and even Fibromyalgia. The 5-HTP Tryptophan is absorbed 75% better into the body compared to just 3% of regular L-Tryptophan. Once the body has a good supply of Tryptophan then it allows the manufacturing of healthy Serotonin levels that encourage better mental attitude and restful sleep to improve. *Caution:* Do not take 5HTP with other natural herbs like St. John's Wort that also increases Serotonin or Pharmaceutical Drugs that do the same. Toxicity of the environment and fluctuating blood sugar as reviewed in Chapter 6 coupled with GIS are all influences to Mental Illness and Physical disease.

Kava Kava is an herb that supports the production of the body hormones needed to relax, sleep and even lose unwanted weight. Several research studies have confirmed the success experienced by hundreds of participants that used Kava Kava therapeutically to reduce anxiety and improve sleep. The Kava Kava pathway is thought to work by stimulating more production of GABA the amino acid responsible for calming the nerves for a smoother neurotransmission of the Nervous System during times of grief and even panic attacks. Strong support has also been experienced for losing weight surmised by researchers to be from balancing the appetite hormones Leptin and Ghrelin. Kava also seems to be a quick short-term remedy for sleep when feeling anxious about a special event. It can be a mild relaxant during the day without feeling drugged. Kava Kava tinctures are available or in combination with other herbs and supplements.

St. John's Wort is an herb that has been used for centuries to treat mild depression, mood disorders and also contains anti-viral activity. The active ingredient is Hypericin which functions to inhibit the reuptake of various neurotransmitters including; Serotonin, Dopamine, GABA and Glutamate. In other words if they go backwards they lose impact instead of forward to promote the desired effects of relaxation and good mood. By St. John's Wort inhibiting the reuptake of the neurotransmitters it works similar to the modern antidepressants including Prozac, Paxil and Zoloft. St. John's Wort works to maintain healthy levels of Serotonin without the same side effect of medication. The drawbacks of the herb are that some people require higher doses to create the relaxation but it may cause a slightly dulled somewhat "dingier" mentality. Another consideration is that St. John's Wort may possibly prevent birth control pills from being as effective. Lastly, it supposedly can cause UV light sensitivity in the higher amounts however this one seems to be a very rare occurrence. One study was halted because of rashes and skin conditions that became problematic at higher dosing. The daily amounts that people found effective by using St. John's Wort for uplifting mild depression in children was 300 mg, teens approximately 300 mg twice per day and adults 600 mg in the morning and 300 mg at night.

Valerian is known for its sedative qualities because it allows a person to relax the Central Nervous System. Over 120 constituents are found in this herb and remarkably it has not been found to have any negative side effects with moderate use. Most people find it calming without being too heavy of a sedative and basically non-addictive. Two double blind studies have shown Valerian truly shortens the time it takes for people to fall asleep. The active ingredient called Valepotriates has regulatory effect on the Autonomic Nervous System; calming for agitation and stimulating for fatigue. Valerian is especially helpful as an anti-spasmodic for menstrual cramps, migraines and even helps with Rheumatic Arthritic pain. It has been useful as a mild tranquilizer for emotional stress and exhaustion for special needs. Follow the directions on a product and call or write the company with any individual concerns. Also, review Chamomile for a milder relaxant as desired.

Melatonin is a hormone the body is designed to make on its own in the Pineal Gland of all mammals including humans. The Pineal is a light sensitive gland located in the brain that only secretes Melatonin in the darkness. Research has shown that at about 20 years of age the body may begin to decline in the amount that it makes. Melatonin is responsible for sleep, body temperature and growth and development. Symptoms of low Melatonin includes; depression, insomnia, Fibromyalgia and even seizures. Recent research has shown that Melatonin is also produced in healthy gut tissue. Varying potencies of supplements are available to give support on the evenings you may have a particular challenge with getting to sleep. Also, make certain all lights are turned off to allow your own body to function properly. Follow directions that generally suggest you take the Melatonin 30 minutes before sleep.

Understanding the Confusion Surrounding Health

New research in the last 20 years has given light to a greater understanding of how the body and immune system works. It is important to understand that the human body still holds many unanswered secrets. Researchers in both the medical field along with the Nutraceutical Industry may never understand all of the workings of the human body. However, there have been thousands of repeatable scientific studies in the US and around the globe that have proven the following two basic concepts of health!

Research Supports Nutrition

- The importance of nutrition and health for reversing and preventing disease.
- The safety and efficacy of nutritional supplements commonly referred to as vitamins.

The urgency of understanding the impact nutrition and health holds for slowing the aging process along with reversing and preventing disease in the first place cannot be over emphasized. Foods and supplements are a very important step in health insurance!

Our attending medical doctors are not taught extended nutrition in medical school and they are also influenced by the media and drug companies themselves. Physicians are taught in school to focus more on the breakdown of the body and symptoms of a disease instead of preventing illness from developing in the first place.

Both areas of expertise are needed and a few select medical institutions and a minority of doctors understand the critical part health plays in healing. This acknowledgement helps to promote improvements in eating healthier yet many professionals still shy away from supplements and herbs. This I believe is due more to ignorance and fear of liability suits and perhaps some investment interest in people staying sick and dependent on pharmaceutical drugs for follow-up care. There are a growing number of physicians who prescribe to the "Integrative Medicine" model which means they take a wholistic approach to healing through addressing the need for nutrition, required supplements and vitamins, a healthy lifestyle along with responsible pharmaceutical drugs. However, these doctors are a rare breed and may not be available in your community.

Gradually the group insurance plans have begun to offer more preventative health care programs for certain diseases. For the masses and for people already living with chronic health diseases diet alone can be too slow and not able to target the nutritional deficiencies covered in the complete GIS Program. The sick body often requires an aggressive supplement program. By using supplements including herbs, vitamins, minerals, essential fats, protein and vegetable supplements the body receives therapeutic nutrition that works faster and compliments the diet to achieve optimum health support. It may feel unnatural to take a handful of supplements. Yet many of the diseases today are extremely unnatural coming from the polluted world and over indulgences that promote disease. Health is a choice not a natural state of the body that cannot be legislated due to an individual's choice of freedom to make or break one's own life!

The bottom line is supplements are safe to take with very few exceptions. You can have your pharmacist or doctor's office run a report on any dangers taking a special supplement of choice with the medications you decide are necessary for life support. Yet do not take a verbal condemnation towards supplements because your life is at stake! The best advice is to filter out the negative media circulating in the news and often taught in school curriculums about the evils of supplements. Supplements are extensions of food and nature has made them in balance with the body with very few exceptions.

The real health danger lies with the overuse of pharmaceutical drugs and you can learn to be responsible about taking the ones you absolutely need in order to keep your body alive and follow your health program at least 80% of the time. All OTC and prescription medicine including antibiotics have a price to pay by taxing the liver and causing nutritional deficiencies that Tuft's University has at last revealed. In fact, recently the FDA has required a warning on Cipro, a full spectrum antibiotic, to state that it may cause tendons to actually explode in the body if you can believe! People should not be living Guinea Pigs for these drug companies any longer. If a single vitamin or supplement ever created even 1% of the premature deaths and side effects these drugs are responsible for the supplements would be pulled off the market in a heartbeat. Remember my friends that health is for everyone young and older alike – Enjoy!

C H A P T E R   9

Healthy Children Require Parrot Food – What?

On one of my evening walks a neighbor shared with me how fatigued she always was and unable to do daily chores or exercise any longer. In fact she told me that she and her husband had put their house up for sale and were moving into a retirement care facility. I was surprised because she only appeared to be in her late-sixties. I told her what I found helpful in my daily routine to give me more energy which included eating protein, fruits and vegetables, making time for breakfast, lunch and dinner and drinking Aloe Vera juice. Apparently I motivated her to try the Aloe and she went right out and bought the Aloe Life Aloe Vera juice at the local health food store. The next month when I saw her again she thanked me, saying she did feel a lot better drinking the Aloe juice and would be taking it for a while because it was helping her pack up her belongings. I asked her about her diet and she shared that the only one in their house who ate regular meals including vegetables and fruits was her pet green parrot!

What does this story have to do with raising healthy children? Not much yet it is a good example indirectly of how many adults including parents - expect to feel good, have energy, experience health, make healthy babies, raise healthy bright and happy kids and experience healthy aging – but do not put the right fuel in their body!

Thank God that some of you have already learned this common sense life lesson in health about cause and effect. "Truly the food you eat today becomes the body tomorrow." Unfortunately, many of you have still remained in the dark or denial about your daily actions affecting your health. The reasons are plentiful yet the fact is - for you and your family to reap the benefits of health your lives need to revolve around applying the health principles at least 80% of the time.

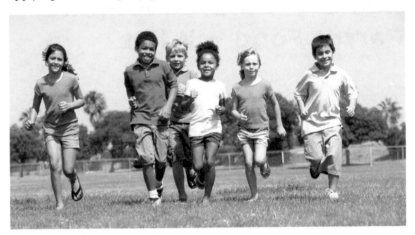

Healthy Children Facts

- A Healthy Child Requires Nutrition and a Healthy Lifestyle 80% of the time.
- The Health of a Child is Only Effected by Heredity Factors 20% of the time.

Another good saying goes like this, "You either spend time in the kitchen to start with or a lot more time in the doctor's office later!" Research supports the guidelines in this book 100% - to eat healthy foods and live a healthy lifestyle if you are to experience health. I realize that learning about GIS puts another facet into your health goals. However, this book lays the groundwork to help you understand the urgency of incorporating the GIS guidelines in order to reach your health potential and avoid disease. As you read the first few chapters I hope you will come to understand how valuable it will be to not only reduce gluten in your diet but also in your children's diet. It is not only important to choose low gluten or gluten free foods but also to reduce and avoid the other

GIS triggers including refined sugar and excessive milk, milk solids and ice cream from the diet. Make certain to be even more stringent on the program if you have a diagnosed illness or conditions in your family as listed in Chapter 5 that relate directly to GIS. The best goal in today's world is to live preventatively with some flexibility!

Health is Scientifically Grounded

50 years ago *Prevention* magazine was started by Irving Rodale and was the first major health periodical. It was "In" reading for the latest breakthroughs and studies in health. At that time before the internet and before cancer, heart disease and the deluge of other diseases began to skyrocket, people who read *Prevention* and health books were viewed as "Health Nuts". Today the facts prove that the majority of U.S. citizens have been heading down the wrong health path for many years. Most people are unaware that the US has dropped to 42nd place in its world health status - behind all the other developed countries according to the World Health Organization (WHO).

In the quest for answers to disease over the past half-century more and more health and scientific magazines have emerged to tell the public the truth. They contain an abundance of published studies conducted from all over the world that support the concept that health and nutrients that are found in foods do indeed prevent disease. Because of the truth slowly but surely reaching the masses, people are gradually joining the health ranks. Living a healthy lifestyle is at last being viewed in a growing segment of our society as a virtue.

Another great resource besides health magazines and books, for the curious health minded individual, is to go online and search through the peer reviewed research for instance on the PubMed website. This one website provides thousands of studies on health topics you may be particularly interested in from cancer, heart disease, allergies and more. The voluminous amount will make your head spin to view the repeatable research papers that have been completed by major universities and scientists in the US and abroad.

The taboo that health can prevent disease of the mind and body is gradually lifting. Yet the falsehood that only prescription medicines can help the aging process and disease including fertility will persist until the last segment of our culture, our physician's, embrace the truth, "Disease in the body or mal-functions occur when the opportunity of mal-nutrition and abuse weakens the host!" Why have our doctors been left behind you ask? The reason is that an "Integrative Health" class that would teach therapeutic nutrition - is still not taught in most medical schools!

So you must continue your individual self-study into health perhaps making a family folder to include the information that is most pertinent. Purchase a few more reference books on health and nutrition that come recommended. There are a handful of MD's that are developing a following such as Dr. Sears, MD, pediatrician www.askdrsears.com. He and other like-minded physicians are gaining respect because they embrace more of a foundational health philosophy and keep medications for times of absolute necessity!

The Gluten Tale

Many books have now been written to share about gluten but no other book is revealing the bigger picture for families as in *Beyond Gluten Intolerance - GIS*. Each book written has value and you can always learn from an author if they share real life experiences and or pertinent studies. It is important to receive support as you challenge the status quo's diet and lifestyle. Support from all sources will help you feel more confident in your health actions around friends, family and co-workers. As you apply health in your life you will build a belief that will not be shaken easily.

In addition to the extended family - other social situations can also be challenging in regards to diet improvements such as pre-school, birthday parties, and extra-curricular activities for your children. A little extra planning ahead for healthy snacks and meals is required yet it does become easier and more accepted by all of the people in your life. Also, health becomes contagious to others as they see the health benefits in your life. Learning new recipes and snacks for children and family from the low and no gluten foods is an ongoing search from books, magazines, TV and on the internet. However, many sources are not telling the whole story of reducing all of the inflammatory agents to avoid their repercussion!

The fact about Gluten and the Gluten Inflammatory Syndrome (GIS) triggers is that when they are eaten in combination and in excess – they significantly impact the health of the body even in regards to a couple's fertility success. The impact of GIS may also set up more challenges during pregnancy and the health of the infant at birth because it affects the hormones of the body. Also, keep in mind that some family members including Mom or Dad may require the strictest protocol in the GIS program Zone 3 to feel their very best. This may entail omitting all grains, flours or breadstuff regardless of it being from wheat, rice, oats or tapioca. As a person applies the GIS supplements and diet for a period of time the body gets healthier and begins to reduce symptoms. As similar as we each are as humans we also develop differences especially in regards to GIS. Reducing Gluten and following the other GIS guidelines in your family's diet will insure a healthier pregnancy and be an important step forward towards a healthier life for the entire family.

Greater GIS Symptoms in Children Result from Genetic Weakness

GIS genetic weakness from one or both parents' will result in more symptoms in your infant or child's body. As presented in the first few chapters all humans have a certain degree of gluten sensitivity and then each child can receive more potential through heredity factors. Each parent may contribute an extra 10% possibility of greater symptoms through their heredity.

If both parents have a strong heredity line for advanced GIS, physically and or mentally, then a 20% greater potential above the average gluten intolerance may develop in your off-spring. Especially when there has been a history of diagnosed mental illness or diagnosed bowel disease a child may experience advanced symptoms of Celiac disease, Crohn's or diagnosed Mental Illness as described in Chapter 2 and 5. Please remember that Mental Illness is the most common disease world-wide and unfortunately it just isn't talked about. Therefore, many families have a chain of diagnosed or undiagnosed relatives that have exhibited Mental Disorders. The history of digestive ailments on the other hand is extremely common from one or both sides of the family. The good news is by applying the GIS Program it will reduce or totally eliminate all the symptoms both mentally and physically.

Along with sparking countless symptoms as listed in Chapter 5 the GIS is directly connected to ulcers developing in the stomach and throughout the digestive tract. This information is important because the condition is being diagnosed in more and more children and teens today. The mal-absorption and malnutrition that occurs with GIS is linked to improper Vitamin A metabolism and other nutrients especially when Diabetes and/or Thyroid disturbances are present. Vitamin A is essential to build healthy lining tissue in the GI tract and every cell of the body including the brain. The "Performed Vitamin A" from fish oil and the GIS Protocol work together to reverse ulcers.

Many parents are unaware of the relationship of the intestinal tract to GIS and view ulcers as just too much stress in a child's life. A young woman I recently worked with noticed blood in her stool. After an intense examination she found she had a bleeding ulcer. The interesting fact is she experienced no pain with it. She had been striving to be a healthy teen and became a Vegetarian. She ate all the whole grains she could and also had a growing sugar addiction as well. Her doctor tested her for gluten intolerance which resulted in a negative reading therefore no dietary restrictions had been made. After following the GIS Diet her body healed and in fact she felt better than ever before. This example demonstrates how the GI tract can be very unhealthy yet show no obvious warning of pain. Review Chapter 4 that covers the testing for Gluten and this will explain why children and adults are often given a "False Negative" from a medical laboratory blood test for gluten intolerance.

A pertinent fact to reflect on is that the entire digestive tract often does not receive the health and nutritional support it requires to function well. In fact according to the American Cancer Society the entire Digestive Tract is the most common system to develop cancer vs. any other single sight for cancer including; lung, breast, prostate and colon! People must strive for a healthy digestive tract to experience health!

GIS Symptoms from Infancy to Teens

The Gluten Inflammatory Syndrome (GIS) can be observed in infants at birth and remain a factor with children to some degree right on through to becoming a teen and then as an adult. The type of symptoms experienced may change yet as I have mentioned in previous chapters adults who finally come to understand that their poor health is connected to GIS remark that they can trace it back to early childhood.

Any nutritional deficiencies and genetic weakness that are present in the parents and especially from the mother effects the health of the infant. One of the more common symptoms of GIS at birth is a colicky infant. "Colic" is a digestive condition experienced by infants with symptoms of gas, constipation, pain and fussiness. Be aware that each sibling can experience different GIS symptoms due to the genetic pool plus the health support they receive during gestation.

Even with the best situation infants are always born with a rather undeveloped digestive system to begin with. Low Hydrochloric Acid (HCL) in the stomach is very common causing some gas and at times it can even be a challenge to properly digest Mother's milk. Also, the types of food the mother is eating, as she nurses the infant, can contribute to symptoms of Colic. With this in mind it is best to follow a stricter hypo-allergenic (low allergy) GIS Diet during the first few months of nursing your infant. Besides keeping gluten and gluten triggers low from grains, sugar and milk products consider toning down eggs, onions, garlic, spices and chocolate. Several natural remedies are available to help with slight to medium digestive upset in the newborn to include; homeopathic bitters, gripe water and even quality Aloe Vera works well for this. Only a small amount of quality

Aloe Vera just a few drops into the baby's mouth before a feeding can stop unwanted gas, irritability and upset. The Aloe drops can also encourage bowel regularity for the infant which is sometimes a challenge as well.

A healthier parent(s) upon conception and especially the mother's health throughout gestation will determine several important outcomes one being the "Term Length" of the pregnancy which is critical to the infants development and health. How well the mother eats and supports her health before pregnancy and during the (potential) 9 month period will also determine the "Mother's Health Status" during the pregnancy. And lastly the mother's health status is a critical factor affecting the "Health of the Infant" at birth including; digestive distress, dermatitis and overall physical and mental well-being.

A Healthy Conception & Building a Healthy Baby Starts 3 Years Before Pregnancy!

The study of healthy children begins with the review of what it takes to attain fertility and to have a healthy conception. Some of you may chuckle that have no challenge getting pregnant yet a healthy conception does take special preparation from both partners; the man and the woman and I believe this section will provide some good information for all couples as you build your family.

Unfortunately, for many eager couples fertility has become a major obstacle. Documented by medical statistics (1) in 6 couples or about 5 million seek the help of a fertility specialist yearly. Even more couples have challenges today without having the funds to work with a specialist. Fertility has declined over the past 50 years and the reason seems to involve both partners.

With regards to the man a review of 61 research papers since 1932 points to the male sperm count declining 42%! This has definitely led researchers to look at everything that may contribute to male infertility from all lifestyle and environmental factors that include; pollution, nutritional deficiencies and addictions.

Factors Lowering the Male Sperm Count
- Toxic Pollutants including Endocrine Disrupters
- Ionizing Radiation
- Zinc, Vitamin E & Nutritional Deficiencies
- Sexually Transmitted Diseases
- Alcoholism & Smoking
- Anabolic Steroid Use
- General Health of the Man

The woman's most common reason for not conceiving is involved in "Ovulation" which is the production of eggs and implantation regulated by the glands in the brain. The Hypothalamus, Pituitary and Thyroid glands all three must be functioning properly for ovulation and fertility success. Some adults are also choosing to start their families in their middle to late thirties and because of experiencing early Menopause the woman must rely on fertility drugs. However, "Orthomolecular" health experts understand that for most people it can flat-out be related to unhealthy parents.

Factors Lowering Female Fertility
- Glandular Health; Hypothalamus, Pituitary & Thyroid
- Ovulation, Eggs & Implantation
- Late Pregnancy Early Menopause
- General Health of the Woman

The question to answer first is what is causing the poor glandular health and what is the solution besides expensive fertility drugs? In today's world the two areas that pose the greatest challenge to achieving overall health is the environment and diet. Research has shown that environmental pollution, and toxicity contributes a major cause of infertility. Review Chapter 6 on Toxicity. As explained in Chapter 6 an adults body may absorb upwards of two hundred or more different chemical toxins from the environment that remain in the body until a person detoxifies. Some of the chemicals are cancer causing, others may disrupt growth and development such as the "Endocrine Disrupters" found in softer plastics which affect glandular health. Many of the chemicals cause DNA damage. The DNA Chromosome damage is connected to birth defects including both mental and physical impairments. Just Google Proposition 65 in California to view the avalanche of chemicals that every person's body must cope with in today's world.

Glandular health in the body is critical for successful conception. It takes a healthy body to support a robust glandular system that is needed to produce hormones and specialized proteins. The Thyroid gland is not always directly associated with fertility yet it is an important gland responsible for many functions of the body and is paramount to conceive. Thyroid function is involved in regulating body temperature significant in weight maintenance and metabolic function, energy, mood and more. Toxicity coming from public drinking water, food, air and consumer products has left not only the Thyroid gland under-functioning but has also impacted a man's body from making plentiful and healthy sperm required for the fertility connection. Focusing on the healthy GIS Diet and making healthier choices in daily life will not only begin the detoxification of the body but will also give the body the critical ECN's required to build healthy glands.

Steve and Sharon's Conception Success by Applying the GIS Program

A couple in their thirties from Southern California had been trying to conceive for many years. Out of desperation and frustration they sought out nutritional counseling. As I began our session I explained to the couple how important getting off sugar and eating a nutritious diet was in helping the body reach its goal. It puzzled Sharon yet she followed my advice even though she was concerned that eating regular meals might cause her some weight gain. She was modeling on the side of her office job and relied on this extra income to afford having a family. I explained how important the Thyroid gland was for fertility which hers was under-functioning. A full proof method to check the Thyroid is to take the body's temperature which is supposed to read 98.6 during waking hours. If your body's temperature tests low, your body requires Thyroid support as outlined in Chapter 6 Glandular Health. Sharon was running a couple of points low so I encouraged her to add the GIS essential core nutrients in a comprehensive Multiple, 50 mg B-Complex, 400 IU of Vitamin E (1 – 2 per day), Minerals to include Zinc 30 mg (1 daily) plus Wheat Germ Oil (1) tablespoon for three months plus Iodine from seaweed and a good Probiotics. They regularly ate fatty fish like salmon and sardines so I did not add the fish oil to their program. As she got onto the complete program as described in Chapter 7 she began detoxification from the Candida Albicans yeast and remarked how much better she was feeling even if she wasn't pregnant yet. Sharon really battled the acne break out period that lasted during her cleansing for about three months and then to her amazement it cleared up. I encouraged her husband to follow suit and Steve also began to feel more energy and overall healthier. We completed our work through the clinic and I told them that they could now get to work. I tearfully received a baby shower invitation that following spring! The need for detoxification and therapeutic nutrition is essential to optimize conception potential!

A Full-Term Healthy Pregnancy Requires a Good Diet Plus Supplements!

The next important goal of the parents-to-be is achieving a "Full-Term Birth" and a healthy baby. Premature births have become ever increasing with (1) in 8 babies or half a million Preemies born each year. 40 weeks is considered Full-Term and less than 37 weeks is Pre-Term. Pre-Term births are the leading cause of death in newborns. Some are so small they can fit into the palm of your hand. Being born before the fetus has fully developed the brain, skeleton and other organs, puts these innocent lives at risk from a variety of birth defects that the CDC relates to poor nutrition and addictions!

A recent study just completed at the University of Davis in California was presented at the 10th International Meeting for Autism Research. This ground breaking study showed the highest incidence of infants born with Autism Spectrum Disorder (ASD) was due in large part to the poor health of the mother. ASD has recognizable symptoms of neurological learning and behavior disabilities and delay which includes Autism. The study revealed that the highest percentage of children that developed ASD was in children from mothers diagnosed with Diabetes, Obesity and Hypertension during their pregnancy. A multiple birth was viewed as the exception however all experts agree multiple births do require "Super Nutrition" during pregnancy to avoid disabilities.

This study accentuates the requirement for all young adults to take responsibility for their health. How you prepare for and support your health during a pregnancy truly reflects on the unborn child at this very critical point of life. Stop looking for the magic bullet from the medical community to prevent birth defects. The answers you are searching for 99% of the time lies in health!

Pregnancy Success Guidelines

- GIS Program for Renewal of Glands
- Detoxification to Eliminate Toxic Waste
- Repair DNA Damage
- Optimize Nutrition for a Healthy Fetus

To optimize your health and increase the chances for a successful conception, a healthy pregnancy and to give birth to a healthier child requires a good detoxification program before conception. Give yourself as much time as you feel is needed. Following the GIS Program for at least 18 - 36 months or longer is suggested, highlighting the Special Needs Supplements (SNS) in Chapter 6 and 8 for Detoxification. You will also want to include the important Foundational Essential Core Nutrients (ECN) that do come in a comprehensive Pre-Natal supplement plus a few extras and get plenty of Antioxidants (from fruits and vegetables) in your diet and or supplements. The GIS Detox Program will help you feel your best to enjoy your pregnancy like an athlete preparing for a good competitive performance.

Research has proven that applying health actually helps to repair the DNA that holds the genetic factors. Antioxidants and Essential Core Nutrients help greatly in this process. DNA is found in the nucleus of almost every cell in the body. The DNA contains two sets of Chromosomes one from the mother and one from the father. The DNA is involved in cell replication. When the time is right the double DNA spiral breaks into two strands and makes two brand new cells. Interestingly, scientists have found that only some of the DNA contains the actual genetic information called your "Genes" holding the newborns blueprint. Focusing on health will provide a strong foundation for the entire family to experience a full and healthier life together while keeping any medical care cost down!

Pregnancy: Nutritional Requirements, Health Risks & Corresponding Nutrients

Nourishment for the fetus comes from the mother through the umbilical cord. It is not an optional feature to build the baby's body it is a requirement. Just how much nourishment the baby receives determines how well the DNA genetic blueprint can be fulfilled!

A Full-Term baby is born with a complete skeleton containing all the bones of an adult and some extras that merge as the baby grows. The fetus demands extraordinary nutrition including Calcium and fifteen other minerals that a Pre-Natal supplement alone does not even contain. To absorb the minerals and make bones Vitamin D and other essential co-factors are required. The other nutrients include Vitamin C, Vitamin A, B-Complex plus Protein that work together to also build the collagen that comes before the bone development.

Requesting a 25 Hydroxy - Vitamin D blood test will take the guess work out of whether the mother's level of Vitamin D is adequate. Vitamin D along with the other core nutrients is vital to meet the mother's and the baby's nutritional needs and is often found extremely low these days in all adults. Vitamin D is tied to mental health. Pregnancy is very demanding both physically and mentally especially with women often working during their pregnancy and taking care of the rest of the family. Be diligent to build up the emotional stamina through extra prenatal nutrition (review Ch. 5)!

A pregnant woman's digestion is another important consideration and often needs improvement. Good digestion is needed for proper absorption of the valuable nutrients from your foods and supplements. Review what good digestion includes in Chapter 3. Also read the Highlight of Chapter 4 that explains the value of including a quality Aloe Vera juice or tablet to optimize digestion and regularity during the pregnancy. Properly processed Aloe juice is 100% safe to drink during pregnancy and postnatal and contains many other benefits like decreasing nausea and constipation especially with the StomachPlus Formula by *Aloe Life* and increasing natural energy so appreciated during gestation.

Diet, Supplements & Healthy GIS Guidelines for Pregnancy

- *Eat Nutritious Foods* - Chapter 7 reviews the diet (3 x daily) and focuses on healthy GIS snacks.
- *Pre-Natal Multiple Vitamin & Mineral*
- *Pre-Natal DHA (EFA)* by *Nordic Naturals* or eat sardines, stop taking any Vitamin A from fish oil source during pregnancy and nursing.
- *Vitamin C* – take an extra 500 - 1,000 mg, (Ester type is buffered).
- *Daily Greens* - increase greens and vegetables in the diet and/or add a supplement to increase minerals including Iron required for building a baby.
- *Last 3 Months Kick Up E & Protein* - extra Vitamin E 200 - 400 IU, Protein 85 grams as tolerated.
- *Exercise, Skip Caffeine and Alcohol, Drink Quality Water and Don't Smoke!*
- *Support Daily Bowel Regularity* (see Aloe Vera & FiberMate Chapter 7) however do not detoxify while pregnant, wait until after weaning your child.

- **Rest** - even for 5 minutes at a time putting your feet up or taking cat naps during the day!

The body's "Pregnancy Nutritional Requirements" increase approximately 15 - 30% over the mother's non-pregnant status. This is an average of 20% more of the required 92 different essential nutrients (Ch. 8) which includes the valuable *DHA* Essential Fatty Acids required by each cell of the body especially for the Nervous System including the brain. Also, in the last trimester of pregnancy an *extra Vitamin E* and *Vitamin C*, in addition to a Pre-Natal Multiple Vitamin and Mineral, is required along with adding more protein to prevent Toxemia. Adding an *extra B-Complex* can also be helpful with energy after making certain your Iron and protein is sufficient. See B-Complex in Chapter 8 for a good description. More vegetables and a few fruits like bananas and organic apples in the diet are also required for the increased need of vitamins and minerals during this period of growth. Keeping a good supply of carrots, celery, apples and greens will help Mom relax and will maintain more regularity of the bowels. To encourage healthy regularity *Aloe Life* makes the StomachPlus Formula and the FiberMate products both are very popular with pregnant women to decrease nausea and support regularity!

How to Avoid Dangerous Health Risks during Pregnancy

During the last three months (Third Trimester) the fetus experiences such rapid growth of the brain and other organs that nutritional requirements spike. Because of the extra nutritional demands a condition called Toxemia is commonly experienced. It may evoke high blood pressure, fluid retention and protein in the urine. Protein in the urine means the body is breaking down muscle to give the baby its increased nutritional requirements. This condition can be reduced or prevented by increasing your pregnancy nutrition as suggested in the GIS Pregnancy Guidelines.

Toxemia symptoms are swollen ankles, headaches, nausea and or vomiting that will alert women of this toxic state. Call the doctor immediately if it does not improve within 24 hours. This condition relates to dietary factors that cause a circulatory reduction in blood vessels which is experienced more often with auto-immune conditions. Following the GIS Pregnancy guidelines and the doctor's advice will reduce the occurrence because this health protocol supports good circulation. Keeping the blood pressure in a healthy range requires minerals from vegetables and fruits especially accenting *Potassium* rich ones like bananas, apples, Kiwis, orange, carrot and prune juice, radishes, beans and fish.

All of the GIS supplements and foods are 100% safe to continue during pregnancy with the exception to stop taking any Fish Oil - Vitamin A supplements and monitor the Vitamin D level. A small amount of fish oil Vitamin A is not a challenge for example below 25 IU or any that might come through eating fish in the diet. Yet because the baby receives the nutritional stores even before the mother the fish oil Vitamin A of any large quantity from supplementing can potentially build up in the liver of the tiny fetus causing them to receive too much. Also, pregnancy is not the time to do any extra detoxification. The mother can safely conduct more detoxification after weaning the baby.

Mothers must be cautious not to take too high of Vitamin D. To side on safety it's a good idea to reduce the daily amount down to a reasonable limit of no more than 1,000 IU until further discussed with the pediatrician who needs to check the Vitamin D level. No other fat soluble vitamin holds any risk to the fetus or infant while nursing not even the extra *Vitamin E.* Taking an additional Vitamin E supports healthy circulation and immune function. Women want to also increase *Protein* intake to approximately 85 grams per day during the last 3 months. Eating an abundance of green and orange vegetables will give sufficient *Beta-Carotene Vitamin A* (non-toxic) and to help reach these nutritious goals carrying snacks like hard-boiled eggs, cheddar cheese, humus dip and veggie sticks - they really come in handy!

Eating healthy and taking an extra *B-Complex 25 – 50 mg or Nutritional Yeast* can help reduce nausea, experienced in the first trimester of the pregnancy or any time. Review Chapter 8 Nutritional Brewer's

Yeast and B-Complex. Most experts agree that this queasy stomach is due to natural hormone changes in the body and eating healthy vs. eating a lot of salty crackers and chips is a much better remedy. Also, very relaxing and soothing is sipping a little Chamomile or Ginger Tea with honey!

Hypoxia is another condition sometimes experienced during pregnancy. This is a state of oxygen imbalance in the blood stream and is potentially very dangerous to the fetus. This low level of oxygen is directly related to poor nutrition, excessive sugar in the diet and smoking cigarettes. Increasing Vitamin C and B-Complex plus eating a good supply of vegetables including *Daily Greens* and a couple of *Fruits* each day (Organic Raisins are high in Iron and Potassium) will all help to reduce your chances of this malady. The greens also supply a good amount of extra *Magnesium* and *Folic Acid* one of the B-Complex needed in higher amounts for a healthy pregnancy and a variety of other vitamins and minerals including *Iron*. Also, include bell peppers; citrus; lemon, limes and oranges, papaya and Kiwi fruit all great sources for *Vitamin C* which are so important for oxygenation. If possible include an extra 500 -1,000 mg of Vitamin C in the Ester type which is lower in acidity, as tolerated, to give more nutritional support for oxygenation. *Avoid refined Sugar, Junk Food* and *processed foodstuff* in the diet and *"Don't Smoke"* because it reduces oxygenation in the body!

Protein is reviewed in Chapter 7 and the World Health Organization states that eating fish while pregnant is so advantageous, for the unborn child, that even with the fear of mercury it is good idea to include it in the diet. Eating fish 1 – 2 times per week to include Salmon, Shrimp, Sardines and other fatty fish like Ocean Cod fish gives your baby some of the valuable Omega-3 Essential Fatty Acids which includes the DHA. Shark, Swordfish and Tuna have been found to contain the higher levels of mercury and it is best to only partake of these varieties once per month as desired and never more than once per week. Chicken, Turkey and even Beef are also good protein sources. Beans contribute excellent protein, not as high as in meat, yet do contain vitamins, minerals, EFA's and fiber. See Healthy

TIPS section for combining Vegetarian protein sources like beans and dairy in Chapter 7.

Highly debated at one time Eggs are a very good source of protein as well if tolerated and the yolk contains the valuable B12 especially viable in poached, over-easy cooked eggs and somewhat in boiled eggs. B12 is part of the B-Complex required for a healthy Nervous System along with *DHA* (EFA's) and EPA Omega-3 fractions from cold water fish and supplements. Olive and Flax oil are also good oils to use in the kitchen and both contain a variety of Omega-3 and Omega-6 EFA's but not the important DHA fraction. See Highlights of Chapter 5 Fish Oil and Essential Fatty Acids for All.

THINK Certified Organic!

One of the goals in motherhood is to reduce the exposure of environmental toxins to the unborn baby as much as possible. Striving to eat Certified Organic fruits and leafy vegetables along with organic apple juice or others is certainly a big first step. Organic peanut butter, raisins and dairy products are all much safer than their commercial counter-part. These foods in the regular or commercial type, according to the FDA standards, contain higher levels of toxic pesticides, higher than some other commercially grown foods. Everyone must balance their budgets with the risk vs. benefit and shopping around people can many times find good savings on Certified Organic foods.

Also, consider using health food store Personal Care products which have shown in testing to be safer than many mainstream lotions, soaps and children's toiletries. The skin absorbs all chemicals both good and bad into the bloodstream. It appears that the larger corporate owned companies are not always as discerning with the ingredient safety standards in regards to personal care products as smaller health minded companies. Laundry soaps and floor cleaners can also potentially bring dangerous toxins into your families bodies. Especially dangerous are the "Perfumed Laundry Detergents" and "Dryer Sheets" that contain chemicals that no one in the family deserves to be contaminated from that have been associated to liver toxicity! Just think if people are advocating these Dryer Sheets to kill insects what more proof do you need in realizing that they are not good for your family?

Ice Cream is Packed Full of GIS Triggers

A Prenatal Multiple Vitamin and Mineral is valuable however it is NOT a replacement for a healthy diet. Good solid nutrition is critical for building a healthy baby. The mother must strive to eat three good meals a day with healthy foods while keeping the GIS Triggers down in the diet. By following through Mom will feel better during the pregnancy and if nursing the baby its digestive system which can pick up irritants through the milk will experience minimal upset. Also, eating healthier will support healthy weight loss after giving birth much more quickly. Following the GIS Diet guidelines allows the Pancreas and Thyroid glands to function healthier to find a Healthy Weight reviewed in Chapter 6. So often a women's view of pregnancy is eating whatever she has a craving for from pickles to ice cream, pizza, soda and junk foods. Indulging occasionally doesn't rock the boat but remember the objective here is to build a healthy baby and feel good while doing it!

Before refrigeration became a common luxury in homes enjoying ice cream was truly a special occasion made from scratch with imported ice. Now-a-days families often eat ice cream every week-end and some individuals eat it every day. Ice cream is a sure way to ignite inflammation in the body triggering many GIS symptoms and poor health!

Most ice cream today is made from milk, sugar and extra thickeners like carrageenan, guar gum and added stabilizers and chemicals. Ice cream is loaded with excess calories from sugar and fat which may increase allergies even Asthma, pain in the joints, Herpes, digestive upset, hyperactivity, moodiness and even depression. "Gestational Diabetes" has become a common occurrence in pregnant women of today. Check-out the recipes for fresh fruit Sorbet and or frozen banana and fruit Smoothies in Chapter 7 – Delicious! Also, introducing your children to the delicious natural desserts of seasonal fruits is a valuable, delicious and fun exercise. Fruit sugar and honey (not for infants) are both non-inflammatory sweeteners on the GIS Diet and great for satisfying the sweet tooth. *Note:* It is important to monitor how much fruit, fruit juice or honey is consumed in regards to Diabetes, high and low blood sugar as reviewed in Chapter 6. At times even one piece of fruit can cause a hypoglycemic reaction. However, there is no other dessert that can compare to a fruit salad with perhaps a little Greek yogurt and a squirt of whip cream on top!

Pizza-man-i-a is a GIS Bombshell

The challenge with Gluten, which is isolated from wheat and other whole grains along with the other Gluten Triggers found in foodstuff, is the body's inability to digest their complex carbohydrate structure. This poor digestive process is due to a deficiency of the required digestive juices. Review Chapter 3 Digestion. Not digesting the gluten from grains and the other triggers, especially refined sugar and milk, causes the body to react with inflammation. An increase in inflammation causes further reduction in the digestive process, causing mal-absorption of nutrients, constipation and or diarrhea.

During the 2nd and 3rd Trimester of pregnancy digestion is impaired even more-so and it requires healthy choices to optimize it. The baby begins growing at a rapid pace and all of the abdominal organs are pushed around which may cause extra gastritis and constipation. The cascade of reactions if not eating properly coupled with the normal pregnancy challenges can exasperate mood disorders and leave an otherwise remarkable experience of pregnancy difficult and at times even traumatic. If women take care during pregnancy to focus on health they build a healthier baby and also avoid the difficult condition called "Post-Partum Depression (PPD)" after delivery.

A wonderful doctor who has addressed the mental stability during pregnancy and PPD after giving birth is Dr. Shoshana Bennett, PhD, Clinical Psychologist. She can be contacted at www.drshosh.com. Dr. Shosh as she is called is experienced in Post-Partum Depression herself with two pregnancies and went onto take PPD out of the closet, helping thousands of women all over the world and couples to understand the dynamics that may occur after childbirth and more. Her books are comprehensive and include some healthy guidelines (that includes the value of fish oil) to also help women during their transition from taking drug therapy when they wish to start a family! Keep in mind that the more junk food eaten during pregnancy, that contain the higher levels of processed Omega-6 oils, the more the body requires Omega-3 oils from fish and flax oil to compensate in order to support health and mental stability. B-Complex is also required in higher amounts during pregnancy and a deficiency is associated with depression and Mental Illness as also reviewed in Chapter 5.

Pizza contains not only Omega-6 oils but also wheat flour and now-a-days added Gluten flour to hold a better pizza shape. Most mass produced pizzas also contain the low grade processed cheese ingredients containing milk solids. Being that the general public is 50 – 70% lactose intolerant, with most people unaware of this sensitivity, eating processed cheeses escalates the GIS reactions adding to allergies and GIS symptoms. The other insults coming from pizza includes the added tomato sauce and sweeteners. To avoid the often sour tomato taste the addition of high fructose corn syrup or cane sugar is added to mellow the pH acidity taste. Lastly, the toppings of sausage or pepperoni is often sprinkled about which is laced with wheat gluten fillers and an array of chemical toxicity mentioned in the book *Diet for a Poisoned Planet* by Freedom Press. Can the pizza taste good? Yes. Is it good for people? In any quantity the answer is emphatically NO! Review Addictions in Chapter 6 to understand more about sugar and other food addictions and also pH Balance.

People do not have to give up all of the fun foods. Making your own pizza with gluten alternative flours can be a family affair and with healthier toppings Umm – Delicious! Frozen low gluten pizza is also available yet they are still quite pricey so be prepared for a sticker shock. Keep in mind serving pizza and the traditional spaghetti including boxed macaroni and cheese, regularly to your kids and family is just asking for GIS trouble, unwanted weight gain and possibly lower test scores in school. Check out the Healthy Tips section in Chapter 7 to learn some kitchen short cuts and become a better label reader to avoid the GIS pitfalls. Remember this; SUGAR in any processed form especially in high quantity is bad news for the body and the baby. Besides causing the kids to turn into spinning tops and even show aggression, it has been found to actually reduce the body's immune system. Drinking a regular soda or eating a candy bar has enough sugar to lower White Blood Cell (WBC) function, in less than 30 minutes!

Do You Drink Milk or Sugary Sodas?

It may come as a surprise to some of you that both milk and soda can be harmful during pregnancy and also to young bodies. In most cases but not all it is better to drink milk vs. soda for the protein value if you do not have any obvious allergy symptoms but not in excess. However, because milk is the number one allergy and a primary trigger in GIS symptoms for many people milk may be more harmful to the body than drinking an occasional sugary soda! Reviewing the Healthy TIPS section in Chapter 7 will give several milk alternatives for children and adults. Chapter 6 goes into depth on the value of drinking filtered water to hydrate the body.

As reviewed in Chapter 3 the Epicenter for GIS is first aggravated by both milk sugar and refined sugar. They are both considered disaccharides and double bonded sugars that require a functioning digestive system to cleave or separate the two part sugar during digestion. It is later in a child's life upon the introduction of grains into the diet that Gluten begins to create more of an inflammation disaster because of the starch complex sugars.

Believe it or not, even though sodas are made from filtered water with high sugar or sugar substitutes, phosphates, sometimes caffeine and other chemicals, some parents raise small children drinking soda and even put it into baby bottles for their infants. Of course the discerning parent would never do this yet indirectly when a pregnant or nursing mother is ingesting a high quantity of soda the baby is getting the aftermath of high circulating glucose! High Fructose Corn Syrup or Cane Sugar found in sodas and other foodstuff are very destructive to the mother's health which affects the infant indirectly. Soda is definitely not a health drink and may contain 3 – 14 tsp. of sugar at times. Many children develop rotten teeth and experience the undermining of metabolic health from the excess refined sugar. Besides being responsible for kicking up the GIS symptoms soda brings "Empty Calories" that contribute to the body's glandular shut down called Metabolic X Syndrome of the young and commonly seen in adults these days. This is reviewed in Chapter 6 along with the Anti-Nutrients that include Sugar Substitutes in the Toxicity section. A handful of enlightened physicians are recognizing that Sugar Substitutes may actually be as dangerous as sugar is to the body because of the chemical reaction they create associated with auto-immune disease. As bizarre as it may seem for many people the use of sugar substitutes stimulate the appetite and people using them often find themselves eating far more calories during their day and gaining weight!

Perhaps due to cow's milk causing extreme allergy reactions in so many children and adults, soda has become a second beverage choice. However, filtered and purified water is actually the best beverage of choice and the protein and minerals one might receive from milk can be better sourced from a healthy nutritionally balanced diet that includes; beans, raw nuts and seeds, a variety of vegetables (including green leafy ones) and a reasonable amount of healthy yogurt and or cottage cheese. People definitely do not need to drink cow's milk to be healthy!

As reviewed in Chapter 7 Healthy Tips section, cow's milk is ideal for baby cows and Mother's Milk is the correct formula ratio of nutrients for the human infant. Truthfully adults were not designed to drink cow's milk! The recipe section gives easy to follow directions to make your own nut or seed milks in a blender from blanched Almonds or Sesame butter that tastes delicious! These milk substitutes or diluted Half n Half (tolerated by most lactose intolerant people) or Lactaid milk can be used in many recipes to include poured over low gluten cereals.

In regards to nursing, the body will make plenty of your own breast milk without drinking a drop of cow's milk. Encouraging milk production only requires healthy hormones, a good supply of protein in one's diet and to drink at least 2 -3 quarts of water each day if not more. Glandular Health is essential to support all of the hormonal processes to function properly including milk production which is strengthened by following the GIS Pregnancy guidelines and diet. The discussion of milk leads us into the decision of whether or not to nurse your child. The healthiest choice and in tune with the natural design for the humans to thrive is Breast Feeding!

Do I give my children milk?

I breast fed both of my children for 22 months and 18 months. The value of nursing, besides the unmatched nutrition that nursing gives a newborn, is the convenience - what a time saver! It also saves a lot of money compared to expensive formulas - that comes in handy for many young families.

Looking back on those first years of motherhood they were the easiest and least stressful especially once the learning curve of how to nurse and what to expect was understood. Most Pediatric nurses are very willing to teach the basics of Breast Feeding these days. The challenge for me came later with how to wean my children and what would be the best solid foods to start them on? I decided to follow the old fashion suggestion of cooked cereal. This was in the eighties so I went with whole grains over refined cereals. I didn't realize what a mistake I was making. I also didn't have a clue that both of my children were Lactose Intolerant to cow's milk!

Out of my motherly responsibility and County Health's advice I decided to give them a small amount of milk. The health officials firmly stated that growing children need milk after weaning. County health's rule of thumb for cow's milk was (1) ounce of milk per year of the child twice per day until around the age of 10. In hindsight I have learned that a good Greek yogurt or one of the "Baby Yogurts" on the market today or better yet homemade yogurt would have been a much better alternative than the straight milk. In fact in those days I was buying the certified raw milk for my family that might have been a little easier for my children to digest however they still developed allergies.

The fermented milk that turns into yogurt is better tolerated by far than any straight milk. This is explained in the Chapter 1 Highlight section. It helps you understand how the friendly bacteria predigest the sugar in milk breaking the double bonded sugar molecule as it converts the lactose. By lowering the lactose it reduces the inflammation that comes from drinking straight cow's milk. Also, because yogurt is concentrated the child does not need to eat as much in ounces as with milk - perhaps 1/3 less. Keep in mind it is still cow's milk and the GIS goal is to get a variety of other proteins and minerals from the daily food selections for each child and the entire family.

A second consideration is when is the best time to drink milk or eat yogurt? Because dairy is a complex food consisting of a complete protein, carbohydrate and fats with some vitamins and minerals the best time to eat it is alone at a separate meal. It makes a great mini meal snack perhaps with some seasonal fruit and a little honey as desired. *Note:* Honey can be dangerous for babies and only given to a baby over the age of (1) year. Remember that milk is the most common allergy in foods. If a child develops GIS or allergy symptoms to milk or yogurt stop it and give the child a Multiple Vitamin and Mineral supplement that includes a good level and variety of minerals to include calcium and even a vegetable supplement if possible. A good practice is to serve a variety of vegetables that contain vitamins and minerals at mealtimes for the parents and to introduce important foods to your young children.

As a young mother I was totally unaware that my children were lactose intolerant and continued to give them as much milk as they desired therefore we battled constipation, skin disorders, headaches, ear infections, frequent colds, extreme shyness and slower learning for years. Once reducing the milk, oatmeal and keeping sugar lower in my children's diet they began to excel in school and the bowel issues improved. Slowly I was unraveling the allergy mystery yet little did I know, even while working as a clinical nutritionist, that the entire family was also gluten intolerant!

To Breast Feed or Not to Breast Feed that is the Question?

More and more women chose bottle feeding over Mother's milk in the 20th century. As you read in Chapter 3 about the History of Bowel Disease you learn that giving infants and children cow's milk has been linked directly to the increase of digestive ailments and the Gluten Inflammatory Syndrome around the globe. Fortunately, another social revolution was sparked during and after the Vietnam War, a getting back to nature trend that supported women to once again reevaluate their social roles and many began to breast feed their children in higher numbers once again.

Benefits of Breast Feeding

- Superior Nutrition to Formulas
- Contains hundreds of Nutrients and Compounds
- Supporting Health and Immunity
- Emotional and Physical Pay-Off
- Saves Time and Money
- Working Moms May Utilize Breast Pumps for Success!

The benefits a baby receives from breast milk cannot be matched by any modern formula of today. As mentioned, scientists have isolated hundreds of nutrients and compounds that support the infant's body coming from the mother that makes a big difference in survival and optimizing the baby's full potential in life. Besides the value of Colostrum received by the infant in the first couple of weeks through nursing that significantly helps immune function, the baby has the potential to receive all 91 essential nutrients available from foods and supplements supplied through the mother and then some. The perks for the mother includes the ease of having no preparation or extra expense for formula. The natural act of nursing is also one that lends emotional and affectionate bonding with the child as mother breast feeds and it brings about a hormonal pay-off too.

The act of nursing stimulates hormones that help Mom's body actually renew itself back to her pre-pregnancy shape. This begins within the first day of nursing the newborn by immediately signaling the Uterus to start shrinking! Women who breast feed actually regain their pre-pregnancy shape of toner muscles significantly faster! Plus through nursing the woman expends a higher amount of calories which also assists in the weight loss process. Another perk almost miraculously via the Nervous System is the act of nursing stimulates a feel-good hormone that's released into the mother's blood called Serotonin that helps initially with preventing post-partum blues. You can think of this like a special pleasurable compensation to help balance out the extra work that definitely comes with motherhood. Along with good nutrition, some exercising and nursing new moms can stay pretty relaxed and get back in shape!

The *La Leche League* www.llli.org has been established for over 50 years answering questions and encouraging women to nurse their newborns. This worldwide organization supports nursing for as long as possible, anywhere from 2 months to 12 – 18 months. Many cities have a La Leche office and some even hold meetings open to the public to give more support for nursing mothers. Unfortunately, many mothers are opting out of breast feeding because of their over-packed full lives. My hope is that women will consider this more advantageous choice in motherhood. Using a Breast Pump to fill mother's milk into bottles has helped many uninspired and/or working women join the ranks of nursing moms. Breast feeding holds lots of perks for both the mother and the newborn. A Pediatrician generally has instructional information and staff that teaches the basics of nursing and sometimes a group situation is also available.

My grown daughter, Loree, mother of three, has nursed each of her babies. What specifically helped her was the advice to use the breast as if it was a bottle. Using her hands to direct the breast into the newborn's mouth worked like a charm. An infant is born not knowing how to nurse and must learn in the first few days of practicing. That takes both mother and child working together once the technique is acquired.

Dawn, my other daughter, also mother of three children found nursing to be an amazing successful experience. She made it work even while holding down a demanding job. She was able to bring her young infants to the workplace and as they became 12 months old she pumped milk to continue mother's milk for Day-Care, her husband and others who helped with the babies. She diligently pumped during the day while at work in the privacy of her office to build a supply for the following day.

What dedication it truly takes for busy women however you only get one chance with each child. The business climate has become more tolerant of nursing moms toward the end of the 20th century. Discuss your choices clearly with your husband and communicate with your employer to develop a workable plan. Some families have not been accustomed to nursing and it can take several discussions to make the case of why nursing is so important. One idea is for both husband and wife to discuss breast feeding with the doctor or nurse at a pregnancy check-up appointment. Also, reading out-loud the sections in this book may open up some good discussion especially about the help it brings for increasing immunity for your child.

Another friend and co-worker found she had a challenge with her baby's ability to nurse as a newborn. Her solution was to use the breast pump practically around the clock to fill a special bottle easier for her baby to latch onto. She also supplemented with a baby formula suited to her infants needs for times she ran short. This demonstrates true commitment and other family friends have had similar experiences. As time consuming as her schedule was she told me she would do it again because of the superior nutrition breast milk gave her son.

To nurse your child, honors the design of the body and lessens the incidence for allergies including gluten intolerance. As mom eats a variety of nutritious foods the baby receives the Smorgasbord of nutrients through the milk as nature intended. As mentioned it is important for the mother to avoid allergens in her diet for the first three months until it is clear that the baby is or is not reacting to foods including; wheat, gluten triggers, milk, eggs, chocolate and sometimes onions and garlic or spicier foods. Nursing your baby is the most valuable "Birthday Present" a Mom can give!

Some situations do arise that prevents nursing from being an option. Fortunately, baby formulas have improved from years ago from just using cow, goat or soy milk with fortification. Yet, even with the gluten and lactose free products available they are still limited in nutrition compared to the hundreds of nutritional compounds scientists have isolated from Mothers Milk! One of the litmus tests to compare the value of a breast fed baby vs. a formula fed baby is by just picking the child up. It may sound a little odd yet simply put the dense weight of a breast fed baby has a totally different feel than a bottle fed child. Building a baby is serious business regardless of the path you choose.

Any extra nutrition that an infant or child can receive is stored in the young baby's liver, bones and other tissue, to act as a sort of emergency nutritional reserve. When children receive only the minimum or less than their requirement they can come up short in nutrition that the body requires to function optimally. As you will read in the vaccine section eight out of ten babies diagnosed with disabilities were not breast fed. That is a very shocking statistic and important as you weigh the pros and the cons of how you are going to feed your new baby!

Immunity from Breast Milk

If the mother does choose to breast feed it is especially valuable within the first year of life because it helps to build up the infants Immune System. The mother produces antibodies that circulate into the breast milk that together with the superior nutrition gives the child constant health support. Also, when the infant first begins to nurse, within the first few days, the baby receives an almost clear fluid called "Colostrum".

It contains nutrients that have been found to significantly heighted the infant's immune system for life.

Fortunately, if a child was not nursed Colostrum supplements are available to give a child later on and/or take as an adult. See Chapter 8 Special Needs Supplements. The Bovine Colostrum products have been highly researched for their value of Proline Rich Polypeptides (PRP). The studies have been impressive from the intake of the Bovine Colostrum products to support immune response in relationship to cancer, inflammatory conditions (including bowel disease) and even helping as an anti-aging supplement for adults! The research has shown that the PRP from cows is very similar to that of humans. Yet, as remarkable as the PRP products have shown in hundreds of research papers they still do not provide the same value compared to receiving the immune support from being nursed as an infant.

The decision to breast feed or not is one to make before the baby is born. The mother and father can then inform the other support family members to avoid any feelings of awkwardness. By making a commitment to nurse your child you also influence other people as well besides the immediate value it holds for your own family.

As mentioned previously the Breast Pump as many women know has really been a wonderful convenience in nursing. It has allowed the modern woman who intends to go back into the workforce to give her infant a great head start with Mother's Milk. It has helped all families including stay at home moms to share feeding times with Dad and other support people (including Day-Care staff) by feeding the baby the "Good Stuff" from a bottle. I encourage parents to fight for the right and opportunity to give your child Mother's Milk no matter what your challenges may be!

17% of Children Born Today Have Disabilities!

Children that are born with Autism or develop Autism Spectrum Disorder (ASD) or other mental and physical disabilities, greatly benefit by following the GIS Program. By lowering inflammation and optimizing health and building up the digestive system of the body many families have found that their children diagnosed with ASD improve.

One in 150 children is born with Autism today in the U.S. and California has a higher rate of (1) in 90 children. The statistics increase to (1) in 63 born with ASD a broader group of disabilities which includes all of the neurological related disorders. In fact 17% of all children born today have some form of disability!

This includes mental retardation 9.7 per thousand infants, 2.8 Cerebral Palsy, hearing loss (1) in a thousand and vision impaired (.9) per thousand births. You must be made aware that all infant disabilities have increased in unprecedented figures and the facts will answer the question of why.

What is Autism Spectrum Disorder (ASD)?

- *Asperger Syndrome* exhibits impaired body functions yet better language skills than Autism.
- *Autism* is generally observed by 18 months of age with children having social, verbal and non-verbal communication challenges, difficulties with pretend play and social interactions.
- *Rett Syndrome* is a brain abnormality dominant in females effecting all neuromuscular function of varying levels of speech, motor skills (sometimes tip-toeing and flopping of arms and legs is observed) , learning difficulties and abnormal body development (including a smaller head and/or scoliosis and more).
- *Childhood Disintegrative Disorder or Pervasive Developmental Disorder* includes any non- specified behavior that is out of the normal growth and development of an infant or toddler. Seek professional support with any of the above symptoms for infants or toddlers before the age of 2 is best or any age!

Why are the statistics increasing? The answer appears to be from two main factors coupled with the health of the mother and father which includes; Chemical Toxicity from the environment and Vaccinations. Toxicity in the world has infiltrated every facet of people's lives to some degree from what we eat, drink, clothing that we wear, our daily personal care products, the cars we drive and even the very air that we breathe. The vaccine debate may not be settled for some time if ever because of it being such a political, bureaucratic and emotionally charged topic however some factors have improved.

The idea of pollution and toxicity affecting our health is easier to understand than vaccines because it has been an ongoing surface issue. However, few people have learned the full impact toxicity has on the world today including it being a factor that seems to be sending couples to the fertility doctor. See Chapter 6 Environmental Toxicity.

Toxic Environment

Besides acknowledging the importance of nutrition some experts are siding with toxicity being the unfortunate reason for so many childhood disabilities with perhaps a secondary health risk coming from vaccinations. When you gather all the facts, toxicity has already been linked to birth defects for many decades so to consider it as a factor for more Autism is not very far-fetched.

Collectively the toxic chemicals from the environment found in adults and newborns of today (see Chapter 6) may share responsibility of birth defects with mercury and antigens from the vaccines. In the book titled, *Diet for a Poisoned Planet* by David Steinman, who by the way is a father, he shares in his book a relevant study. This 1976 research conducted with mammals was published in the *Journal of Food Science* and the object was to observe how the animals reacted to chemicals commonly found in the environment at that time and these chemicals are still present over thirty years later. The team of scientists used (3) chemicals on the group of rats. The chemicals were first used (1) at a time on each rat and it showed no obvious ill effects. When they gave (2) chemicals at a time their health declined. Lastly and dramatically, when they gave all (3) chemicals at the same time 100% of the rats died within 2 weeks! This was a powerful study showing how important it is for scientists to test the combination of chemicals in a safety analysis - to responsibly monitor the effects chemicals in our environment have on the human body.

Today's world is a potential health disaster since the amount of chemical pollution has quadrupled in the last 30 years! The Environmental Protection Agency (EPA) is well aware of this fact. The shocking truth is that the EPA found that if you total up the amount of chemical hits an individual may receive in just one day it can be more than 500 percent above safety levels!

History, Facts and Current Standing of Vaccinations

Frankly, the topic of vaccinations for parents is a challenging one because it gives busy and often over-stressed men and women just one more responsibility that demands a critical decision about their child's welfare. Weighing the pros and cons of vaccinations is often just too big a burden and challenge to dig for the truth especially when you hear from both our government and the American Pediatrics Association that vaccines are necessary and safe. Also, very unsettling is the rhetoric coming from our trusted and trained physicians who have not understood themselves the history and present situation including the safety vs. risks of vaccinations. When the facts are reviewed you can see that doctors have been handed an ideology surrounding vaccines and untruths funneled through their medical media. My hope is that some truthful facts will help you get your heads out of the sand and encourage you to dig a little deeper for your own good. Maybe as physicians have their own children or grandchildren it will stimulate their interest to learn the truth about vaccines.

The science behind vaccinations is complex however the principle of how it works is pretty simple. What has happened in our society unfortunately is the "Inferred Value" of vaccinations that has been highly perpetuated in advertisements, that they are responsible for building the immune system. In fact they are referred to as an "Immunization" and this is a falsehood. This couldn't be further from the truth. To settle this misunderstanding you must first realize that vaccinations do not build the immune system. What actually builds the immune system is nutrition and a healthy lifestyle both equally responsible for this important job.

What a vaccination actually does is injects a part of the disease, either alive or dead, itself into the host, the infant, child or adult. This is done to promote a reaction of the immune system to fight against a chosen "Antigen". The object is to have the body make antibodies for any future attack. However, researchers have found that often people do not make the antibodies to the vaccines as desired. What occurs in life is that most of the microbes being vaccinated against are present in the living and working environment and people naturally make a certain level of antibodies as they have casual exposure to a wide variety of microbes. Through vaccines the individual receives potent strains of hepatitis, measles, whooping cough, polio, influenza and a conglomerate of other potentially dangerous microbes in a concentrated form. The concern with vaccines is three fold; the Antigen microbe or toxoid (disease), the Preservative System and the Substrate that it is grown on plus other excipients. The FDA's website made the important reference to the preservative Thimerosal (mercury) being one concern with vaccinations but also gave testimony of how dangerous a vaccination can be even without the preservative!

The researchers are supposed to know how to safely process the Antigens used in the vaccinations yet people do have reactions, sometimes very severe, especially when they have a weak immune system as with babies and seniors. I mention seniors because all you need to do is talk with a nurse in a care facility and they will confirm the fact that it is fairly common for one of their resident seniors to get sick after receiving a "Flu Vaccination" for example. Why is it so difficult to admit that babies and toddlers also develop reactions to vaccinations at times?

The facts prove that thousands of reactions have taken place every year within the young population and some have been deadly. Research and hard data has proven these reactions have a relationship to both the preservatives in the vaccines and/or the "Antigen" that it contains. It is important for every person to question the safety of vaccines. In fact in the book *Vaccines – Are They Really Safe & Effective?*, written by Neil Z. Miller, it states that in 1995 the *New England Journal* published a study that stated children who received the Polio vaccine had an 8 times more likelihood to develop Polio! Learning the truth about vaccinations may feel a little uneasy yet it brings such a settling calm about the subject as well.

The Vaccination Controversy - Dr. Andrew Wakefield, Gastroenterologist

The recent vaccination battle began on foreign soil in the United Kingdom. A medical researcher and Gastroenterologist specializing in bowel disease by the name Andrew Wakefield found that many Autistic children suffered from acute digestive symptoms. After researching over 200 Autistic children his research team focused on 12 children which they conducted an intestinal biopsy on among other tests. Their work launched the safety debate of vaccinations into a more visible arena resulting in many parents opting out of vaccinating their children. He published his findings from 1988 in the *Lancet* in the 1997 issue. He and his colleagues concluded "The Possibility" that the MMR Multi-Dose vaccination may be the culprit in children developing Autism. Because of his research he also encouraged the Single-dose vaccines vs. Multi-dose as a safer choice and all together his research sent shock waves around the globe.

Wakefield stated that most of the children he focused on did not have the digestive issues or neurological disorders until after receiving the MMR vaccine therefore he warned that more research in this relationship must be done to rule out the vaccine factor. The British General Medical Council (GMC) did not find Wakefield's work ethical which resulted in his disbarment from the legal right to work in medicine. The GMC felt environmental causes could have been at work and that the researchers had not endorsed this other possibility. They also felt the research team conducted unnecessary tests on the children that were not coinciding with acceptable medical practices. The researchers had also received some payment for their work that surfaced in the review which seemed to be outside the earlier parameters of the *Lancet's* criteria for published work. Dr. Wakefield did not recant any of his work or statements about the safety of vaccinations being in question. Later in 1993, after the controversy was in full force, Britain ruled against the Multi-dose vaccination and began offering only the Single-dose vaccines as Andrew Wakefield had promoted. His work led him to design a protocol for children to treat their digestive illnesses like Crohn's with anti-inflammatory agents and a custom diet that reduces diarrhea, pain and symptoms very similar to the GIS Program.

Later, once the controversy began to heat up, the *Lancet* insisted on a retraction of his published work because they felt he made the statement that vaccinations caused Autism. Wakefield was unrelenting in his reply that no retraction was in order because he only printed the truth of his research that opened the possibility of the link to vaccine. Nine of the twelve people involved in the research printed a retraction that they could not say MMR caused Autism. Andrew Wakefield's latest book, *Calleous Disregard* is sure to be a tell-all book about his struggle to protect the children from an out of control medical witch hunt. His in-depth research into the weak testing procedures of vaccines of yesterday and today will help citizens gather more understanding of the reckless nature that has allowed too many injured children and adults to be used as living Guniea Pigs.

Infants as with seniors have weak immune function and can be more vulnerable to the side effects of vaccinations. The poor health status of some infants and toddlers coming into the world may also be part of the cause because mal-nourishment may lead to the "Undeveloped Brain Barrier" of the baby. The theory postulates that when this natural barrier is not working as efficiently as it does in an older child - it cannot prevent contaminants such as mercury (a lethal nerve toxin) present in high amounts of past vaccines and other toxins from entering the brain. *Note:* Ask for vaccines without the mercury preservative and ask for proof that you are receiving the correct one.

Even older toddlers have a more vulnerable immune system

especially when they have not received quality wholesome nutrition or are living with health challenges. This leaves the child unable to protect themselves against the side effects from the vaccines potent strains of Antigens. Health ailments have soared in infants, toddlers and even teens today yet our children are being given four times more vaccinations today than they received 60 years ago. By the time a child reaches 16 years of age during the 21ˢᵗ Century, following the recommended vaccination schedule, they would receive 40 vaccinations!

This is why Dr. Sears, MD, pediatrician has taken the stance to not jump the gun with infant vaccinations. He supports parents to consider the option of starting them later when a child is older which makes more biological sense considering all the ramifications of today's vaccination debate. This is called a modified vaccination schedule. This is not an endorsement of Dr. Sears's protocol of vaccinations or giving into his suggested Multi-dose vaccines. It is an example to illustrate how parents are being assertive with their right to choose what they decide is best for their child. Especially with the pressure the government is voicing to vaccinate for everything. Please understand YOU as an American citizen have the right to say NO!

The question of whether or not to vaccinate your child and when - is a big question for parents today. Regardless of where your decision lands for now the fact that a spike in the incidence of Autism and the Autism Spectrum Disorders and other Disabilities exists. In just the past 14 years childhood disabilities have increased 15 times between the years of 1984 to 1999. This is a 1500% increase!

The Facts Concerning Vaccinations

The use of "Mercury" in vaccines began in the 1940's as the main part of the preservative called "Thimerosal". The mercury content in Thimerosal is reported to be 49.6 percent of the total ingredients. The type of mercury that was chosen to keep the batches of vaccines from growing microbials was the highly absorbable type called Methyl-Mercury.

It worked beautifully for the Eli Lilly pharmaceutical company who started researching this preservative system in 1920. They went with it because of the lethal action mercury has on living tissue however they by-passed the critical fact that the government had classified mercury as a hazardous substance if it was swallowed. Mercury poisoning is directly associated with nerve damage and results in a variety of challenges of the Nervous System to include; certain cardiovascular disease, seizures, mental retardation, hyper-activity, dyslexia, a strong link to ASD besides the adult epidemic of Alzheimer's Disease!

What has occurred in the last two decades to coincide with the sharp increase of disabilities seen in childhood statistics is the doubling of the number of childhood vaccinations being given to our youth. In fact, in 1940 only 3 vaccinations were given to children through age 2. At that time the cases of Autism were only (1) in 10,000 children. In 2000 children receive a total of 22 vaccinations by age 2 combined in multiple vaccines given at the same time. The incidence of Autism in 2000 was (1) in 150 children. Could this be just a coincidence? Researchers did not think so and they attempted to tell the truth to the CDC from reviewing the CDC's own database but that didn't seem to satisfy the government!

Because of the outrage of parents whose children developed ASD coming from all ethnic and economic sectors of our society the FDA first released some information data to the public which heightened the controversy leading to a review board by the CDC. In 2000 the Center of Disease Control (CDC) held an invitation only forum to gain professional opinions on the rise in ASD and Vaccinations addressing the citizen's concerns. The highlights of the meeting truly pointed to vaccinations being problematic.

However, after the meeting was over the CDC decided to have another medical review board do more investigation called the Institute of Medicine (IOM) which took another year. After this somewhat cooling off period of the hot debate the IOM issued a ruling that even Robert F. Kennedy Jr. called a "White Wash" that said they did not find that vaccines contributed to ASD and they did not find that they didn't! What absurd political mumbo jumbo was contrived on such an important topic that affects the health of our children!

2000 – 2001 CDC Data Review of ASD vs. Vaccination Revealed a True Association

- Epidemiologists Tom Verstraeten reviewed the CDC's data in their possession and voiced his opinion that the increase in Autism was associated with the Thimerosal in the vaccinations. He also stated earlier studies indicated a strong connection of the vaccinations to the incidence of delayed speech and Attention Deficit Disorder (ADD).

- American Academy of Pediatrics spokesperson Dr. Bill Well and Dr. Richard Johnson, MD, Immunologist and Pediatrician from Colorado both in high standing in their professions gave similar testimony to the CDC review board.

- Despite the overwhelming testimony of the experts during the 2000 CDC meeting they made the decision to financially pay another medical review board called the Institute of Medicine (IOM) to form a Safety Review Committee on the subject of vaccinations. The IOM stated that the connection between the vaccinations including the Thimerosal and the symptoms of neurological disorders was biologically plausible yet they went on to say that the research neither proved it nor disproved it and was inconclusive!" The IOM later voiced that it would be prudent to remove the mercury and or lower the content in vaccinations. **Most pharmaceutical companies are now offering alternative vaccines with lower or mercury-free however confirm this with your nurse before the vaccination appointment.**

Vaccination Facts

- 1943 was the year Leo Kanner, child psychiatrist, labeled the development of a new childhood illness never before seen was the result from brain damage and he called it Autism. The symptoms were neurological affecting the child's mental and physical behavior. The cases began to pop-up occurring shortly after the Pertussis vaccine was becoming increasingly available. Europe received the vaccine in 1950 and the first Autism developed there during the following decade. By 1962 the National Society for Autistic Children was established in Britain.

- 1984 – 1999 revealed the big increases of ASD by 1500% and sparked the search for answers to include the relationship to childhood vaccinations and toxicity.

- 1988 Dr. Andrew Wakefield conducted research on Autistic children and their acute digestive symptoms that appeared to develop after receiving vaccinations and published his work in the *Lancet* in 1997. His research was later rejected on formalities more than any credible rationale and he maintains that his research has integrity. Two other researchers have duplicated his work in the U.S. successfully.

- The Hepatitis B Vaccine was started in 1991 and was mandated for infants and children to be given before they are permitted to leave the hospital. The shot originally contained 12.5 mcg of Mercury per dose! This one shot was 100 times the EPA's upper limit standard for Mercury in infants. The Mercury is supposedly reduced or eliminated at present however the safety of giving an infant this antigen is in question with many parents opting out for good reasoning. The U.S. does not have a significant Hepatitis B health challenge and in accordance to the World Health Organization (WHO) standards it is not necessary for infants and young children unless parents are carriers.

- France outlawed the Hepatitis B Vaccine after 15,000 citizens filed a class action suit against the government.

- 1996 the DTP vaccine was altered to change the "P" the Pertussis (Whooping Cough) from a whole cell active type to a-cellular type providing reduced side effects from that "Toxoid Antigen" and now it is called DTaP. This improvement and others must be attributed to the citizens out-cry for higher safety standards in vaccines. Make certain you ask for the vaccine insert of any shot you are considering for your child. With this preventative step you will be prepared for any side effects or risks seen in your child once vaccinated. <u>If a child does have acute or severe reactions take this as a sign to re-evaluate any further vaccinations as they could be in a high risk population for potential harm as suggested in literature review.</u> As per Dr. Robert Sears, M.D. in his book *The Vaccine Book*, severe reactions tend to become even worse with subsequent shots. He also rates the reactivity of vaccines he has had experience with as a pediatrician on page 186 of his book. <u>He cautions to not continue with shots if your child experiences severe reactions without a thorough review!</u>

- 1999 revealed Multi-dose vaccines such as MMR and DPT contain Antigens not fully tested for safety in the combination Multi-dose delivery to infants within the first 12 months of life. They had contained 62.5 mcg of Mercury per vaccination - 100 times the safe dose by Federal Environmental Protection Guidelines until just recently. <u>Some shots used today even with reduced Mercury still contain up to 5 combinations of microbial Antigens (toxoids) that have not been tested for safety in combination.</u>

- Only (1) country in Europe still mandates the DPT – Diphtheria, Pertussis and Tetanus shot to even be given whereas the U.S. requires 4 separate doses of them. The MMR – Measles, Mumps and Rubella are now given in single dose in the U.K. where the U.S. continues in Multi-dose.

- American Pediatrics continues their campaign that vaccines are all safe and necessary even though children have experienced results of ASD, brain damage and even death. Safety considerations are essential for the future safety of vaccines of all of the ingredients to include; the preservative system, the Antigen (type of vaccine) and the substrate (what the Antigen is grown on) plus the other ingredients used in a particular vaccine. A reference that will open your eyes even wider is the book, *The Virus and the Vaccine - Contaminated Vaccine, Deadly Cancers and Government Neglect* by D. Bookchin and J. Schumacher.

- The "Thimerosal" Mercury preservative was banned in many countries years ago included; Russia (for 20 yrs.), Japan, United Kingdom, Denmark, Australia and the Scandinavian countries and only due to the grass-root advocacy in the U.S. did the citizens achieve some change.

- Consumer pressure has led the U.S. government to mandate for the pharmaceutical companies to develop vaccinations that are Mercury Free or low in Thimerosal, less than (1) mg. However, make certain you request them if choosing any vaccinations. The actual amount of preservative (if any) in the vaccines still remains questionable from past records of the vaccine companies.

- Adult vaccines still contain mercury in higher levels. You must request Mercury Free shots before you stand in line at a facility or through your doctor's office. Reports indicated that a Senate Mandate in 1999 told pharmaceutical companies they must decrease the amount of Mercury in their vaccinations because of the potential for harm yet Merck Co kept selling their stockpiles of products until they were forced to comply several years later.

- Merck's top scientific advisor in 1991 sent a memo to top executives alerting them that infants receiving their vaccinations at 6 months of age were receiving 87 times the considered safe amount of mercury - recommending the elimination of Thimerosal as reported in the Los Angeles Times (source from an internal leak). In today's reappraisal of the lethal nature of Mercury it actually equated to 400 times the safety standards.

- In 2003 when GlaxoSmith Kline (pharmaceutical company) hired Tom Verstraetea to work for them he changed his professional opinion that he had previously voiced strongly against the Thimerasol in the 2000 CDC review meeting. It was later reported that he still thinks that a connection may be found with Autism and vaccinations in the future. This just illustrates the pressure "Big Pharma" exerts on good scientists.

- In 2000 Dr. V. Singh researcher from the Dept. of Pharmacology at the Univ. of Michigan repeated the original work done by Dr. Wakefield in England who associated the Antigens of the MMR vaccine (Measles, Mumps and Rubella) to the development of Autistic children. Other doctors have also repeated this work.

- Scientists from Maryland, Dr. Mark Geier expert genecist and vaccinologist, reviewed the CDC data with colleagues and concluded the 5,000 articles written on the relationship of Thimerosal and ASD had a strong basis and that the CDC ignored the science.

- Recently the CDC made an attempt to prevent further access to their extensive file on the controversy of ASD and vaccinations by selling their complete stash of documents to a private firm to prevent any further access allowed by the Freedom of Information Act of 1966 and amended in 2007.

- The *National Vaccine Information Center* was launched in 1982 to help educate citizens and families about the questions to ask about vaccinations, informed consent information in the public health system and to form a database for vaccine safety. In 1996 alone there were 872 serious adverse events experienced from children 14 years or younger, after having the Hepatitis B vaccine alone. The reactions included emergency room visits with life threatening symptoms, hospitalization and or a disability injury. *Note:* If you choose vaccinations make sure to download the questionnaire on the website to review with your physician. Even with the levels of Mercury being reduced in 2011 the "Antigens" in the vaccines themselves can be problematic for certain children causing brain swelling and even permanent brain damage and other miscellaneous symptoms you will want to discuss with your doctor as needed – www.nvic.org.

- The U.S. Government established reporting of harmful side effects from vaccines due to public pressure in 1991 which confirms the back seat concern for People vs. Profits of the pharmaceutical companies. Vaccination history side effects are not new to the CDC, FDA or the NIH government agencies. Their files hold an abundance of historic reports of injury or disease occurrence.

- Children living with ASD disabilities today number above 500,000.

- Statistics showed 8 out of 10 children who developed ASD were not Breast Fed which truly underlines the value of nursing the young providing an opportunity of "Natural Immunity".

- Over 4,200 lawsuits have been filed for injured children who developed side effects after receiving their childhood vaccines. The government and court systems have protected the pharmaceutical companies from responsibility by several out-dated loop holes and protests even though sources have testified to their knowledge of responsibility. The lawsuits that have most frequently been allowed are against Eli Lilly the makers of the Thimerosal preservative. From Lilly and other companies billions of dollars have been awarded to families by the courts or arbitration.

- In present day an onslaught of vaccines is in the pipeline seeking fast track approval from the FDA and the government is making mandates to put pressure on families to vaccinate. It is not true that the unvaccinated child carries more disease in fact it is quite the contrary. This is why pregnant women are not supposed to be around children that get their MMR shots because the vaccinated child can become a carrier and infect a pregnant woman! The Polio vaccine is a good example of this fact and in 1992 the CDC published an admission that the Polio vaccine was the dominant cause for Polio in the United States! In fact, they stated that every case of Polio since 1979 was due to the vaccine itself. The live vaccine could live in the throat and intestinal tract for an extended period of time. Both the active and inactivated Polio vaccine has been connected to thousands of serious problems and even deaths as reviewed in the CDC's own database.

This time-line is a condensed but accurate over-view surrounding the vaccine subject that will be debated for some time to come. It gives key events of important information without telling the entire story. Supposedly, children's vaccines are now being offered in the Mercury-Free option which is good yet you must have more conversations within your family about the safety of the Antigen part of the vaccines and how they are being delivered in Multi-dose. My six grandchildren have not been vaccinated and they have been by far healthier than most of their playmates. Recently, they all came down with the latest winter viruses with deep coughs with lung congestion that demanded antibiotics. Their pediatricians scolded them for not receiving their vaccines and ran all the tests for meningitis, whooping cough and other potential childhood diseases which all came back negative. I vaccinated my two daughters however I waited until they were older toddlers and parents please keep in mind that was 30 years ago. The amount of vaccines the government now wants to give children today has more than tripled! The occurrence of a baby or child developing a childhood disease from the vaccine has always been a risk ever since vaccines became a practice in modern medicine. Parents in my day were asked to sign waivers before a child was vaccinated because of the risk that has always existed. If you read the inserts on vaccines and the waiver release for instance on the Hepatitis B vaccine today you will also read about the potential physical harm and even possible death to your child.

One of the promotional lines used by medical professionals in defense of vaccinations is that we do not have Polio anymore! Hello - it might surprise you to find out that Polio was decreasing in numbers and not an out-of-control epidemic back in the 50's at the time when the Polio vaccine was first introduced. In fact, what occurred as they began the inoculations is a definite increase in cases of childhood Polio. So many new cases popped up in the vaccinated children that at one point the public health department's own officials refused to vaccinate their own children and ordered the Polio shots to be stopped.

The Truth behind the Polio Vaccine

Doctors and scientists within the National Institute of Health (NIH) during the 1950's were well aware that the Salk vaccine was causing Polio. Dr. Jonas Salk himself viewed the vaccine as a gamble stating once you inoculate your child you cannot sleep for weeks afterwards for concern. Read more yourself in the highly referenced book called *Vaccines – Are They Really Safe?* This book fills in the gaps about the Polio vaccine and the many others that have been added to the list to explain inoculations. The author Neil Z. Miller states that it was obvious at that time that intense pressure coming from investors and pharmaceutical companies all but forced the U.S. Public Health Service to falsely proclaim the vaccine's safety and effective.

As you step back and look for the truth about our medical system and what their agenda is really about, then and only then, can you pick and choose to seek the appropriate medical assistance you need or desire. My husband and I have not received any vaccinations since our early teens. Neither one of us have experienced more than a few colds or flu while maintaining a pharmaceutical free life and we feel good 95% of the time! Truly this is not an easy lesson about health with vaccines yet an important one for children and adults.

The fact is the entire world has been brain-washed to think that the body is dependent on "Big Pharma's array of drugs" including the growing plethora of vaccines. The health movement seeking to understand the vaccination frenzy and who some are rejecting the mandatory path that has slowly developed into the 21st Century are not radical Anti-American Conspirators. It is quite the opposite and the largest segment of these people not going along with the status quo - consists of parents and individuals who are well educated professional men and women. They embrace the design of the body and are beginning to understand you cannot walk blindly any longer thinking our government is working in our best interest. Unfortunately, their track record has spoken and the government has often placed "Profits before People". Wake up citizens – and take the time to inform yourself!

Take the Time to Learn About Vaccines

I think the topic of vaccines deserves pause and an in-depth look of not only the vaccines but also a decision to avoid chemical pollution in the environment for all the reasons. The question has gone unanswered as to why the government has not insisted that the drug companies complete full comprehensive testing to support the safety of the vaccines especially in the Multi-dose? Parents have documented the many ASD disabilities often occurring directly after a Multi-dose vaccine was administered! Secondly, ask yourself does my child even need to be vaccinated? Reading the brochure about possible side effects and perhaps a couple of small books on vaccines will give you the knowledge to make informed decisions and to be pro-active in case a child experiences a reaction.

The take away point I want to reinforce to parents is no matter what your decisions are about vaccines there is the need to invest in your child's health the way nature intended - vaccinated or not. Give their bodies the core nutrients through natural unprocessed foods and a few key supplements to build a healthy developed functioning body with a hearty immune system. It is the children who are vulnerable or populations that are living in unhealthy hygienic living conditions that experience the high incidence of disease as this fact has been confirmed by the World Health Organization the WHO. Junk food builds a junky body and healthy foods build a healthy child with a bright future!

Healthy Food Guidelines & Supplements from Birth through Childhood Endorsed by the WHO – Who?

Another decision in parenthood is when to begin giving solid food to your infant. Some disagreement does exist as to the best time to start. However, you can watch for signs from your child to give you the best clue. First, observe what interest your little one may have in the foods around them. Next, contemplate if their body is requiring extra nutrition by a simple observation. When your baby is requiring more nutrition he or she will begin to wake more often during the night to eat. They will display very similar behavior as when they were just a newborn. If you have double checked your nutrition to make certain you are eating enough for two when breast feeding then begin the introduction of more solid food at the evening dinner meal for baby.

Your child may have some interest in food even at four months yet as long as you are feeding them every 2 ½ – 3 hours their body will be getting adequate nutrition without solid food. You don't have to rush this step. However, anywhere between 4 – 6 months you can begin giving tastes remembering at this age an infant has no teeth and has not yet learned how to chew or swallow even the mashed or pureed baby food.

Six months or older is a better time to teach your baby how to chew. Their digestive juices will be functioning better as they grow and that will also help the food to digest better. The World Health Organization (WHO) agrees that 6 months is the best time to begin adding regular complimentary foods with continuing to Breast Feed and or Formula until 24 months. To give grains as the first food, as in white rice cereal, is not required. Fruits have simpler mono-saccharide sugars and are the easiest to digest. Many begin with a ripe banana, applesauce and pears and next add a vegetable like strained carrots or green beans and even mashed avocado may be enjoyable. Making your own infant baby food is tedious but a possibility. Be cautious to dilute the baby food with distilled water, mixed well into a liquid but firm texture to avoid choking. Commercial baby foods are strained to avoid the potential for problems in consistency.

Foods to Introduce at 6 - 12 Months

- Breast Milk / Formula
- Fruits & Vegetables (baby food consistency)
- Soft Cooked Meat & Fish (8 – 12 months)
- Low Gluten White Rice Grain Cereal (if desired)

Experts agree to avoid the common allergy foods until your child is older including; whole grains, eggs, cow's milk, yogurt, chocolate and be cautious with fish. Some infants enjoy butternut squash, sweet potatoes or yams in their first foods too. You do not have to introduce grains until 8 – 12 months or older. White rice cereal is the most gentle on the stomach to give some extra variety. Higher protein foods may be introduced at 8 - 12 months as well to include; meats, fish and eggs. It is a good idea to only add one new food at a time for three days to see if any reactions occur like a rash, diarrhea or other symptom that you may want to discuss with your pediatrician or nutritionist.

During this time a little "Baby Yogurt" can also be introduced yet cautiously and not in large amounts to avoid any allergy reaction. Most yogurts made today, even the Greek style yogurt, still contain lactose sugar and other thickeners that may cause indigestion and allergy upset. Homemade yogurt, see directions in Chapter 7, converts the lactose sugar almost 100% and is the best for all people to avoid lactose (milk sugar) intolerance.

Frequency of Adding Complementary Foods for Infants & Toddlers by the WHO

- 6 – 8 months add foods 2 – 3 times per day.
- 9 – 11 months add foods 3 – 4 times per day.
- 12 – 24 months add 2 healthy snacks to 3 meals per day.

Use good hygienic food preparation techniques to avoid any food poisoning with your young child just as you would with older family members. Do not feed your baby directly out of a baby food jar unless directions on a container directs otherwise. Take the portion out of the jar for each individual meal and properly refrigerate the remainder. Also, do your best to keep refined sugar and cow's milk, biscuits and cookies out of your baby's diet until you begin to wean them at about 12 - 18 months. Wait until a child is older to start more complex starches of whole grains and with eggs too. Eggs are a very common allergy food and many toddlers find eggs delicious so beware.

Fortunately, "Organic Baby Food" is more reasonably priced for today's economy and "Baby Food Grinders" also make a terrific quick meal for older babies and toddlers starting at around 10 – 12 months. When the baby is more interested in eating and requiring more sustenance I found a food grinder indispensable. Easy to use, just place food from the dinner table into the little cylinder and giving it a few twists and the addition of a little water – "Dinner is served!" Truly it is best to wait until teeth arrive.

Introducing solid foods has its challenges but it can also be such an entertaining and enjoyable experience to share with your baby and toddler as they begin to eat. Do your best to make it fun and healthy!

Honey & Dirt Can Be Dangerous to Infants

Honey as a sweetener cannot be given to an infant until they are at least 12 months old. It can carry microscopic amounts of Botulinum Bacteria Spores that germinate toxins in the gastrointestinal tract of the baby due to an immature immune system. According to the *Journal of European Epidemiology*, Nov. 1993 even a pacifier sweetened with honey can bring about this life threatening infection. The Botulinum Toxin is the most poisonous natural substance known to man. Just a tiny amount of toxin in the blood stream can cause death within minutes through paralysis of the muscles used in breathing. It has been seen most commonly in California, Utah and Pennsylvania. It has been suggested that Botulinum Toxin is responsible in about 10% of the SIDS deaths that occurs most frequently in the first 6 months of life.

Another important threat to mention is the potential of a toxic spore that is commonly found in soil and dust and therefore present in vacuum cleaner bags. Take extreme precaution to safely empty your vacuum bag outside away from your infant.

Healthy Calories & Adequate Protein Are Required to Build a Healthy Body!		
Age	Calories	Protein Grams
0 – 6 months	770	14
6 – 12 months	900	14
1 – 3 years	1100	23
4 – 6 years	1600	30
7 – 10 years	2200	34
11 – 14 Girls	2300	46
Boys	2800	46
15 – 18 Girls	2300	46
15 – 18 Boys	3000	56
25 – 50 Women	2000	44
Pregnant	2300	74
Lactating	2800	102
25 – 50 Men	2600	56

As your child grows it is important to understand that growing bodies require healthy calories (fuel) and adequate protein to build cells and systems of the body as reviewed in Chapter 7. The vitamins and minerals come from the fruits and vegetables including grains, potatoes, beans, nuts and seeds and some from meats and eggs as with Iron. You also need to make certain you are giving your growing child adequate protein for their age especially once you wean your child from breast milk or formula. You will find that when their bodies have adequate protein and other essential nutrients they naturally calm down and optimize their health and growth potential.

As a child grows their focus and success for healthy development is dependent upon nutrition, exercise and their level of GIS coupled with a loving and caring home environment the best you can provide. Be prepared that toddlers or older children with GIS may experience slow growth or behavior symptoms to include; dyslexia, hyperactivity, Attention Deficit Disorder (ADD) or Attention Deficit Hyperactivity Disorder (ADHD). Even aggressive and manic behavior with periods of withdrawal or depression can be experienced by some children. Review Chapter 5 GIS A Factor in All Disease; Mental & Physical. Definitely follow the GIS Program before going to medication and counseling unless the situation dictates immediate professional care. Many children and adults have been able to reduce or eliminate current pharmaceutical drugs once they have stayed on the GIS protocol for a period of time.

The good news is that parents across the globe are seeing behavior challenges and even ASD symptoms improve anywhere from 40 – 100% through applying health and proper parenting. If you are seeking parenting support on a particular topic there are many great books available. Good tips and guidelines can also be found by searching on the web. One such website is www.babycenter.com. Another is The Thoughtful House when more professional behavior protocols are required. That is accessed through their website at www.johnson-center.org. Learning and applying health becomes fun and rewarding especially after you go through the initial transitional 3 months period. It takes some time to get the required nutrition into the body and affect the biology and actions of the human body yet you the parent will personally benefit following the program and can rest assured that you are giving your child the healthiest head start possible!

The Family Dynamics: Schedule Time for Health & Happiness

The family dynamics in the U.S. and other developing countries has been constantly changing. At the turn of the century in America many women began to slowly enter the workforce as the industrial revolution impacted rural country life. Women also won the "Right to Vote" and WWI and WWII drew more women into the workforce including the military. Through achieving a closer autonomy with men women changed some of their fundamental familiar responsibilities including switching from the breast to the bottle for their infants. An ever growing percentage of women also spent less time in the home during the day leading to designate new family roles for both women and men.

Any changes in society's social norms have never come easy throughout history. The last 100 years has shown no exceptions. With many families having both mom and dad working (often the case with the current economy) trading traditional roles has not been easy. For a while women had morphed into "Wonder Women" attempting to do it all including; work, housework and ultimately raising the kids. This lifestyle has taken its toll on working families with the divorce rate skyrocketing, more illnesses for both adults and children and an overall decline in the quality of family life.

With the attempt to achieve happiness the current generation has attempted to do things better with shared parenting and child raising, shared housework yet the food issue has still not been resolved in many households. Daily health is continuing to be a struggle with the temptation of fast foods and convenience stores on practically every corner in some communities. The toll is seen by the enormous numbers of people experiencing Obesity and Mental Illness in the 21st Century. Over 75% of Americans are overweight and one in four people are living with some form of psychosis leading to experimenting with mood enhancement medications. Families must really work overtime literally to keep quality in their lives and focusing on health and communication to promote happiness in daily life!

Family Focus for Health & Happiness
- Follow the GIS Guidelines at least 80%
- Shop for Nutritious Foods Weekly
- Prepare Healthy Meals Together (at least 3 times per week)
- Share in Dishes & Clean Up
- Eat Out Only Once a Week (and eat leftovers from previous meals)

- Create Family Outings and Projects
- Give Thanks!

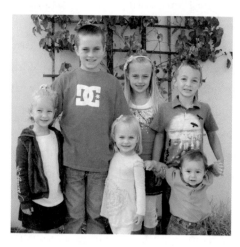

I challenge each of you to re-evaluate your family life together. Place the emphasis on health and nutrition the way God intended people to live striving for a healthy and balanced lifestyle. Look for joy in your work at home or on the job regardless of what you do. Plan your family outings to enjoy the beauty of nature, music, the arts and or sports. Families that stay together create an atmosphere that each family member has a valuable role and is a part of the whole. This is accomplished through family projects and playtime (special events and or family vacations) and giving each family member household responsibilities for their age.

Dad and Mom are leaders of the pack and are to instill respect of elders and others setting the ground rules (always with certain flexibility) and boundaries for the children (and each other). Give appropriate consequences for actions (praise and discipline) to create security in a child's life that they crave growing up. Remember parents that even with the weight of parental responsibility to always "Give Thanks" and keep joy in the family with laughter and fun regardless of the economic state. It is so easy to lose sight of the fact that truly the best gifts in life are free – Love and Time from a parent!

Pick the Lead Person Responsible for Shopping, Food Prep and the Clean Up Co-Coordinator!

To keep the focus on health in the family one adult in the home must be held responsible for meals and purchasing the food and supplies for the household. "Shopping" can be a shared task yet ultimately one person is in the driver seat and often the wife takes this position. A family shopping list can be posted anywhere in the house as desired yet often the kitchen area is a good spot on a clip or wipe-off board. In this way it will simplify a shopping trip to the store with a final look about before heading off. The fact is ladies men make great shoppers and it is important to have the family share in this necessary household job whenever possible. Stock up on non-perishables and keep enough frozen foods and some canned food items that allow for a quick defrost and meal prep on busy days. See suggestions in Chapter 7.

The second step is "Food Preparation" and this can be a shared responsibility as well. If both parents work together they can put a healthy meal on the table in only 30 - 45 minutes. Either the husband or the wife must be in the driver seat to plan the meals and make certain of the follow through. Ask the other spouse or older children for input and help. This is good because it creates a collective mind and a family spirit. Encourage older children to help choose one meal each week giving them at least two choices to pick from and this will nurture their interest in meal planning.

Even though food preparation takes some planning and a lot of work remember fixing food for your family and friends is an act of LOVE! The job of meal planning is often the wife's responsibility however men make great cooks and I encourage all women and/or men to open up the kitchen to their spouse. This was one of the best moves I ever made in my own life. My only regret was that I didn't do it sooner. Each person can excel as they desire and it pays off with more time for each other. Cooking with my husband has broadened our relationship experimenting with new foods and having fun. I learned that it was more of my own fear to relinquish control that had kept him out of the kitchen – better late than never!

Share in the Meal - Share in the Clean Up

Once the meal is enjoyed who is going to help with the clean up afterwards? I started doing family dishes at 5 years old having some direction from older siblings of course. You get to decide who does what chores in your house but teamwork is what a family is about! If I cook my husband cleans up and visa-versa. Girls and boys need to help in all the chores in the house including in the kitchen. *Note:* Remember safety must always be taught along with the chores! Working together as a family deepens the bonds of each member at every age. I was washing dishes with my 2 year old grand-daughter at a recent family function and it was one of my highlights during that day. The setting and cleaning off of the table are great chores for younger family members. I personally stayed with unbreakable dishes to relax with the kids helping until my children were in their teens!

Enjoying the tastes of nutritious and tasty foods made in your own home is a pleasure beyond words. Some meals will be enjoyed more than others and just like life you cannot get everything you want at all times! As it has been said many times a family needs to sit down at the dinner table, pray together to bless the bounty and discuss ups and downs appropriate for mealtimes. Set your family goals to revolve around nutrition and the family will have these bonding moments to recharge their batteries. You will find as you simplify and refocus on priorities in life that you create a healthier and more enjoyable life for your entire family!

CHAPTER 10

Pets Eating Gluten Free Stay Healthier

Taking your furry family members to the Vet without Pet Insurance can be a costly experience no matter what the cause. These days Vets are seeing more and more pets of both cats and dogs developing a long list of ailments linked to Gluten Intolerance! If you have noticed more skin conditions, allergies, behavior concerns, illnesses and bouts of vomiting from your special furry companion perhaps you need to switch them to a Gluten Free Diet. With diet changes and the addition of a few GIS Pet Supplements you'll have them back feeling better and on top of their game in no time at all!

Any mammal can have problems with their digestive system and that includes the common family pet be it cat or dog. Cats and dogs by nature are scavengers in the wild and were designed to eat meat as the main component of their meal. A wild dog's diet includes many different foods to provide their needed calories with the exception of grains. Wild cats and dogs have never grazed on grains as elk, cows and sheep do. The traditional mainstay of natural foods in the diet for cats and dogs is high protein, high fat and water with relatively very little carbohydrate.

What has evolved over the centuries of domesticating wild animals and is even recommended in today's protocol for cats and dogs is the complete opposite of what nature intended and that consists primarily of grains! When you read the ingredients of most mainstream products for your beloved furry friends it consists of high carbohydrate, low protein and fat and practically no moisture. It is no wonder that cats and dogs develop so many ailments these days and frankly don't live to their potential - due to cancer, diabetes and other diseases that are associated to their poor nutritional state!

Commercial Diets for Cats and Dogs are Loaded with Glutinous Grains!

The facts show that most commercial pet foods which always describe their product as the best food you can feed your pet - are high in carbohydrate "Grain-Based" and low in meat that eventually leads them to poor health symptoms. The optimum diet for cats and dogs needs to

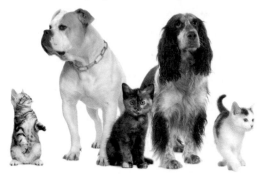

resemble the natural diet they were used to in nature being primarily meat, fat with some vegetables contributing core vitamins, minerals, moisture and fibers.

A Healthy Diet for Cats and Dogs

- Meat including; Lamb, Beef, Fish or Fowl (some dogs do best on Lamb)
- Higher Fat Content including EFA's: Omega-3's, 6's plus DHA and EPA from Flax or Fish Oil.
- Fiber from Vegetables (not grain sources); carrots, potato, sweet potato, yam, greens and some white rice and eggs are allowable.
- Avoid: Whole Grains including; Wheat, Oats, Barley, Rye, Brown Rice and Corn.
- Sufficient Fresh Filtered Water

Gluten is found in whole grains to include; wheat, oats, barley, rye, brown rice and even corn as described in Chapter 1. The Gluten molecule is composed of both protein and carbohydrate tightly bound together that is very difficult for animals to digest. As described in Chapter 3 the small intestine is where the body rebels resulting in inflammation from failed attempts to digest and absorb the gluten through the microscopic villi. The inflammation that develops leads to damage of the villi and once scarred or missing they lack the ability to properly absorb the nutrients from the foods.

This mal-absorption leads to many nutritional deficiencies within the animal and allows disease to develop which includes more allergies, skin irritations and even cancer. Do cats and dogs need any grains in their diet? Most experts agree that they can eat some carbohydrates yet they do not require grains to be healthy and as mentioned they are actually problematic. Some of the low gluten diet formulas for cats and dogs will contain some rice. Most animals do alright with rice because it is the lowest source of common inflammatory agents especially in the "white" rice form. The exception would be in animals having major yeast over-growth. In this case you may want to omit any grains for a period of time and consider a special zero grains formula you make or buy.

Common Gluten Inflammatory Syndrome (GIS) Symptoms in Cats & Dogs

- *Low to Medium Inflammatory Conditions*; Arthritis, Epilepsy, Changes in Behaviors, Sneezing and Allergies.
- *Advanced Inflammatory Conditions;* Weight Loss, Failure to Thrive, Pancreatitis, Hepatitis, Kidney Ailments, Auto-Immune & Low Immune System Function.
- *Chronic GI Upset;* Gas, Loss of Appetite, Diarrhea, Constipation, Mucus in Stool & Vomiting.
- *Skin Conditions;* Itchy Skin, Licking or Chewing the Paws and Pads, Inflamed Paws, Hot Spots, Dermatitis and Scaly Skin, Dry Skin, Hair Loss, Bumps, Rashes & Redness.

• *Yeast Conditions;* Skin Conditions, Ear Inflammation and Infections with Smelly Wax Build-Up and Head Shaking. *Note:* High grain-diet converts to carbohydrate sugars and causes the over-growth of the yeast that can also be accompanied by low Thyroid function.

How to Reverse Gluten Intolerance or GIS in Pets

As with people, to reverse the Gluten Intolerance in animals ultimately requires applying the Gluten Inflammatory Syndrome (GIS) principles for your pets. Just tailor the diet program to their more natural diet in the wild. To be healthy your pet requires the correct nutritionally dense foods omitting the grains other than a small amount of low gluten rice, corn or potato. Make certain you apply the foundational basics giving your cat or dog filtered water (not tap) to avoid Fluoride and other toxic chemicals especially if the pet is living with Advanced GIS. Sunshine and daily exercise are a must. How can you expect pets to relax and not act up if they don't get some time to run, jump and play working off their pent up energy? Public water today is flat out dangerous admitted the Environmental Protection Agency (EPA). Your animals require the same health factors as the rest of the family to avoid disease and be well. Also, to reduce their stress which reduces your stress as an owner domesticated animals require some attention and appreciation on a daily basis. Neglect is a horrible situation for people to endure and our beloved pets, even if they do tend to drive their owners a little crazy from time to time, need a little love directed their way! The unconditional Love that is returned from a pet is worth its weight in gold. Another perk that statistics support show that people who live alone but have a pet live much longer!

The GIS Pet Renewal Program includes Supplements & Love for our Furry Friends!

• Low Gluten / Gluten Free Diet - Meat Based
• Exercise, Water & Sun
• Detoxification & Balancing Immunity; Regular Bowels – Aloe

Vera, Probiotics, DetoxPlus Formula & Daily Greens (see Chapter 7). Chinese Mushrooms and Aloe have both been used to support mammal's Immune System.

- Supplements – Consult a Vet and or Pet Store including; Core Nutrients in a Multiple Vitamin & Mineral plus Nutritional Yeast (see Ch. 8), Healthy Oils (fish oils or other) and any herbal tonic or homeopathic remedies. *Note:* Avoid capsules or soft gels.
- Love, Appreciation & Grooming!

Observe how well your pet responds to applying the new GIS Pet Renewal Program and make certain they are having daily elimination of stool and urine. If your kitty or dog is not - give them more Aloe Vera by *Aloe Life* (1 to 4 ounces) for dogs in their water or wet food separated into two separate doses. For small dogs or cats Animal Aloe by *Aloe Life* can be squirted directly into the food for regularity which reduces both hair balls and Kidney ailments. If they experience loose stool then reduce the Aloe Vera until you see soft but formed bowel movements. StomachPlus Formula by *Aloe Life* is another very valuable herbal tonic for people and pets for occasional digestive issues, vomiting or other obvious allergies and nervous disorders. *Note:* Consult a Vet with chronic health challenges. Pets also thrive on Nutritional Yeast, Daily Greens, Fish and Flax Oils, Probiotics and Essential Core Nutrients that you can purchase from your Vet, Pet Store or Health Food Store found in a good Multiple Vitamin and Mineral product. The *Nordic Naturals* company makes superior healthy oils for people and one specifically for your pet called Pet Cod Liver Oil following the Scandinavia recommendations for family pets. Remember no capsules for your furry girls and boys either if you can possibly avoid them! Another ailment is ear aches and also itchy ears. They can be experienced by both cats and dogs and both have responded brilliantly using a natural herbal product called Ear Drops by *Aloe Life* used by pet groomers and owners across the globe! Check out *Aloe Life International* on the internet at www.aloelife.com and in the Reference.

These supplements coupled with the natural diet and healthier lifestyle choices will address the majority of complaints experienced by your pets. Once you get your pet exercising along with the dietary improvements the glandular insufficiencies begin to improve including the Thyroid that affects hair loss, fertility, arthritis, auto-immune and immune function. Occasionally a Vet will suggest adding a pharmaceutical drug temporarily to address chronic challenges like Thyroid, Yeast infections or appropriate conditions. Be assured you can blend prescription medicines with your natural health regimen called Complimentary Medicine.

Each modality helps greatly and whether you make your animals food from scratch as some owners do every 1 – 2 weeks freezing portions to prevent spoilage or buy it from a specialty pet shop (that deals in low gluten and gluten free diets for animals) the important point is to follow through with a healthier meat-based diet. You may try a few different ones before settling on the formula that gives your pet what it truly needs. Recipes are available to make your own pet food and some other terrific healthy treats for your pet that can save you money in the long run. Check out a do-it-yourself website at www.doityourself.com/stiy/gluten-free-dog-food-recipes. Cats are a bit fussier and I have found Friskies offers a very low gluten line of canned meats in the shredded variety and the dry food by Friskies at least contains meat in the ingredients. They also have a dry snack that can help reduce tarter on teeth to some degree. Keeping your pets teeth in good shape is another important factor of pet health.

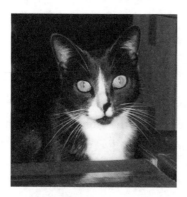

"Cinco" the Furry Girl

The testimony of my 17 year old Furry Girl (kitty) named "Cinco" (named because of her 5 digits on each paw) includes the endorsement of why I gave her Friskies. She also received the Animal Aloe, Daily Greens and Nutritional Yeast daily in her canned food carefully mixed to disguise it. After dealing with a scratched eye condition from her tree climbing I had three separate Vets do blood work from A – Z and they could not find any disease in her whatsoever even though I never inoculated her. My Cinco was a healthy kitty!

Do your best during the detoxification and renewal process because it can become a little confusing at times to understand the difference between the healing process and any disease condition the pet may have. One fact for certain is if your pet has chronic symptoms "Yeast" is always a common occurrence. Through detoxification the yeast dies and that can spike all symptoms temporarily of the original illness from the yeast die-off. It is very important that you support your pet's daily regularity. You can review the section on Detoxification of humans to understand the process in Chapter 6. Exercise and following the basics are important in fighting yeast and as mentioned you may wish to work with a Vet using a few pharmaceutical medications to get you through some difficult health challenges.

Having a 3 month goal to assess the improvement of your pet gives a better viewpoint and helps to develop more patience. I know you will see improvements as millions of pet owners who take these steps do. It may require the expertise of an experienced Vet to give you a more concrete diagnosis through blood work and examinations expanding the bigger health picture along the way. With applying more health through a low gluten diet and the GIS Pet Program you will hopefully have many more wonderful years to enjoy with Your Best Buddy!

CHAPTER 11

Bio-Snapshots of Undiagnosed Gluten Intolerance

1. Mental Imbalance & Brilliance

TBK grew up in Washington State in the "Apple Capital" of the U. S. An ideal childhood some would say living in a quaint American agricultural community where trips to the lake were a regular childhood activity with his sisters and brother for swimming and fun.

A gorgeous homeland was shared with fruit orchards surrounded by national forests and breath-taking rivers and lakes. The family ate well maintaining their seasonal vegetable garden yet they did get their share of sweets. Even during the WWII Era, late 40's and 50's that imposed economic pressures on most families, desserts including pies and confections were always available. Memories of the sweet treats almost daily prevailed because the fruits were seasonal and his father's profession was trucking baked goods all over the region and the family received a variety of day old items absolutely free.

The History

Looking back now with a GIS health perspective – TBK can see what set him up to experience his rebel like view of the world. Always a hard worker from a young child he followed a different beat of the drum. It was obvious that he was his own person from his boyish pranks, his love of mechanics, cars and planes, a cynical view of school and his independent ways. His independence led him to enlist early as a young teen into the Navy - hopeful to see the world. Living with an exceptionally "High IQ" he excelled in the Navy however only spent one enlistment and went on to develop his own business later on building yachts.

Relationships weren't as successful as his business endeavors and he experienced two failed marriages. The highlight was fathering two remarkably bright children with higher than average IQ's as well. Heredity cut the path for both children to model after Dad in many ways including living with highs and lows of depression mixed with manic behavior and unsuccessful relationships. As TBK was on the brink of another failed marriage the puzzle pieces began to slowly come together revealing that he had been living with undiagnosed Gluten Intolerance – GIS that heightened his Bi-Polar events.

Factors for GIS Bi-Polar (Manic Depression) Imbalance

- Diet; Milk, Sugar & Whole Grains develop inflammation > Psychosis (see Ch. 5).
- Toxic Chemicals; Congest the Liver Reducing Hormones Needed to Balance Moods.
- Herpes Simplex Virus; Contribute to GIS, Low Blood Sugar and Mood Fluctuations.
- Blood Sugar Imbalance; Eating Poorly Contributes to Reduced Emotional Control, Hyperactivity and High & Low Moods.
- Heredity Factor; Higher Percentage of Potential to Mental Illness Experienced in Families.

The GIS plot thickened as he reflected on his diet during his third marriage. In an attempt for the family to eat healthier they had kicked up whole grains. He loved eating bread especially whole wheat toast with peanut butter however the problem was that bread didn't love him back. With the addition of oatmeal and granola bars and brown rice he felt bloated a lot of the time and began to gain weight. The clincher was that

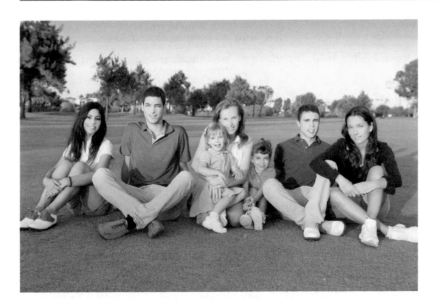

eating the whole grains made TBK's behavior worsen to the point of alienating his entire family from his life.

He loved eating healthy foods but ice cream and an occasional Snickers candy bar would sneak in that had always been life-long favorites. Orange juice was another choice in the morning along with coffee, milk and sugar. Looking back one could track the pattern of inflammation that seemed to escalate with the inclusion of chocolate and eggs especially if the eggs weren't cooked thoroughly enough. If he ate a healthy breakfast with eggs over-easy and wholegrain toast with orange juice and coffee a herpes outbreak either HSVI or HSVII would often show up a day or two later. The inflammation factor from eating the bread mixed with high Arginine containing foods (see Chapter 6) especially when the night before included a bowl of ice cream with chocolate or caramel syrup was a recipe for disaster! The cascade of inflammation is text book material described in Chapter 3, 4 and 5. It would start at breakfast and then lunch foods would increase the inflammation and then dinner GIS triggers could bring about an emotional outburst that didn't have a lot of restraint.

Lunch foods were typically tuna fish or peanut butter and jelly sandwiches. For dinner the family would sometimes have chicken or turkey with brown rice, tofu and vegetables at least once a week. Occasionally whole grain pasta with tomato sauce, meat or beans, vegetables and salad. The foods tasted absolutely delicious but it kept emotional turmoil in the house! Potatoes were kept to just once per week because of the strong accent for increasing the whole grains and little did anyone know that the family's diet was keeping everyone especially TBK from feeling mentally and physically well!

A closer look into TBK's family history revealed his dearly beloved mother also lived with periods of Mental Illness. His other siblings showed similar symptoms and nieces and nephews the like. Besides the family having all the milk and sweets a child could dream about and of course bread was always in the diet because that was the American way - another GIS factor came to light. The city he grew up in that was famous for their fruit orchards had been heavily spraying the orchards with toxic chemicals!

In 1998 a few years after this awareness which happened to be the same time TBK was giving up cow and soy milk (that in turn stopped his reflux and sleep apnea), a "60 Minute" TV special aired about the little town that he grew up in. Amazingly this city had more residents taking Prozac than any other city in the U.S. It had to be associated to the chemicals from the orchards he thought. Perhaps some impact also came from the leaded gasoline that people used to use in their cars years ago that now could be affecting the town's mental health? The valley that was so perfect for growing fruit trees developed an inversion level in the atmosphere that would hold the local air pollution captive whatever the source. It had to be partially responsible why so many people experienced poor mental health – much higher than the average across the nation.

The Solution

The profile of a manic personality is heightened senses including; thought processes, smell, hearing, taste, body sensations and often exaggerated animation to include excessive talking. When the manic behavior would start he could talk non-stop until the listener found a good excuse to change the topic or politely leave. At one point his narcissistic attitude took on a role of TBK against the world - be it family, friends or any authority figure whatsoever!

Life got complicated and he and his wife separated to avoid the constant battles. During the separation a psychiatrist shared that Lithium is the only chemical he had seen help Bi-Polar (manic-depressant) patients over the years. The challenge he shared about using Lithium even though it is a natural chemical is its potential for liver damage and with that warning he wrote out the prescription. Even though his wife told the doctor about the GIS Program he didn't understand the full potential of dietary restrictions and how it might help the psyche and he just wished everyone the best. TBK met with his wife and they reviewed the options and both decided to give the GIS Program blended with some healthy relationship boundaries and better communication skills a few months.

Once the family began to put the GIS Program into practice the dark cloud that had kept him captive began to lift. He first stopped eating oatmeal for breakfast and whole grain sandwiches for lunch and included more salads. The family stopped buying ice cream and cookies and kept more fruit and yogurt on hand. That seemed to lower TBK's grouchiness with family members and fighting with his wife right away. Slowly but surely as he gave up the Gluten and Gluten Triggers and added the ECN supplements that are outlined in Ch. 8 improvement followed. Next he followed the Detoxification Program and blended in the brain support supplements helping with the brain chemistry. The 5HTP is one of the impressive supplements he added to the ECN list described in Chapter 8. *Note:* Read Chapter 5 to review the importance of learning new improved communication skills for the entire family once the body is not dictating the exaggerated behaviors. Now after nearly a decade TBK can share with others - how the GIS Program Really Works for Mental Wellness!

2. Ulcerative Colitis & Poor Glandular Health

KKC was born in 1975 in the greater Southern California region and grew up in a large Italian-Cuban family that believed in natural health.

She always had lots of encouragement to do well in school, participate in sports and she developed a strong drive to make something of her life. After graduating college she found herself in many different management positions from law firms to restaurants yet found herself drawn to work in health radio communications because of a deep interest in natural healing. The ironic underlying truth was through her relentlessness - she became successful in health radio but her own health was nearly destroyed and she became trapped in poor glandular health.

The History

In her younger years she loved to swim and this appeared to bring about chronic ear infections. That demanded tubes in the ears and also went hand in hand with repetitive antibiotics. KKC seemed to be fairly healthy other than normal childhood colds except for one important challenge. Her bowels were stubbornly slow and often her mother was giving her remedies or laxatives to help her with regularity. No one likes having to spend extra time in the bathroom with such a personal body function especially as an active teen involved in school activities, sports and fun-time with her friends!

The bowels took a second seat as a teen and the doctor said it was normal with some people. So it just became accepted to make time for her weekly date in the bathroom. Later in her twenties Thyroid function began to require some attention and because that is also pretty common these days no one paid too much attention. During college when stresses are normally high that can spark more digestive distress - it didn't seem so odd that she developed bleeding ulcers. She took more antibiotics to help with the pain and in an attempt to heal them. That always helped for a little while then boom the pain and symptoms were back. The doctors would give her a variety of different prescriptions all the while she battled with colitis symptoms of diarrhea intermittent with her chronic constipation. It just seemed to her that no matter what she ate it didn't help so she might as well just eat what she enjoyed and that became pizza and soda, pizza and soda and more pizza!

Factors for GIS – Ulcerative Colitis & Glandular Deficiency

- Milk Intolerant from Infancy KKC was not Breast Fed; Reflects on the health of the mother.
- Diet; Wheat (Whole Grains), Sugar & Milk Solids (Lactose hidden in foods) affects regularity of the bowels.
- Antibiotics & Chronic Constipation; leads to poor gut and skin health.
- Mal-Nutrition & Toxicity Reducing Glandular Function; Low Thyroid, Liver and all glands lead to weight gain, depression, hyperactivity and agitation.

As described in Chapters 2, 3, 4 and 5, the inflammation process can remain silent for many years causing Nervous System irregularities like constipation and reducing glandular function. After a while mal-nutrition also affects the glands of the body interrupting a woman's menses schedule, allowing for endometriosis, depression, weight gain and irregular sleep patterns from under-functioning Liver and Thyroid glands. This is reviewed in Chapter 6 called "Glandular Health" and it is dependent on keeping GIS low in the body.

The Solution

With all the trips to the doctor's office during childhood and increasing into her 20's and 30's the doctors never mentioned a possibility of Gluten Intolerance. As the GIS Program was unveiled to her and she began to apply it in her life one product and one new food at a time – her body began to heal. That was 7 years ago and along the way through only using natural and healthy foods (leaving wheat pasta and most grains alone) and using the supplements outlined in the GIS Program her ulcers resolved along with the long list of other health challenges. Even her skin renewed itself to be youthful once again. She got her natural energy back and through exercising and her new found delicious diet - she lost over 70 pounds and has kept it off. KKC just completed her yearly physical and her physician of five years gave her a 100% pass on all of her tests.

She also admitted to her that she has been amazed to watch her fragile health return so extraordinarily. Candidly she stated to KKC that she did not expect her to have lived past age 50 with all the health challenges she had five years ago. KKC's life has been given back to her as she made the effort and with it feeling 99% excellent - 7 days a week; mentally, spiritually and physically!

3. Childhood Fast Transit, Asthma, Allergies & OCD

AJG was born in San Diego County in 1978 and had an active childhood with balancing school work and lots of sports. He went on to receive a full football scholarship and graduated with a double major which he has reflected on as a miracle since he was a slow learner in elementary education. Marrying his high school sweetheart he went on to graduate the police academy excelling in every segment of his work.

The History

Throughout childhood his health seemed fairly normal other than growing up with a lot of allergies. This included having an Asthma condition that was coupled with "Fast Transit". The definition of Fast Transit is food(s) that irritate(s) the bowel, as with an allergy, bringing about loose stool or diarrhea in a short period of time after eating. *Note:* The normal transit time of food is about 6 – 8 hours as outlined in Chapter 3 Understanding Digestion. With Fast Transit a bowel movement generally occurs within 30 minutes or less accompanied with gas, bloating and often a watery elimination. This occurs frequently with milk intolerance and other food triggers including; milk, milk solids, wheat, whole grains to include oatmeal, corn, eggs, chocolate, nuts, soy and other starches especially pizza and French fries because they contain a lot of Omega 6 oils.

Even though the digestive battle was a chronic on-going health challenge doctors never suggested to the family that their son may be Gluten intolerant. This is understandably a very challenging condition that affects millions of people yet it is especially difficult for a child who was so active throughout childhood into his teens, college years and young adulthood. Besides the inconvenience of living with this condition the health challenge the Fast Transit brings is the loss of valuable nutrients that the body requires to maintain physical and mental health. Fast growing GIS children as with AJG commonly experience slow learning, dyslexia and developmental challenges. Boys may experience a challenge 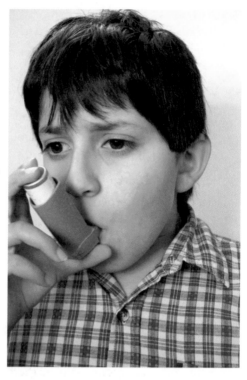 developing muscle mass and weight gain where girls on the other hand may have a delay in developing breasts and are late starting their menses.

Developmental challenges can be accentuated from medications and chemical toxicity including steroid use by children with Asthma and antibiotics that affect the body systemically. A diet higher in refined sugar will also cause more inflammation in the body increasing allergy symptoms and contributing to the GIS inflammation in the gut with or without the consumption of wheat. *Note:* The value of increasing the Omega-3 Fatty Acids from all sources is paramount with AJG's history to include (as tolerated) Salmon, shrimp, sardines or Fish Oil, Flax Oil, Algae and Green Leafy and other vegetables (see Chapter 7). Consumption of the Omega-3 Fatty Acids are significant in both lowering the associated inflammation of the bowel and also instrumental to mental well-being that includes; Obsessive Compulsive Disorder (OCD) tendencies and even periods of Manic – Depression.

Factors for GIS - Fast Transit, Asthma, Allergies & OCD

- Diet; Milk Intolerance, Refined Sugar & High Omega 6's Increasing Inflammation.
- Allergies; Milk Solids, Grains, Soft and Processed Cheese, Seafood, Molds, Dust Mites and Animals.
- Mal-absorption; GIS Affect from Steroids, Refined Sugar and Candida Albicans Overgrowth.
- Mal-Nutrition; Mono-Diets, Lack of Minerals, Poor Absorption leading to slow developmental or Imbalances in Growth (Hormones) and Mental Health.
- Blood Sugar Imbalances; Diet & Viral Connection.

The Solution

People are not machines and they have complex lives that change from one day to the next based on many factors. What is known based on science and clinical findings is how a person's reactions to foods can truly effect emotions, pain in the body and physical symptoms. This is outlined in Chapter 5 Glossary of Conditions and Chapter 6 Healthy Focus Factors under Addictions including sugar addiction. In AJG's life as he stayed away from Grains, Milk and Milk Solids and Fried Foods including Pizza he witnessed a big improvement in his bowel health. He also gradually added the full GIS ECN supplements as outlined in Chapter 8 which he took for a period of time when he felt the best. However, he is still contemplating for himself about the true value of supplementing taking them sporadically. My hope is that he will continue the full GIS Program to reap all of the benefits for mental well-being.

Some major victories have been conquered by AJG! Some other health challenges still remain to be addressed that possibly may be due to secondary GIS triggers. Lower on the inflammation trigger list yet not to be overlooked include; processed corn products, gelatin from supplements and or pharmaceutical prescriptions, hormone imbalance and blood sugar metabolism. Herpes Simplex I (HSVI) as mentioned in several chapters is tied to tricky blood sugar (review Ch. 6 Viruses). It is a major consideration affecting one's health status and attitude with symptoms to include; frequent headaches, mood disorders, OCD and ultimately relationships. All people learn in layers and my hope is that the rest of the program will be embraced in the future to allow even greater victory in health!

4. Colitis, Cystic Acne, Asthma & Weight Gain

LMS was born in beautiful Washington State in a small rural city where most of the children belonged to the 4H club - learning about agriculture, horses and other farm animals. The seasons are extreme in this part of the world and fortunately she had a mother who understood the importance of nutrition and the planning of family meals year round.

The relatives grew lots of fresh vegetables and fruits and her family shared in caring for their own garden and farm animals. Fondly, she remembers driving the family truck around the property even before she had her license. The long cold winters brought on more baking of bread and squelching the family's sweet tooth with confections as in most average American families. Growing up was full of fun and games with an older brother and a younger sister who truly loved playing every game imaginable from scrabble to card games and the whole family read lots of books. Academics had a strong push in the family with LMS taking part in many spelling bees and singing competitions that developed her voice career.

The History

Looking back at how she excelled in academics and extracurricular activities in her youth takes on an even greater significance once you know that throughout growing up she was battling a long list of health challenges. She recalls spending many a cold evening on the front porch drinking coffee with her mother just to ease her Asthma flare-ups. Knowing she had Allergies her mother switched her to lactose-free milk at an early age and her colitis improved. Even though it helped she still battled gas, bloating and bouts of diarrhea and constipation throughout her childhood, teen years and after college.

The teen years were a constant uphill trek for LMS with skin problems leading her to try multiple pharmaceutical drugs to help her Cystic Acne including antibiotics. The deep scars left from years of acne along with more flare-ups she endured (even while in college) - seemed extremely unfair and left her wondering when would her skin challenges cease? Besides her migraine headaches that came on fairly regularly her weight gain bothered her the most. It seemed as if nothing she did made any difference. In and out of doctor offices left her knowledgeable about her chronic Anemia, fluctuating Thyroid and always searching for the best Iron supplement. Gluten intolerance was questioned yet the testing she had completed as a youngster resulted in a negative reading! *Note:* Read Chapter 4 Testing Methods for GIS that explains the common false negatives that people receive from blood tests.

Factors for GIS – Colitis, Cystic Acne, Asthma & Weight Gain

- Diet; Milk and Milk Solids in soft and processed cheese, Refined Sugar and Grains plus High Omega-6 Fatty Acids leading to bowel distress.
- Inflammation and Mal-Nutrition; leads to Anemia and TMJ jaw tightness, headaches and more.
- Pharmaceutical Drugs and Antibiotics; Increase Yeast Overgrowth and mal-nutrition.
- Constipation, Candida & Liver Congestion; Leads to Lazy Liver reducing Fat Soluble Skin Vitamins A, E, Fatty Acids (Om3's) and Vitamins C, D, B-Complex and Minerals; Zinc, Calcium, Magnesium and more.
- Inflammation Reduces Glandular Function; Pancreas, Liver and Thyroid developing improper Weight gain.
- Hormonal Deficiency Increase; Migraine Headaches, Acne Flare-Ups, Emotional Ups and Downs, along with Connective Tissue Breakdown Increasing Chemical Allergies and Headaches.

The Solution

As LMS applied the GIS Program one day at a time - with one new food and one new supplement at a time – her health began to return. That was 9 years ago and she is a beautiful young woman who rarely has a headache, Asthma is of the past and only rarely does she experiences GI upset. If it does occur it is generally because she has eaten something on the GIS Trigger list or just fighting a little Flu bug. Just recently LMS had her annual blood test and all of her glandular and chemistry markers came back in the normal range - the healthiest she has ever tested. Her energy is great even with a young toddler, a husband, working outside the home at least 30 or more hours per week and a baby on the way. Her weight came off before the baby over 40 unwanted pounds and will again because her glands are working well now. She also has received a renewed complexion and by the use of the topical Aloe Vera Skin Gel by *Aloe Life* the body reversed all of her deep scars from childhood to the present. It is truly miraculous to see how the body heals when it is given the opportunity. The GIS Program works for everyone who decides to make the effort regardless of whether or not you get a positive Gluten intolerant diagnosis or not!

Home Health Practices 101

Looking for ways to assist the body to heal at home has inspired the following practices to be included in this chapter. Some have been taught over many centuries such as enemas and colonics and others have developed out of the need to give the modern man and woman fast relief from pain and other symptoms. Learning to close the "Ileocecal Valve" for example is an exercise that can stop pain very quickly in the abdomen and it only takes seconds to complete.

If your child was choking on a piece of food I think you may use the Heimlich maneuver – Right? Well, similar to removing a foreign object from the throat of your toddler is learning to do "Cross-Crawl". This is a great way to remove a static energy blockage and balance the right and left brain (electrical transmission) so a person can think more clearly, reduce dyslexia and calm down.

There are other great healing tools for the body not included in this chapter such as "Massage" however it is mentioned in Chapter 6 under relaxation. Simply massaging your ears, feet, back and hands while adding more pressure and attention to the painful areas - can soothe a headache, ease an upset stomach and even promote a bowel movement when needed. Most children and spouses love touch when given in a non-sensual way. Intimacy between adults is healthy yet it deserves a chapter of its own in another book, perhaps on longevity.

Human touch as with hugging is extremely healing. My grandson just learned a song in kindergarten that is called, *4 Hugs is Not Enough* – the world definitely needs more HUGS!

1. Colon Cleansing, Enemas & Colonic Irrigation Therapy

People have been giving themselves "Enemas" for centuries long before the advent of rubber by using a type of bamboo reed as did the Essenes. The Essenes lived during the 2nd Century BC and advocated the health of the body and purification as noted in the Dead Sea Scrolls. The goal of "Colon Cleansing" is to remove feces and nonspecific toxins from the colon and intestinal tract thereby reducing; gas, bloating, nausea and microbial agents. The accumulation of waste may include; bad bacteria, yeast, mucus, parasites and infection trapped in pockets. The challenge with poor elimination especially chronic constipation is that the food waste enters into the 9 feet of large intestine to further break down and if not evacuated properly it promotes putrefication leading to "Auto-Intoxication" of the entire body and undermines health.

The Egyptians believed in the common sense cleansing of the bowel for health along with the ancient Greeks right into the 19 Century. Even though modern medicine has been reluctant to embrace the value of colon cleansing it is done prior to many surgeries and colonoscopies. Working in a Geriatrics care facility as a young woman it was a routine practice to give patients with irregularity soap enemas.

The negative comments that have been made concerning colon cleansing through the media and by physicians are unfortunate because the value to assist the body to evacuate is of utmost importance. The doctors certainly don't waste time in writing up a prescription for a stool softener or laxative if they understand the weeks some people go without a bowel movement! Infants, children and adults all feel better and experience better health with bowel regularity that is daily not weekly. Once the bowels are moving regularly it allows the Liver, the Lymph and the Blood to purify and renew which increases one's health and sense of well-being!

Overeating and eating the wrong foods including glutinous foods and triggers have been highlighted as the common reasons that lead people to Colon Cleansing. As discussed in Chapter 2 Learning about Bowel Disease after years of having bowel problems the intestines may actually develop blockages requiring medical attention. In rare cases even a tumor may be stopping the elimination and must be diagnosed and surgically removed as required. Do not delay in seeking medical assessment - if you see blood, red or black color in the stool or have acute pain in the abdomen or experience constipation that will not right itself for longer than 10 days! Action must be taken because beyond this time period becomes dangerous and in some people sepsis poisoning or gangrene infection can set in which in some cases might end a person's life from complications!

Steps for a Successful (Coffee) Enema

- Supplies Needed Include; enema bucket or bag, rubber tubing, clip to control water flow, lubricating jelly, filtered warm water (not hot or cold) plus coffee. Enema supplies can be purchased through a pharmacy or on the internet.
- 3 – 4 cups of water, (1) cup coffee made just like brewing it or purchasing a cup (optional). Coffee is safe to use and makes the enema more successful. If acute hyper-tension only use ½ cup of coffee per enema even though it does not affect the Nervous System the same as drinking coffee.
- Lay in bathtub or on the floor in the bathroom if possible on a plastic sheet or towel to protect against any spills.
- Place liquid in enema bucket or bag filling the tube with water, secure clamp and place on a steady stool or hang it 1 ½ feet above your body as you lay down. Gravity is needed to allow the flow of liquid into the intestine.
- Experts agree to carefully lay on the left side if possible, with a pillow under your head for comfort, lubricate your rectum with a hygienic lube and while breathing in and out your

nostrils (this allows your abdomen muscles to relax) slowly let the enema liquid flow into your body releasing the clamp yet regulating it at about (1) cup per minute.

- If the enema becomes too stimulating to the bowels, to the point that you must get up and use the toilet, just clamp off the enema and carefully pull yourself up and evacuate.

- If possible return to the down position and take the remainder of the enema continuing to breathe slowly. The object is to take the full 4 cup enema then remove the tubing and hygienically wrap it with a paper towel.

- Roll from left side to your back and then to your right side breathing slowly and eliminate when the urge comes.

- Do not feel terribly disappointed if all the water absorbs into the bowel at first. This happens fairly often when just beginning enemas and shows the need to hydrate the intestines. You can repeat the process to encourage elimination. It will help regularity through hydrating yet you may require taking extra cleansing supplements (See Chapter 8) in addition to the enema to achieve regularity.

- A successful routine develops within a rather short period of time and the result is a healthier colon and better health!

Caution: If you have any physical limitation that prevents you from lying down safely and taking an enema then check with your physician for other options. Review Irregular Bowel Conditions in Chapter 6 to prevent constipation. Once you begin to apply the GIS Program many people start to eliminate better. However, for some people they still experience "Lazy Bowel". This stubborn condition of the bowel lacking normal peristalsis may improve. Yet for some people the function of the colon to properly remove waste requires the addition of a daily or weekly enema.

Another option is the professional "Colon Irrigation" available by an experienced and highly trained technician. The person administers the therapy by using an FDA approved Colonic Irrigation (CI) piece of equipment. This CI machine holds water and has the appropriate tubing to encourage evacuation of the intestinal waste and the toxic contents from the colon through controlled water pressure and a slight vacuum motion. This procedure does have some cautions yet when done correctly it is a valuable modality for speeding up the cleansing process.

Colonic Irrigation Therapy Questions

- Best to ask for a referral from a Chiropractor doctor or health food store.
- Ask to see the operator's certification and also ask the length of time in practice to confirm the experience and ask any other questions you may have. You should be properly sheeted and made to feel as comfortable as possible with the insertion and removal of the disposable tube.
- This modality is more thorough because the equipment holds a larger amount of water vs. an enema. It cautiously reaches further up into the colon rather than just an enema for hydration purposes and elimination success.
- Do not be disappointed if the first couple of treatments do not expel a large quantity of waste. Often feces become impacted and dry almost resembling tar. There is a viewing tube so an operator will point out different types of discharge if you desire.
- Often an operator will suggest different supplements to take temporarily so the detoxification and cleansing will be more beneficial.
- Results can include; a lessening of pain including headaches, reduced gas, bloating, more energy and improved overall health!

Note: High Calcium can also promote constipation so make certain you have your Para-Thyroid Hormone tested along with Calcium levels in blood and urine. If you find this to be the case then seriously consider surgery to remove a couple of the Para-Thyroid glands or as the surgeon recommends that will help remedy the over production of the hormone. Toxicity in the environment is pointed to as one of the culprits for Para-Thyroid malfunction and it is not easily rebalanced naturally. Review this condition on the internet to read the entire description and results of the suggested protocol.

2. Slant Board Magic

This modality is very remarkable when you understand how it works. The facts reveal that during life once you grow into an adult most people do not place themselves in an upside down position very often!

The slant board allows the body to be positioned in a slight declining head down position. Any board with one end mounted higher than the other (that can safely hold a person's weight) may be used. You can make your own, constructed out of a piece of heavy duty board (10 – 12 inches in width) and cover it with padding and material. Yet the quickest board to have access to, that is if you are not overweight, is collapsing a large ironing board and placing one end on two large books about 6 inches off the ground to start.

Slant Board Therapy

- With an empty stomach lay on the board with your feet about 6 inches above your head. About every month you can raise the slant board another inch to a final 12 inches if you desire.
- Start out by spending only 5 minutes on your slant board per session. You can do a second session later in the day if you desire.
- It gives the body passive exercise from altering the gravity we live with and it gives a gentle massage to the entire colon both small and large intestine as they shift position.
- If you have had a history of diverticulitis pay special attention to what happens after the treatment.
- Several people have remarked having a discharge of fluid fairly soon after their treatment that contains a foul odor.
- Make certain you are taking both the Aloe Vera juice and

Probiotics recommended in Chapter 7 and 8 to combat any side effects from the discharge. Paramount to staying well is drinking 6 – 8 glasses of filtered water each day.

- What apparently takes place is captive fluid, containing miscellaneous toxins from the diverticula pouches in the intestines, is allowed to exit. After the elimination of the fluid the individuals feel exceptionally better than they have in recent years!

3. Closing the Ileocecal Valve

The Ileocecal Valve is a sphincter muscle located at the junction of the small intestine called the ileum and the large intestine. It comes before the appendix in the lower right side of the abdomen in most people. The main purpose of this muscle group is to limit the back flow from the large intestine waste material from going back into the small intestine.

Approximately, two quarts of liquid waste may flow through the Ileocecal Valve into the large intestine daily. Scientists have also found that this area in the colon is where the greatest amount of B12 is supposedly absorbed along with bile acids and it contains a higher than normal amount of lymphatic tissue required for detoxifying and fighting infection in the body .

When the valve does not function properly a host of gastrointestinal problems and other symptoms occur in the body to include; gas, pain, nausea, diarrhea, migraine headaches, an increase in blood pressure besides a higher incidence of colds and flu. When an individual is experiencing symptoms it is suggested to go through the exercise of closing the valve with your open hand.

Steps to Gently Close the Ileocecal Valve

- Locate the valve area that can be slightly different from person to person on the right side of the abdomen. As mentioned it is rare but can be located on the left side.

- Place your left thumb on your belly button and your right thumb on your right pelvic hip bone. Next place your right pointer finger in the middle of those two points and go down 3 – 4 inches. That spot is your Ileocecal Valve area.
- Now that you know where the spot is place your open hand fingers together on the spot and push in with about 5 pounds of pressure (firmly) and pull up towards your right pelvic bone.
- Repeat this motion 3 or 4 times and that will complete the closing. You may feel tenderness in the area from inflammation which generally decreases as you apply the GIS Program and regularly close the valve.

Massaging the area using a circular motion to the right is a good way to relax all of the muscles in the area that can become tight. With extra visceral fat it can be a little challenging however using oil or a light lotion can help in the process of locating the area and giving yourself a treatment. Chiropractors have used this modality for many years to encourage the healing of the body from sickness and bouts of irritable bowel syndrome IBS and IBD. See Chapter 2 to review the big picture of bowel disease. *Note:* Pain that does not resolve or that may increase after following the GIS Program for a period of 3 months needs to be evaluated by a medical professional for more diagnostic testing as required. Children and adults respond excellently to closing the Ileocecal Valve and will be healthier from this practice at any age!

4. Cross-Crawl Exercise

Some health professionals consider the Cross-Crawl exercise as a way to organize your mental coordination. It really works and why it does is because of the support and balance it gives to the Nervous System. When you hear this exercise presented in this fashion it is easier to understand why it can help an individual's walking, talking, reading, self-confidence and even optimizing one's IQ.

Cross-Crawl Supports the Nervous System's "Out-of-Balance" Symptoms

- Learning Disabilities
- Poor Balance
- Dyslexia
- Clumsy and Accident Prone
- Emotional Imbalance
- Stuttering
- Dropping Objects
- Body Toning

Science has confirmed that that the human body runs on a type of electrical energy similar to an integrated circuit. The cells of the body generate energy likened to other simple electronic devices having positive and negative charges. The body also has a more complex electronic system that is described in Acupuncture Medicine as Meridian energy that can be measured with an electrical monitor. The Hormonal System of the body is a separate factor that also influences energy by creating changes in the body through Biorhythms and metabolic function. The underlying goal to successfully execute any of the Cross-Crawl exercise options is to move opposite limbs at the same time the way the body was designed to walk for instance. There is an exercise that fits just about anyone's lifestyle - you only need to do it to reap the benefits of clearer thinking and better body functions!

Cross-Crawl Exercise

- *Marching* in place or moving forward you are lifting the right leg bending at the knee and the left arm folds across the torso to even touch the knee if possible - opposites. The left leg comes up next with right arm crossing over to meet it.
- *Laying* down on a mat or bed and lifting opposites is a more passive warm up for the physically impaired or as desired.
- *Sitting* in a chair at home or in an office setting you can very

easily bring your knee up and over toward your opposite hand and arm alternating sides for 10 – 20 seconds. This works if you are stopped at a red light or stop sign if you can secure the car from going forward while you take this quick break to Cross-Crawl.

The Cross-Crawl exercise is effective in helping the brain send the correct messages to the correct body part required for the job of movement or thought. The harder it is for an individual to correctly perform this exercise reveals how much they require the GIS Program for renewal that includes the nutrition and lifestyle foundations. The core nutrients as explained in Chapter 8 and drinking purified water are paramount to getting balance back in the body's Nervous System for health!

5. Liver & Gallbladder (LG) 2-Day Flush

The liver is the largest organ in our body and perhaps the hardest working, responsible for hundreds of activities including digestion and the cleansing of toxins. Many health challenges that occur in our body can be linked to a toxic liver. The gallbladder resides right next to the liver and they actually rest upon each other. They work as a team for supplying bile to the small intestine for digestion and pH balancing. Both organs can become sluggish and store excess waste that includes the development of stones that may disrupt their function. Over time people have developed several types of medicinal flushes that allow the organs to rest and encourage waste products to be cleansed from them - a requirement for rejuvenation. This is not a painful procedure expelling gallstones when they are eliminated through the stool. It is not to be confused with eliminating Kidney stones. Epsom Salts are recommended in the LG Flush and it is safe to drink. It consists primarily of Magnesium Sulfate used as a cathartic to move the bowels and reduce inflammation.

For best preparation for the flush it is suggested to reduce meat intake and any other fats coming from fried or processed foods three days before the flush. Also, because apples contain malic acid that is very supportive in helping to increase bile flow include at least (1) quart of organic apple juice daily with a good amount of water (as tolerated) and or eat several apples to help the body cleanse due to the many properties they contain including good non-irritating fiber for the body. Individuals that follow through and complete the flush as outlined reap the beneficial effects of feeling better faster. It is possible to repeat this LG Flush as desired customizing it to your own body's needs. Read the entire section to understand what it entails and the necessary items you will need including the health caution.

Steps of the 2 Day LG Flush

- *Breakfast Day One:* Eat a good size breakfast including proteins, fruits even carbohydrates as you like and a light lunch. Restrict yourself from eating any fat like butter, oil, mayonnaise, nuts and seeds or fried foods.
- *2 pm Day One:* Stop eating all food no snacking of any kind. Allow your digestive system to empty and rest completely. Water and herbal teas are recommended throughout the afternoon. Mint, Chamomile and even a delicious Japanese Hojicha (roasted green tea or other) are good selections. Fresh lemon and honey is OK if kept to a minimum, apple juice and lots of water to hydrate well is important. Once you drink the "Epsom Salts" it tends to dehydrate a person if you are not drinking enough water.
- *8 pm Day One:* Mix (1) teaspoon of Epsom Salts in (1) cup of apple juice. Stir thoroughly and drink quickly. Some people find drinking this through a straw is helpful because of the strong taste.
- *10 pm Day One:* Repeat another cup of mixture and follow it with (1) cup of water.
- *12 Midnight Day One:* Be totally ready for bedtime around midnight. Have your sleepwear on and be ready to lie down after drinking the olive oil and lemon juice preparation (see recipe).

Also, have a few items in your bathroom ready for the next morning when you eliminate the gallstones to catch the stones.

Recipe for the Olive Oil / Lemon Juice Preparation: ½ cup olive oil with 1 – 2 fresh lemon(s) juiced is enough for one person weighing approximately 110 pounds. Use twice the amount for a person weighing 200 plus pounds around (1) cup olive oil to 4 lemons juiced. Place in a large glass and stir for about 60 seconds to blend. A variation can be made by replacing lemons with grapefruit juice and it is OK to drink up to equal amounts of the citrus as per the olive oil in this recipe. A straw may be helpful for some people or to sip from two separate cups containing both oil and citrus juice with the juice being the chaser. The consistency or taste may cause slight nausea yet do the very best you can to finish the drink.

Once you drink the preparation you can brush your teeth and lie down on your RIGHT SIDE to optimize the release of gallstones. Bend at the knees and tuck your feet as in the fetal position(pillow between the knees for comfort) to facilitate the flush the best you are able staying still for about 20 minutes before changing positions. It is OK to move about changing positions and sleep for as long as possible throughout the night.

- *Morning 7 am Day Two*: This morning take the 3ʳᵈ Epsom Salts drink DOUBLING the strength to 2 teaspoons of salts per (1) cup of apple juice. You will start having bowel movements generally during the morning hours between 9 a.m. – 12 Noon. The first elimination can be regular with the second being a greenish color followed with some loose stool. This is expected so it is best not to plan to go anywhere on this second day.
- *10 a.m. Day Two:* ONLY if you have not had any bowel movement by 10 am consider a 4ᵗʰ Epsom Salts drink. Everyone is different in the amount of Epsom Salts that are required to move the bowels. If you are aware of the stubborn nature of your

body's peristalsis then you may increase it to 3 teaspoons in (1) cup of apple juice and follow with (1) cup of warm water.

- *12 Noon Day Two:* It is normal to feel a little weak during the LG Flush. Rest and don't eat any solid food until you have a bowel movement. With some people that have a history of slow bowels it may take giving yourself an enema to have a bowel movement. See the section on "Enemas" and be prepared with the required equipment or purchase a Fleet Enema (green type or oil) from the pharmacy just in case you require this.

After having a bowel movement you may enjoy some fruit or soup for lunch to continue the restful state for the digestive system. Later in the day about 3 – 4 hours later you may enjoy solid foods again but it is best to keep it vegetarian for one more day if possible. After the second day it is OK to resume eating fish and or meat as per the GIS Program. This is a great time to eat healthier foods if your diet was lacking. People who go through the LG Flush generally experience better digestion at mealtimes and less symptoms of gas, bloating and even pain in the abdomen.

Note: As the authors of this regimen Awaken.com suggest if you have a sensitive and Fast Transit GI tract already you can modify the steps and reduce the Epsom Salts to very low or eliminate them all together. The original flush by Edgar Cayce consisted of just eating apples and drinking the olive oil and lemon juice mixture. It did not include the salts however so many people live with constipation that it seems to be the most effective protocol for the masses. As desired you can follow the steps only eating apples, drinking apple juice and or prune juice especially after drinking the olive oil preparation.

Caution: This is not a program for Diabetics, people with fragile health or children under 18 years of age. Consult your physician if pain or symptoms persist.

This modality is not intended to diagnose or treat any disease or replace advice given by any medical personnel.

6. Fasting for Health

The modality of Fasting has been used to heal oneself for thousands of years long before the advent of medicine and drugstores. Fasting can consist of one, two or even a three day fast. It is recommended to seek professional supervision during a fast that lasts longer than a week. Many modern day health professionals promote the one day a week fast to rest the body's digestive system taking in just water or vegetable juice or eating extremely light with just vegetable salads, soups and perhaps a little fruit. Others more skilled in this area suggest a two to three day fast especially if a person has been suffering with a lot of health challenges using water, vegetable juices, Aloe Vera juice and herbal teas. This longer fast allows the natural detoxification pathways to clean the cells from toxic debris that builds up in the tissues and systems of the body.

Different Fasting Modalities

* *One Day Fast;* water, juices or eating lightly.
* *2 – 3 Day Fast;* water, juices and herbal teas and take enemas as needed.
* *Longer Fast;* Supervision is suggested.

Many books are available that give detailed information for fasting including the protocols that have been used successfully in fasting by doctor, Joel Fuhrman, M.D., in his book called *Fasting and Eating for Health – A Medical Doctor's Program for Conquering Disease.* The introduction in this book gives the best description from the author himself.

He states, "Therapeutic fasting accelerates the healing process and allows the body to recover from serious disease in a dramatically shorter period of time. In my practice I have seen fasting eliminate lupus and arthritis, remove chronic skin conditions such as psoriasis and eczema, heal the digestive tract in patients with ulcerative colitis and Crohn's disease and quickly eliminate cardiovascular diseases such as high blood pressure and angina. In those cases the recovery was permanent. Fasting enabled longtime disease sufferers to unchain themselves from their multiple toxic drugs and even eliminate the need for surgery which was recommended to some of them as their only solution!"

A supporter of this work, Michael Klaper, M.D. says, "Dr. Fuhrman's book places the ancient healing practices of diet and fasting into the hands of modern practitioners – and their patients. Thought provoking and sure to be controversial, this guide will be seen as one of the mileposts on society's journey towards sane, affordable health care, based upon simpler and more natural methods. It will be valued by anyone seeking more vitality, a greater understanding of the body and aid in overcoming a personal health challenge."

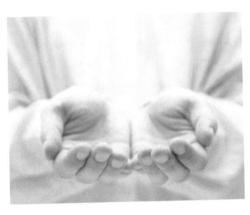

7. Prayer & Healing Touch

Many studies have demonstrated the beneficial health effects that "Prayer" has when directed towards people or animals. Another type of healing that has also shown success is "Energetic Healing" some refer to it as the Healing Touch. The Laying-On of Hands used in Healing Touch, Reiki Therapy and other similar practices is an ancient practice of healing. The word Reiki is from two Japanese words. "Rei" (ray), meaning from God's Wisdom or Higher Power and "Ki" (key) meaning Life Force Energy. Reiki is originally a Japanese technique that today is provided in many "Wholistic" health practices. It is used for stress reduction and relaxation and to promote healing. The variables involved in these healing arts are many including; the human belief system, attitudes and other psychological factors that are difficult to control. The *Examiner* magazine brought the following research studies together for your enlightenment.

Studies to Support Healing Through Prayer & Touch

- The National Institute of Mental Health issued a grant to a group of scientists at the University of Jackson in the U.S. to study prayer. In 2006 their study was published in the peer reviewed journal called *Alternative Therapies* providing an overwhelming body of evidence to support the effectiveness of prayer. Primates called "Bush Babies" were used in this unique study that avoided the human variables. The Bush Babies tend to over-groom themselves in captivity from boredom and stress to the point of causing wounds that are painful and life threatening. Some researchers have likened this to humans that develop Obsessive Compulsive Disorder (OCD). The study was very well controlled using 22 primate babies and divided them into two equal groups based on the size and complications of their wounds. The only difference in the groups was that one was prayed for by distance healers and the other group was not. In only 4 weeks the healing was significantly faster in the prayed for group. Blood measurements showed a marked increase in red blood cells and hemoglobin that the researchers attributed to greater oxygenation resulting in faster healing!

- Researchers from several countries including the U.S. have confirmed that people do have varying amounts of energy referred to as light streaming from their hands. In 2005 a team of photonic scientists in Japan confirmed that all people have varying degrees of light emitting from their fingernails, fingers and palms of the hands which they measured with a photon counter.

- A team of researchers in 2006 from the International Institute of Biophysics in Germany submitted their findings that a person's health level is directly correlated to the amount of emission of photons from the hands. They stated that the weaker the immune system of an individual the less emission of photon light was discharged through the hands of an individual. They also made a fascinating discovery measuring Reiki practitioners. As these professionals demonstrated the therapeutic touch on a client using their hands - surges of both light and electrostatic charges emerged from 1 to 12 seconds in duration. The voltage of electricity coming from their hands was measured varying from 4 to 221 volts!

• Ohio State University researchers recently utilized equipment on campus to measure the results of Laying-On of Hands healing. They observed consistent and dramatic fluctuations in all ten subjects resulting from their treatment through testing the gamma rays that respond with high frequency electromagnetic energy. This research provided very strong evidence for the healing force directed through touch and prayer to activate the cellular and molecular processes beneficial to healing and health.

Trained Reiki or Healing Touch professionals can be located in your city through referrals or going on-line. Individuals and families can always provide healthy touch and prayer for oneself and each other uplifting the quality of daily life!

Resources

Gluten & Health Organizations
The Celiac Disease Foundation
www.celiac.org

Celiac Disease and Gluten-Free Diet Support Center
www.celiac.com

The University of Maryland Center for Celiac Research
www.celiaccenter.org

National Eating Disorders
www.nationaleatingdisorders.org
www.eatingdisordersinfo.org
One in five women struggle with eating disorders - Take Action!

Forever Young Radio
www.fyradio.biz
Listen regularly and receive support to choose a healthier path honoring the Divine Design of the body! Easy to read articles on Health topics; Gluten, IBS & Reflux, Detox & Cleansing, The New Immune System, Weight Loss for Losers and more!

Food Friendzee Radio

www.foodfriendzee.com

Recipes for Gluten Free diets and low Gluten plus facts about Organic Foods and gourmet tips for busy people!

Local Harvest – National Food Search

www.localharvest.org

This is your opportunity to find out who is growing and selling healthier food and food products in your area for freshness and Certified Organic!

Looking for Organic Products

www.theorganicpages.com

From corn products to any other specialty organic grain check out this reference for success.

Testing Laboratories

Doctors Data Inc. - Hair Analysis

www.doctorsdata.com

www.inquiries@doctorsdata.com

www.integrativepractitioner.com

Over 30 years of experience, certified independent clinical laboratory sends kit for testing heavy metal burden, nutritional deficiencies and detoxification from metabolic and environmental origins. At Home Hair Test Kit - takes about one month for analysis results.

EnteroLab – Gluten & Allergy Testing

www.enterolabs.com

Easy stool kit for specimens to send back to their experienced labs to quantify. Their research reveals 4 in 10 Americans have advanced sensitivity to Gluten.

Omega 3 Test
At Home Blood Test Kit - takes about one month for analysis results.
www.omega3Test.com
Tests Total Om 3 Fatty Acids & Fractions plus gives individuals placement in the national and world percentages. Don't guess test – Know Your Numbers!

NSF - Water Testing for Safety
www.nsf.org
A non-profit organization to provide safer water for you and your family look for the NSF Seal!

Health Therapies
Healing Touch
www.healingtouchprogram.com
Find a practitioner in your area by clicking on the prompts. Benefits include reducing; pain, anxiety, depression and trauma. Increases healing time, mobility and immune function. Supports the dying process and deepens spiritual awareness of daily living.

International Association for Colon Hydrotherapy
www.i-act.org
homeoffice@i-act.org

Nutritional Supplements
Aloe Life International Inc.
1-800-414-2563 www.aloelife.com
Quality Organic Aloe Vera Products; Supplements, Juices, Herbal Blends, Pet Products, Bug Spray & Personal Care.

Bach Flower System
www.bachcentre.com

38 Remedies plus Rescue Remedy Dr. Edward Bach (1931) believed in People healing themselves!

Dr. Ohhira's Probiotics

www.drohhiraprobiotic.com

Award Winning – 12 Strains, Aged for 3 years, includes the Potent TH10 Strain plus other products.

Herb Pharm

info@herb-pharm.com

www.herb-pharm.com

Liquid Herbal Extracts & Herbal Healthcare Products.

Kyolic

Aged Garlic Extract

www.kyolic.com

Wakunaga Nutritional Supplements Full line of health products that include the famous "Aged Garlic".

Nordic Naturals

Pure and Great Tasting Omega Oils

www.nordicnaturals.com

info@nordicnaturals.com

One-Stop shopping for the whole family to include products for Pets, Pregnancy DHA, Children's Omegas, Adults and Seniors plus Specialty Blends, Multiples and more.

Prevagen - Clearer Thinking!

www.prevagen.com

The Calcium Regulating Jellyfish Protein – Apoaequorin. Great for People and Pets for a Healthier Brain & Sharper Mind!

Sovereign Silver Hydrosol

www.sovereignsilver.com

Natural-Immunogenics Corp. High Quality Liquid Silver used for internal and topical application.

Xlear Inc

www.Xlear.com

Nasal Spray for infants, children and adults plus xylitol chewing gum and bulk powder and other dental hygienic products.

Food Manufacturers

Authentic Foods – Baking Needs

It is not just Gluten Free its better!

www.authenticfoods.com

1-800-806-4737

Great flours, mixes, pasta (corn) and other baking needs plus Gluten Free Cook Books to order direct or found in quality health food stores - Delicious!

Food for Life – Only Use Select Products!

www.foodforlife.com

Attention consumers: A corporate decision made in recent years changed the bread recipe to include gluten flour. I no longer recommend the bread or their Gluten Free muffins. However for Zone 1 and 2 the English muffins Ezekiel 4:9 and 7 Sprouted are good! The tortillas I find also have too high of Fiber and evoke GIS symptoms.

Thai Kitchen – Rice Noodles

Stir Fry Rice Noodles and more!

www.thaikitchen.com

Look for these products which are marked Gluten Free 99% accurately!

Ancient Harvest Quinoa Flakes

www.quinoa.net

Quinoa Corporation Gluten Free Alternative and Organic for a healthy replacement for oatmeal.

La Tortilla Factory

www.latortillafactory.com

Sonoma Gluten Free Teff Tortillas and Flatbreads for Wraps – ask for these by name – Delicious!

Kaia Foods – Snack Foods

www.kaiafoods.com

Gluten Free, sprouted and dried; granola, spiced sunflower seeds & fruit leather – Delicious!

The Sprout People - Sprouting Supplies

www.sproutpeople.org

Make your own sprouts! Beautiful pictures of sprouts on the web site that are Delicious and Nutritious! 19 years in business a very trustworthy company supporting optimal health!

Nancy's - Dairy Products

www.nancysyogurt.com

www.nancyscottagecheese.com

Look for Nancy's great Low Lactose, Fermented and some Organic Dairy products -65% Lactose Free.

Horizons - Dairy Products

www.horizonsdairy.com

Partnering with hundreds of Organic Dairies across the USA they have excellent cream cheese and sour cream using only locust bean thickener - Delicious!

Bragg's - **Live Food Products**

www.bragg.com

Bragg's Liquid Aminos are in a spray bottle, sourced from soy however does not contain wheat – Delicious!

Farmers Cheese or Dry Curd Cottage Cheese

www.scdiet.org

Locating Dry Curd Cottage Cheese (DCCC) can be difficult so check out Whole Foods Market or Trader Joe's that may be able to order it for you or go online to the above website to find a source in your area. No milk is added after the fermentation process takes place so lactose intolerant people can use this cheese and it can be frozen before using – bonus!

San – J International - **Seasoning**

www.san-j.com

Organic Tamari – Gluten Free Soy Sauce & Reduced Sodium – No MSG Added!

Marukan Vinegar USA Inc. - **Seasoning**

www.marukan-usa.com

Genuine Brewed Rice Vinegar is Low on allergic response for; salad dressings, soups, dips and great taste when lemon is not available.

The Spice Hunter – **Organic Seasoning**

www.spicehunter.com

Wonderful full flavor spices, spice blends, & Salt free picks. The website has many great recipe suggestions. Read ingredients to make certain recipes are gluten free before making them.

De Boles - **Organic Pasta Products**

www.deboles.com

Whole grain and Gluten Free varieties have something for the whole family! Zone 1 and 2 can enjoy the Spinach Jerusalem Artichoke Flour variety and Zone 3 can often eat the rice flour or corn pasta.

Tropics Best - Coconut Products

www.tropicsbest.com

A variety of coconut products to use in baking and food preparation are all Gluten-Free. Cooking with Coconut Flour by Bruce Fife, N.D. Piccadilly Books

Kinnikinnick Foods – Cookies

Gluten free has never tasted so good!

www.kinnikinnick.com

A variety of products to select from yet be aware that not all of these products are free of secondary GIS triggers. The cookies can give a wheat free choice and you may wish to experiment with a few other products.

Crown Prince - Natural Sea Foods

www.crownprince.com

Wild caught Salmon and a variety of Sardine products are excellent. Look for the line in health food stores and mass merchandising outlets as well.

References

Introduction References

1. Fenech, M., 2003. "Nutritional Treatment of Genome Instability: A paradigm shift in disease prevention and in the setting of recommended dietary allowances", CSIRO Health Sciences and Nutrition/Cooperative Research Centre for Diagnostics/ Genome Stability Project, Australia. Published 2003, Nutrition Research Reviews. DOI: 10.1 079/NRR.200359 16, 109-122.

2. Sorsa, M., 1994. GENOTOXIC CHEMICALS, Overview article referencing world conference IARC – Cancer and DNA; Damage of DNA Proceeds the Development of Cancer. Exposure > DNA Damage > Mutation > Cancer or Heritable Disorder. IARC Technical Pub. No 24. http://www.ilo.org/safework_bookshelf/ English?content&nd=857170303.

3. Simons, J.A., Irwin, D.B., Drinnien, B.A., 1987. "Psychology-The Search for Understanding", A review of Abraham Maslow's theory of human needs. West Publishing Co., N.Y., USA. Maslow's paper was written about his work in 1943, "A Theory of Human Motivation", which came from a broad study interviewing people who reached their full potential in life including Albert Einstein.

4. Avery, O.T., MacLeod, G.M., McCarty, M., 1944. "Study of the Chemical Nature of the Substance Inducing Transformation of Pneumococcal Types: By a Desoxyribonucleic Acid Fraction Isolated from Pneumococcus Type III", Review of conclusion

states this work identified the molecule responsible for inheritance patterns of transformation as DNA. Journal of Experimental Medicine,79(2): 137. DOI:10.1084/jem.79.2.137, PMID 33 226.

5. Ogura, Y., Bonen, D.K., Inohara, N., 2001. "A Frame Shift Mutation in NOD2 Associated with Susceptibility to Crohn's Disease." Nature, 411(6837): 603-606. DOI: 10.1038/35079114. PMID 11385577.

6. Peppercorn, M.A. MD, Odze, R.D. MD, 2010. "Colorectal Cancer Surveillance in Inflammatory Bowel Disease", UpToDate. Patients with IBD are at increased risks for colorectal cancer. Risk is related to the duration and anatomic extent of the disease. Mortality is higher from Colorectal cancer with IBD than sporadic Colorectal cancer incidence. http://www.uptodate.com/home/content/topic.do?topicKey=inflambd/8300.

7. Hays, J., 2010. "Rice Agriculture in China", States most people in China eat white rice. China is the top producer and consumer of rice with about 200 million tons eaten per year. The average life span of a Chinese man is 69 yrs. and a woman 73 yrs.

Chapter 1 References

1. Sameer, Z., Benson, M.J., Kumar, D., 2005."IBS/Gluten Referencing Spastic Colon; Food-Specific Serum IgG4 and IgE Titers to Common Food Antigens in Irritable Bowel Syndrome." *American Journal of Gastroenterology;* 100: 1550-1557.

2. Mayo Clinic Staff, 2009. "Irritable Bowel Syndrome Definition," http://www.mayoclinic.com/health/irritable-bowel-syndrome/DS00106/DSECTION=symptoms.

3. Sinatra, Stephen T. MD, F.A.C.C., 2005. "The Sinatra Solution: Metabolic Cardiology". Covers relationship of silent inflammation at work tested by C-Reactive Protein (CRP) and the relationship to heart disease via plaque build up from all factors. Basic Health Pub., 2008. "Reverse Heart Disease Now:

Stop Deadly Cardiovascular Plaque Before It's Too Late!" Wiley Pub., 2006.

4. Gorman, P., 2004. "The Secret Killer – The Surprising Link Between Inflammation and Heart Attacks, Cancer, Alzheimer's and Other Diseases & What to do to fight it!" *TIME*, pg. 39-45. Sources; Dr. Moses Rodriguez of Mayo Clinic, Dr. Gailen Marshall of Univ. of Texas-Houston, Scientific American, May 2002.

5. Host, A., 1994. "Cow Milk Protein Allergy and Intolerance in Infancy." Pediatric Allergy-Immunol., 5: 1-36.

6. Niggemann, B., et al., 2001. "Prospective Controlled Multi-Center Study of the Effect of an Amino Acid Based Formula in Infants with Cows Milk Allergy / Intolerance and Atopic Dermatitis."

7. Gray, G., 1982. "Intestinal Di-Saccharidase Deficiencies and Glucose – Galactose Malabsorption." *The Metabolic Basis of Inherited Disease*, 5th ed., McGraw-Hill, N.Y., Stanbury, J.B., Wyngarden, J.B., Fredrickson, D.S., Goldstein, J.S., Brown, M.S..

8. Cluysenaer, O.J.S., VanTongeren, J.H.M., 1977. "Malabsorption in Coeliac Sprue." Martinus Nijhoff Medical Division, Hague.

9. Hadjivassiliou, M. MD, Royal Hallamshire Hospital, Sheffield, U.K., 2002. "Gluten Ataxia (loss of balance) is a Common Neurological Manifestation of Gluten Sensitivity." Research revealed patients with ataxia had antibodies against Purkinje cells output neurons of the cerebellum and also against gluten anti gliadin antibodies. Scientific journal of the *American Academy of Neurology*, April 23, 2002.

10. Phelan, J.J., Stevens, F.M., Cleere, W.F., McNicholl, B., McCarthy, C.F. and Fottrell, P.F., 1978. "The Detoxification of Gliadin by the Enzymic Clearage of a Side-Chain Substituent." In *Perspectives in Celiac Disease*, Univ. Park Press, Baltimore, MD.

11. Baker, P.G. and Read, A.E., 1976. "Oats and Barley Toxicity in Celiac Patients." *Post Graduate Medical Journal*, 52: 264-268.

12. Maki, M., 2010. "Gluten Intolerance in Finland Has Doubled." *Science Daily*, March 5, 2010. Professor Markku Maki states that 3 out of 4 people are living with gluten intolerance and not diagnosed. Cases have doubled in the last twenty years along with similar trends in allergies and autoimmune conditions. Maki is head of a research project in the Academy of Finland's Research Programme on Nutrition, Food and Health referred to as ELVIRA.

13. Heaton, K.W., 1990. "Dietary Factors in the Etiology of Inflammatory Bowel Disease." Inflammatory Bowel Diseases, Eds. Allan, R.N., Keighley, M.R.B., Alexander-Williams, J. and Hawkins, C.F.. Churchhill Livingston, NY.

14. Loftus, E.V., Schoenfeld, P., Sandborn, W.J., 2002. "The Epidemiology and Natural History of Crohn's Disease in Population - Based Patients Cohorts from North America: A Systematic Review." Alimentary Pharmacology & Therapeutics, 16 (1): 51-60. DOI: 10.1046/j.1365-2036. 2002. 01140.X. PMID 11856078.

15. Nesbitt, M., 2001. "Wheat Evolution: Integrating Archaeological and Biological Evidence." *Wheat Taxonomy: The Legacy of John Percival*, pgs. 35-59, edited by Caligari, P.D.S. and Brandham, P.E.. London: Linnean Society, Linnean Special Issue 3.

16. Gayla, J. and Kirschmann, J.D., 1996. Grains; Section VIII, pgs. 367-369. *Nutrition Almanac*, McGraw Hill, NY.

17. Shang, H., Wei, Y., Long, H., Yan, Z., Zheng, Y., 2005. "Identification of LMW Glutenin – Like Genes From Secale Sylvestre host." Genetika 41 (12): 1656-64. PMID 16396452. http://www.ncbi.nlm.nih.gov/pubmed/16396452.

18. Mazzeo, M., De Giulio, B., Senger, S., Rossi, M., Malorni, A., Siciliano, R., 2003. "Identification of Transglutaminase-Mediated Deamidation Sites in a Recombinant Alpha-Gliadin

by Advanced Mass Spectrometric Methodologies." Protein Science, 12 (11): 2434-42. DOI: 10.1110/ps.03185903. PMID 14573857 pubmed/14573857.

19. Allaby, R.G., Banerjee, M., Brown, T.A., 1999. "Evolution of the High Molecular Weight Glutenin Loci of the A, B, D and G Genomes of Wheat." *Genome*, 42: 296-307.

20. Dvorak, J., Luo, M.C., Yang, Z.L., Zhang, H.B., 1998. "The Structure of the Aegilops Tauschii Gene Pool and the Evolution of Hexaploid Wheat." *Theoretical and Applied Genetics*, 97: 657-670.

21. Thompson, L.U., 1993. "Potential Health Benefits and Problems Associated with Anti-Nutrients in Foods." *Food Research International*, 26: 131-149.

22. Hitchcock, 1950. " "Reactions in the Human Eating Grasses Not Related to Evolution of the Grain: Classified Into Tribes." Review relates Tribe 3; wheat, rye, barley, Tribe 4; Oats, Tribe 9; Rice, Tribe 10; Wild Rice, Tribe 11; Millet, Tribe 13; Sorghum, Tribe 14; Corn. *Manual of Grasses*, U.S.

23. Wrigley, C.W., Bekes, F., Bushuk, W., 2006. "The Gluten Composition of Wheat Varieties and Genotypes." *AACC International*.

24. Stepankova, R., Tlaskalova-Hogenova, H., Fric, P., Trebichavsky, I., 1989. "Enteropathy Induced in Young Rats by Feeding with Gliadin-Similarity with Celiac Disease." *Folia Biol.* (Praha) 35 (1): 19-26. PMID 265 3886.

25. Mamone, G., Ferranti, P., Rossi, M., et al 2007. "Identification of a Peptide from Alpha-Gliadin Resistant to Digestive Enzymes: Implication for Celiac Disease." DOI: 10.1016/j.jchromb.2007.05.009. PMID 17544966.

26. I.N.Cognito, 2009. "Bread Dread: Are You Really Gluten Intolerant? " A biography of a bread maker from Brisbane, Australia of 1950 and he shared how bread making changed from the 8 hours of fermenting (bread rising) to brewing in just

2 hours! The case was made that if properly raised the breads of modern day will not cause the flare of gluten inflammation. The article mentioned it was rare to ever allow bran to be left in the finished bread! *Nourished Magazine*, Australia.

Chapter 2 References

1. Cyril, P., Brian (translator), 1930. *The Papyrus Ebers.* Original date of book is 1500 BC, London: Bles, G., England.

2. Lawless, J., Allan, J., 2000. *Aloe Vera Natural Wonder Cure.* Pg. 2, Sumerian clay tablets note digestive ailments addressed with herbs in ancient times. City of Nippur of ancient Mesopotamia was the site where the writings were found and dated 2,000 BC, Thorsons Pub, London, UK.

3. Hell, J., 2008. "Useful Known and Unknown Views of the Father of Medicine, Hippocrates and His Teacher Democritus." *Nucl Med,* Jan – April; 11(1): 2-4. U.S. National Library of Medicine, National Institutes of Health, PMID: 18392218.

4. Goodyer, J., (translator), 1934. *The Greek Herbal of Dioscorides, 60 AD - De Materia Medica.* Oxford Univ Press & Hafner Pub. Co., 1968: 257.

5. Heinemann, W., Jones, W.H.S., (translator) 1949-1962. *Natural History – Pliny.* 10 Volumes, pgs. 399-401, Harvard University Press, USA.

6. DeLacy, P., 1972. Review of Galen's work: "Galen's Platonism", *American Journal of Philosophy*, pgs 27-39, Cosans, C., 1997, "Galen's Critiques of Rationalist and Empiricist Anatomy", *Journal of Biology*, 30: 35-54, and Cosans, C., 1998, "The Experimental Foundations of Galen's Teleology", *Studies in History and Philosophy of Science*, 29: 63-80.

7. Adams, F. (translator), 1856. "Coeliac Affection". *The Extant Works of Aretaeus – The Cappadocian, Sydenham Society, London.* http://web.archive.org/web/20070311164628/http://www.chlt.org/

sandbox/dh/aretaeusEnglish/page.102.Retrieved on 2006-09-04. [7A & 7B Questions]

8. Gottschall, E., B.A., M.Sc., 1995. *Breaking the Vicious Cycle – Intestinal Health Through Diet."* Pgs. Foreword iii, The Kirkton Press, Ontario, Canada.

9. Merck, Sharp & Dohme Corp., 2009-2010. *The Merck Manual of Geriatrics,* Ch. 107, Lower Gastrointestinal Tract Disorders, Whitehouse Station, N.J.. http://www.merck.com/mkgr/mU.S.A.. IBS/mg/sec 13/ch107/ch107f.jsp.

10. Merck, Sharp & Dohme Corp., 2009-2010. *The Merck Manual of Geriatrics,* Ch. 107, Lower Gastrointestinal Tract Disorders, Whitehouse Station, N.J.. http://www.merck.com/mkgr/mU.S.A.. IBS/mg/sec 13/ch107/ch107f.jsp

11. Merck, Sharp & Dohme Corp., 2009-2010. The Merck Manual Home Edition, Ulcerative Colitis: Inflammatory Bowel Diseases (IBD), Whitehouse Station, N.J., U.S.A. http://www.merck.com/mmhe/sec09/ch126/ch126c.html.

12. Merck, Sharp & Dohme Corp., 2009-2010. The Merck Manual Home Edition, Proctitis: Anal and Rectal Disorders, Whitehouse Station, N.J., U.S.A. http://www.merck.com/mmhe/sec09/ch130/ch130j.html.

13. Merck, Sharp & Dohme Corp., 2009-2010. Merck Manual Professional, Crohn's Disease: Inflammatory Bowel Disease (IBD), Whitehouse, N.J., U.S.A.. http://www.merck.com/mmpe/sec02/ch018/ch018b.html.

14. Merck, Sharp & Dohme Corp., 2009-2010. Merck Manual Professional, Celiac Sprue: Malabsorption Syndromes, Whitehouse, N.J., U.S.A. http://www.marck.com/mmpe/sec02ch017/ch017/ch017d.html.

15. World Health Statistics, 2008. www.who.int/entity/whosis/whostat/EN_WHS08_Full.pdf.

16. Balch, J. F., MD and Walker, M, MD, 1998. *Heartburn and What To Do About It,* pg 10. Avery Pub. Group Inc., N.Y.

17. Fasano, Alessio, MD, 2009. "Surprises from Celiac Disease. *Scientific American*, pgs 54-60, August 2009.

18. American Osteopathic College of Dermatology, 2010. "Dermatitis Herpetiformis." http://www.aocd.org/skin/ dermatologicd disease/dermatitisherpet.html.

19. Mayo Clinic, 2009. "Celiac Disease." http://www.mayoclinic.com/ health/celiac-disease/DS00319.

20. Hedin, C., Whelan, K., Lindsey, J.O., 2007. "Evidence for the Use of Probiotics and Prebiotics in Inflammatory Bowel Disease; A Review of Clinical Trials", *Proc Nutri Soc,* Nutritional Science Division, King's College London, London SE1 9NH, UK. Abstract: Probiotics and Prebiotics have been investigated in clinical trials as treatment for IBD especially in Pouchitis and Ulcerative Colitis. Some of the data was not as convincing in Crohn's however many factors must be reviewed. Mounting evidence suggests in both animal and human studies that the relationship of Microbiota and Inflammatory Bowel Disease are due to the important balance.

21. Ewaskchuk, J. B., Dieieman, L. A., 2006. "Probiotic and Prebiotic in Chronic Inflammatory Bowel Disease", *World J Gastroenterol,* Centre for Excellence for Gastrointestinal Inflammation and Immunity Research, University of Alberta, Edmonton, Alberta, T6G 2X8, Canada. Abstract: Disturbance in the symbiosis of the colon cells can result in inflammatory bowel disease. Although not fully understood as to the etiology Crohn's, Ulcerative Colitis and Chronic Pouchitis are a result of an over active immune response to the commensal intestinal flora in genetically susceptible people. Understanding the role of micro flora and modifying the bacterial load to improve health has arisen.

22. University of North Carolina, 2004. "Therapeutic Manipulation of the Enteric Microflora in Inflammatory Bowel Diseases: Antibiotics, Probiotics and Prebiotics." *Gastroenterology,* May, 126 (6): 1620-33. Selected probiotics prevented relapse of quiescent

ulcerative colitis and relapsing Pouchitis. Stated in documents that these agents will likely become an integral component of treating IBD in combination with anti-inflammatory and immunosuppressive agents. Dept. of Medicine, Microbiology and Immunology, Center for gastrointestinal Biology and Disease, Chapel Hill, North Carolina, 27599-7032, U.S.A.. PMID:15168372, [PubMed-Indexed for MEDLINE]

23. Haas, S.V., Haas, M.P., 1951. *Management of Celiac Disease.* J.B. Lippincott Co., P.A.

24. Metchnikoff, E., 1908. *The Prolongation of Life.* G.P. Putnam's Sons, N.Y...

25. Quigley, E.M., 2007. "Probiotics in Irritable Bowel Syndrome: an Immuno-modulating Strategy?" *J. Am. Coll. Nutr.,* 26(6): 684 S, Dec...

26. Geier, M.S., Butler, R.N. Howarth, G.S., 2007. "Inflammatory Bowel Disease: Current Insights into Pathogenesis and New Therapeutic Options; Probiotics, Prebiotics and Symbiotic." *Int. J. Food Microbial,* 115(1): 1-11, April.

27. Gaxella, K.A., Hoffman, R., MD, 2008. "Impressive Allies: Probiotics + Prebiotics = Symbiotic." Reviews the work of Dr. Ohhira, Eamonn Quigley, MD president of Am. College of Gastroenterology and the NIH Gut Microbiome Project, discovering the unique "bacterial fingerprint" that people are born with. Health requires balance of bacteria in the gut and entire body. *Better Nutrition Mag, Probiotics,* Active Interest Media, Inc., CA...

28. Kuwaki, S., Ohhira, I., Takahata, M., Murata, Y., Tada, M., 2002. "Antifungal Activity of the Fermentation Product of Herbs by Lactic Acid Bacteria Against Tine." *J. Biosci Bioeng,* 94(5): 401-5.

29. Lesbros-Pantoflickova, D., Corthesy-Theulaz, I., Blum, A.L., 2007. "Helicobacter pylori and Probiotics." *J. Nutr.,* 137 (3 Suppl. 2): 812 S-8S, March.

30. Heaton, K.W., 1990. "Dietary Factors in the Etiology of Inflammatory Bowel Diseases." *Inflammatory Bowel Diseases*, Eds. Allan, R.N., Keighley, M.R.B., Alexander-Williams, J., Hawkins, C.F... Churchill Livingston, N.Y.

31. Struthers, J.E., Singleton, J.W., Kern, F., Jr., 1965. "Intestinal Lactase Deficiency in Ulcerative Colitis and Regional Ileitis." *Annals of Internal Medicine*, 63: 221-228.

32. Write, R., Truelove, S.C., 1965. "Review Study Therapeutic Trial of Various Diets in Ulcerative Colitis." *British Medical Journal*, 2:138-141.

33. Cady, A.B., Rhodes, J.B., Littman, A., Crane, R.K., 1967. "Significance of Lactase Deficit in Ulcerative Colitis." *Journal of Lab and Clin Med*, 70: 279-286.

34. Kirschner, B.S., Defavaro, M.V., Jensen, W., 1981. "Lactose Malabsorption in Children and Adolescents with Inflammatory Bowel Disease." *Gastroenterology*, 81: 829-832.

35. Haas, S.V., MD, 1924. "The Value of the Banana in the Treatment of Coeliac Disease." *Am J Dis Child*, 24: 421-37.

36. Losowsky, M.S., 2008. "A History of Coeliac Disease." *Dig Dis*, 26(2): 112-20. DOI:10.1159/000116768.PMID 18431060.

37. Balch, J.F., MD, Walker, M., MD, 1998. *Heartburn and What To Do About It*, pgs 7-10. Avery Pub. Group, Inc., N.Y..

38. Tong, J.L., 2007. "Et al. Meta-Analysis: the Effect of Supplementation with Probiotics on Eradication Rates and Adverse Events with H. Pylori eradiation therapy. *Ailment Pharmacol Ther*, 25(2): 155-68, Jan..

Chapter 3 References

1. Brandt, L.J., et al., 2002. "Systemic review on the management of Irritable Bowel Syndrome in North America", *American Journal of Gastroenterology*, 97, 11, Supplemental: 57-526.

2. Spanier, S.A., et al. 2003. "A Systemic Review of Alternative

Therapies in the IBS-Psychiatric Treatment", *Archives of Internal Medicine*, 163 (3): 265-274.

3. Gonsalkorale, W.M., 2003. "Long-term Benefits of Hypnotherapy for Irritable Bowel Syndrome", Gut, Nov; 52(11): 16239.

4. Shen, Y.H.; Nahas, R., 2009. "Complimentary and Alternative Medicine for Treatment of Irritable Bowel Syndrome". Study reviewing the Brain-Gut relationship. *Canada Family Physician*, 55 (2): 143-8. PMID 19221071.

5. Lynn, R.B., Friedman, L.S., 1993. "IBS – Psychosocial Factors Effect the Clinical Expression of Symptoms". New England J Med; 329: 1940-1945.

6. Jackson, J., O'Malley, P., Tomkins, G., Balden, E., Santoro, J., Kroenke, K., 2000. "Treatment of Functional Gastrointestinal Disorders with Antidepressant medications: Meta-Analysis", Am J. Med, 108 (1): 65-72. PMID 11059442.

7. Binion, D.G., 2010. "Clostridium Difficile and IBD". *Inflamm Bowel Dis Monit; 11 (1): 7-14.* Latent symptoms of C.Diff., often mimic some flu-like symptoms and symptoms of bowel disease in IBD patients including colitis. C.Diff. is the most common cause of serious Antibiotic Associated Diarrhea (AAD).

8. Talley, N.J., 2006. "A Unifying Hypothesis for the Functional Gastrointestinal Disorders: Really Multiple Diseases or One Irritable Gut?" *Gastroenterological Disorders*, 6 (2): 72-8. PMID 16699476.

9. Mayo Clinic, 1998-2011. "Prednisone and Other Corticosteroids: Balance the Risks and Benefits". States that growth rate of children is slowed by these anti-inflammatory drugs. Individuals are encouraged to supplement to compensate for induced deficiencies and help to avoid osteoporosis and other dangerous side effects to include; visceral fat gain, increased blood pressure, reduced immune function, hormone irregularities, reduced adrenal function, vision challenges, thinning skin, etc.

Weigh the benefit to risk ration of the medication. http://www. mayoclinic.com/health/steroids/HOO1431.

10. Saag, K.G., 2010. "Major Side Effects of Systemic Glucocorticoids". http://www.update.com/home/index.html.

11. Cannon, G.W., 2007. "Immunosuppressive drugs including corticosteroids", In: Goldman, L., et al. *Cecil Medicine, 23rd ed.*, Philadelphia, PA.: Saunders Elsevier.

12. Gottschall, E., B.A., M.Sc., 1999. *Breaking the Vicious Cycle – Intestinal Health Through Diet, pg. 36.* The Kirkton Press, Canada.

13. Steinman, D, 2007. *Diet for a Poisoned Planet*, Avalon Publishing Group, New York, N.Y. 10011.

14. Kirschmann, G.J., 1996. *Nutrition Almanac, Fourth Edition*, pgs. 19-387, McGraw-Hill, New York, N.Y., 10011.

15. Pugh, M.B., 2000. Stedman's Medical Dictionary, 27th ed., pg. 65, Lippincott, Williams & Wilkins, Baltimore, MD, U.S.A.

16. Florkin, M., 1957. "Discovery of Pepsin by Theodor Schwann." Rev Med Liege (French), 12 (5): 139-44.

17. Evans, W., PH.D, Rosenberg, I.H., M.D., Thompson, J., 1992. *BIOMARKERS-The 10 Keyes to Prolonging Vitality, You Can Control the Aging Process!*, pg. 246, Fireside, New York, N.Y., 10020.

18. Goldstein, R., Braverman, D., Stankiewicz, H., 2000. "Carbohydrate Malabsorption and the Effect of Dietary Restriction on Symptoms of Irritable Bowel Syndrome and Functional Bowel Complaints". *Israel Medical Assoc. Journal*, Aug, 2 (8): 583-7. Gastroenterology Institute, Shaare Zedek Medical Center, Jerusalem. Results: Only 7% of IBS patients absorbed food sugars normally. 61% displayed significant malabsorption. 56% of patients experienced a marked improvement in absorption with dietary restriction of the problematic sugars in the diet.

19. Mayo Clinic, Picco, Michael, M.D., 2010. "Stool Color: When

to Worry?" Factors for a healthy stool and unhealthy stool were reviewed. All shades of brown considered normal. Any change for any length of time including mucus is a reason to talk to your doctor. http://www.mayoclinic.com/health/stool-color/an00772.

20. Quigley, E.M., 2006. "Germs, Gas and the Gut; the Evolving Role of the Enteric Flora in IBS", Am J Gastroenterology, 101 (2): 334-5. Discussing the role of Probiotics in bowel health.

21. Merck Sharp & Dohme Corp, a subsidiary of Merck & Co., Inc, 2009. "Introduction: Lymphatic Disorders", Merck Manual Home Edition, Whitehouse Station, N.J., U.S.A. http://www.merckmanuals.com/home/sec03/ch0371ch037a.html.

22. Mendyk, H., 2010. "The Prescription Drug Industry Exposed: Part I", Buffalo Women's Health Examiner, August. Referenced Journal of General Internal Medicine, 79% of doctors used brand name terminology in prescriptions even when generic counterpart was available at a much lower price. Seems as though there is an intentional mandate to promote the more expensive medications.

23. Senator Feinstein, Senate Rules and Administration Committee for Ethics & Lobbying Reform, 2007. "Ethics & Lobbying Reform Legislation" passed into law on September 14th. The reform provision attempts to slow the revolving door between Congress and lobbyists; requiring disclosure of lobbyists who bundle campaign contributions; and increased transparency in the legislative process. http://www.Feinstein.senate.gov/public/index.cfm?title=legislative.

24. Adams, K.M., Lindell, K.C., Kohlmeier, M., Zeisel, S.H., 2006. "Status of Nutrition Education in Medical Schools", Am J Clin Nutr., April; 83 (4): 9415-9445. Dept. of Nutrition, School of Public Health, School of Medicine, University of North Carolina at Chapel Hill, NC, 27599-7461. CB#7461. Study: 126 U.S. medical schools accredited were surveyed to determine the amount and type of nutrition education the medical students received. Conclusion: The amount of nutrition

education available in the medical schools, remain inadequate. Manuscripts available upon request.

25. Kirschner, B.S., Defavero, M.V., and Jensen, W., 1981. "Lactose Mal-absorption in Children with IBD", Gastroenterology, 81: 829-832.

26. Vernia, P., Ricciardi, M.R., Frandina, C., Bilotta, T., Frieri, G., 1995. "Lactose Malabsorption and Irritable Bowel Syndrome - Effect of a Long-term Lactose Free Diet". The Italian Journal of Gastroenterology, 27 (3): 117-21. PMID 7548919. http://www. ncbi.nlm.nih.gov/pubmed/7548919.

27. Whorwell, P.J., 1994. "Bran and Irritable Bowel Syndrome: Time for Reappraisal", *Lancet*, July 2; 344(8914): 39?40.

28. Williams, R.D., Stehlin, I., 2011. "Breast Milk or Formula?", 10 pgs, survival of infants greater when breast fed, Mother's milk contains over 100 unique nutrients over formula milk and cow's milk chemistry is in significant contrast to Mother's milk for the infant. http://pregnancy.about.com/cs/breast feedinginfo/1/ blbreastorbottl.

29. Nutrition MD, 2011. "Irritable Bowel Syndrome: Nutritional Considerations; Medical, Nutritional and Behavioral". Reference study stopped milk, wheat, eggs, sugars and added Probiotics intestinal flora and peppermint, etc and found symptoms reduced in approximately half of the subjects. http://www. nutritionalmd.org/consumers/gastrointestinal/ibs_nutritional_.html.

30. Hoyle, T., 1997. "The Digestive System: Linking Theory and Practice", *Br J. Nurse*, 6 (22): 1285-91. PMID9470654.

31. VanEys, J., 1977. "Nutritional Therapy in Children with Cancer", *Cancer Research*, 37: 2457-2461.

32. U.S. National Library of Medicine, 2010. "Congenital Sucrase-Isomaltase Deficiency", *Genetics Home Reference*. Lack of essential enzymes usually becomes apparent after an infant is weaned and begins to eat fruit, juices and grains resulting with gas, bloating, cramps and diarrhea. The children often outgrow the deficiency

of enzymes. http://ghr.nlm.nih.gov/condition/congenital-sucrase-isomaltase-deficiency.

Chapter 4 References

1. North, M., 2002. "The Hippocratic Oath", National Library of Medicine – National Institutes of Health, http://www.nlm.nih.gov/hmd/greek/greek-oath. Retrieved 2009-02-02.

2. Seigworth, G.R., M.D., 1980. "Blood-letting Over the Centuries", http://www.wikipedia.org/wiki/Bloodletting.

3. AMA, American Medical Association, 2007. "AMA: After One-Year Increase, AMA Membership Declines Again", htt;://www.medpagetoday.com/MeetingCoverage/AMA/6006.

4. AMA – American Psychiatric Association, 2001. "Federal Repository Ethics: The Principles of Medical Ethics with Annotations Especially Applicable to Psychiatry". The first revision document since 1957. Gives the review boards the power of directing content and behavior. http://www.ama-assn.org/ama/pub/physician-resources/medical-ethics/about-eithics-group.

5. Adams, K.M., Lindell, K.C., Kohlmeler, M., Zeisel, S.H., 2006. "Status of Nutrition Education in Medical Schools", *Am J Clinical Nutrition, April; 83(4): 9415-9445.* Univ. of North Carolina at Chapel Hill, NC, 27599-7461. CB#7461. Study: 126 U.S. accredited Medical Schools were surveyed to determine the amount and type of nutrition education the medical students received. Conclusion: The amount of nutrition education available in medical schools remained inadequate even though many had the desire to attain more knowledge in this area. Manuscripts are available upon request.

6. FDCA, Federal Drug and Cosmetic Act, 1938. Section 201 (g) (B) and (C), sites the definition of a drug. http://www.fda.gov/RegulatoryInformation/Legislation/FederalFoodDrugandCosmeticActFDCAct/FDCActC.

7. Gorman, P., 2004. "The Silent Killer-The Surprising Link Between Inflammation and Heart Attacks, Cancer, Alzheimer's and Other Diseases & What to do to fight it!" *TIME*, pg. 39-45. Sources; Dr. Moses Rodriguez of Mayo Clinic, Dr. Gailen Marshall of Univ. of Texas-Houston, *Scientific American*, May 2002.

8. Algert, S. J., Stubblefield, N.E., Grasse, G., Shragg, P., Conner, J.D., 1987. "Assessment of Dietary Intake of Lysine and Arginine in Patients with Herpes Simplex", *Journal of the Amer. Dietetics Assoc.* 87 (11): 1560-1561. Conclusion: Whole grains including brown rice, whole-wheat bread, whole-wheat tortillas, oats and barley are high in the amino acid Arginine and Gluten that may trigger Herpes Simplex.

9. Lowe, C., 2009. "Can Bread Give You Herpes?" *Birmingham Family Health Examiner (BFHE)*. Result: Several studies have confirmed the trigger of grains and herpes; (A) Research at Southern Illinois Univ. at Carbondale, 2005, *Journal of Athletic Training*, Oct-Dec; 40 (4): 365-369, (B) Mammals eating wheat had an Immune Response Stimulating the Herpes Simplex Virus to Activate, *Cancer Letters*, 1982, Nov-Dec; 17 (2): 175-185. (C) Personal testimony of author in BFHE, found outbreaks of Herpes Simplex on mouth and lips correlating with eating grains which significantly declined after stopping bread, cookies, crackers, cakes and other wheat products. Conclusion: Scientists speculate the high Arginine in wheat causes the imbalance of Lysine resulting in outbreaks of HSV.

10. Maroon, J.C., M.D., Bost, J., P.A.C., 2006. *FISH OIL – The Natural Anti – Inflammatory; Nature's Safest Most Effective Anti-Inflammatory*, pgs. 48-57. Basic Health Publications, Inc., Laguna Beach, CA., U.S.A. Conclusion: The general public is deficient in Omega 3 essential fatty acids and receive too high of levels in the Omega 6 EFA's from over consumption of vegetable oils, grain fed beef and processed foods also high in trans-fats.

11. Mayo Clinic Staff, 2010. "Rosacea-Causes". Lists a number of factors to include spicy foods that aggravate the facial skin, increasing inflammation. http://www.mayoclinic.com/health/rosacea/DS00308/DSECTION=causes.

12. Kagnoff, M.F., M.D., 2011. FAQ, "I think I have Celiac Disease, but the blood tests are negative. What do I do"? Wm. K. Warren Medical Research Center for Celiac Disease, University of California San Diego (UCSD), 9500 Gillman Drive, LaJolla, CA, 92073-0623. http://www.celiaccenter.ucsd.edu/aboutcdadults.shtml.

13. Korn, D., 2006. *Living Gluten Free for Dummies*, pgs. 37-43. Wiley Publishing, Inc., 111 River St., Hoboken, N.J., 07030-5774.

14. Kagnoff, M.F., M.D., 2011. FAQ, "I think I have Celiac Disease, but the blood tests are negative. What do I do"? Wm. K. Warren Medical Research Center for Celiac Disease, University of California San Diego (UCSD), 9500 Gillman Drive, LaJolla, CA, 92073-0623.

15. EnteroLab, Dr. Kenneth Fine, M.D., 2010. Stool Testing for Gluten Intolerance and Other Allergens. http://www.enterolab.com/StaticPages/TestInfo.aspx.

16. Koch, K. M., C.N., 1999. *Gift of Nature Whole Leaf Aloe Vera*, Clinical Observation and Applications, pgs. 35-55, Total Health Science Press, Santee, CA, 92072.

17. Koch, K. M., C.N., 1999. *Gift of Nature Whole Leaf Aloe Vera*, Clinical Observation and Applications, pgs. 21-22, Toxicity Study Revealed 100% Safe to drink, Total Health Science Press, Santee, CA, 92072.

18. IASC, International Aloe Science Council, 2011. Scientific Research Center: Numerous scientists, doctors and other researchers around the world are conducting significant and repeatable research on the properties and benefits of Aloe.

Hundreds of published papers support the value of the Aloe Vera plant. http://www.iasc.org/articles.html.

19. Koch, K. M., C.N., 1999. *Gift of Nature Whole Leaf Aloe V*era, Clinical Observation and Applications, pgs. 9-10, Total Health Science Press, Santee, CA, 92072.

Chapter 5 Reference

1. Feingold, B. F., M.D., 1982. "The Role of Diet in Behavior", *Ecology of Disease,* 2 (213): 153-165. Review: Implementing a nutritious, low allergen diet, low processed foods, chemical free showed dramatic results in children's behavior. PMID6090095, http:11www.ncbi.nlm.nih.gov./pubmed/6090095.

2. Lesser, M., M.D., 2002. *The Brain Chemistry Diet,* Penguin Putman Inc., New York, NY, 10014. Review: Michael Lesser, M.D. is a pioneering Orthomolecular Psychiatrist trained at Cornell University Medical College, New York, and the Albert Einstein Medical Center in Bronx, NY. Focusing on nutritional and vitamin therapy to regulate brain function he founded his Orthomolecular Medical Center in 1975. He testified before the U.S. Senate in 1977 on the value of nutrition for mental health.

3. Pheiffer, C.C., PhD., M.D., 1987. *Nutrition and Mental Illness-An Orthomolecular Approach to Body Chemistry,* Healing Arts Press, Rochester, Vermont, 05767.

4. Feingold, B. F., M.D., 1982. "The Role of Diet in Behavior", *Ecology of Disease,* 2 (213): 153-165. Review: Implementing a nutritious, low allergen diet, low processed foods, chemical free showed dramatic positive results in children's behavior. PMID6090095, http:11www.ncbi.nlm.nih.gov./pubmed/6090095.

5. Haidemenos, A., Kontis, D., Gazi, A., Kallai, E., Allin, M., Lucia, B., 2007. "Plasma Homocysteine, Folate, and B12 in Chronic Schizophrenia". *Prog Neuropsychopharmacol Bio-Psychiatry,* Aug 15; 31(6): 1289-96. Epub 2007 June 2, PMID:

17597277. Review: Homocysteine designates inflammation in the brain plasma. Research found that the inflammation did not correlate to a lack of folate and B12 with these patients but was coming from other causative factors (perhaps diet).

6. Snider, L.A., Swedo, S. E., 2003. "Post-Streptococcal Autoimmune disorders of the Central Nervous System", *Current Opinion Neurology*, 16: 359-365. Review: Clinical and research findings in both immunology and neuropsychiatry have established the existence of post Streptococcal Neuropsychiatric Disorders including O.C.D. This work is beginning to shed light on the possible pathological processes that may develop from infection. Researchers state that molecular mimicry is just one possible mechanism by which post-infectious auto-immune disorders can occur (affecting mental illness). Pediatrics and Devel. Neuropsych, Branch, National Institute of Health and Human Services, Bethesda, MD, 20892, USA.

7. Firestein, G. S., M.D., Sorkin, L., PhD, 2006. "Mind-Body Connection: How Central Nervous System Regulates Arthritis", University of Calif. San Diego, School of Medicine Research Team, USA. Review: The research suggests that the CNS can profoundly influence immune response, and may even contribute to the understanding so-called placebo effects and the role of stress in inflammatory diseases, states *Science Daily*. http://www.sciencedaily.com/releases/2006/09/060905084830.htm.

8. Human Nervous System Defined, 2011. New World Encyclopedia, http://www.newworldencyclopedia.org/entry/central_nervous_system.

9. Bruno, J., PhD, 2009. "Neurotransmitters", *Child Wisdom*, Peninsula Child & Youth Assessment Clinics, Pacifica, CA, 94044. A review of the requirements of the body to build the required neurotransmitter chemicals for health and wellness. http://www.nutritionpsych.com/neurotransmitters.

10. Seaman, D., DC, MS, DABCN, 2003. "Magnesium Deficiency,

Inflammation and the Nervous System hyper-excitability", Dynamic Chiropractic, March 24, Vol. 21, Issue 07. Article referenced: Elin, K.J., 1994. "Magnesium: the fifth but forgotten electrolyte", Am. J. Clinical Path, 102: 616-22.

11. Nevilly, S., (France), 2004. "Clinical Forms of Magnesium Depletion with Hyper Function of the Biological Clock", 8th Europeans Magnesium Congress, May 25, 2004, Romania.

12. Nechifor, M., Vaideanu, C., Mindreci, I., Borza, C., 2004. "Variations of Magnesium Concentrations in Psychosis", Dept. of Pharmacology, University of Medicine and Pharmacy, "Gr. T. Popa", Iasi, "Socola" Clinical Psychiatric Hosp. Iasi, Biophysics Dept, Univ. of Medicine and Pharmacy, Romania. Review: Magnesium plays important roles in CNS functioning states the researchers. Plasmatic and cellular magnesium concentrations are modified in psychosis. Magnesium levels significantly measure lower in patients suffering with depression vs. the controls without depression.

13. Singh, V.K., PhD. 1997. "Immunotherapy for Brain Diseases and Mental Illnesses", *Progress in Drug Research*, Vol. 48, pp. 129-146.

14. Haidemenos, A., Kontis, D., Gazi, A., Kallai, E., Allin, M., Lucia, B., 2007. "Plasma Homocysteine, Folate, and B12 in Chronic Schizophrenia". *Prog Neuropsychopharmacol Bio-Psychiatry*, Aug 15; 31(6): 1289-96. Epub 2007 June 2, PMID: 17597277. Review: Homocysteine designates inflammation in the brain plasma. Research found that the inflammation did not correlate to a lack of folate and B12 with these patients but was coming from other causative factors.

15. American Heart Association, 2007. "Homocysteine, Folic Acid and Cardio-Vascular Disease", *Learn Online*, Review: The AHA will not promote the science of Homocysteine levels in the blood even though they are associated with greater levels of plaque build-up in the arteries leading to CVD - even though good

evidence suggests this fact. The AHA goes on to state that B-Complex including Folic Acid, B6 and B12 is required in the body in higher levels to reduce the Homocysteine (inflammatory marker) levels successfully. They also state that evidence reveals that low blood levels of folic acid are linked to higher risk of fatal Coronary Heart Disease and Stroke. http://www.americanheart. org/print_presenter.jhtml:jhtml:jsessionid=3QEDHCJEA02G GCQFC.

16. Snider, L.A., Swedo, S. E., 2003. "Post-Streptococcal Auto-immune disorders of the Central Nervous System", *Current Opinion Neurology*, 16: 359-365. Review: Clinical and research findings in both immunology and neuropsychiatry have established the existence of post Streptococcal Neuropsychiatric Disorders including O.C.D. This work is beginning to shed light on the possible pathological processes that may develop from infection. Researchers state that molecular mimicry is just one possible mechanism by which post-infectious auto-immune disorders can occur (affecting mental illness). Pediatrics and Development. Neuro-psych, Branch, National Institute of Health and Human Services, Bethesda, MD, 20892, USA.

17. Tang, Y. W., Mitchell, P. S., Epsy, M. J., Smith, T. R., Persins, D. H., 1999. "Molecular Diagnosis of Herpes Simplex Virus (HSV) Infection in the Central Nervous System", *American Society of Microbiology*. Division of Clinical Microbiology, Dept. of Medicine and Pathology, Mayo Clinic, Rochester, MN, 55905. Review: Specific diagnosis of HSV of an 18 year old woman showed symptoms including: headache, fever, mild confusion, severe pseudo-bulbar palsy.

18. Conrady, C. D., Drevats, D. A., Carr, D. J., 2009. "Herpes Simplex Type 1 (HSV1) infection of the Nervous System: is an immune response a good thing? " *Journal of Neuro-Immunology*, Vol. 220, 1 SSN: 1872-8421, March. Review: Hosts response to infection may also play a pathogenic role; involved in pathogenesis

of several diseases in humans to include inflammatory disorders and auto-immune. While immune response is necessary to quell viral replication collateral damage causes tissue damage in the CNS (especially in brain tissue) from release of inflammatory mediators including reactive oxygen species. Therapeutic intervention is needed to reduce unwarranted inflammation from viruses.

19. Blaybock, R., L., M.D., Neurosurgeon, 1997. *Excitotoxins- The Taste That Kills,* Health Press, P.O. Box 1388 (drawer), NM, 87504, USA. Review: Important resource reveals that many if not all synthetic chemical sweeteners and some other chemicals are very reactive in the human body and for some people may pose a big danger within their chemistry with high quantities.

Index